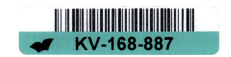
KV-168-887

The ISLETS
of LANGERHANS

Biochemistry, Physiology, and Pathology

Contributors

S. J. H. Ashcroft

G. Eric Bauer

Dorothea Baxter-Grillo

Enrique Blázquez

S. J. Cooperstein

William E. Dulin

Suad Efendić

Donald J. Fletcher

Piero P. Foà

Brian Furman

W. Gepts

John Gerich

T. Adesanya I. Grillo

Robert L. Hazelwood

A. Herchuelz

Mitsuyasu Itoh

Paul E. Lacy

Rolf Luft

Michael L. McDaniel

Noel K. Maclaren

W. J. Malaisse

B. L. Munger

Bryan D. Noe

M. Alan Permutt

Philip Raskin

Elliot J. Rayfield

Gerard Reach

R. P. Robertson

Janove Sehlin

A. Sener

Jean-Claude Sodoyez

Francoise Sodoyez-Goffaux

Manuel G. Soret

Dudley Watkins

Ji-Won Yoon

NY2/ MKD/LIB

38·80

DATE DUE FOR RETURN

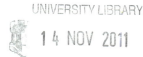

UNIVERSITY LIBRARY

14 NOV 2011

GML 02

Any
is c

UNIVERSITY LIBRARY

14 APR 2014

GGL 27

Tw
used

UNIVERSITY OF NOTTINGHAM

TELEPEN

6 20 022265 7

WITHDRAWN

FROM THE LIBRARY

The ISLETS of LANGERHANS

Biochemistry, Physiology, and Pathology

Edited by

S. J. COOPERSTEIN
DUDLEY WATKINS

Department of Anatomy
The University of Connecticut School
of Medicine and Dental Medicine
Farmington, Connecticut

1981

ACADEMIC PRESS

A Subsidiary of Harcourt Brace Jovanovich, Publishers
New York   London   Toronto   Sydney   San Francisco

√c

MEDICAL LIBRARY
QUEEN'S MEDICAL CENTRE

Class	WK 800
Fund	605 - 001
Book No.	9830707/000/01

COPYRIGHT © 1981, BY ACADEMIC PRESS, INC.
ALL RIGHTS RESERVED.
NO PART OF THIS PUBLICATION MAY BE REPRODUCED OR
TRANSMITTED IN ANY FORM OR BY ANY MEANS, ELECTRONIC
OR MECHANICAL, INCLUDING PHOTOCOPY, RECORDING, OR ANY
INFORMATION STORAGE AND RETRIEVAL SYSTEM, WITHOUT
PERMISSION IN WRITING FROM THE PUBLISHER.

ACADEMIC PRESS, INC.
111 Fifth Avenue, New York, New York 10003

United Kingdom Edition published by
ACADEMIC PRESS, INC. (LONDON) LTD.
24/28 Oval Road, London NW1 7DX

Library of Congress Cataloging in Publication Data
Main entry under title:

The Islets of Langerhans.

Includes index.
1. Islets of Langerhans. 2. Islets of Langerhans--
Diseases. I. Cooperstein, S. J. II. Watkins, Dudley.
[DNLM: 1. Islets of Langerhans--Physiology. 2. Islets
of Langerhans--Pathology. 3. Diabetes mellitus--Etiology.
WK 800 I82]
QP188.P26I77   612'.33   81-10895
ISBN 0-12-187820-1   AACR2

PRINTED IN THE UNITED STATES OF AMERICA

81 82 83 84   9 8 7 6 5 4 3 2 1

Contents

I. Morphology and Development of Islet Tissue

1. Morphological Characterization of Islet Cell Diversity

B. L. MUNGER

2. Functional Development of the Pancreatic Islets

DOROTHEA BAXTER-GRILLO, ENRIQUE BLÁZQUEZ,
T. ADESANYA I. GRILLO, JEAN-CLAUDE SODOYEZ,
FRANCOISE SODOYEZ-GOFFAUX AND PIERO P. FOÀ

II. Synthesis and Secretion of Islet Hormones

3. Transport Systems of Islet Cells

JANOVE SEHLIN

4. Biosynthesis of Insulin

M. ALAN PERMUTT

5. Interactions of Cell Organelles in Insulin Secretion

MICHAEL L. McDANIEL AND PAUL E. LACY

9. Biosynthesis of Glucagon and Somatostatin

BRYAN D. NOE, DONALD J. FLETCHER, AND
G. ERIC BAUER

10. Secretion of Glucagon

MITSUYASU ITOH, GERARD REACH, BRIAN
FURMAN, AND JOHN GERICH

11. Somatostatin and Its Role in Insulin and Glucagon Secretion

SUAD EFENDIĆ AND ROLF LUFT

III. Pathology of the Islets of Langerhans

15. Action of Toxic Drugs on Islet Cells

S. J. COOPERSTEIN AND DUDLEY WATKINS

16. Role of Viruses in Diabetes

ELLIOT J. RAYFIELD AND JI-WON YOON

17. Autoimmunity and Diabetes

NOEL K. MACLAREN

**18. Insulin, Glucagon, and Somatostatin
    Interaction in Diabetes**

PHILIP RASKIN

List of Contributors

Numbers in parentheses indicate the pages on which the authors' contributions begin.

S. J. H. Ashcroft (117), Nuffield Department of Clinical Biochemistry, John Radcliffe Hospital, Headington, Oxford OX3 9DU, England

G. Eric Bauer (189), Department of Anatomy, University of Minnesota Medical School, Minneapolis, Minnesota 55455

Dorothea Baxter-Grillo (35), Faculty of Health Sciences, University of Ife, Ile-Ife, Nigeria

Enrique Blázquez* (35), Instituto Gregorio Marañón, Velázquez, 144, Madrid-6-Spain

S. J. Cooperstein (387), Department of Anatomy, University of Connecticut Health Center, Farmington, Connecticut 06032

William E. Dulin (357), Diabetes and Atherosclerosis Research, The Upjohn Company, Kalamazoo, Michigan 49001

Suad Efendić (257), Department of Endocrinology, Karolinska Sjukhuset, Stockholm 60, Sweden

Donald J. Fletcher (189), Department of Medicine, Medical College of Virginia, Richmond, Virginia 23298

Piero P. Foà (35), Department of Physiology, Wayne State University School of Medicine, Detroit, Michigan 48201

Brian Furman (225), Departments of Medicine and Physiology, Endocrine Research Unit, Mayo Clinic, Rochester, Minnesota 55901

W. Gepts (321), Dienst Anatomo-Patologie, Academisch Ziekenhuis, Vrije Universiteit Brussels, Laarbeeklaan, 1090 Brussel, Belgium

John Gerich (225), Departments of Medicine and Physiology, Endocrine Research Unit, Mayo Clinic, Rochester, Minnesota 55901

T. Adesanya I. Grillo (35), Faculty of Health Sciences, University of Ife, Ile-Ife, Nigeria

* Present address: Departamento de Fisiología, Facultad de Medicina, Oviedo, Spain.

Robert L. Hazelwood (275), Department of Biology, University of Houston, Central Campus, Houston, Texas 77004

A. Herchuelz (149), Laboratoire de Médecine Expérimentale, Université Libre de Bruxelles, 1000 Bruxelles, Belgium

Mitsuyasu Itoh (225), Departments of Medicine and Physiology, Endocrine Research Unit, Mayo Clinic, Rochester, Minnesota 55901

Paul E. Lacy (97), Department of Pathology, Washington University School of Medicine, St. Louis, Missouri 63110

Rolf Luft (257), Department of Endocrinology, Karolinska Sjukhuset, Stockholm 60, Sweden

Michael L. McDaniel (97), Department of Pathology, Washington University School of Medicine, St. Louis, Missouri 63110

Noel K. Maclaren (453), Department of Pathology, University of Florida College of Medicine, Gainesville, Florida 32610

W. J. Malaisse (149), Laboratoire de Médecine Expérimentale, Université Libre de Bruxelles, 1000 Bruxelles, Belgium

B. L. Munger (3), Department of Anatomy, The Milton S. Hershey Medical Center, Hershey, Pennsylvania 17033

Bryan D. Noe (189), Department of Anatomy, Emory University School of Medicine, Atlanta, Georgia 30322

M. Alan Permutt (75), Department of Internal Medicine, Washington University School of Medicine, St. Louis, Missouri 63110

Philip Raskin (467), Department of Internal Medicine, The University of Texas Health Science Center at Dallas, Dallas, Texas 75235

Elliot J. Rayfield (427), Diabetes Research Laboratory, The Mount Sinai Medical Center, Mount Sinai School of Medicine, New York, New York 10029

Gerard Reach (225), Departments of Medicine and Physiology, Endocrine Research Unit, Mayo Clinic, Rochester, Minnesota 55901

R. P. Robertson (173), Department of Medicine, Division of Clinical Pharmacology, University of Washington School of Medicine, Seattle, Washington 98195

Janove Sehlin (53), Department of Histology, University of Umeå, S-901, 87 UMEÅ, Sweden

A. Sener (149), Laboratoire de Médecine Expérimentale, Université Libre de Bruxelles, 1000 Bruxelles, Belgium

Jean-Claude Sodoyez (35), Department of Internal Medicine, Université de Liège, 4020 Liège, Belgium

Francoise Sodoyez-Goffaux (35), Department of Pediatrics, Université de Liège, 4020 Liège, Belgium

Manuel G. Soret (357), 7400 S. W. 112th Street, Miami, Florida 33156

Dudley Watkins (387), Department of Anatomy, University of Connecticut Health Center, Farmington, Connecticut 06032

Ji-Won Yoon (427), Laboratory of Oral Medicine, National Institute of Dental Research, National Institutes of Health, Bethesda, Maryland 20205

Foreword

Because diabetes is one of the most prevalent disorders suffered by mankind, it has always attracted large groups of investigators among clinicians, physiologists, pathologists, and biochemists. The progressive steps by which the mechanisms operative in this disease have been steadily uncovered have had and continue to have important influences on discovery in a wide sweep of biomedical problems, greatly aiding their elucidation.

Consider the following facts gleaned from the last hundred years of research into the diagnosis, etiology, course, and biochemical derangements of diabetes. Minkowski, amply confirmed by Hedon, offered the first clear proof of the endocrine role of a gland (the pancreas and the regulation of the blood sugar). Removal of its secretion led to the production of a permanent, severe disorder. This prompted a histological study of the islets, which soon established the multiendocrine nature of this dispersed gland. The biochemical derangements of diabetes were a powerful stimulus to the rapid development of our knowledge of the intermediary metabolism of food stuffs catalyzed by the intracellular enzyme systems. Insulin was the first of the 'peptide'' hormones to be fully purified and chemically characterized. Protein sequencing began with Sanger's demonstration of the primary structure of insulin, followed soon by the elucidation of mutational variations in the amino acid pattern in various species and genera. The precise regulation of insulin secretion and biosynthesis by glucose has served as a model for substrate–hormone interaction. Perhaps no single technique has so influenced modern endocrinology (as well as other fields) as has the immunoassay, a method first devised by Berson and Yalow for the measurement of circulating insulin levels. The study of specific hormone and drug receptors owes much to investigators in the diabetes field, as does the growing awareness of the subtle control of enzymatic events (in the liver) exerted by electrical and chemical messages from the central nervous system.

These reflections were prompted by the reading of the thoughtful and well-documented reviews comprising the present volume. The chapter titles and the authoritative quality of their several authors attest to the wide usefulness of the volume. Useful to whom? In the first place to all scientists and clinicians who work in the myriad highways and byways of clinical and experimental diabetes; to the graduate students embarking on a research career in the field; to workers in endocrinology interested in the functions of ductless glands and their behavior; and to physiologists, biochemists, and histologists endeavoring to understand the biosynthesis, storage, secretion, and actions of hormones.

No single person is able these days to encompass the sea of literature that surrounds him and threatens to engulf him, nor is he able to examine critically the ever more complex techniques of modern day biological research. It is thus a positive and needed service which the authors and editors have provided, by their sifting of the literature and by their knowledgeable way of steering us through the difficult methodological waters toward the comparative safety of available landing places.

Rachmiel Levine

CITY OF HOPE MEDICAL CENTER
DUARTE, CALIFORNIA

Preface

This volume is an attempt to bring together in a coherent, coordinated form current knowledge of the complex phenomena involved in the functioning of the multiendocrine organ, the islet of Langerhans, and of the various influences that can lead to its abnormal functioning; in all cases recent developments are stressed. It is also intended to point up the major gaps in our knowledge and to indicate the directions of current research designed to understand its functioning and to explain at the molecular level the defects in this organ that lead to its major pathology, diabetes mellitus. Although several excellent symposia on the islets of Langerhans have been published, these tend to consist of a somewhat disconnected series of articles emphasizing the contributions of the individual authors. In contrast, this book is designed to produce an integrated picture of the islet organ compiled from the work of many laboratories. As such it should be of interest primarily to research workers in endocrinology, particularly those interested in pancreatic hormones, graduate students in endocrinology, and medical endocrinologists interested in diabetes; it should also be of interest to those many physiologists and biochemists studying peptide synthesis and secretion.

This book starts with a section designed to provide the necessary background information on the nature and development of the islet of Langerhans. The first chapter describes, from a historical perspective, the evolution of our knowledge of the ever-increasing number of cell types found in islet tissue. In this connection, no attempt has been made to artificially enforce uniformity on the variety of terms used by different groups for these different cell types; thus, in this and subsequent chapters the insulin-secreting cells are variously referred to as B, beta, or β cells, the glucagon-secreting cells as A, alpha, α, or α_2 cells, the somatostatin-secreting cells as D, delta, or α_1 cells, and the pancreatic polypeptide-secreting cells as PP or F cells. The second chapter of this section follows with a description of the fetal development of the functional capacities of the islet cells, relating this to the changing metabolic needs and capacities of the fetus.

The second section is devoted to the synthesis and secretion of islet hormones, and begins with a chapter on the membrane transport systems of islet tissue as a prelude to subsequent examination of their role in the regulation of these processes. There then follows a chapter (Chapter 4) on the mechanism of insulin synthesis, its control, and the ways in which it might go awry, and another (Chapter 5) on the role of different cell organelles in insulin secretion. Chapter 6 provides an extensive discussion of the metabolic pathways of islet cells, particularly as they relate to control of insulin secretion, and Chapter 7 deals with the role of ions in this process. Although the roles of different cell organelles, metabolic pathways, and ions are dealt with separately, they are clearly interrelated, as witnessed by the possible role of Ca^{2+} in organelle functioning and interaction discussed in Chapter 5, and the link between metabolism and ion flux indicated in Chapters 6 and 7; additionally, the two different major models of control of insulin release—the glucoreceptor model and the metabolic model—are pointed up. Finally, some interesting new perspectives on the possible role of prostaglandins, compounds of great current interest in insulin secretion and diabetes, are set forth in Chapter 8.

In contrast to the chapters on insulin secretion which emphasize almost solely information on the biochemical mechanisms of control as garnered from *in vitro* work, the state of knowledge about the control of glucagon and somatostatin secretion dictated a different approach; in these areas we have only recently begun making the transition from the physiological to the biochemical level. Thus, following a chapter on the synthesis of these two hormones (Chapter 9), the following two chapters on control of secretion (Chapter 10 and 11) place more emphasis on correlating physiological *in vivo* and biochemical *in vitro* studies. Still less is known about pancreatic polypeptide, and Chapter 12 reflects this in emphasizing almost solely physiological studies. Additionally, in contrast to the well-known physiological roles of insulin and glucagon, the uncertainty about the roles of somatostatin and pancreatic polypeptide in the economy of the organism is reflected in the discussion in Chapters 11 and 12.

The final section is devoted to examining the effects of deleterious conditions and agents on the morphology and function of islet cells. Beginning with a description of the pathological changes in the islet in human diabetes in Chapter 13, there follows a discussion (Chapter 14) of the morphological and functional changes in various animal models of spontaneous diabetes, pointing up the usefulness of these models in achieving a better understanding of human diabetes. Chapter 15 describes the actions of certain toxic drugs, with particular emphasis on the use of these drugs to further our understanding of B cell physiology and diabetes. The examination of the actions of various viruses in Chapter 16 includes analysis of both clinical studies in humans and experimental studies in animal models, and the discussion of the possible role of autoantibodies in Chapter 17 provides interesting insights as well into possible explanations of the complex genetics of diabetes. The volume then concludes with Chapter 18 on the exciting new area of the interaction of insulin, glucagon, and somatostatin in the diabetic syndrome.

Diabetes mellitus is a major public health problem. It is estimated that there are 10 million Americans with the disease, and that this number is increasing at the rate of 6% per year. It is one of the leading causes of death by disease, and under present circumstances an American born today and living to age 70 has a one in five chance of developing diabetes. The seriousness of this problem has been recognized by the Congress of the United States, which has mandated a special emphasis on diabetes research, and also by the numerous private organizations supporting research in this field; an estimated $200 million is being spent this year on diabetes research by the Federal government, pharmaceutical companies, foundations, voluntary health agencies, etc. These funds support a great many investigators carrying out studies designed to understand the functioning of the islets of Langerhans and to understand, cure and/or prevent diabetes mellitus. It is hoped that by providing a clear picture of the current state of the field, this book will help further that goal.

S. J. Cooperstein
Dudley Watkins

I

MORPHOLOGY AND DEVELOPMENT OF ISLET TISSUE

1

Morphological Characterization
of Islet Cell Diversity

B. L. MUNGER

I. INTRODUCTION

The pancreatic islets consist of anastomosing cords of cells that abut a prominent vascular connective tissue stroma (Fig. 1). The anastomosing cords of cells constitute the typical endocrine pattern of cells in that each cell has direct access to at least one capillary and in many cases the cells abut a capillary on two opposing poles. The cells tend to be cuboidal or columnar, and the nucleus is present in the base of the cell if the surface facing the capillary is considered the secretory pole (Figs. 1 and 2). The secretory pole of islet cells contains abundant secretory granules, and the

3

The Islets of Langerhans
Copyright © 1981 by Academic Press, Inc.
All rights of reproduction in any form reserved.
ISBN 0-12-187820-1

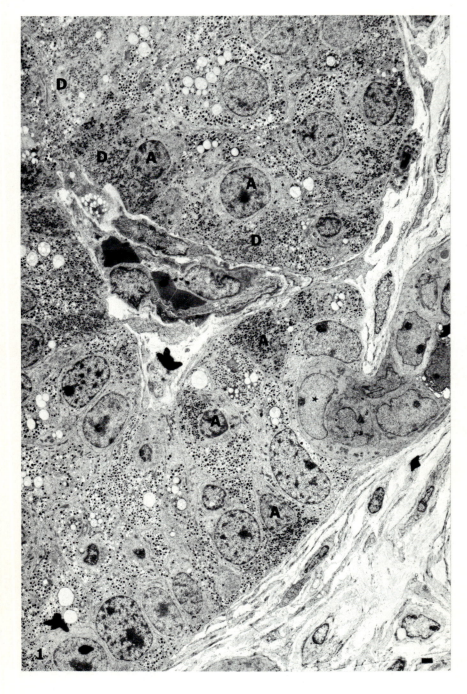

cytoplasm around the nucleus often has fewer secretory granules. This polarization of islet cells is most convincingly demonstrated at survey magnification, as in Fig. 1. These secretory granules are unique biochemically and structurally for each specific islet cell type, as first convincingly noted by Lane (1907) on the basis of relative solubility. The literature on pancreatic islets since the time of Lane (1907) reflects the problems posed by the identification and characterization of specific secretory cell types.

The electron microscope has played a key role in the evolution of our understanding of the biology of pancreatic islets. In most tissue systems, basic cellular composition had been defined by the light microscopic studies of the past century. However, only with the use of the electron microscope has the variety of cell types comprising the pancreatic islets been appreciated. In contrast, the cell types of tissues as complex as the central nervous system were characterized adequately with the light microscope. The technology of preparing tissues for microscopic analysis has been the limiting factor in assessing the cellular composition of islets.

Bensley (1911) confirmed Lane's (1907) report that multiple cell types were present, based on tinctorial properties of islets stained with a neutral dye (neutral gentian–acid fuchsin). Bensley (1911) used the terminology proposed by Lane (1907) based originally on the fact that A cells were fixed by alcohol and B cells by chrome sublimate. Bensley (1911) in turn added to the alphabetical list by describing C cells in the guinea pig pancreas as agranular (non-endocrine-secreting?) cells.

A new cell type was described by Bloom in 1931. He was in the process of studying human autopsy tissues which had been removed a short time after death and stained with Mallory–azan following Zenker–Formol fixation. In one pancreatic islet (subsequently confirmed in three other autopsies) he saw an infrequent cell that stained differently from A or B cells. The drawing of this islet became the color plate for the 1931 paper describing D cells in human islets. This drawing has since been used in each edition of Maximow and Bloom's and subsequently Bloom and Fawcett's "A Textbook of Histology" (1975).

Fig. 1. Normal human pancreas. This low-magnification electron micrograph illustrates the direct continuity of a pancreatic islet to the left with duct cells (★) to the right. Even at this low magnification, it is possible to discriminate the angular secretory granules of B cells (unlabeled) from those of A and D cells (A and D), as well as to evaluate the quality of preservation. The A cells have secretory granules that are more electron-opaque than those of the adjacent D cells, and both types of secretory granules are round, lacking the angular profiles of the B-granule core. The relatively round, large, irregularly electron-lucent spaces within the cytoplasm of all islet cells are masses of lipofuscin. The duct cells (★) lack secretory granules in the cytoplasm and, when examined at higher magnification, intervening basal lamina was not found between the duct cells and the contiguous B cells. This duct cell appears in the other plane of section as an ungranulated islet cell or C cell. × 2200.

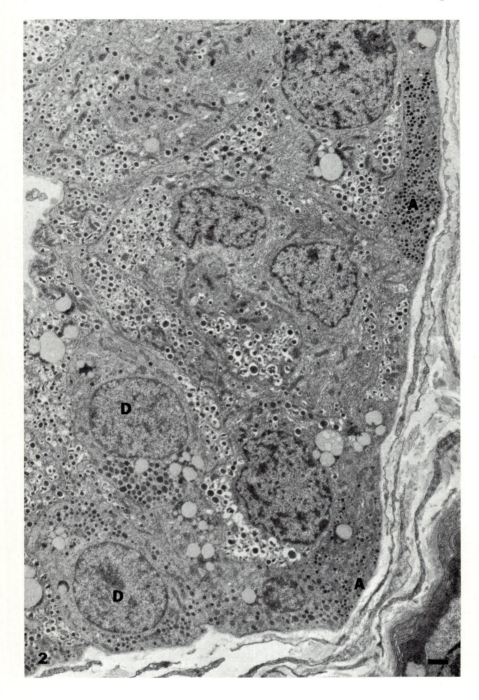

The logical letter sequence of A, B, C, and D cells thus became established during the 1930's. Thomas (1937, 1942) subsequently confirmed Bloom's work by defining at least three different cell types in a variety of mammalian and reptilian pancreatic islets. Thomas's paper on mammalian islets was derived from his doctoral dissertation and unfortunately was illustrated only with semidiagrammatic representations of islet cell distribution. Convincing photomicrographs of mammalian D cells were not provided by either Bloom (1931) or Thomas (1937). Thus, unfortunately both these studies were all but forgotten, largely as a result of the development of aldehyde fuchsin (AF).

The development of specific staining sequences for islet cells as described by Gomori (1939a,b, 1941, 1950) had a significant impact on prevailing attitudes regarding the identification of islet cells. Gomori (1939a), working in the Department of Medicine at the University of Chicago, surveyed the effects of various stains including neutral stains as described by Bensley, azan variants as used by Bloom, and "single basic stains or successive complex stains having an acid and a basic component" (Gomori, 1939a). He was critical of the specificity of neutral stains as well as procedures such as the azan method that required overstaining and a differentiation step to obtain specific staining. The same year, Gomori (1939b) published a technique for chrome alum hematoxylin phloxin (CAHP) staining of A and B cells. The specific component of this stain is the hematoxylin, and the phloxin is merely an acidic dye counterstain. The CAHP stain was most specific in Bouin-fixed tissue where the acetic acid destroys mitochondria but apparently stabilizes A and B granules. Using CAHP as well as azan and phosphotungstic acid hematoxylin (PTAH) methods on human autopsy tissue Gomori (1941) subsequently noted the specific staining of B cells with CAHP and of A cells with PTAH. The D cells could be demonstrated only with the azan technique, and he estimated that they comprised approximately 2–8% of islet cells. In CAHP-stained sections, D cells were counted as A cells, and in PTAH-stained sections they were unstained and thus usually counted as B cells (Gomori, 1941). Gomori (1941) then reached the conclusion that "D cells are probably aged alpha cells." Since D cells could resemble A or B cells depending on the staining method, the development of AF as a preferential stain for B cells by Gomori (1950) further prejudiced attitudes that islets contained only A and B cells because all

---

Fig. 2. Normal human pancreatic islets. This electron micrograph illustrates the difference in contrast and the shape and electron opacity of the secretory granules of A cells (A) as contrasted to those of D cells (D). Both A and D granules are easily distinguished from the agranular paracrystalline core of B-cell granules. The A cells are somewhat variable in appearance in terms of the number and size of secretory granules, but both examples indicated differ significantly from pancreatic D cells whose secretory granules are more electron-lucent. × 4500.

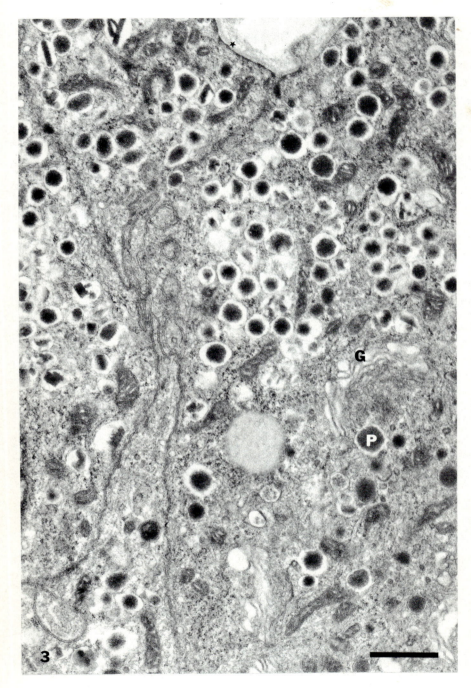

non-B cells stained with the counterstain. The specificity of AF stain for B granules is considerable (Hartroft and Wrenshall, 1955), though even it can be variable (Mowry, 1978, 1980). Mowry (1978, 1980) has eliminated much of this controversy by describing the use of AF on Formalin-fixed tissue without prior oxidation and blocking sulfate staining with alcian blue pretreatment. Mowry's method of preparing and using AF is now the preferred technique in our laboratories.

Based on the extremely precise cytochemical delineation of B cells provided by AF, the prevailing weight of opinion by the time I became involved in cytological studies on the pancreatic islets was that there were only two specific islet cell types, A and B (Munger, 1958). Exceptions to prevailing opinion appeared in the studies of Manocchio (1960) and Manocchio and Caramia (1962) who identified cells in the pancreatic islets, with metachromatic or argyrophilic staining characteristics, that they regarded as different from either A or B cells. Similar silver-positive cells were considered to be a type of A cell by Hellerström and Hellman (1960). Coincident with our study, Caramia (1963) subsequently documented the existence of a third granular cell type in rat pancreatic islets by electron microscopy. I began a collaborative effort with Caramia and Paul Lacy, documenting a diversity of cell types in pancreatic islets including the criteria for identifying Bloom's D cell (Caramia et al., 1965; Munger et al., 1965). Fujita (1964) independently concluded that D cells constituted an independent type of islet cell. Considerable resistance to the concept that D cells were, indeed, a unique population of islet cells was encountered at that time, in part due to the problem posed by the presence of more cells than hormones. With the advent of immunocytochemical techniques for the localization of islet hormones (Erlandsen et al., 1976; Larsson et al., 1976a,b; Orci et al., 1976; Rhoten and Smith, 1978), remaining doubts as to the diversity of islet cells have been dispelled, although the role of islet hormones, other than those produced by the A and B cells, is still speculative. The present goal is to review the morphological basis of islet cell diversity or cell specificity, and we will conclude that there are still more islet cells than functionally defined islet hormones.

Fig. 3. Normal human pancreatic islets. The cytoplasm of these B cells contains an abundance of secretory granules, many of which contain agranular, irregular, electron-opaque paracrystalline cores. The cores of some secretory granules are spherical and appear to be homogeneous rather than paracrystalline. In the region of the Golgi apparatus (G), secretory granules often have homogeneous cores of low electron opacity identified as presumptive prosecretory granules (P). Scattered granular endoplasmic reticulum, mitochondria, and other typical organelles fill the cell. A distinct basal lamina (★) is present facing the vascular connective tissue stroma. × 19,500.

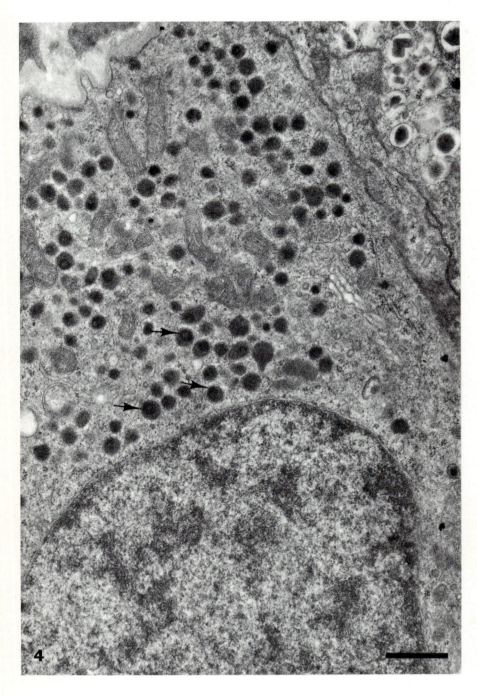

II. B CELLS (β CELLS)

The micrographs in this chapter are grouped by species to permit internal characterization of cell types from human, monkey, and canine tissue. Cross-species differences will also be pointed out using these three examples. Figures 1–5 are from normal human islets, Fig. 6–8 are from a squirrel monkey, and Fig. 9–14 from a dog pancreas. The human and monkey tissue was fixed by immersion, and the canine tissue by vascular perfusion.

B cells are the easiest cells to identify in electron micrographs in that they usually have very distinctive cytological characteristics (Figs. 1 and 2). Lacy (1957a,b, 1962) provided the first documentation of the paracrystalline nature of the granule core of B-cell secretory granules and correlated this characteristic appearance with the staining characteristics of adjacent thick sections stained with AF. This correlation was established in several different animals and established the basic criteria for differentiating B cells from A cells. Munger (1958) used Lacy's criteria to study the embryological development of mouse A and B cells.

B cells of most animals studied to date, such as humans (Figs. 1–4), monkeys (Fig. 6), and dogs (Figs. 9–11), are characterized by the presence of an electron-opaque paracrystalline granule core. This electron-opaque usually somewhat angular mass is separated from an agranular limiting membrane by an electron-lucent space. The diameter of the granule (the limiting membrane) is in most animals 300 ± 50 nm. These characteristic secretory granules are usually massed toward the secretory pole. In states of relative degranulation secretory granules are preferentially located immediately subjacent to the plasma membrane (Merlini and Caramia, 1965; Munger and Lang, 1973). The cytoplasm of B cells between the numerous secretory granules contains the usual complement of organelles including the Golgi apparatus, rough and smooth endoplasmic reticulum, scattered mitochondria, microtubules, and cytoplasmic microfilaments. The Golgi apparatus varies in prominence from animal to animal; in examples such as the guinea pig it tends to be prominent, whereas in animals such as the dog

---

Fig. 4. Normal human pancreas. A typical pancreatic A cell (center) is compared to a B cell (upper right). Human and other primate pancreatic A cells are characterized by an eccentric bull's-eye profile within the secretory granule core (arrow). Many of the granules are also somewhat elliptical or teardrop-shaped. The Golgi apparatus is relatively small in this instance, although other areas of human A cells resemble the canine A cells depicted in Fig. 12. Delicate wisps of granular as well as agranular endoplasmic reticulum are present throughout the cytoplasm, as are scattered mitochondria. A distinct basal lamina is present abutting the vascular connective tissue stroma. A portion of A-cell cytoplasm is illustrated at higher magnification in Fig. 5. × 19,500.

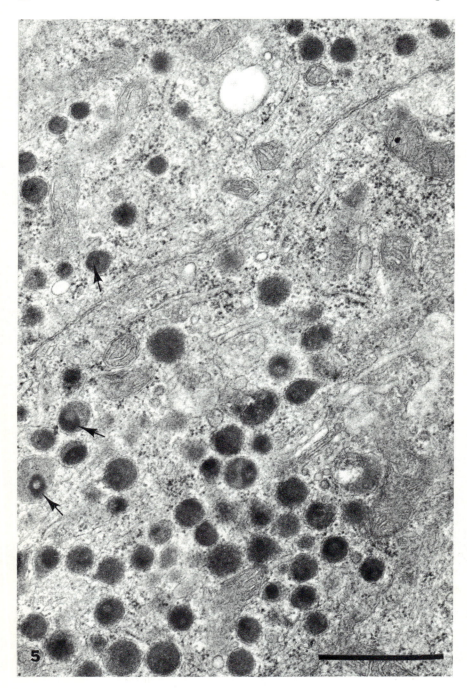

and primate it is not as prominent. Presumptive prosecretory granules (Munger, 1958) or condensing vacuoles (Jamieson and Palade, 1967) are often present in the region of the Golgi apparatus and are characerized by a homogeneous finely granular core of moderate electron opacity that will presumably subsequently crystallize (Fig. 3). The concept that condensing vacuoles or prosecretory granules represent the packaging of secretory material in the Golgi apparatus destined for secretion by the cell is now accepted. The use of the term "prosecretory granules" as proposed by Munger (1958) is consistent with the older literature, whereas the term "condensing vacuole" as proposed by Jamieson and Palade (1967) on the basis of biochemical studies is more descriptively accurate. While typical human B-cell granules are distinctive, one can see differences even in a related primate, for example, by comparing Figs. 1–3 with Fig. 6. In this monkey B cell, many B granules lack a paracrystalline core (Wages and Munger, 1977, Abstr.). More consistent crystallization is seen in dog B granules (Figs. 9–12) in that most granules have an angular paracrystalline core. The species differences noted here can be extended to other animals as well. With experience a microscopist can often name a species by examining the ultrastructure of only a B cell.

Exceptions to the general rule that B cells are characterized by the presence of granules with paracrystalline cores are most notable in the case of the guinea pig (Munger *et al.,* 1965; Munger and Lang, 1973) and the rat and rabbit as noted originally by Lacy (1962). In these animals a homogeneous granule core can be round in the rat and rabbit or kidney bean-shaped as in the case of the guinea pig (Caramia *et al.,* 1965; Munger and Lang, 1973). As has been repeatedly documented, guinea pig insulin is different from other insulins and thus apparently does not crystallize in the same pattern. This perhaps accounts for the fact that the secretory granules of guinea pig B cells differ from those of other species rather significantly in terms of normal ultrastructure (Caramia *et al.,* 1965; Munger and Lang, 1973). The guinea pig is also unique in other respects, not the least of which is its apparent susceptibility to disorders of carbohydrate metabolism (Munger and Lang, 1973; Lang and Munger, 1976). In pancreatic islets of nonmammals, as documented in studies on fish by Brinn (Brinn, 1973, 1975; Brinn and Epple, 1976), on birds by Smith (1973, 1974, 1975a,b) and on reptiles by Rhoten (1971a,b, 1973, 1974), distinctions in granule core morphology may become blurred as compared to mammalian examples;

Fig. 5. Normal human pancreatic islets. A portion of the cytoplasm of two contiguous A cells illustrates the eccentric bull's-eye of the secretory granule cores (arrows). In the background cytoplasm, elements of the Golgi apparatus, granular and agranular endoplasmic reticulum, and numerous microtubules, microfilaments, and other typical cytoplasmic organelles are present. × 37,500.

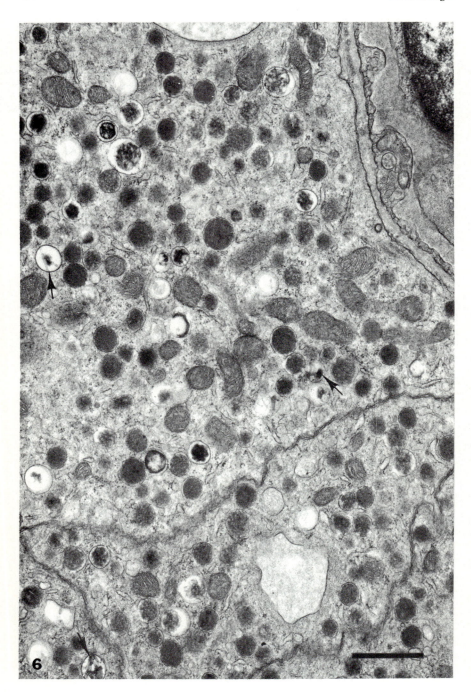

6

but the tendency is still for the B cell granules to have a paracrystalline core permitting accurate identification of B cells by electron microscopy.

The relationships between secretory granules and the plasma membrane assume special importance in the case of pancreatic islets, since the plasma membrane is presumably not only the receptor for glucose but also the structural barrier limiting the egress of insulin from the cytoplasm of the cell. In most cells bulk secretion of material that occurs following fusion of a cytoplasmic sac with the plasma membrane is referred to as *exocytosis*. In the case of pancreatic islets the term emiocytosis was used by Lacy and Hartroft (1959). The former is a more generic term and would be preferable for consistency to refer to all secretory activities of cells characterized by the presence of fusion of the limiting membrane of the secretory granule with the plasma membrane as exocytosis. Exocytosis has been observed infrequently in pancreatic islets with conventional transmission electron microscopy (Orci *et al.*, 1969, 1969–70, 1973a). Orci *et al.* (1973a) and Orci *et al.* (1977) have documented the presence of pits in the plasma membranes of B cells by electron microscopy in freeze-etched islet cells after exposure to glucose in high concentration in culture. The documentation of an exocytotic event in B cells in freeze-etched preparations thus provides conclusive evidence that this release mechanism of B granules is a verified hypothesis as proposed by Lacy and Hartroft (1959) and Lacy (1968). The uptake by islet cells of horseradish peroxidase as described by Orci *et al.* (1973c) is further confirmation of the reality of this cellular process. Based on our knowledge of other systems, especially acinar pancreatic cells, exocytosis would appear to be the general mechanism of cellular protein secretion. An exception may well be the case of thyroid C cells as described by Fortney (1975, 1978).

A closely related intracellular phenomenon to the process of exocytosis is the mechanism of cytoplasmic motility. As proposed by Lacy *et al.* (1968) and amplified in numerous other studies (Malaisse *et al.*, 1971; Malaisse-Lagae *et al.*, 1971; Malaisse, 1973), the microfilaments and microtubules that are ubiquitous in cells play a critical role in the movement of

---

Fig. 6. Squirrel monkey pancreatic islets. These B cells from a normal squirrel monkey pancreatic islet illustrate the diversity of B cells within primates and should be compared with Figs. 1–4 from human pancreatic islets. The secretory granule cores in many instances appear agranular and somewhat irregular but in others are very uniformly homogenous. The stubby paracrystalline cores of human B granules are seen only infrequently (arrows). Subsequent electron micrographs of A and D cells from the same species are strikingly similar to those observed from humans (Figs. 7 and 8). The background cytoplasm is identical to that observed from human pancreatic islets in that it contains scattered granular and agranular endoplasmic reticulum, elements of the Golgi apparatus, and numerous microfilaments, microtubules, and scattered mitochondria. A portion of the capillary with a fenestrated endothelium is present on the right. × 19,700.

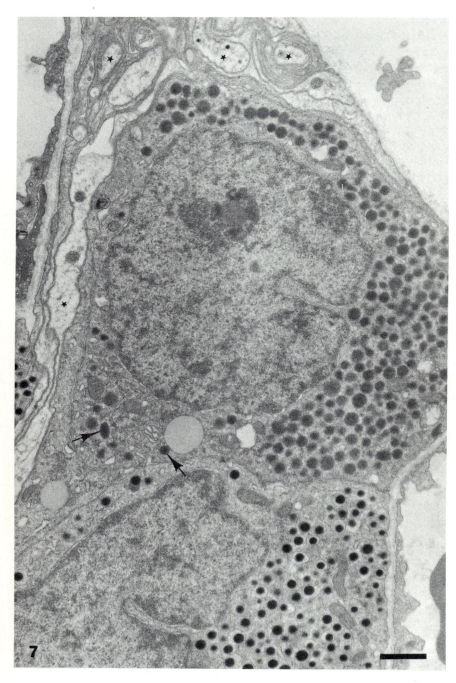

cytoplasmic organelles including secretory granules. Thus the events of B cell secretion involve the utilization of contractile organelles to move B granules to a position subjacent to the plasma membrane where the abutting membranes fuse and rupture releasing the insulin in the granule core into the intercellular or extracellular compartment. Insulin gains access to the blood vascular compartment by free diffusion through the stroma, a process that could be compromised by the fibrosis and scarring of the vascular stroma as seen in diabetes (Munger and Lang, 1973).

III. A CELLS (α CELLS, α_2 CELLS)

A cells as contrasted to B cells were originally characterized as having a uniform population of extremely electron-opaque secretory granules (Figs. 1, 2, 9, 10, and 12) (Lacy, 1957a,b, 1962). This generalization has been reaffirmed in virtually all ultrastructural studies to date on mammalian pancreatic islets including human islets (Sato *et al.,* 1966; Like, 1967; Greider *et al.,* 1970; Wellman *et al.,* 1970; van Assche and Gepts, 1971; Deconinck *et al.,* 1972; Munger, 1972a). In most animals studied to date, A and B secretory granules are roughly the same size (300 ± 50 nm), the only distinguishing feature being the nature of the core.

A fascinating question relative to A cells involves the unique appearance of A-cell secretory granules in the primates studied to date, including humans (see previous list above). In all primates studied the granule core of A cells has two characteristic components, an extremely electron-opaque central spherical mass located asymmetrically with respect to the limiting membrane (Munger, 1972a,b) and granular material of moderate electron opacity filling the compartment between the electron-opaque component and the limiting membrane (Figs. 4, 5, 7, and 8). Thus the granule of

Fig. 7. Squirrel monkey pancreatic islet. This electron micrograph illustrates a portion of a D cell (above) and an A cell (below) from squirrel monkey pancreatic islets. The D cell is similar to that illustrated in human pancreatic islets in Figs. 1 and 2. The A cell has a typical eccentric bull's-eye with a finely granular material filling the secretory granule between the opaque core and limiting membrane. These A granules resemble the eccentric bull's-eye seen in the human material depicted previously. The D cell in the region of the Golgi apparatus has several secretory granules (arrows) that are more irregular and more electron-opaque than typically seen throughout the cytoplasm. This is a constant feature of well-fixed pancreatic islet D cells. These are presumptive prosecretory granules that have a greater electron opacity than the secretory granules found throughout the cytoplasm. Surrounding both these A and D cells are elements of the autonomic nervous system. The axons are indicated by stars. The cytoplasm between the axon and the D and A cells is that of a Schwann cell. In this instance the Schwann cell and its enveloped axons are within the basal lamina of the islet epithelium, which can be seen both to the left and to the right of this epithelial complex. A portion of a vascular capillary is present at the upper left. × 13,700.

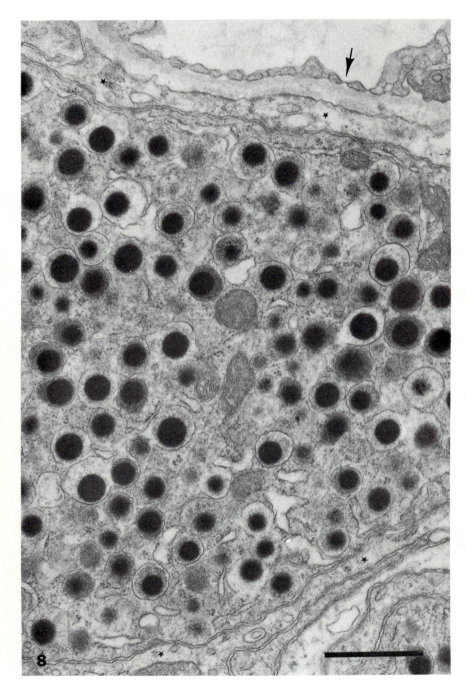

primate A cells resembles an eccentric bull's-eye. Even the secretory granules of presumptive glucagon-secreting cells from human and primate gastrointestinal mucosa have this unique appearance (Kobayashi *et al.,* 1970). Other mammals have A cells characterized by a clearly demarcated, spherical, electron-opaque core and an electron-lucent space separating the core from the limiting membrane (Figs. 9, 10, 12, and 13) (Munger *et al.,* 1965). These examples from canine pancreas closely resemble the ultrastructure of other mammalian A-cell granules (Munger, 1972b). As described by Smith (1974, 1975a) in birds, Rhoten (1970, 1971a,b, 1973a,b) in reptiles, and Brinn (1973, 1975, 1976) in fish, A cells do not follow the mammalian model or the primate exception as described above (Munger, 1972b). The granule size also differs significantly in submammalian species. In contrast to the variability encountered in nonmammalian species, the similarities of A cells from a diverse group of nonprimate mammals is surprisingly constant. Caramia *et al.* (1965) previously has noted a variability in the diameter of secretory granules of A cells in guinea pigs, although this could not be confirmed on the basis of the quantitative studies of Bencosme and Lechago (1968). Using statistical methods they were not able to document discrete populations of A cells based on granule size, and the problem posed by secretory granules of small diameter as described subsequently has not been satisfactorily answered in the guinea pig on the basis of more recent studies by Munger (1972b) and Munger and Lang (1973).

The other cytoplasmic organelles present in pancreatic A cells are similar to those of pancreatic islet B cells with minor exceptions. Clusters of granular endoplasmic reticulum are commonly observed in A cells (Figs. 9 and 12). The Golgi apparatus of all animals studied to date often contains small masses of accumulated secretory material in the cisternae (Fig. 12). This presumptive prosecretory material or condensing secretion product is consistently observed in A cells and is only rarely present in other cells of the pancreatic islets, as in Fig. 10 in a B cell. Munger (1962, 1972b) has observed small electron-opaque particles on the plasma membrane of A cells, and similar densities can occasionally be seen on plasma membranes

---

Fig. 8. Squirrel monkey pancreatic islet. A portion of an A cell with a typical primate core illustrated at higher magnification. The cores have an eccentric, electron-opaque portion that is elliptically or eccentrically placed within the limiting membrane. The A cell in this instance is completely enveloped by Schwann cell cytoplasm which is indicated by stars. Other areas have axons of the autonomic nervous system similar to those seen in Fig. 7. The Schwann cell cytoplasm is within the epithelium of the endocrine pancreas, thus the basal lamina is outside the Schwann cell proper and there is no basal lamina material between the Schwann cell and the A cell. A portion of a capillary at the top of the micrograph demonstrates prominent diaphragms covering the fenestrae (arrow). × 28,700.

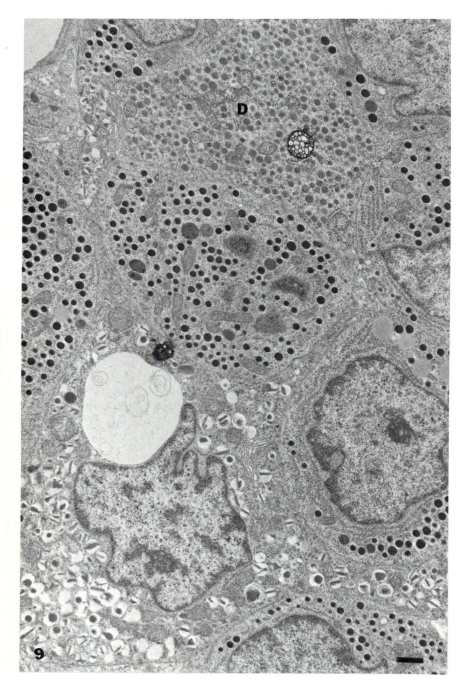

of a variety of cells and are thought by some to be a fixation artifact (Munger, 1962). These densities nonetheless are present and have been consistently observed in ultrastructural studies to date (Munger, 1972b). Their nature still remains to be elucidated. Another incidental finding by electron microscopy of pancreatic islet A cells is their association with peripheral ganglia (Munger, 1972b), forming what has been referred to as neuroinsular complexes on the basis of light microscopy (von Campenhout, 1927; Simard, 1937). As noted in this isolated case, the intimate association of developing endocrine cells within peripheral ganglia can indeed be confirmed by electron microscopy, and the interrelationship between neuronal somata and islet cells is a topic deserving future study. Many A cells, as in Figs. 7 and 8, are intimately associated with nerve fibers and Schwann cells, and A cells are responsive to sympathetic stimulation or the administration of sympathomimetic drugs (Esterhuizen and Howell, 1970; Porte, et al., 1975).

IV. C CELLS

C cells were identified as ungranulated cells in guinea pig pancreatic islets by Bensley (1911). Caramia et al. (1965) described cells lacking cytoplasmic secretory granules in guinea pig pancreas in electron micrographs studied at that time. Since 1965, however, the appearance of degranulated or agranular cells in pancreatic islets is suspect because many animals including the guinea pig (Munger and Lang, 1973; Lang and Munger, 1976) can evidence spontaneous diabetes mellitus with degranulated B cells. Thus the identification and characterization of agranular cells or undifferentiated cells in pancreatic islets can be done only on a presumptive basis. The micrograph illustrating a presumptive C cell published originally by Caramia et al. (1965) thus could have several interpretations other than confirming Bensley's (1911) characterization of agranular cells. Cells in the pancreatic islets often have characteristics of ductal elements, since pancreatic islets develop by budding from small ductules, as depicted in Fig. 1. Any ductal cytoplasm directly contiguous with the islet parenchyma (with no intervening basal lamina) could in turn be interpreted as being part of

Fig. 9.   This and Figs. 10–14 illustrate portions of the dog pancreatic islet. This particular electron micrograph is from the left lobe and illustrates a portion of a D cell (D) surrounded by A cells which have very electron-opaque secretory granules and obviously crystalline B-cell granules at the lower left. The irregular electron-opaque masses of material within the cytoplasm of all islet cells are lipofuscin. The A cells at the right have masses of granular endoplasmic reticulum, an observation common in A cells. × 7800.

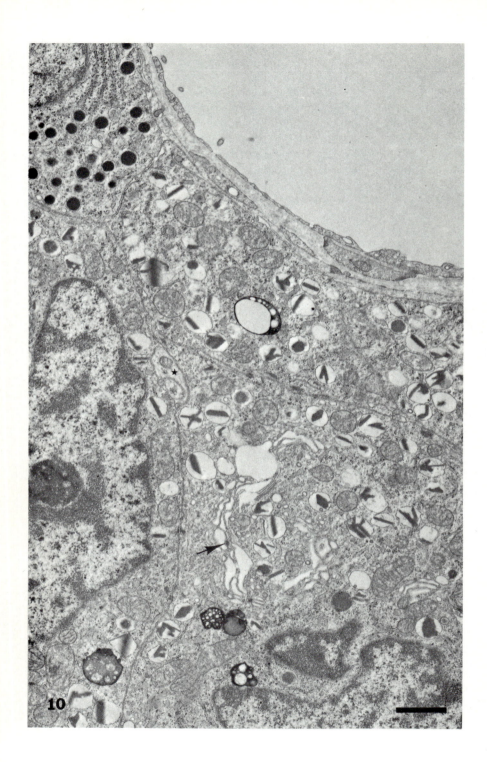

10

the islet but in reality represents only cells intimately associated with the islet. A similar situation exists in neuronal somata and associated satellite cells of a neuroinsular complex (Munger, 1972b). The normal innervation within the islet epithelial compartment, as in Fig. 7, 8, 10, 11, 13, and 14, also illustrates the same point (see Section IX). On the basis of these considerations, it is my opinion that the question of C cells be held in abeyance and that any proposal to characterize C cells as a distinct cellular population should be done with extreme care. Based on our present understanding of islet cells, any nondifferentiated cell could qualify as a C cell.

V. D CELLS (α_1 CELLS)

As noted in Section I, the third granulated cell of pancreatic islets was characterized on the basis of staining characteristics as a D cell by Bloom in 1931. Other staining parameters including argyrophilia and metachromasia were noted by Manocchio (1960) and Manocchio and Caramia (1962). The acceptance of a D cell as a discrete cell type in pancreatic islets awaited the advent of electron microscopy (Caramia, 1963; Fujita, 1964; Caramia *et al.*, 1965; Munger *et al.*, 1965; Sato, Herman and Fitzgerald, 1966; Forssmann, 1976). With the use of a specific type of silver impregnation for light microscopic study, it was possible to identify a distinctive population of cells of specific distribution having common ultrastructural characteristics. Again as noted above with respect to A and B cells, the situation in non-mammalian vertebrats is different, but among the mammals studied to date the similarity of D cells is striking. These cells are characterized by a uniform population of moderately electron-opaque secretory granules that tend in most animals to be somewhat smaller than A-or B-cell granules (Figs. 1, 2, 7, 9, and 13), usually ~ 250 nm in diameter. In primates including humans, this distinction is striking because of the density differences between electron-opaque secretory granule cores of A cells and the more modest but uniform electron opacity of D-cell granules. Since some

---

Fig. 10.   Dog pancreatic islet, left lobe. Portions of several B cells are present in the center of the micrograph and a small portion of an A cell at the upper left. Contrast in the electron opacity and secretory granule core in this instance is striking in that the B cells in most instances have agranular paracrystalline arrays for the secretory granule core. Presumptive secretory material is indicated by the arrow in the area of the Golgi apparatus. As in the case of the squirrel monkey indicated previously, components of the nervous system are indicated by a star identifying a portion of Schwann cell cytoplasm. The adjacent profile is that of a small axon of the autonomic nervous system. The background cytoplasm contains abundant but scattered endoplasmic reticulum, numerous vesicular profiles, and scattered mitochondria. A portion of a fenestrated capillary is present at the upper right. × 14,000.

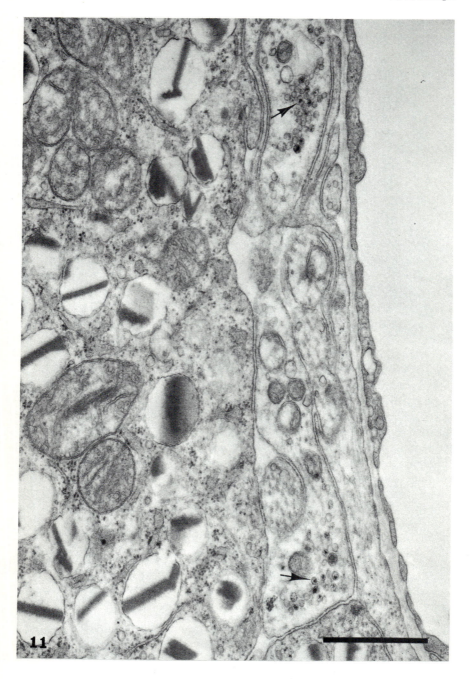

B-cell granules can also be homogenous, that is, not have a paracrystalline central core, the problem of identifying B cells as contrasted to D cells can be difficult in animals where many B-cell secretory granules are homogeneous in appearance. This particular problem is especially prominent in perinatal primate pancreatic islets. At high-magnification electron microscopy it might be impossible to identify a given small segment of cytoplasm of a cell with any degree of certainty. Low magnification or survey electron microscopy is not only necessary to identify a reasonable extent of cytoplasm but also to ensure the quality of cytoplasmic preservation. Much of the early controversy regarding the identification of D cells was the result of a fixation artifact, specifically the relatively poor fixation that resulted from direct osmium fixation (Munger, 1958). Under some conditions of fixation the secretory granule core of D cells becomes extremely electron-lucent, appearing washed out. Fixation artifacts are a current problem in the characterization of F cells, as noted below.

Other cytoplasmic characteristics of D cells are in many ways relatively undistinguished. Granular endoplasmic reticulum is scant, mitochondria are small, and the Golgi apparatus is relatively small and at times difficult to identify. Some granules near the Golgi body appear more electron-opaque than usual (Fig. 7) and may represent prosecretory granules similar to those of thyroid parafollicular cells as described by Fortney (1975, 1978). In this cell, unlike the situation in other islet cells, the prosecretory granules are more electron-opaque than the mature secretory granules. Masses of electron-opaque material identified as lipofuchsin are present scattered throughout the cytoplasm of D cells. Exocytosis has been observed rarely in D cells to date. The other charactristics of pancreatic D cells are their shape and distribution in islets. They tend to be stellate in form, having long cytoplasmic processes, and tend to be sandwiched between A and B cells.

With the use of immunocytochemistry methods evidence has been accumulating that D cells contain somatostatin (Erlandsen et al., 1976; Larsson et al., 1976a,b; Orci et al., 1976; Rhoten and Smith, 1978). The localization of somatostatin within neural as well as nonneural tissues raises several interesting questions with few answers. The major question concerns the normal functional role of this hormone.

Fig. 11. Dog pancreatic islet. The electron micrograph illustrates the intimate association between elements of the autonomic nervous system and cells of the pancreatic islet. The extremely small electron-opaque centers of the synaptic vesicles (arrow) indicate that this axon is an adrenergic terminal adjacent to a B cell at the left. The diaphragms covering the fenestrae of the fenestrated capillary at the right are prominent. × 31,500.

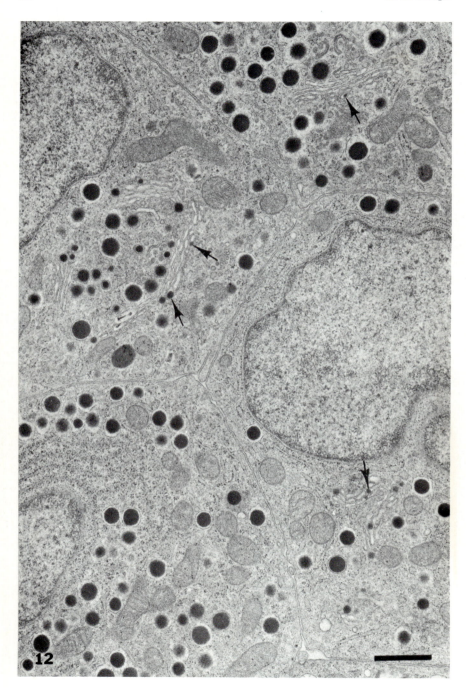

VI. E CELLS

E cells were first reported in the opossum by Thomas (1937) who described very large granules in cells at the margin of the pancreatic islets almost reaching the dimensions of acinar cell zymogen granules. In logical letter sequence this new cell type was thus called an E cell. Munger *et al.* (1965) confirmed this description by identifying large granule cells distinct from A, B, and D cells in opossum pancreatic islets as studied by electron microscopy. Since that time opossum islets have not been studied in detail, and this work should be reconfirmed using immunocytochemical as well as ultrastructural techniques. In the opossum, fortuitously, pancreatic islet A cells contain glycogen particles. The E cell, by way of contrast, never contained cytoplasmic glycogen, and thus ultrastructural differentiation of A from E cells was convincing. The E-cell granules were indeed larger than those of any other islet cell type in this species, and the relationship of this cell to the F cell described below certainly needs to be reevaluated.

VII. F CELLS (PP CELLS)

Bencosme *et al.* (1958) correlated the glucagon content of the dog pancreas with the presence or absence of A cells, noting the absence of glucagon from the right lobe of the pancreas, often incorrectly referred to as the uncinate process (Munger *et al.*, 1965). While the left (or splenic) lobe of the dog pancreas contains a typical amount of glucagon, the right (or duodenal) lobe does not contain a significant amount. Bencosme and co-workers identified a cell they characterized as being distinct from B cells in the right lobe, and not knowing the nature of this cell they called it an "X cell." Munger *et al.* (1965) identified islet cells with unique secretory granules in the dog that were somewhat irregular in profile, were electron-opaque, and had uniform dark cores as differentiated from B and D cells of the pancreatic islets in the right lobe. The letter sequence described above was extended to include this cell as an F cell. Since the pancreatic islets in the right lobe of the dog pancreas are relatively small and infrequent, ultrastructural study is at best difficult. Sporadic attempts by the present author to repeat this work have always resulted in questionable fix-

Fig. 12. Dog pancreatic islets, left lobe. The A cells of the dog pancreatic islet as illustrated in this electron micrograph frequently contain masses of prosecretory material within the Golgi apparatus (arrows). The electron-opaque secretory granules are scattered throughout the cytoplasm, separating masses of granular endoplasmic reticulum and other typical cytoplasmic organelles as noted previously. The presence of prosecretory material within the cisternae of the Golgi apparatus is well illustrated in this micrograph, although equivalent areas can be found in A cells of other animals. × 14,000.

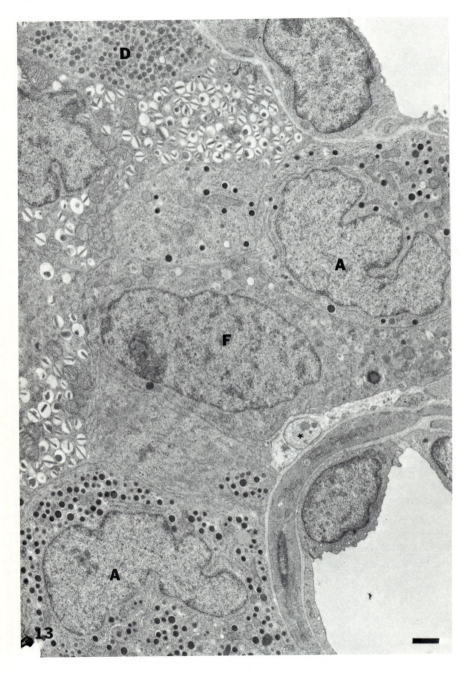

ation, with secretory granules appearing empty as if the result of a fixation artifact (similar to that originally described in D cells) (Figs. 13 and 14). Recently we have had an opportunity to study the dog pancreatic islets following vascular perfusion with techniques that usually result in superb islet preservation, and empty granules have again been consistently observed as in Figs. 13 and 14. Thus when techniques known to result in good fixation are used, this particular cell responds in a special way to the preparative procedures used for ultrastructural analysis. The recent observations of Forssmann *et al.* (1977) and Larsson and co-workers (1976a,b) confirm the existence of pancreatic polypeptide in these cells in the right lobe of the dog pancreas. Thus the F cell of the dog is a cell that contains pancreatic polypeptide. The role of this cell in the function of the islet is a subject deserving further study. In purely ultrastructural terms we are left with a series of unanswered questions. Does the F cell or pancreatic polypeptide cell (PP cell) of the dog resemble those of other animals? The answer to this question is certainly not apparent in the current literature or from the extant studies of this author's laboratory. Smith (1975b) has also observed a peculiar reaction to the fixation of these cells in the right lobe of the dog pancreas. It thus appears that F cells are extremely labile to aldehyde fixative, not responding in a manner typical of other endocrine-secretory cells.

VIII. OTHER ISLET CELLS

In addition to the list of cells cited above, other cells have been observed in pancreatic islets to date (Forssmann, 1976). In humans (Munger, 1972a) small granule cells can be observed in the adult as well as in embryonic specimens. The existence of small granule cells can also be verified in human embryonic pancreatic islets (Wages and Munger, 1977, Abstr.). In this study we also have observed cells with large secretory granules, also the nature of which is not known. Whether these are related to pancreatic polypeptide secreting cells, analogous to F cells, has not been determined,

---

Fig. 13. Dog pancreatic islet, right lobe. All four cell types of the dog pancreatic islet are illustrated in this fortuitous electron micrograph. A portion of a D cell (D) is present at the top of the micrograph, and a portion of an F cell (F) is present in the center surrounded by several B cells and three A cells (A). In most islets of the right lobe, A cells are only infrequently present, and this example is useful in providing a contrast between the ultrastructure of A as compared with F, D, or B cells, The secretory granules of the F cell are poorly defined, having an irregular finely granular core of low electron opacity. This is quite different in appearance from the homogeneous moderate electron opacity of B-cell granules visible at the top of the micrograph. A small axon (★) surrounded by Schwann cell cytoplasm directly abuts the F cell. A portion of a small arteriole is present at the lower right. × 7350.

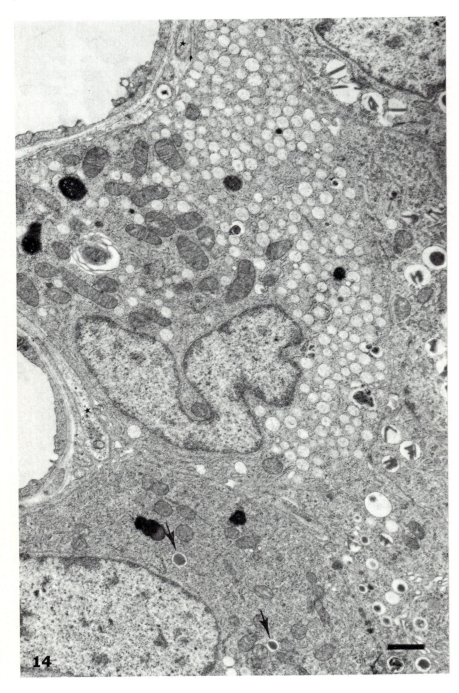

in that immunocytochemical studies to date have been consistently negative for hormones other than insulin and glucagon in embryonic rhesus monkey pancreatic islets.

Clearly cells containing small secretory granules resembling catecholamine-containing cells that might well be silver-positive are present in primate, including human, pancreatic islets. Other cell types as defined by electron microscopy may well indeed be present, and thus caution should be exercised in evaluating the hormonal interactions and functional parameters of pancreatic islets.

IX. INNERVATION

Pancreatic islets of all animals studied to date are well innervated with presumptive components of the autonomic nervous system. The identification of small unmyelinated axons in electron micrographs is impossible without resorting to cytochemical techniques. However, axon profiles and associated Schwann cells are variably prominent components of pancreatic islets. In some animals, such as the dog and cat, axon terminals can be seen frequently (Figs. 11, 13, and 14). Unmyelinated axons thus are found in the vascular connective tissue stroma infiltrating the islet. In some cases Schwann cells and associated unmyelinated axons are present within the islet parenchyma proper, as in Figs. 7 and 8. In this instance there is no intervening basal lamina between the Schwann cell and islet tissue. This latter arrangement is that of a neuroinsular complex as described previously in the dog (Munger, 1972b). In other species such as the human (as illustrated in this chapter) and the guinea pig, a neural component within the pancreatic islet parenchyma is not very prominent, although it is consistently observed if many electron micrographs are carefully examined. Distinguishing catecholamine-containing components of the sympathetic nervous system from parasympathetic fibers is tenuous at best, depending upon fortuitous preservation of the small electron-opaque component in the synaptic vesicles of catecholamine-containing axon terminals as in Fig.

Fig. 14. Dog pancreatic islet right lobe. A portion of F-cell cytoplasm is illustrated at higher magnification and can be compared with the F cell in Fig. 13. At the right is a B cell, and a small portion of F-cell cytoplasm is present at the bottom of the micrograph that has more electron-opaque secretory granules (arrows). The variability in electron opacity of secretory granules is illustrated in this example of two contiguous F cells, one containing almost exclusively electron-lucent, empty-appearing granules and the bottom cell containing scattered secretory granules of greater electron opacity. In other F cells, the more electron-opaque secretory granules were consistently observed in the region of the Golgi apparatus, suggesting their prosecretory nature. A small adrenergic terminal is indicated by the star. × 10,800.

11. The examples provided from monkey pancreatic islets in terms of inner-vation (Figs. 7 and 8) are somewhat unusual in that prominent nerve fibers are not usually observed in primate pancreatic islets.

X. VASCULATURE

The vascular connective tissue stroma of the pancreatic islets plays an important functional role in removing biologically active secretory products from these endocrine cells. The capillary endothelium is fenestrated, and these fenestrae are covered by a small, delicate diaphragm (Figs. 10 and 11). Arterioles can usually be identified at the margins of islets (Fig. 13), and in most cases a double basal lamina can be seen, one associated with the vascular endothelium and the other with the islet parenchyma proper (Fig. 10). The processes of cells insinuating themselves between the vascular capillary endothelium and the islet parenchyma are in most cases identified as pericyte in nature or as small processes of fibroblasts elaborating small amounts of collagen fibrils that can usually be identified in this compartment. Nerve fibers are usually embedded in the vascular connective tissue stroma (Fig. 14) although, as noted previously, they can in turn be found within the islet parenchyma. In some cases a single basal lamina appears to be the result of fusion of the basal lamina of the epithelial compartment and that of the epithelium (Fig. 11). The vascular connective tissue stroma in turn evidences age-related changes as seen in the examples of human pancreatic islets in Figs. 1 and 2. The degree of pro-liferation of connective tissue elements, fibroblasts, and bundles of col-lagen are all indicative of age-related scarring in this case. Examples of scarring in the vascular connective tissue stroma can also be seen in states related to diabetes mellitus (Munger and Lang, 1973) (See Chapter 13).

ACKNOWLEDGMENTS

This study was supported in part by U.S. Public Health Service contracts NIDR72–2401 and HD4–2869 and research grant HD11216 and AM11407.

REFERENCES

van Assche, F. A., and Gepts, W. (1971). *Diabetologia* **1**, 434–444.
Bencosme, S. A., and Lechago, J. (1968). *Lab. Invest.* **18**, 712–720.
Bencosme, S. A., Mariz, S., and Frei, J. (1958). *Lab. Invest.* **7**, 138–145.
Bensley, R. R. (1911). *Am. J. Anat.* **12**, 297–388.

Bloom, W. (1931) *Anat. Rec.* **49**, 363–37 .
Bloom, W., and Fawcett, D. W. (1975). "A Textbook of Histology," 10th ed. W. B. Saunders, Philadelphia, Pennsylvania.
Brinn, J. E., Jr. (1973). *Am. Zool.* **13**, 653.
Brinn, J. E., Jr. (1975) *Cell Tissue Res.* **162**, 357.
Brinn, J. E. Jr., and Epple, A. (1976) *Cell Tissue Res.* **171**, 317–329.
van Campenhout, E. (1927). *Arch. Biol. (Liege)* **35**, 45–88.
Caramia, F. (1962). *Folia Endocrinol.* **15**, 804–811.
Caramia, F. (1963). *Am. J. Anat.* **12**, 53–64.
Caramia, F., Munger, B. L., and Lacy, P. E. (1965). *Z. Zellforsch.* **67**, 533–546.
Deconinck, J. F., van Assche, F. A., Potvliege, P. R., and Gepts, W. (1972). *Diabetologia* **8**, 326–333.
Erlandsen, S. L., Hegne, O. D., Parsons, J. A., McEvoy, R. C., and Elde, R. P. (1976). *J. Histochem. Cytochem.* **24**, 883–897.
Esterhuizen, A. C., and Howell, S. L. (1970). *J. Cell Biol.* **46**, 593–598.
Forssmann, A. (1976). *Cell Tiss. Res.* **167**, 179–195.
Forssmann, W. G., Helmstaedter, V., Metz, J., Greenberg, J., and Chance, R. E. (1977). *Histochemistry* **50**, 281–290.
Fortney, J. A. (1975). "A Cytological Study of the Thyroid Parafollicular Cells of the Opossum, *Didelphis virginiana*." Ph.D. Thesis, The Pennsylvania State Univ., Pennsylvania.
Fortney, J. A. (1978). *Gen. Comp. Endocrinol.* **36**, 119–132.
Fujita, T. (1964). *Arch. Histol. Jpn.* **25**, 189–197.
Gomori, G. (1939a). *Anat. Rec.* **74**, 439–459.
Gomori, G. (1939b). *Am. J. Pathol.* **15**, 497–499.
Gomori, G. (1941). *Am. J. Pathol.* **17**, 395–406.
Gomori, G. (1950). *Am. J. Clin. Pathol.* **20**, 665–666.
Greider, M. H., Benscome, S. A., and Lechago, J. (1970). *Lab. Invest.* **22**, 344–354.
Greider, M. H., Gensell, D. J., and Gingrich, R. L. (1978). *J. Histochem. Cytochem.* **26**, 1103–1108.
Hartroft, W. S., and Wrenshall, G. A. (1955). *Diabetes* **4**, 1.
Hellerström, C., and Hellman, B. (1960). *Acta Endocrinol.* **35**, 518–532.
Jamieson, J. D., and Palade, G. E. (1967). *J. Cell Biol.* **34**, 597–615.
Kobayashi, K., Fujita, T., and Sasagawa, T. (1970). *Arch. Histol. Jpn.* **31**, 477–494.
Lacy, P. E. (1957a). *Anat. Rec.* **128**, 255–268.
Lacy, P. E. (1957b). *Diabetes* **6**, 498–507.
Lacy, P. E. (1962). *Diabetes* **11**, 509–513.
Lacy, P. E., and Hartroft, S. W. (1959). *Ann. N.Y. Acad. Sci.* **82**, 287.
Lacy, P. E., Howell, S. L., Young, D. A., and Fink, C. J. (1968). *Nature (London)* **219**, 1177.
Lane, M. A. (1907). *Am. J. Anat.* **7**, 409–422.
Lang, C. M. and Munger, B. L. (1976). *Diabetes* **25**, 434–443.
Larsson, L. I., Rehfeld, J. F., Sundler, F., and Håkanson, R. (1976a). *Nature (London)* **262**, 609–610.
Larsson, L. I., Sundler, F., and Håkanson, R. (1976b). *Diabetologia* **12**, 211–226.
Like, A. (1967). *Lab. Invest.* **16**, 937–951.
Malaisse, W. J. (1973). *Diabetologia* **9**, 167–173.
Malaisse, W. J., Malaisse-Lagae, F., Walker, M. O., and Lacy, P. E. (1971). *Diabetes* **20**, 257–265.
Malaisse-Lagae, F., Greider, M. H., Malaise, W. J., and Lacy, P. E. (1971). *J. Cell Biol.* **49**, 530–535.
Manocchio, I. (1960). *Z. Allg. Pathol. Anat.* **101**, 1–4.

34 B. L. Munger

Manocchio, I., and Caramia, F. (1962). *Sperimetale* **112**, 1–27.
Merlini, D., and Caramia, F. (1965). *J. Cell Biol.* **26**, 245–261.
Mowry, R. (1978). *Stain Technol.* **53**, 141–154.
Mowry, R. (1980). *Stain Technol.* **55**, 91–103.
Munger, B. L. (1958). *Am. J. Anat.* **103**, 275–297.
Munger, B. L. (1962) *Lab. Invest.* **11**, 885–901.
Munger, B. L. (1972a). *In* "Handbook of Physiology" (F. Steiner and N. Freinkel, eds.), Vol. I, pp. 305–314. Amer. Physiol. Soc., Washington, D.C.
Munger, B. L. (1972b). *In* "Glucagon" (P. J. Lefebvre and R. H. Unger, eds.), pp. 7–25. Pergamon, Oxford.
Munger, B. L., and Lang, C. M. (1973). *Lab. Invest.* **29**, 685–702.
Munger, B. L., Caramia, F., and Lacy, P. E. (1965). *Z. Zellforsch.* **67**, 776–798.
Orci, L., Stauffacher, W., Beaven, D., Lambert, A. E., Renold, A. E., and Rouiller, C. (1969). *Acta Diabetologica Latina* **6**, 271–374.
Orci, L., Lambert, A. E., Kanazawa, Y., Renold, A. E., and Rouiller, C. (1969–70). *Chem.-Biol. Inter.* **1**, 341–359.
Orci, L., Amherdt, M., Malaisse-Lagae, F., Rouiller, C., and Renold, A. E. (1973a). *Science* **179**, 82–84.
Orci, L., Amhert, M., Malaisse-Lagae, F., Rouiller, C., and Renold, A. E. (1973b). *Science* **179**, 82–84.
Orci, L., Malaisse-Lagae, F., Ravazzola, M., Amherdt, M., and Renold, A. E. (1973c). *Science* **181**, 561–562.
Orci, L., Baetens, D., Ravazzola, M., Stefan, Y., and Malaisse-Lagae, F. (1976). *In* "Endocrine Gut and Pancreas" (T. Fujita, ed.), pp. 73–88. Elsevier, Amsterdam.
Orci, L., Perrelet, A., and Friend, D. S. (1977). *J. Cell Biol.* **75**, 23–30.
Rhoten, W. B. (1970). *Anat. Rec.* **167**, 401–423.
Porte, D., Woods, S. C., Chen, M., Smith, P. H., and Ensinck, J. W. (1975). *Pharm. Biochem. Behav.* **3**, Suppl. 1, 127–133.
Rhoten, W. B. (1971a). *Gen. Comp. Endocrinol.* **17**, 203–219.
Rhoten, W. B. (1971b). "The Histophysiology of Reptilian Pancreatic Islets." Ph.D. Thesis, The Pennsylvania State Univ., Pennsylvania.
Rhoten, W. B. (1973a). *J. Exp. Zool.* **184**, 313–320.
Rhoten, W. B. (1973b). *Am. J. Pathol.* **227**, 993–997.
Rhoten, W. B., and Smith, P. H. (1978). *Am. J. Anat.* **151**, 595–601.
Sato, T., Herman, L., and Fitzgerald, P. J. (1966). *Gen. Comp. Endocrinol.* **7**, 132–157.
Simard, L. C. (1937). Les complexes neuro-insulaires du pancréas humain. *Arch. Anat. Microsc. Morphd. Exp.* **33**, 49–64.
Smith, P. H. (1973). "Histophysiology of the Pancreatic Islets in the Quail, *Coturnix coturnix japonica*." Ph.D. Thesis, The Pennsylvania State Univ., Pennsylvania.
Smith, P. H. (1974). *Anat. Rec.* **178**, 567–586.
Smith, P. H. (1975a). *Gen. Comp. Endocrinol.* **26**, 310–320.
Smith, P. H. (1975b). *Am. J. Anat.* **144**, 513–518.
Thomas, B. (1937). *Am. J. Anat.* **62**, 31–57.
Thomas, B. (1942). *Anat. Rec.* **82**, 327–345.
Wages, D. W., and Munger, B. L. (1977). *Anat. Rec.* **187**, 739 (Abstr.).
Wellmann, K. F., Volk, B. W., and Brancato, P. (1970). *Lab. Invest.* **25**, 97–103.

2

Functional Development of the Pancreatic Islets

D. BAXTER-GRILLO, E. BLÁZQUEZ,
T. A. I. GRILLO, J SODOYEZ,
F. SODOYEZ-GOFFAUX, and P. P. FOÀ

I. INTRODUCTION

Our interest in the embryological development of islet function began about 20 yr ago when epididymal fat pad assay and radioimmunoassay were not yet available and we had joined in the search for an *in vitro* insulin bioassay. Our tool was the chick embryo heart and, although its sensitivity turned out to be insufficient for the intended purpose, we found that, while during the early stages of development the rate of intracellular phosphorylation controlled glucose uptake by the myocardium, an insulin-sensitive glucose transport system became rate-limiting on the seventh day of incubation (Guidotti and Foà, 1961). Evidence that this event may coin-

35

The Islets of Langerhans
Copyright © 1981 by Academic Press, Inc.
All rights of reproduction in any form reserved.
ISBN 0-12-187820-1

cide with the appearance of beta granules in the pancreas (Lièvre, 1957; Thommes, 1960) stimulated our interest in the ontogeny of the islets and of certain hormone-dependent enzymes and in their relationship to the type of nutrients and to the manner in which they are obtained by the developing organism. Since then much work has been done on these matters, and a review of the published data, no matter how superficial, would turn this chapter into little more than a voluminous annotated bibliography. For this reason, rather than summarizing the evidence, we will attempt to weave the conclusions of our work and that of many other investigators into a coherent story, using morphological information mostly as an aid in interpreting biochemical and physiological data. Furthermore, we will attempt to show that development of the hormones of islet and other cells, and of the hormone-sensitive enzymes concerned with the regulation of metabolism, proceeds uniformly throughout embryogenesis, although abrupt changes may be brought about by modifying the nature and the supply of nutrients.

II. STAGES OF METABOLIC ONTOGENY

Metabolic ontogeny may be divided into several nutrition-dependent periods. During the first period, representing about one-third of development, glucose and other substrates are utilized for energy and growth; they need not be stored by the embryo, since they are provided in continuity by egg yolk or placental transfer. During the second period, corresponding to the development of the liver and adipose tissue, there is an accumulation of glycogen and fat. This accumulation prepares the developing organism for the third period—that of "physiological fast" between birth and the start of oral feeding. During the third period, in part as a result of a high glucagon/insulin ratio, these deposits are mobilized, providing the endogenous substrates necessary to sustain the high metabolic activities of the newborn and the glucose required by the brain and other glucose-dependent tissues. During this period the newborn may lose weight, and the preservation of euglycemia takes precedence over growth which resumes when the emergency is over and milk or other foods become available.

While birds appear to reach metabolic maturity at this point, mammals must go through a period of nursing during which, even though the secretion of insulin increases, the glucagon/insulin ratio remains relatively high; at this time the animal is consuming a high-fat, low-carbohydrate diet and obtains fuel and glucose from lipolysis and gluconeogenesis. This is followed by a fifth or weaning period during which the glucagon/insulin ratio decreases, lipolysis gives way to lipogenesis, glycogenolysis to glycogen synthesis, and gluconeogenesis to protein synthesis. This is an age of accelerated growth leading to the sixth and final period when the animal becomes adapted to the mixed diet typical of an adult. We hope that readers will accept these conclusions as a reasonable working hypothesis, and we urge them to fill in the gaps in our narrative and to correct our bias by reading at least a few of the many available reviews (Adam, 1971; Anderson *et al.*, 1975; Andreani *et al.*, 1980; Blazquez *et al.*, 1972; Borchard and Münterfering, 1969; Foà *et al.*, 1976; Girard *et al.*, 1975a,b; Greengard, 1975; Grillo, 1965; Hellman, 1956; Jost and Picon, 1970; Pictet and Rutter, 1972; Shelley *et al.*, 1975; Villee, 1969).

III. DEVELOPMENT OF THE PANCREAS

The classical description of the development of the pancreas assumes that this organ derives from the embryonic endoderm. However, Golosow and Grobstein (1962) and Wessels (1964) have shown that rudiments of dorsal pancreas do not differentiate *in vitro* unless mesodermal cells are present, while Pearse (1969) has suggested that the neural crest cells derived from the ectoderm might contribute to the development of the pancreatic islets, possibly by giving rise to APUD cells. While it has been established that the neural crest gives rise to a host of tissues, e.g., the adrenal medulla, dorsal root ganglia, sympathetic ganglia, and pigment cells (Hörstadius, 1950), there is no conclusive evidence of their migration into the pancreas or into other tissues where "pancreatic" hormones are produced (Dieterlen-Lièvre and Beaupain, 1976). Indeed, it has been demonstrated that one can separate chick embryo splanchnopleura from somatopleura before the migration of neural crest cells, graft it onto the coelom of quail embryos, and obtain insulin- and glucagon-producing pancreatic tissue. Pictet *et al.* (1975) have confirmed these results in rats. One should note, however, that the exact timing of this migration has not been established. Thus a neural crest origin must still be considered a possibility for some islet cells. Perhaps this uncertainty about the time of migration is one of the reasons why the results of much of the work on the embryological development of the islets are not uniform, which is perhaps not surprising if one considers the variety of animal species and techniques used.

As mentioned above, Thommes (1960) found evidence of beta granules in the pancreas of chick embryos on the seventh day of incubation, that is, one day before the time when Lièvre (1957) could demonstrate the first organized islets. Other workers found islets, consisting mostly of A cells, on the twelfth day of embryological development, or about 9 days after glucagon could be detected in the tissue and 1 day before the appearance of islets composed primarily of B cells (Lièvre, 1957; Beaupain and Dieterlen-

Lièvre, 1972). These and other findings led to the suggestion that A cells may play a role in early embryogenesis (Rall *et al.*, 1973) and in B-cell differentiation (Lambert *et al.*, 1970), a chronological and functional relationship which may or may not prove to be correct in other species. Indeed, although there is evidence that in the early stages of organogenesis the rat pancreas contains primarily alpha granules and produces about 100 times more glucagon than insulin (Rall *et al.*, 1973), most investigators believe that both glucagon (Assan and Boillot, 1973; Benzo and Stearns, 1975; Jarousse *et al.*, 1973) and insulin (Asplund, 1973; Benzo and Green, 1974; Clark and Rutter, 1973; Freie *et al.*, 1975; Heinze *et al.*, 1975; Rall *et al.*, 1979; Schaeffer *et al.*, 1973) appear by midgestation and increase as gestation progresses. In addition, the fact that biologically active insulin can be extracted from the rat pancreas on the fourteenth day (Grillo, 1965), while the A cells do not differentiate until the eighteenth day (Orci *et al.*, 1969) or thereafter (Hellman, 1965), suggests that the chronological relationship may actually be reversed.

In the human fetus, islets have been detected at the 54-mm stage, the presence of insulin at the 80-mm stage, and the first beta granules at the 90-to 110-mm stage (Rastogi *et al.*, 1970; Schaeffer *et al.*, 1973). Not too long thereafter, toward the middle of the third trimester of pregnancy, cells containing alpha and beta granules have been identified and significant amounts of insulin extracted from the pancreas (Wellman *et al.*, 1971), while glucagon-like materials have been found in the pancreas at about the sixth week and in the blood toward the fifteenth week (Assan and Boillot, 1973; Assan and Girard, 1975; Schaeffer *et al.*, 1973). At the 130-mm stage A cells appear to be more abundant than B cells, although at term the latter represent about 60% of the islet cell mass and A cells about 30% of it (Ville, 1969). Complicated by methodological difficulties, the matter becomes even more complex when one considers that hormone biosynthesis is not synonymous with hormone secretion. Indeed, it appears that even though insulin biosynthesis and total pancreatic insulin content may increase throughout fetal life, and even though appropriate stimuli may cause a rapid hormone release during early embryogenesis, perhaps in response to the developing adenylate cyclase system (Burr *et al.*, 1971; De Gasparo *et al.*, 1975; Grill *et al.*, 1975; Milner *et al.*, 1971), the mechanism for insulin release does not become fully mature until the end of gestation or after birth (Asplund, 1973; Blázquez *et al.*, 1975; Cohen and Turner, 1972; Fiser *et al.*, 1974a; Lernmark and Wenngren, 1972; Sodoyez-Goffaux *et al.*, 1979, in press). In spite of this relative immaturity, the prenatal plasma insulin levels are high and drop abruptly as soon as the umbilical cord is cut, probably because the transplacental nutrient and a specific placental secretagogue provide constant stimulation to the B cells (Blázquez *et al.*, 1972, 1974b, 1975; Felix *et al.*, 1971; Sodoyez-Goffaux *et al.*, 1971, 1979).

The importance of nutritional factors in the regulation of fetal insulin secretion is demonstrated also by the fact that exogenous secretagogues, including the high glucose levels of a diabetic mother (Obenshain *et al.*, 1970), can stimulate the fetal pancreas (Asplund *et al.*, 1969; Bassett *et al.*, 1974; Blázquez *et al.*, 1975; Davis *et al.*, 1971; Kervran and Girard, 1974; Phillips *et al.*, 1979; Sodoyez-Goffaux *et al.*, 1971). The mechanism of this stimulation and, in particular, the metabolic reactions required for insulin synthesis and release by the developing pancreas are not clear. However, information obtained using mature (Ashcroft, 1980) as well as fetal tissue (Andersson *et al.*, 1975; Asplund and Hellerström, 1972) suggests that the effectiveness of nutrients depends upon the ability of B cells to metabolize them, and that other factors such as the adrenal cortical hormones (Bassett *et al.*, 1973), ACTH (Jack and Milner, 1975; Milner and Jack, 1975), and growth hormone (Hoet *et al.*, 1975) may act as modulators. As in the case of insulin, the biosynthesis of glucagon is not synonymous with its release. Thus, although glucagon can be found in the fetal pancreas by midgestation or before (see above), in most cases a full response of A cells to secretagogues or their suppression by insulin and glucose cannot be observed until the end of gestation or after birth (Jarrousse and Rosselin, 1975; Lernmark and Wenngren, 1972; Massi-Benedetti *et al.*, 1974; Sodoyez-Goffaux *et al.*, 1979; Sperling *et al.*, 1974; Wise *et al.*, 1973). This maturation of the release mechanism manifests itself with a pronounced surge in plasma glucagon levels immediately after birth, when, as we have seen, the release of insulin is suppressed and therefore the glucagon/insulin ratio rises (Blázquez *et al.*, 1972, 1974b; Di Marco *et al.*, 1975, 1978; Girard *et al.*, 1972, 1975; Grajwer *et al.*, 1977; Jarrousse and Rosselin, 1975; Jarrousse *et al.*, 1973; Rogers *et al.*, 1974; Sperling *et al.*, 1974). It has been suggested that these endocrine changes are facilitated by the neonatal activation of the alpha-adrenergic system (Eliot *et al.*, 1978; Grajwer *et al.*, 1977; Wood and Porte, 1974), resulting in decreased B-cell sensitivity to insulinogenic stimuli (Blázquez *et al.*, 1975), increased A-cell sensitivity to amino acids (Wise *et al.*, 1973), decreased A-cell resistance to the inhibitory effect of glucose (Luyckx, 1974; Luyckx *et al.*, 1972), or actual A-cell stimulation by glucose (Fiser *et al.*, 1974b).

A survey of the embryological development of the endocrine pancreas is not complete without citing studies on the presence of somatostatin in fetal rat pancras (Doi *et al.*, 1979; McIntosh *et al.*, 1977; Mueller *et al.*, 1978), on the secretion of somatostatin by monolayer cultures of neonatal rat pancreas (Patel *et al.*, 1979), on the inhibitory effect somatostatin has on the A and B cells of newborn animals (Duran Garcia *et al.*, 1976; Grajwer *et al.*, 1977; Sodoyez-Goffaux *et al.*, 1979; Sperling *et al.*, 1977), and on the development of pancreatic polypeptide (PP) cells (Paulin and Dubois, 1978; Rahier *et al.*, 1979).

IV. DEVELOPMENT OF RELATED ENDOCRINE FUNCTION

In view of the direct and indirect relationships among pancreatic islets, growth hormone, ACTH, and glucocorticoids, a brief mention of the ontogeny of these hormones is in order. Growth hormone is found in fetal rat pituitary and plasma on the nineteenth day of gestation, declining thereafter only to rise again after weaning (Blázquez *et al.*, 1974a; Rieutort, 1974), while somatomedin appears long before term in the lamb (Gluckman *et al.*, 1979) and in the rat (Drazin *et al.*, 1979; Rechler *et al.*, 1979). In man, the anterior pituitary and plasma content of growth hormone increases from weeks 10–14 to weeks 35–40 of gestation and then again between the ages of 1 and 9 yr (Kaplan *et al.*, 1972; Pronina and Sparonova, 1976). Although a response to arginine can be demonstrated at birth, even if the infant is premature (Ponté *et al.*, 1972), a sleep–wake cycle appears only after the third month of life (Vigneri and D'Agata, 1971).

In the rat, adrenocorticotropic activity appears to start between the seventeenth and the eighteenth days of gestation (Milkovic *et al.*, 1973), whereas the level of glucocorticoids increases significantly only toward the end of gestation, reaching a maximum 1 or 2 days after birth (Di Marco *et al.*, 1978; Villee, 1969). Nevertheless the fetal rat liver is sensitive to the glycogenic action of cortisol (Dawes and Shelley, 1968; Eisen *et al.*, 1973; Greengaard and Dewey, 1970; Shelley *et al.*, 1975). Ultrastructural and histochemical evidence for the development of serotonin and enteroglucagon in the developing chick duodenum has been published (Baxter-Grillo *et al.*, 1973).

V. DEVELOPMENT OF TARGET SYSTEMS

Although hormone biosynthesis and release are necessary steps for hormone action, the latter cannot be carried out unless the target tissues are endowed with the necessary hormone receptors and mediator enzymes. Indeed, insulin and glucagon binding have been demonstrated in fetal rat liver (Bláquez *et al.*, 1976; Sodoyez-Goffaux *et al.*, in press), while enzymes for glycogen synthesis and breakdown (Baer and Hahn, 1971; Ballard, 1971; Blázquez *et al.*, 1972, 1974b; Boxer *et al.*, 1974; Dawes and Shelley, 1968; Devos and Hers, 1974; Eisen *et al.*, 1973; Girard *et al.*, 1972, 1975a; Greengard, 1975; Grillo, 1965; Grillo and Baxter-Grillo, 1966; Grillo *et al.*, 1964a,b; Kirby and Hahn, 1974; Linarelli *et al.*, 1974; Mersmann *et al.*, 1972; Mintz *et al.*, 1973; Novák *et al.*, 1972; Okuno *et al.*, 1964a,b; Plas and Nunex 1976; Schaub and Becker, 1972; Schwartz *et al.*, 1975; Shelley *et al.*, 1975) and for glycolysis, gluconeogenesis, lipogenesis, and lipolysis have been demonstrated in fetal liver and adipose tissue (Adam *et al.*, 1975; Girard *et al.*, 1976; Koler *et al.*, 1969; Langslow, 1972; Novak and Monkus, 1972; Philippidis and Ballard, 1970; Schaub *et al.*, 1972; Taylor *et al.*, 1967; Willgerodt *et al.*, 1975). These enzymes are hormone-sensitive and can be activated by the administration of insulin or glucagon. For example, exogenous insulin stimulates glucose uptake and glycogen synthesis (Manns and Brockman, 1969; Rabain and Picon, 1974) by the liver of the rat fetus and glycogen synthetase activity in the skeletal muscle of the chick embryo (Leibson *et al.*, 1974), inhibits the normal development of hepatic glucose-6-phosphatase and phosphoenolpyruvate carboxykinase (Girard *et al.*, 1973a,b), and stimulates glucose and amino acid uptake and protein synthesis by fetal rat heart (Vinicor *et al.*, 1975) and glucose uptake and lipogenesis by chick embryo heart (Guidotti and Foà, 1961; Foà *et al.*, 1965). On the other hand, exogenous glucagon stimulates the activity of hepatic adenylate cyclase (Linarelli *et al.*, 1974), phosphorylase (Pines *et al.*, 1975), and gluconeogenetic enzymes (Garcia Ruiz *et al.*, 1973; Girard *et al.*, 1973a,b; Hanson *et al.*, 1973; Philippidis and Ballard, 1970) and consequently stimulates glycogenolysis and gluconeogenesis (Adam, 1971; Adam *et al.*, 1975; Chiu and Phillips, 1974; Swiatek, 1971). Little is known about the activities of other glycogen-degrading enzymes, such as amylo-1,6-glocosidase (a debranching enzyme) and lysosomal α-glucosidase, except that in the rat they increase toward the end of gestation (Vaillant, 1975).

VI. ROLE OF NUTRITION

Although the time of these embryological developments appears to vary from species to species, the overall picture suggests that, as the embryo undergoes early development in a protected environment, its metabolic requirements are fulfilled through pathways regulated primarily by the facilitated transfer of nutrients through the placenta (Alexander *et al.*, 1955; Davies, 1957) which, in the words of Bernard (1859), serves as a "transitory liver." Sudden changes seldom occur, although mechanisms for rapid adaptation already exist in the form of maturing endocrine and enzymatic systems. As time goes on, these become more important and the embryo becomes more dependent upon its own hormones, since the placenta appears to be impermeable to those of the mother (Adam *et al.*, 1972; Alexander *et al.*, 1973; Chez *et al.*, 1975; Jost and Picon, 1970; Schwartz, 1975; Wolf *et al.*, 1969). This process corresponds to a gradual takeover of the placental glycogenic function by the liver, so that, as the end of gestation approaches, the fetus, having practiced "a rigid glycogen economy at the expense of its mother's dextrose" (Windle, 1940) and driven by the prevailing action of insulin, begins to accumulate glycogen and fat (Ballard, 1971; Blázquez *et al.*, 1972; Dawes and Shelley, 1968; Harding, 1970; Shelley, 1960; Windle, 1940) in anticipation of the relative independence of life after birth.

Changes in maternal metabolism also contribute to this fetal adaptation: For example, during the last third of pregnancy the mother tends to utilize more fat and, perhaps as the result of an increased secretion of growth hormone, cortisol, and placental lactogen (Adam, 1971; Chez *et al.*, 1975; Mintz *et al.*, 1969; Spellacy *et al.*, 1973), develops a relative insulin resistance, sparing glucose for fetal energy requirements and glycogen synthesis. This relative abundance of hepatic glycogen reveals itself during birth, when a sudden release of catecholamines (Eliot *et al.*, 1978; Korman, 1973) and glucagon stimulates glycogenolysis, raises neonatal plasma glucose, and erases the maternofetal gradient characteristic of earlier times. This neonatal hyperglycemia is of short duration, and almost immediately after birth the plasma glucose decreases, remaining at relatively low levels throughout the period of fasting which precedes the start of oral feeding. During this period, which lasts several hours in the rat and about 12–24 hr in man, the metabolic substrates needed by the newborn and, in particular, the glucose necessary for the function and development of the central nervous system, must be obtained from the nutrients stored during fetal life. This retrieval is controlled by glucagon, epinephrine, and glucocorticoids, and by the hormone-dependent enzyme systems which, as we have seen above, lead to (1) increased glucose production from hepatic glycogen (Adam *et al.*, 1975; Jost and Picon, 1970; Snell and Walker, 1973) and lactic acid production from muscle glycogen (Shelley, 1960; Shelley *et al.*, 1975), (2) decreased lipogenesis from glucose (Hahn and Skala, 1972; Novak *et al.*, 1973; Taylor *et al.*, 1967), (3) an increased supply of fatty acids, glycerol, and ketone bodies (Alexander *et al.*, 1969; Aranda *et al.*, 1973), and (4) relative glucose intolerance and insulin resistance (Blázquez *et al.*, 1975; Dawes and Shelley, 1968; Falorni *et al.*, 1974).

The survival value of these endocrine and metabolic occurrences is self-evident. Indeed, the risk of neonatal hypoglycemia is great in infants of diabetic mothers who secrete large amounts of insulin and, in some cases, insufficient amounts of glucagon (Bloom and Johnston, 1972; Foà, 1979; Shelley and Neligan, 1966) and in whom the normal reversal of the insulin/glucagon ratio fails to occur. By the fourth hour after birth, as the supply of hepatic glycogen dwindles, gluconeogenesis supplants glycogenolysis as the major supplier of glucose in the rat pup, and both substrate (protein) and energy source (fatty acids) are provided by maternal milk (Adam, 1971; Ballard, 1971; Beaudry *et al.*, 1977; Girard *et al.*, 1975a,b; Haymond *et al.*, 1974). The immediate cause of this neonatal switch from nutrient conservation to nutrient mobilization appears to be an abrupt change in the secretion of regulating hormones and consequent activation of the necessary enzymes. Indeed, the switch can be accelerated by the injection of glucagon into a rat fetus and retarded by the injection of insulin.

But what causes this sudden change in the "impressive stability of the fetal hormonal milieu" (Schwartz, 1975)? We believe that the reasons may well be the composition of the diet and the change from a continuous to an interrupted mode of nutrition. This hypothesis is supported by evidence that prenatal abnormalities in nutrient supply, such as may occur in prematurity (Grasso et al., 1973), in postmaturity (Portha et al., 1976), in infants of diabetic mothers (Andreani et al., 1979; Luyckx et al., 1972; Shima et al., 1966; Sosenke et al., 1979), in maternal starvation (Shanbaugh, 1977), or as a result of other manipulations of early feeding, can cause profound and possibly permanent endocrine, enzymatic, and metabolic changes (Asplund, 1972; Bertrand et al., 1977; Hahn and Kirby, 1973; Johnson et al., 1973; Lemonnier, 1972; Spellacy et al., 1973).

The major sites of these neonatal metabolic changes are the liver, the white adipose tissue, and the skeletal muscle, while other tissues, which in the adult are glucagon-sensitive, at birth appear to be relatively resistant. Thus the brown adipose tissue of newborn rabbits continues to accumulate triglycerides, as if under the preponderant influence of insulin (Hardman and Hull, 1970), while the cyclase system of rat myocardium does not respond to glucagon until the animal is 4 weeks old or older (Vinicor et al., 1975), although glucagon receptors are present at term (Windenthal and Wakeland, 1973). Given the vital function of myocardium and the important role of brown adipose tissue in thermogenesis, the protection of these tissues from the lipolytic and glycogenolytic action of glucagon during the neonatal period may have survival value. At weaning, when the nature, size, and frequency of meals change to those characteristic of adult life, many of the endocrine and metabolic processes are again reversed: The insulin/glucagon ratio gradually increases, glycogenolysis gives way to glycogen synthesis, gluconeogensis decreases, protein synthesis increases, and lipogenesis, no longer inhibited by the high-fat diet (Susini et al., 1979; Taylor et al., 1967), overtakes lipolysis. As in the adult animal, the endocrine system in now capable of responding "on demand."

REFERENCES

Adam, P. A. J. (1971). Adv.. Metab. Disord. 5, 183–275.
Adam, P. A. J., King, K. C.. Schwartz, R., and Teramo, K. (1972). J. Clin. Endocrinol. 34, 772.
Adam, P. A. J., Glazer, G., and Rogoff, F. (1975). Pediatr. Res. 9, 816–820.

Alexander, D. P., Andrews, R. D., Huggett, A. St. G., Nixon, D. A., and Widdas, W. F. (1955). *J. Physiol. (London)* **129,** 352–366.
Alexander, D. P., Britton, H. G., Cohen, N. M., and Nixon, D. A. (1969). *Biol. Neonat.* **14,** 178–193.
Alexander, D. P., Assan, R., Britton, H. G., and Nixon, D. A. (1973). *Biol. Neonat.* **23,** 391–402.
Andersson, A., Grill, V., Asplund, K., Berne, C., Agren, A., and Hellerström, C. (1975). *In* "Early Diabetes in Early Life" (R. A. Camerini-Davalos and H. S. Cole, eds.), pp. 49–56. Academic Press, New York.
Andreani, D., Fallucca, F., Russo, A., Maldonato, A., Caccamo, C., Lamalfa, G., De Gado, F., and Pachi, A. (1979). *J. Annu. Diabétol. Hôtel-Dieu* pp. 93–101.
Andreani, D., Lefebvre, P. J., and Marks, V., eds. (1980). "Current Views on Hypoglycemia and Glucagon." pp. 11–511. Academic Press, New York.
Aranda, A., Blázquez, E., and Herrera, E. (1973). *Horm. Metab. Res.* **5,** 350–355.
Ashcroft, S. J. H. (1980). *Diabetologia* **18,** 5–15.
Asplund, K. (1972). *Diabetologia* **8,** 153–159.
Asplund, K. (1973). *Eur. J. Clin. Invest.* **3,** 338–344.
Asplund, K., and Hellerström, C. (1972). *Horm. Metab. Res.* **4,** 159–163.
Asplund, K., Andersson, A., Jarrousse, C., and Hellerström, C. (1975). *Isr. J. Med. Sci.* **11,** 581–590.
Assan, R., and Boillot, J. (1973). *Pathol. Biol.* **21,** 149–155.
Assan, R., and Girard, J. R. (1975). *In* "Early Diabetes in Early Life" (R. A. Camerini-Davalos and H. S. Cole, eds.), pp. 115–126. Academic Press, New York.
Baer, H. P., and Hahn, P. (1971). *Can. J. Biochem.* **49,** 85–89.
Ballard, F. J. (1971). *In* "Diabetes" (R. R. Rodriguiz and J. Vallance-Owen, eds.), pp. 592–600. Excerpta Medica Found., Intern. Congr. Ser. No. 231, Amsterdam.
Bassett, J. M., and Madill, D. (1974). *J. Endocrinol.* **61,** 465–477.
Bassett, J. M., Thorburn, G. D., and Nicol, D. H. (1973). *J. Endocrinol.* **56,** 13–25.
Baster-Grillo, D. L., Amakawa, T., and Ito, R. (1973). *Histochemie* **33,** 281–286.
Beaudry, M. A., Chiasson, J. L., and Exton, J. H. (1977). *Am. J. Physiol.* **233,** E175–E180.
Beaupain, D., and Dieterlen-Lièvre, F. (1972). *C. R. Acad. Sci. Ser. D (Paris)* **275,** 413–415.
Benzo, C. A., and Green, T. D. (1974). *Anat. Rec.* **180,** 491–496.
Benzo, C. A., and Stearns, S. B. (1975). *Am. J. Anat.* **142,** 515–518.
Bernard, C. (1859). *C. R. Soc. Biol. (Paris)* **11,** 101–107.
Bertrand, H. A., Masoro, E. J., and Yu, B. P. (1977). *Nature (London)* **266,** 62–63.
Blázquez, E., Sugase, T., Blázquez, M., and Foà, P. P. (1972). *Acta Diabetol. Lat.* **9,** 13–35.
Blázquez, E., Simon, F. A., Blázquez, M., and Foà, P. P. (1974a). *Proc. Soc. Exp. Biol. Med.* **147,** 780–783.
Blázquez, E., Sugase, T., Blázquez, M., and Foà, P. P. (1974b). *J. Lab. Clin. Med.* **83,** 957–967.
Blázquez, E., Lipshaw, L. A., Blázquez, M., and Foà, P. P. (1975). *Ped. Res.* **9,** 17–25.
Blázquez, E., Rubalcava, B., Montesano, R., Orci, L., and Unger, R. H. (1976). *Endocrinology* **98,** 1014.
Bloom, S. R., and Johnston, D. I. (1972). *Br. Med. J.* **4,** 453–454.
Borchard, F., and Münterfering, H. (1969). *Virchows Arch. Pathol. Anat. Physiol.* **346,** 178–198.
Boxer, J., Kirby, L. T., and Hahn, P. (1974). *Proc. Soc. Exp. Biol. Med.* **145,** 901–903.
Burr, I. M., Kanazawa, Y., Marliss, E. B., and Lambert, A. E. (1971). *Diabetes* **20,** 592–597.
Chez, R., Mintz, D. H., and Epstein, M. F. (1975). *In* "Early Diabetes in Early Life;" (R. A. Camerini-Davalos and H. S. Cole, eds.), pp. 141–163. Academic Press, New York.
Chiu, H. F., and Phillips, M. J. (1974). *Lab Invest.* **30,** 305–310.

Clark, W. R., and Rutter, W. J. (1972). *Dev. Biol.* **29**, 468–481.

Cohen, N. M., and Turner, R. C. (1972). *Biol. Neonat.* **21**, 107–111.

Davies, J. (1957). *Am. J. Physiol.* **181**, 21–24.

Davis, J. R., Beck, P., Colwill, J. R., Makowski, E. L., Meschia, G., and Battaglia, F. C. (1971). *Proc. Soc. Exp. Biol. Med.* **136**, 972–975.

Dawes, G. S., and Shelley, H. J. (1958). *In* "Carbohydrate Metabolism and Its Disorders" (F. Dickens, W. J. Whelan, and P. J. Randle, eds.), vol. 2, pp. 87–191. Academic Press, New York.

De Gasparo, M., Pictet, R. L., Rall, L. B., and Rutter, W. J. (1975). *Dev. Biol.* **47**, 106–122.

Devos, P., and Hers, H. G. (1974). *Biochem. J.* **140**, 331–340.

Dieterlen-Lièvre, F., and Beaupain, D. (1976). *In* "Evolution of Pancreatic Islets" (T. A. I. Grillo, L. Leibson, and A. Epple, eds.), pp. 37–50. Pergamon, Oxford.

Di Marco, N., Ghisalberti, A. V., Martin, C. E., and Oliver, I. T. (1978). *Eur. J. Biochem.* **87**, 243–247.

Doi, K., Yoshida, M., Utsumi, M., Kawara, A., Fujii, S., Sakoda, M., and Baba, S. (1979). *Excerpta Medica Found. Interr. Congr. Ser.* 1978, No. 468, pp. 432–441, Amsterdam.

Drazin, B., Morris, H. G., Burstein, P. J., and Schlach, D. S. (1979). *Proc. Soc. Exp. Biol. Med.* **162**, 131–138.

Duran Garcia, S., Jarrousse, C., and Rosselin, G. (1976). *J. Clin. Invest.* **57**, 230–243.

Eisen, H. J., Goldfine, I. D., and Ginsmann, W. H. (1973). *Proc. Natl. Acad. Sci. U.S.A.* **70**, 3454–3457.

Eliot, R. J., Lam, R., Artal, R., Hobel, C., and Fisher, D. A. (1978). *Clin. Res.* **26**, 198A.

Falorni, A., Fracassini, F., Massi-Benedetti, F., and Maffei, S. (1974). *Diabetes* **23**, 172–178.

Felix, J. M., Sutter, M. T., Sutter, J. Ch. J., and Jacquot, R. (1971). *Horm. Metab. Res.* **3**, 71–75.

Fiser, R. H., Jr., Erenberg, A., Sperling, M. A., Oh, W., and Fisher, D. A. (1974a). *Pediatr. Res.* **8**, 951–955.

Fiser, R. H., Phelps, D. L., Williams P. R., Sperling, M. A., Fisher, D. A., and Oh, W. (1974b). *Am. J. Obstet. Gynecol.* **120**, 944–950.

Foà, P. P. (1979). *In* "Special Topics in Endocrinology and Metabolism" (M. P. Cohen and P. P. Foà, eds.), Vol. 1, pp. 39–54. Alan R. Liss, New York.

Foà, P. P., Melli, M., Berger, C. K., Billinger, D., and Guidotti, G. G. (1965). *Fed. Proc. Fed. Am. Soc. Exp. Biol.* **24**, 1046–1050.

Foà, P. P., Blázquez, E., Sodoyez, J. C., and Sodoyez-Goffaux, F. (1976). *In* "The Evolution of Pancreatic Islets" (T. A. I. Grillo, L. Leibson, and A. Epple, eds.), pp. 7–19. Pergamon, Oxford.

Freie, H. M. P., Pasma, A., and Bouman, P. R. (1975). *Acta Endocrinol.* **80**, 657–666.

Garcia Ruiz, J. P., Ingram, R., and Hanson, R. W. (1978). *Proc. Natl. Acad. Sci. U.S.A.* **75**, 4189–4193.

Girard, J., Bal, D., and Assan, R. (1972). *Horm. Metab. Res.* **4**, 168–170.

Girard, J. R., Caquet, D., Bal, D., and Guilett, I. (1973a). *Enzyme* **15**, 272–285.

Girard, J. R., Cuendet, G. S., Marliss, E. B., Kervran, A., Rieutort, M., and Assan, R. (1973b). *J. Clin. Invest.* **52**, 3190–3200.

Girard, J., Ferre, P., and Gilbert, M. (1975a). *Diabète Métab.* **1**, 241–257.

Girard, J. R., Kervran, A., and Assan, R. (1975b). *In* "Early Diabetes in Early Life" (R. A. Camerini-Davalos and H. S. Cole, eds.), pp. 57–71. Academic Press, New York.

Girard, J. R., Guillet, I., Marty, J., Assan, R., and Marliss, E. B. (1976). *Diabetologia* **12**, 327–337.

Gluckman, P. D., Uthne, K., Styne, D. M., Kaplan, S. L., Rudolph, A. M., and Grumbach, M. M. (1979). *Ped. Res* **13**, 194–196.

Golosow, N., and Grobstein, C. (1962). *Dev. Biol.* **4**, 242–255.

Grajwer, L. A., Sperling, M. A., Sack, J., and Fisher, D. A. (1977). *Pediatr. Res.* **11**, 833–836.
Grasso, S., Messina, A., Distefano, G., Vigo, R., and Reitano, G. (1973). *Diabetes* **22**, 349–353.
Greengard, O. (1975). *In* "Early Diabetes in Early Life" (R. A. Camerini-Davalos and H. S. Cole, eds.), pp. 9–22. Academic Press, New York.
Greengard, O., and Dewey, H. K. (1970). *Dev. Biol.* **21**, 452–461.
Grill, V., Asplund, K., Hellerström, C., and Cerasi, E. (1975) *Diabetes* **24**, 746–752.
Grillo, T. A. I. (1965). *In* "Organogenesis" (R. L. De Haan and H. Ursprung, eds.), pp. 513–538. Holt, New York.
Grillo, T. A. I., and Baxter-Grillo, D. L. (1966). *Gen. Comp. Endocrinol.* **7**, 420–423.
Grillo, T. A. I., Okuno, G., Guidotti, G., Price, S., and Foà, P. P. (1964a). *In* "The Structure and Metabolism of the Pancreatic Islets" (S. E. Brolin, B. Hellman, and H. Knutson, eds.), pp. 157–171. Pergamon, Oxford.
Grillo, T. A. I., Okuno, G., Price, S., and Foà. P. P. (1964b). *J. Histochem. Cytochem.* **12**, 275–280.
Guidotti, G., and Foà, P. P. (1961). *Am. J. Physiol.* **201**, 869–872.
Hahn, P., and Kirby, L. (1973). *J. Nutr.* **103**, 690–696.
Hahn, P., and Skala, J. (1972). *Comp. Biochem. Physiol.* **41B**, 147–155.
Hanson, R. W., Fisher, L., Ballard, F. J., and Reshef, L. (1973). *Enzyme* **15**, 97–110.
Harding, P. G. R. (1972). *Physiol. Biochem. Fetus, Proc. Int. Symp. 1970* pp. 229–243. Thomas, Springfield, Illinois.
Hardman, M. J., and Hull, D. (1970). *J. Physiol. (London)* **210**, 41P–42P.
Haymond, M. W., Karl, J. E., and Pagliara, A. S. (1974). *N. Engl. J. Med.* **291**, 322–328.
Heinze, E., Schatz, H., Nierle, C., and Pfeiffer, E. F. (1975). *Diabetes* **24**, 373–377.
Hellman, B. (1965). *Biol. Neonat.* **9**, 263–278.
Hoet, J. J., Grasso, S., and v. Assche, F. A. (1975). *In* "Early Diabetes in Early Life" (R. A. Camerini-Davalos and H. S. Cole, eds.), pp. 93–101. Academic Press, New York.
Hörstadius, S. (1950). "The Neural Crest." Oxford Univ. Press, London and New York.
Jack, P. M. B., and Milner, R. D. G. (1975). *J. Endocrinol.* **64**, 67–75.
Jarrousse, C., and Rosselin, G. (1975). *Endocrinology* **96**, 168–177.
Jarrousse, C, Rancon, F., and Rosselin, G. (1973). *C. R. Acad. Sci.* **276**, 585–588.
Johnson, P. R., Stern, J. S., Greenwood, M. R. C., Zucker, L. M., and Hirsch, J. (1973). *J. Nutr.* **103**, 738–743.
Jost, A., and Picon, L. (1970). *Adv. Metab. Dis.* **4**, 123–184.
Kaplan, S. L., Grumbach, M. M., and Shepard, T. H. (1972). *J. Clin. Invest.* **51**, 3080–3093.
Kervran, A., and Girard, J. R. (1974). *J. Endocrinol.* **62**, 545–551.
Kirby, L., and Hahn, P. (1974). *Pediatr. Res.* **8**, 37–41.
Kohrman, A. F. (1973). *Pediatr. Res.* **7**, 575–581.
Koler, R. D., Vanbellinghen, P. J., Fellman, J. H., Jones, R. T., and Behrman, R. E. (1969). *Science* **163**, 1348–1349.
Lambert, A. E., Orci, L., Kanazawa, Y., Jeanrenaud, B., and Renold, A. E. (1970). *Acta Isot.* **10**, 191–204.
Langslow, D. R. (1972). *Comp. Biochem. Physiol.* **43**, 689–701.
Leibson, L. G., Plisetskaya, E. M., and Bondareva, V. M. (1974). *Zh. Evol. Biokhim. Fiziol.* **10**, 433–439.
Lemonnier, D. (1972). *J. Clin. Invest.* **51**, 2907–2915.
Lernmark, A., and Wenngren, B. J. (1972). *J. Embryol. Exp. Morphol.* **28**, 607–614.
Lièvre, F. (1957). *Arch. Anat. Microsc. Morphol. Exp.* **46**, 61–80.
Linarelli, L. G., Bobik, C., Bobik, J., Drash, A. L., and Rubin, H. M. (1974). *J. Clin. Endocrinol. Metab.* **39**, 411–417.

Luyckx, A. (1974). "Sécrétion de l'Insuline et du Glucagon. Etude Clinique et Expérimentale." Masson, Paris.

Luyckx, A. S., Massi-Benedetti, F., Falorni, A., and Lefèbvre, P. J. (1972). *Diabetologia* **8**, 296–300.

McIntosh, N., Pectet, R. L., Kaplan, S. L., and Grumbach, M. M. (1977). *Endocrinology* **101**, 825–829.

Manns, J. G., and Brockman, R. P. (1969). *Can. J. Physiol. Pharmacol.* **47**, 917–921.

Massi-Benedetti, F., Falorni, A., Luyckx, A., and Lefèbvre, P. (1974). *Horm. Metab. Res.* **6**, 392–396.

Mersmann, H. J., Phinney, G., Mueller, R. L., and Stanton, H. C. (1972). *Am J. Physiol.* **222**, 1620–1627.

Milkoviĉ, S., Milkoviĉ, K., and Paunoviĉ, J. (1973). *Endocrinology* **92**, 380–384.

Milner, R. D. G., and Jack, P. M. B. (1975). *In* "Early Diabetes in Early Life" (R. A. Camerini-Davalos and H. S Cole, eds.), pp. 85–92. Academic Press, New York.

Milner, R. D. G., Barson, A. J., and Ashworth, M. A. (1971). *J. Endocrinol.* **51**, 323–332.

Mintz, D. H., Chez, R. A., and Horger, E. O., III (1969). *J. Clin. Invest.* **48**, 176–186.

Mintz, D. H., Levey, G. S., and Schenk, A. (1973). *Endocrinology* **92**, 614–617.

Mueller, P. L., Pictet, R. L., Kaplan. S. L., and Grumbach, M. M. (1978). *Clin. Res.* **26**, 190A.

Novák, E., Drummond, G. I., Skála, J., and Hahn, P. (1972). *Arch. Biochem. Biophys.* **150**, 511–518.

Novak, M., and Monkus, E. (1972). *Pediatr. Res.* **6**, 73–80.

Novak, M., Hahn, P., Penn, D., Monkus, E., and Kirby, L. (1973). *Biol. Neonat.* **23**, 19–24.

Obenshain, S. S., Adam, P. A. J., King, K. C., Teramo, K., Raivio, K. O., Raiha, N., and Schwartz, R. (1970). *N. Engl. J. Med.* **283**, 566–570.

Okuno, G., Grillo, T. A. I., Price, S., and Foà, P. P. (1964a). *Proc. Soc. Exp. Biol. Med.* **117**, 524–526.

Okuno, G., Price, S., Grillo, T. A. I., and Foà, P. P. (1964b). *Gen. Comp. Endocrinol.* **4**, 446–451.

Orci, L., Lambert, A. E., Rouiller, C., Renold, A. E., and Samols, E. (1969). *Horm. Metab. Res.* **1**, 108–110.

Patel, Y. C., Amherdt, M., and Orci, L. (1979). *Endocrinology* **104**, 676–679.

Paulin, C., and Dubois, P. M. (1978). *Cell Tissue Res.* **188**, 251–257.

Pearse, A. G. E. (1969). *J. Histochem. Cytochem.* **17**, 303–313.

Philippidis, H., and Ballard, F. J. (1970). *Biochem. J.* **120**, 385–392.

Philipps, A. F., Carson, B. S., Meschia, G., and Battaglia, F. C. (1978). *Am. J. Physiol.* **235**, E467–E474.

Pictet, R., and Rutter, W. J. (1972). *In* "Endocrine Pancreas. Handbook of Physiology" (D. F. Steiner and N. Freinkel, eds.), Vol. 1, Sec. 7, pp. 25–66. Williams & Wilkins, Baltimore, Maryland.

Pictet, R. L., Rall, L. B., Phelps, P., and Rutter, W. J. (1976). *Science* **191**, 191–192.

Pines, M., Bashan, N., and Moses, S. W. (1975). *Biochim. Biophys. Acta* **411**, 369–376.

Plas, C., and Nunez, J. (1976). *J. Biol. Chem.* **251**, 1431–1437.

Ponté, C., Gaudier, B., Deconinck, B., and Fourlinnie, J. C. (1972). *Biol. Neonat.* **20**, 262–269.

Portha, B., Rosselin, G., and Picon, L. (1976). *Diabetologia* **12**, 429–436.

Pronina, T. S., and Sapronova, A. J. (1976). *In* "The Evolution of Pancreatic Islets" (T. A. I. Grillo, L. Leibson, and A. Epel, eds.), pp. 25–35. Pregamon, Oxford.

Rabain, F., and Picon, L. (1974). *Horm. Metab. Res.* **6**, 376–380.

Rahier, J., Wallon, J., Gepts, W., and Haot, J. (1979). *Cell Tissue Res.* **200**, 359–366.

Rall, L. B., Pictet, R. L., Williams, R. H., and Rutter, W. J. (1973). *Proc. Nat. Acad. Sci. U.S.A.* **70**, 3478–3482.

Rall, L. B., Pictet, R. L., and Rutter, W. J. (1979). *Endocrinology* **105**, 835–841.

Rastogi, G. K., Letarte, J., and Fraser, T. R. (1970). *Diabetologia* **6**, 445–446.

Rechler, M. M., Eisen, H. J., Higa, O. Z., Nissley, S. P., Moses, A. C., Schilling, E. E., Fennoy, I., Bruni, C. B., Phillips, L. S. and Baird, K. L. (1979). *J. Biol. Chem.* **254**, 7942–7950.

Rieutort, M. (1974). *J. Endocrinol.* **60**, 261–268.

Rogers, I. M., Davidson, D. C., Lawrence, J., Ardill, J., and Buchanan, K. D. (1974). *Arch. Dis. Child.* **49**, 796–801.

Schaeffer, L. D., Wilder, M. L., and Williams, R. H. (1973). *Proc. Soc. Exp. Biol. Med.* **143**, 314–319.

Schaub, J., and Becker, I. (1972). *Biochim. Biophys. Acta* **279**, 398–400.

Schaub, J., Gutmann, I., and Lippert, M. (1972). *Horm. Metab. Res.* **4**, 110–119.

Schwartz, A. L., and Rall, T. W. (1975). *Diabetes* **24**, 1113–1122.

Schwartz, R. (1975). *In* "Early Diabetes in Early Life" (R. A. Camerini-Davalos and H. S. Cole, eds.), pp. 127–134. Academic Press, New York.

Shambaugh, G. E., III. (1977). *Clin. Res.* **25**, 624A.

Shelley, H. J. (1960). *J. Physiol. (London)* **153**, 527–552.

Shelley, H. J., and Neligan, G. A. (1966). *Br. Med. J.* **22**, 34–39.

Shelley, H. J., Bassetts, J. M., and Milner, R. D. G. (1975) *Br. Med. Bull.* **31**, 37–43.

Shima, K., Price, S., and Foà, P. P. (1966). *Proc. Soc. Exp. Biol. Med.* **121**, 55–59.

Snell, K., and Walker, D. G. (1973). *Biochem. J.* **132**, 739–752.

Sogoyez-Goffaux, F., Sodoyez, J.-C., and Foà. P. P. (1971), *Diabetes* **20**, 586–591.

Sodoyez-Goffaux, F., Sodoyez, J.-C., De Vos, C. J., and Foà, P. P. (1979a). *Diabetologia* **16**, 121–123.

Sodoyez-Goffaux, F., Sodoyez, J.-C., De Vos, C. J., and Thiry-Moris, Y. M. *In* "Antenetal Factors Affecting Metabolic Adaptation to Extrauterine Life: Role of Carbohydrates and Energy Metabolism" (R. De Meyer, ed.). Nijhoff, The Hague (in press)

Sodoyez-Goffaux, F. R., Sodoyez, J.-C., and De Vos, C. J. (1979b). *J. Clin. Invest.* **63**, 1095–1102.

Sosenko, I. R., Kitzmiller, J. L., Loo, S. W., Blix, P., Rubenstein, A. H., and Gabbay, K. H. (1979). *N. Engl. J. Med.* **301**, 859–862.

Spellacy, W. N., Buhi, W. C., Bradley, B., and Holsinger, K. K. (1973). *Obstet. Gynecol. Surv.* **41**, 323–331.

Sperling, M. A., DeLamater, P. V., Phelps, D., Fiser, R. H., Oh, W., and Fisher, D. A. (1974). *J. Clin. Invest.* **53**, 1159–1166.

Sperling, M. A., Grajwer, L., Leake, R. D., and Fisher, D. A. (1977). *Pediatr. Res.* **11**, 962–967.

Stuart, M. C., Lazarus, L., Moore, S. S., and Smythe, G. A. (1976). *Horm. Metab. Res.* **8**, 442–445.

Susini, C., Lavau, M., and Herzog, J. (1979). *Horm. Metab. Res.* **11**, 694–696.

Swiatek, K. R. (1971). *Biochim. Biophys. Acta* **252**, 274–279.

Taylor, C. B., Bailey, E., and Bartley, W. (1967). *Biochem. J.* **105**, 717–722.

Thommes, R. C. (1960). *Growth* **24**, 69–80.

Vaillant, R. (1975). *FEBS Lett.* **52**, 22–24.

Vigneri, R., and D'Agata, R. (1971). *J. Clin. Endocrinol. Metab.* **33**, 561–563.

Villee, D. B. (1969). *N. Engl. J. Med.* **281**, 473–484, 533–541.

Vinicor, F., Clark, J. F., and Clark, C. M., Jr. (1975). *In* "Early Diabetes in Early Life" (R. A. Camerini-Davalos and H. S. Cole, eds.), pp. 105–114. Academic Press, New York.

Wellmann, K. F., Volk, B. W., and Brancato, P. (1971). *Lab. Invest.* **25**, 97–103.

Wessels, N. K. (1964). *J. Cell Biol.* **20,** 415–255.

Wildenthal, K., and Wakeland, J. R. (1973). *J. Clin. Invest.* **52,** 2250–2258.

Willgerodt, H., Vizek, K., Rážová, M., and Melichar, V. (1975). *Biol. Neonat.* **27,** 88–95.

Windle, W. F. (1940). "Physiology of the Fetus, Origin and Extent of Function in Prenatal Life." Saunders, Philadelphia, Pennsylvania.

Wise, J. K., Lyall, S. S., Hendler, R., and Felig, P. (1973). *J. Clin. Endocrinol. Metab.* **37,** 347–350.

Wolf, H., Šabata, V., Frerichs, H., and Stubbe, P. (1969). *Horm. Metab. Res.* **1,** 274–275.

Wood, S. C., and Porte, D., Jr. (1974). *Physiol. Rev.* **54,** 596–619.

II

SYNTHESIS AND SECRETION OF ISLET HORMONES

3

Transport Systems of Islet Cells

J. SEHLIN

I. INTRODUCTION

During the last two decades methods have been developed for the isolation of pancreatic islets, making it possible to study in detail cellular processes, for example, transmembrane transport. Generally, such experi-

53

The Islets of Langerhans
Copyright © 1981 by Academic Press, Inc.
All rights of reproduction in any form reserved.
ISBN 0-12-187820-1

ments have been interpreted assuming that the data are representative of β cells. Most work has been performed with islets from rats and normal mice, containing 70–80% β cells, or islets from *ob/ob* mice, which are particularly rich in β cells (> 90%: Hellman, 1965). Inherent in this work, however, are two problematic aspects that should be kept in mind in analyzing the data. First, the minority cells may of course interfere significantly with the results and, second, the cellular distribution makes it quite difficult to measure transport processes in these minority cells per se. It is not my intention to draw conclusions about the cellular localization of various transport phenomena further than the authors of the original articles have done themselves.

The purpose of this chapter is to review briefly the basic features of transport mechanisms in pancreatic islet cells without going into detail or mentioning more than a representative selection of the large number of observations made. Aspects of how such transport mechanisms are involved in the regulation of specific islet cell functions, e.g., secretion and synthesis, are dealt with in subsequent chapters.

II. SUGARS

A. Metabolizable Sugars

It was early observed that the D-glucose concentration in islet water was nearly identical to that in serum (Goetz and Cooperstein, 1962; Idahl and Hellman, 1968) and that phlorizin (Coore and Randle, 1964) or nonmetabolizable sugars (Grodsky *et al.,* 1963) failed to inhibit D-glucose-induced insulin release. The interpretation was that the β-cell membrane was freely permeable to D-glucose and that carrier mechanisms were not involved in the transport.

However, experiments aimed at measuring islet transmembrane movement of sugars more directly showed that glucose uptake was stereospecific for the D isomer (Cooperstein and Lazarow, 1969, Hellman *et al.,* 1971a,b) and, indeed, inhibited by phlorizin at both 8°C (Hellman *et al.,* 1971b) and 37°C (Hellman *et al.,* 1972c). The lower temperature was chosen to reduce the rates of transport and degradation of D-glucose. Carrier-mediated D-glucose transport was characterized by a high velocity. At 37°C the half-time for equilibration of labeled D-glucose was less than 45 sec (Hellman *et al.,* 1974), at 20°C this half-time was about 1 min (McDaniel *et al.,* 1974), and at 8°C it was about 5 min (Hellman *et al.,* 1971b). At 8°C the equilibrium concentration of labeled D-glucose (Hellman *et al.,* 1971b) was almost identical with that of labeled urea or 3-*O*-methyl-D-glucose (Hellman *et al.,* 1971c). Since these compounds are thought to be passively distributed across most cell membranes (Marshall and Davis, 1914; Stein, 1967), the data indicate a passive distribution of D-glucose as well. At 37°C the picture was complicated by the lack of a constant equilibrium plateau in studies on time dependence of the D-glucose uptake (Hellman *et al.,* 1974). The probable reason for this is that labeled metabolites of D-glucose were accumulating in the islets. However, even at 37°C there was a rapid initial phase of D-glucose uptake, probably representing the rate of transmembrane influx (Hellman *et al.,* 1974).

Analysis of the concentration dependence of D-glucose influx at 8°C in *ob/ob*-mouse islets revealed an apparent V_{max} of about 400 mmol/kg dry wt islet per hour and an apparent K_m of about 50 mM D-glucose (Hellman *et al.,* 1971b). No such data are available for D-glucose flux at 37°C because the very high flux rate at this temperature made it difficult to estimate the initial influx. However, at 37°C and 5 mM of labeled D-glucose, 4.1 mmol/kg dry wt islet was taken up during the first 45 sec (Hellman *et al.,* 1974), whereas at 8°C and the same D-glucose concentration only 1.4 mmol/kg dry wt islet was taken up during the first 3 min (Hellman *et al.,* 1971b). If these data are assumed to represent the initial rates of D-glucose influx, the values calculated per minute would be 5.4 mmol/kg dry wt islet for the 37°C data and 0.48 mmol/kg dry wt islet for the 8°C data. If the V_{max} had the same temperature sensitivity, this would give a V_{max} for D-glucose uptake at 5 mM and 37°C of no less than 4.5 mmol/kg dry wt islet per hour. This should be compared with the maximal velocity of $^{14}CO_2$ production from 5 mM D-[U-^{14}C] glucose (about 10 mmol D-glucose equivalents/kg dry wt islet per hour; Hellman *et al.,* 1974) or ^3H_2O production from D-[5-^{3}H] glucose (about 50 mmol D-glucose equivalents/kg dry wt islet per hour; Hellman *et al.,* 1975). It is clear from this comparison that D-glucose transport is normally not rate-limiting for D-glucose metabolism in islet cells.

D-Glucose uptake was not affected by its L isomer, was only slightly reduced by D-mannoheptulose (Hellman *et al.,* 1971b), and was not affected by anoxia (Hellman *et al.,* 1975). The two anomers α-D-glucose and β-D-glucose induced similar countertransport of 3-*O*-methyl-D-glucose, suggesting that they may fit the transport site equally well (Idahl *et al.,* 1975). D-Glucose influx was reduced by 5-thio-D-glucose but not by 1-thio-β-D-glucose (Hellman *et al.,* 1973c). The thiol reagents *p*-chloromercuribenzoic acid and chloromercuribenzene-*p*-sulfonic acid reduced D-glucose uptake (Bloom *et al.,* 1972), but iodoacetamide (Hellman *et al.,* 1973a) or alloxan (McDaniel *et al.,* 1975) had no effect. Cytochalasin B, which augments insulin release (Lacy *et al.,* 1973), inhibited the inward transport of D-glucose measured at both 20° and 37°C (McDaniel *et al.*, 1974). Also, potentiators of insulin release, caffeine and theophylline, reduced D-glucose transport (McDaniel *et al.*, 1977).

In contrast to D-glucose transport, *N*-acetyl-D-glucosamine transport is thought to be the rate-limiting step for *N*-acetyl-D-glucosamine metabolism (Ashcroft, 1980). Indirect evidence suggests that *N*-acetyl-D-glucosamine transport in islet cells is inhibited by phloretin (Ashcroft *et al.*, 1978; Williams and Ashcroft, 1978), caffeine (Williams and Ashcroft, 1978), and 3-*O*-methyl-D-glucose (Ashcroft *et al.*, 1980). These characteristics indicate that *N*-acetyl-D-glucosamine may share a transport mechanism with D-glucose.

B. Nonmetabolizable Sugars

1. Transported Sugars

In this group of sugars, the main interest has been focused on islet cell transport of 3-*O*-methyl-D-glucose because it is transported like D-glucose in a variety of other cells without being metabolized (Stein, 1967).

Initial studies showed that labeled 3-*O*-methyl-D-glucose was distributed across islet cell membranes like urea (Hellman *et al.*, 1971c), which is thought to equilibrate in the total tissue water (Marshall and Davis, 1914; Stein, 1967). The unidirectional influx of 3-*O*-methyl-D-glucose was inhibited by D-glucose, phlorizin, phloretin, D-mannoheptulose, and D-glucosamine, strongly suggesting that D-glucose and 3-*O*-methyl-D-glucose share a common transport mechanism (Hellman *et al.*, 1973f). Observations that 3-*O*-methyl-D-glucose transport was inhibited by cytochalasin B (McDaniel *et al.*, 1974) and not affected by alloxan (McDaniel *et al.*, 1975) further support this view. 3-*O*-Methyl-D-glucose was also transported into dispersed islet cells in suspension, the transport characteristics being close to those found in intact islets (Lernmark *et al.*, 1975).

McDaniel *et al.* (1974) reported that islet uptake of labeled 2-deoxy-D-glucose was inhibited by cytochalasin B just like the transport of D-glucose and 3-*O*-methyl-D-glucose. This suggests that 2-deoxy-D-glucose also shares a transport system with D-glucose.

2. Nontransported Sugars

It was suggested by early studies on fish islets from *Opsanus tau* that L-glucose was restricted to a tissue space much smaller than the D-glucose space (Cooperstein and Lazarow, 1969). This was further explored in β-cell-rich islets from *ob/ob* mouse and rat islets. The volume distribution of L-glucose and sucrose was much smaller than that of D-glucose and 3-*O*-methyl-D-glucose, and L-glucose and sucrose reached almost perfect equilibration in the *ob/ob* mouse islets. It was therefore suggested that these sugars did not markedly bind to islet structures and did not permeate to any significant extent the *ob/ob* mouse islet cell membranes (Hellman *et al.*, 1971b,c). Similar results have been obtained with radioactively labeled inulin (Lernmark *et al.*, 1975). In rat islets, McDaniel *et al.* (1975) observed a persistent difference between the volume distribution of L-glucose and sucrose, the L-glucose space being larger and also sensitive to temperature. A few other sugar alcohols, such as mannitol (Watkins *et al.*, 1970; Hellman *et al.* 1971d; McDaniel *et al.*, 1975), sorbitol, and xylitol (Matschinsky, 1972), have been used as markers for the extracellular water space in pancreatic islets.

III. AMINO ACIDS

A. Neutral Amino Acids

Islet cells are equipped with different mechanisms for transmembrane transport of the various classes of amino acids. Neutral amino acids are transported essentially by mechanisms resembling the L and A systems originally described for Ehrlich ascites cells (Oxender and Christensen, 1963). The L system displays the highest affinity for amino acids with bulky side chains. Direct studies on the transport of labeled L-leucine (Hellman *et al.*, 1971e, 1972a; Idahl *et al.*, 1976; Lin, 1977), D-leucine (Hellman *et al.*, 1972a), and the artificial, nonmetabolizable transport analogue 2-aminobicyclo[2.2.1]heptane-2-carboxylic acid (BCH) (Christensen *et al.*, 1971) have been performed. L-Leucine transport was characterized by a high apparent K_m and an estimated distribution ratio (concn.$_{in}$/concn.$_{out}$) of about 4 at 1 mM external L-leucine (Hellman *et al.*, 1972a). It was not dependent on Na$^+$, K$^+$, or Ca^{2+} (Hellman *et al.*, 1971e) and was reduced by external L-arginine (Lin, 1977) and L-isoleucine, L-tryptophan, glycine, L-phenylalanine, or D-leucine (Hellman *et al.*, 1972a), suggesting that these amino acids may share affinity for the carrier sites of the L system. In fact, it apparently was not possible to distinguish between the transport characteristics of D-leucine and L-leucine. Sugars such as D-glucose, 3-O-methyl-D-glucose, and D-mannoheptulose had no effect on the L-leucine or D-leucine transport rate. Neither was this transport affected by glibenclamide or diazoxide (Hellman *et al.*, 1971e, 1972a).

L-Alanine, glycine, and their nonmetabolizable transport analogue α-aminoisobutyric acid (AIB) are transported in pancreatic islet cells by a mechanism similar to the A system of Ehrlich ascites cells (Oxender and Christensen, 1963). The islet transport of these amino acids was Na$^+$-dependent and resulted in a vigorous accumulation of amino acid (Hellman *et al.,* 1971c,e; Sehlin, 1972a). L-Leucine and L-alanine reduced the uptake of glycine (Sehlin, 1972a), but L-leucine had no significant effect on L-alanine (Hellman *et al.,* 1971e) or AIB (Hellman *et al.,* 1971c) uptake. The uptake of L-alanine was inhibited by L-methionine (Hellman *et al.,* 1971e) and L-arginine (Lin, 1977), and the uptake of AIB was reduced by L-lysine or L-methionine (Hellman *et al.,* 1971c), indicating that these amino acids may compete for transport sites of the A system. The transport of L-alanine or glycine was reduced by the insulin secretagogues D-glucose and gliben-clamide, whereas diazoxide had no effect (Hellman *et al.,* 1971e; Sehlin, 1972a).

The amino acid experiments described so far were performed with isolated islets from *ob/ob* mice or rats. The accumulation of amino acids has also been examined in isolated islets from the toadfish after injecting labeled amino acids *in vivo* (Cooperstein and Lazarow, 1977).

B. Dicarboxylic Amino Acids

L-Glutamic acid is thought to be transported into most cells by a transport mechanism specific for dicarboxylic amino acids (Neame, 1968). The islet cell uptake of 5 mM L-glutamic acid showed an estimated distribution ratio slightly above unity at apparent isotope equilibrium and an almost linear concentration dependence at 1–20 mM external amino acid (Sehlin, 1972b). These results indicate a nonconcentrating transport mechanism with a high K_m. The uptake rate was not affected by L-arginine or L-leucine but slightly reduced by L-alanine, which may indicate a slight overlapping of the A system for transport of neutral amino acids and the dicarboxylic amino acid transport system (Sehlin, 1972b). The possibility that L-glutamic acid is transported mainly by the A system was ruled out by the observation that D-glucose slightly increased the uptake of L-glutamic acid, whereas D-glucose reduced uptake by the A system (see Section III,A). D-Galactose or glibenclamide had no effect on L-glutamic acid transport (Sehlin, 1972b).

C. Cationic Amino Acids

L-Arginine was vigorously accumulated in islet cells, resulting in an estimated distribution ratio of about 15 after 2 hr of incubation at 5 mM external L-arginine (Hellman *et al.,* 1971e). The rate of L-arginine oxidation to CO_2 was very low (Hellman *et al.,* 1971f), but the possibility that a significant part of the accumulation was due to L-arginine metabolites should not be overlooked. In view of the D-glucose dependence of the L-arginine-induced insulin release, it is of interest (Table I) that the initial

TABLE I

Effects of Hexoses or Phlorizin on Islet Uptake of L-Arginine[a]

Test substance	Uptake of labeled L-arginine (mmol/kg islet dry wt per 5 min)
None (control)	6.02 ± 0.32 (22)
D-Glucose, 20 mM	4.97 ± 0.26 (16)**
D-Mannose, 20 mM	5.56 ± 1.02 (6)*
D-Galactose, 20 mM	6.59 ± 0.60 (6)
Phlorizin, 10 mM	4.75 ± 0.33 (6)***

[a] Microdissected islets from noninbred *ob/ob* mice were incubated for 5 min at 37°C in Krebs–Ringer bicarbonate buffer (pH 7.4) supplemented with 1 mM L-[^{14}C]arginine and 0.1 mM [^{3}]sucrose. The concentration of test compounds also applied to a 30-min preliminary incubation in nonradioactive media. The values for L-arginine uptake are corrected for labeled L-arginine in the [^{3}H]sucrose (extracellular) space. Results are mean values ± SEM for the number of experiments in parentheses. Significance levels for differences from control values were determined by t test for paired observations. *$p < 0.02$; **$p < 0.01$; ***$p < 0.005$. Unpublished results of B. Hellman, J. Sehlin, and L.-B Täljedal.

uptake of L-arginine was reduced by D-glucose, D-mannose, or phlorizin but not by D-galactose.

The nonmetabolizable, transport-specific cationic amino acid 4-amino-1-guanylpiperidine-4-carboxylic acid (GPA) was accumulated more than five-fold in islet cells (Christensen *et al.*, 1971). Like L-arginine, GPA stimulated insulin release in a D-glucose-dependent manner, supporting the idea that interaction of cationic amino acids with their transport sites may be of importance for their recognition as secretory stimuli (see Chapter 6).

IV. INORGANIC IONS

A. Cations

1. Calcium

Extensive studies on transmembrane and subcellular movements of ^{45}Ca^{2+} support the hypothesis that Ca^{2+} is an essential link in the distal part of the stimulus–secretion coupling in pancreatic β cells. Only a few studies have provided information about the mode of action of Ca^{2+} in islet cells other than β cells. Thus it has been suggested that Ca^{2+} is important for the secretion of pancreatic glucagon (Leclercq-Meyer *et al.*, 1973; Gerich *et al.*, 1974; Wollheim *et al.*, 1976; Ashby and Speake, 1975; Iversen and Hermansen, 1977) and somatostatin (Hermansen *et al.*, 1979) but not pancreatic polypeptide (Hermansen and Schwartz, 1979). Islets enriched in α_2 cells (A cells) by streptozotocin treatment of guinea pigs displayed a lower total content of Ca^{2+} and lacked D-glucose stimulation of $^{45}Ca^{2+}$ uptake, as compared with normal islets (Berggren *et al.*, 1979).

The detailed mechanism of Ca^{2+} action in islet cell stimulus–secretion coupling will be discussed in Chapter 7. Here only a few basic features of transmembrane Ca^{2+} transport will be described.

Pancreatic islet cells are, like most animal cells, thought to possess very low cytoplasmic Ca^{2+} activity. It is therefore generally thought that Ca^{2+} fluxes into the cells down its electrochemical potential gradient (Matthews, 1978, for a review). A large number of articles, starting in the early 1970s (Hellman *et al.*, 1971d, Malaisse-Lagae and Malaisse, 1971), have described in detail how D-glucose and other insulin secretagogues and inhibitors control $^{45}Ca^{2+}$ uptake and efflux. Interpretation of these $^{45}Ca^{2+}$ data is severely hampered by the excessive binding of Ca^{2+} to various cellular components. Attempting to discriminate better between $^{45}Ca^{2+}$ surface adsorption and transmembrane uptake, Hellman *et al.* (1976a) introduced a La^{3+} wash technique in studies on $^{45}Ca^{2+}$ fluxes. These experiments revealed that D-glucose indeed induced net uptake of Ca^{2+} in the La^{3+}-nondisplaceable (intracellular) Ca^{2+} pool (Hellman *et al.*, 1976a, Hellman *et al.*, 1977). D-Glucose also increased $^{45}Ca^{2+}$ incorporation in a La^{3+}-displaceable, probably superficial Ca^{2+} compartment that was very mobile and may be involved in acute regulation of insulin release (Hellman *et al.*, 1976b).

Prior to direct measurements of Ca^{2+} movements in pancreatic islets, Milner and Hales (1970) suggested that, in analogy with ideas about other cells, Ca^{2+} flux might be linked to Na^+ flux by an exchange mechanism. Some evidence for such an exchange has since been obtained. Thus tracer studies have shown that Na^+ deficiency increases long-term basal $^{45}Ca^{2+}$ uptake (Hellman *et al.*, 1978) and reduces $^{45}Ca^{2+}$ efflux (Hellman *et al.*, 1979, 1980; Henquin, 1979a). It has also been suggested that Ca^{2+} and Na^+ compete for transport sites in a Na^+–Na^+ exchange (Sehlin and Täljedal, 1974a). Some data indicate that $^{45}Ca^{2+}$ efflux is engaged in a Ca^{2+}–Ca^{2+} exchange (Henquin, 1979a; Herschuelz *et al.*, 1980). Such mechanisms may be of ultimate importance in the regulation of cytoplasmic Ca^{2+}.

Extrusion of Ca^{2+} from islet cells has been suggested to occur by an ATP-consuming Ca^{2+} pump (Malaisse *et al.*, 1978b). The evidence for such a mechanism is only fragmentary. Islet subcellular particles contain Ca^{2+}-dependent ATPase activities that might be involved in Ca^{2+} transport (Löffler and Kemmler, 1974; Formby *et al.*, 1976a; Levin *et al.*, 1978), and

ATP stimulates $^{45}Ca^{2+}$ transport in subcellular membrane particles (Howell *et al.,* 1975; Sehlin, 1976). However, poisoning of islet cell metabolism leads to a marked increase in $^{45}Ca^{2+}$ efflux (Henquin, 1979a,b) which clearly does not indicate any metabolism-dependent outward transport of $^{45}Ca^{2+}$. However, Fig. 1 shows that $^{45}Ca^{2+}$ uptake in *ob/ob* mouse islets for 10 or 120 min was increased by the metabolic inhibitor antimycin A, as

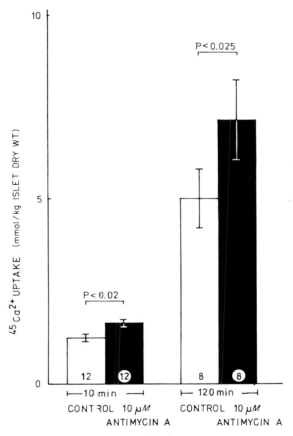

Fig. 1. Effect of metabolic inhibition on $^{45}Ca^{2+}$ uptake. Microdissected islets of noninbred *ob/ob* mice were incubated for 10 or 120 min at 37°C in Tris–HCl-buffered medium (pH 7.4) containing Na^+, K^+, Ca^{2+}, and Mg^{2+} at approximately the same concentrations as in Krebs–Ringer buffer and no anions other than Cl^-. After this incubation, the islets were incubated for another 60 min with 2 mM La^{3+} to wash out extracellular $^{45}Ca^{2+}$ without affecting the intracellular label. Results are mean values ± SEM (top bars) for 8–12 experiments. Significance levels for differences from controls were determined by t test for paired observations. Unpublished results of J. Sehlin and I.-B. Täljedal.

would be expected if Ca^{2+} efflux were metabolism dependent. These two pieces of isotope tracer data are somewhat difficult to reconcile. However, it appears possible to have at the same time a net gain in cellular Ca^{2+} and an increase in $^{45}Ca^{2+}$ efflux if the increase in label release from organelles is greater than the poison-induced inhibition of transmembrane extrusion.

2. Zinc

This cation has been studied because it was found in the 1930s that Zn^{2+} stabilized the insulin crystalline structure (Scott, 1934). It has consequently been thought that the ability of β cells to keep insulin in crystal form in their storage granules might likewise be dependent on Zn^{2+}. This idea is supported by experiments showing covariation in islet Zn^{2+} content and insulin content under various treatments (Maske, 1957; Okamoto and Kawaniski, 1966; Bander and Schesmer, 1970; Berglund and Hellman, 1976).

Experiments with radioactive $^{65}Zn^{2+}$ (Figlewicz et al., 1979; Ludvigsen et al., 1979) showed that in rat islets $^{65}Zn^{2+}$ was taken up without isotope equilibrium being reached within 24 hr. The uptake had complex kinetics, one component being saturated (apparent K_m 1.5 μM) and the other being nonsaturated up to at least 3 mM $^{65}Zn^{2+}$. The saturable uptake component was inhibited by cadmium and probably engaged in a Zn^{2+}–Zn^{2+} exchange across the islet cell plasma membranes. D-Glucose did not exert any clear effect on $^{65}Zn^{2+}$ uptake.

3. Sodium

Evidence suggests that Na^+ is extruded from islet cells by a mechanism similar to the Na^+–K^+ pump. Ouabain as well as 2,4-dinitrophenol inhibited efflux of $^{22}Na^+$ from prelabeled islets (Sehlin and Täljedal, 1974a; Kawazu et al., 1978) and induced net uptake of this ion (Sehlin and Täljedal, 1974b; Kawazu et al., 1978). Efflux of $^{22}Na^+$ was increased by the omission of extracellular Ca^{2+} and decreased by the omission of Na^+ ions. The omission of K^+, however, failed to affect $^{22}Na^+$ efflux significantly, possibly because of a slow washout of K^+ from the islet tissue (Sehlin and Täljedal, 1974a). These data, as well as $^{86}Rb^+$ data (see Section IV,B,4), suggest that Na^+ is extruded from islet cells with a mechanism similar to the Na^+–K^+ pump found in other cells. They also indicate that islet cells may be equipped with coupled transport of Ca^{2+} and Na^+ as well as Na^+–Na^+ exchange. D-Glucose induced a small increase in $^{22}Na^+$ efflux in rat islets (Kawazu et al., 1978) but had no significant effect on this flux in ob/ob mouse islets (Sehlin and Täljedal, 1974a). Attempts have been made to measure Na^+–K^+-stimulated ATPase in islet homogenates. Species variation may exist, because only low activities of this enzyme were found in mouse islets (Formby et al., 1976b; Idahl et al., 1977; Lernmark et al.,

1980), whereas considerable activity was obtained in rat islets (Lernmark *et al.,* 1976; Kemmler and Löffler, 1977; Levin *et al.,* 1978).

The influx of $^{22}Na^+$ in islet cells was time-dependent, with half-equilibration after about 5 min (Sehlin and Täljedal, 1974b; Kawazu *et al.,* 1978). At a low D-glucose concentration, the estimated intracellular Na^+ concentration was about 95 mM in *ob/ob* mouse islets (Sehlin and Täljedal, 1974b) and 50–74 mM in rat islets (Kawazu *et al.,* 1978), as estimated from isotope tracer data. There appears to be some controversy as to what effect the D-glucose concentration has on the intracellular $^{22}Na^+$ concentration and $^{22}Na^+$ influx. Kawazu *et al.* (1978) observed an increase in the $^{22}Na^+$ influx rate and a decrease in the equilibrium concentration of $^{22}Na^+$ in islet cells. On the other hand, Sehlin and Täljedal (1974b) found no effect of D-glucose concentration on $^{22}Na^+$ uptake for 1–25 min, and Gagerman *et al.* (1980) showed a stimulation of $^{22}Na^+$ uptake by D-glucose for 1 hr. The action of D-glucose on Na^+ flux deserves further analysis.

The presence of Na^+ channels controlling the Na^+ uptake in islet cells was suggested by observations that neurotoxins, e.g., veratridine (Donatsch *et al.,* 1977; Pace and Blaustein, 1979) and scorpion venom (Pace and Blaustein, 1979), caused insulin release that could be inhibited by tetrodotoxin. Veratridine increased long-term uptake of $^{22}Na^+$ by isolated islets (Kawazu *et al.,* 1978).

4. Potassium

Most studies on the K^+-transporting mechanism in islets have been done with rubidium, which traces K^+ in a nearly perfect manner (Sehlin and Täljedal, 1974a; Boschero *et al.,* 1977). $^{86}Rb^+$ was accumulated by *ob/ob* mouse islets more than 30-fold, whether the islet cells were maintained in intact islets (Sehlin and Täljedal, 1974a) or isolated in a cell suspension (Lernmark *et al.,* 1975). The half-life of $^{86}Rb^+$ equilibration was about 25 min (Sehlin and Täljedal, 1974a), and the uptake was inhibited by ouabain (Howell and Taylor, 1968; Sehlin and Täljedal, 1974a; Malaisse *et al.,* 1978a; Henquin, 1980), metabolic blockers, Na^+ deficiency (Sehlin and Täljedal, 1974a), and low temperature (Frankel *et al.,* 1978). These results suggest that Rb^+ and K^+ are pumped into islet cells by a metabolism-dependent mechanism similar to the Na^+–K^+ pump. $^{86}Rb^+$ influx was reduced by diphenylhydantoin or chloromercuribenzene-*p*-sulfonic acid (Sehlin and Täljedal, 1974a), alloxan (Idahl *et al.,* 1977), and valinomycin (Idahl *et al.,* 1978). D-Glucose did not affect the unidirectional influx of $^{86}Rb^+$ or $^{42}K^+$ (Sehlin *et al.,* 1974a; Malaisse *et al.,* 1978a) but induced net uptake of these cations (Howell and Taylor, 1968; Malaisse *et al,* 1978a; Henquin, 1980).

The net uptake is probably explained by a D-glucose-induced reduction in

Rb$^+$ or K$^+$ efflux (Sehlin and Täljedal, 1974a, 1975; Boschero *et al.*, 1977; Henquin, 1977, 1978; Malaisse *et al.*, 1978a). The efflux of these ions is probably determined by their ability to permeate islet cell membranes. D-Glucose-induced depolarization of β cells may at least partly be due to a decrease in the K$^+$ permeability (Sehlin and Täljedal, 1975; c.f. Meissner *et al.*, 1979). The efflux of ^{86}Rb$^+$ approximated an exponential function with a rate constant of about -0.036 to -0.042/min in *ob/ob* mouse islets (Sehlin and Täljedal, 1974a; Idahl *et al.*, 1978), -0.035/min in lean C57BL/KsJ $+/+$ mouse islets (Berglund *et al.*, 1978), and -0.055/min in rat islets (Malaisse *et al.*, 1978a). The ^{86}Rb$^+$ efflux resembled Rb$^+$ and K$^+$ flux in voltage-dependent K$^+$ channels in nerve and muscle cells in being inhibited by tetraethylammonium or 9-aminoacridine (Henquin, 1977; Henquin *et al.*, 1979) and stimulated by valinomycin (Henquin and Meissner, 1978; Boschero *et al.*, 1979). This efflux seemed not to be linked to the transport of Ca^{2+} or Na$^+$, because omission of these ions had no effect on the ^{86}Rb$^+$ efflux rate (Sehlin and Täljedal, 1974a; Boschero and Malaisse, 1979). A K$^+$ deficiency, on the other hand, reduced the efflux (Boschero and Malaisse, 1979).

Some evidence has been presented suggesting that pancreatic islet cells also possess a mechanism similar to the Ca^{2+}-activated K$^+$ channel found in other cells. Thus it has been found that islets release ^{86}Rb$^+$ when they are treated with metabolism blockers (Henquin, 1979b) which are thought to increase the cytoplasmic Ca^{2+} level by releasing Ca^{2+} from organelles (Henquin, 1979a,b).

B. Anions

1. Chloride

Pancreatic islets have mechanisms for transmembrane transport of Cl$^-$. Isotope tracer experiments indicate that Cl$^-$ is actively transported into islet cells and that passive, probably electrogenic, efflux is controlled by regulators of insulin release.

Studies on ^{36}Cl$^-$ distribution showed that the estimated intracellular Cl$^-$ concentration was much higher than would be expected for a passive Nernstian distribution (Sehlin, 1978). This indicates that Cl$^-$ is transported into islet cells against its electrochemical gradient. In support of this idea, 2,4-dinitrophenol (Sehlin, 1978) and furosemide (Sehlin, 1980b) reduced both uptake and equilibrium concentration of ^{36}Cl$^-$ in islets. Uphill inward transport of Cl$^-$ is not due to coupling with cation transport, since a deficiency in Na$^+$, K$^+$, or Ca^{2+} did not affect the ^{36}Cl$^-$ uptake and ouabain even increased it (Sehlin, 1978).

Transmembrane Cl^- efflux may be a passive flux determined essentially by an outwardly directed electrochemical gradient and the islet permeability for Cl^-. Efflux of $^{36}Cl^-$ followed a simple exponential function with a rate constant of -0.12 to -0.18/min in *ob/ob* mouse islets (Sehlin, 1978; Berglund and Sehlin, 1980) and -0.14 to -0.17/min in islets from lean C57BL/KsJ $+/+$ mice (Berglund and Sehlin, 1980). Membrane amino groups may participate in the efflux, because the amino reagent 4-acetamido-4′-isothiocyanate-stilbene-2,2-disulfonic acid (SITS) or an increase in pH reduced the $^{36}Cl^-$ efflux rate (Sehlin, 1978).

D-Glucose or D-mannose increased the rate of $^{36}Cl^-$ efflux, whereas L-glucose or 3-O-methyl-D-glucose had no effect (Sehlin, 1978). Other stimulators of insulin release, e.g., L-leucine and glibenclamide, have also been found to increase $^{36}Cl^-$ efflux (Sehlin, 1980b). The D-glucose effect had the same dose dependence as insulin release and was abolished by mannoheptulose. However, it was probably not the result of insulin release, because Ca^{2+} omission and EGTA addition failed to affect $^{36}Cl^-$ efflux at 20 mM D-glucose. Instead, it was suggested that D-glucose-induced depolarization of β cells and possibly insulin release, at least partly, may be due to an increase in Cl^- permeability (Sehlin, 1978, Sehlin, 1980a). This has so far been supported by membrane potential measurements using microelectrodes (Meissner and Sehlin, 1980) or measuring islet cell distribution of the lipophilic $[^3H]$ triphenylmethylphosphonium cation (^3H TPMP$^+$) (Sehlin and Täljedal, 1980). Both types of experiments showed that Cl^- replacement with isethionate led to a reduction in the D-glucose-induced depolarizing electrical activity after 5–10 min of treatement.

2. Phosphate

Freinkel *et al.* (1974) observed that rat islets prelabeled with $[^{32}P]$ orthophosphate released the label transiently in a D-glucose-dependent manner (the phosphate "flush") (also see Chapter 7). This phenomenon has since been scrutinized. The phosphate flush coincides in time with the first peak of insulin release (Freinkel *et al.*, 1974, 1976). It is elicited not only by D-glucose but also by other insulin secretagogues (Freinkel *et al.*, 1974, 1976; Asplund *et al.*, 1979) and the D-glucose effect shows dose dependence and anomeric specificity for the insulin-releasing α anomer (Pierce and Freinkel, 1975; Pierce *et al.*, 1976). The phosphate flush is not abolished by the omission of Ca^{2+} or the addition of Ca^{2+} transport inhibitors, suggesting that it may be involved in β-cell recognition of secretory stimuli or some proximal step in the stimulus–secretion coupling (Freinkel *et al.*, 1974).

Studies on phosphate movements in cells are made difficult by the fact that phosphate is incorporated in many cellular compounds and structures.

However, evidence has been obtained for the view that labeled phosphate in the phosphate flush originates essentially from labile pools of tissue orthophosphate and not from degradation of phosphorylated compounds (Freinkel *et al.*, 1978; Pierce *et al.*, 1978; Bukowiecki *et al.*, 1979). On the other hand, the D-glucose-induced radiophosphate efflux is markedly reduced by Na^+ depletion, K^+ depletion, or the addition of ouabain (Asplund *et al.*, 1981). This may indicate a coupling to ouabain-sensitive cation transport.

The basal efflux of labeled phosphate was inhibited by SITS, whereas the phosphate flush was not (Asplund *et al.*, 1979). This is in contrast to the $^{36}Cl^-$ efflux, where the D-glucose augmentation of the $^{36}Cl^-$ efflux rate was totally abolished by SITS (Sehlin, 1980b). The difference seems to rule out the possibility that D-glucose affects these two anionic fluxes by the same mechanism.

3. Sulfate

$^{35}SO_4^{2-}$ was rapidly taken up by islets from *ob/ob* mice. Figure 2 shows that apparent isotope equilibrium was reached within 30 min. The efflux shows complex kinetics. The rapid first component may represent washout from the extracellular islet compartment, and the later component may represent transmembrane efflux of $^{35}SO_4^{2-}$. This interpretation is supported by the inhibitory effect of low temperature or SITS on the later efflux. D-Glucose did not affect the efflux of $^{35}SO_4^{2-}$ but slightly accelerated the uptake (Sehlin, 1980b).

V. BIOGENIC AMINES

Biogenic amines may participate in the regulation of insulin release (cf. Lebowitz and Feldman, 1973) (see Chapter 8). Most of the work on biogenic amine action in islet cells has been done by using precursors. The main reason is that early work involving the injection of biogenic amines *in vivo* failed to show uptake of the amines in islets when fluorescence measurements were used (Cegrell *et al.*, 1964; Gagliardino *et al.*, 1971). A number of later studies, however, have shown that serotonin indeed is accumulated by pancreatic islet cells (Hellman *et al.*, 1972d; Mahoney and Feldman, 1977; Gylfe, 1978; Lindström *et al.*, 1980). The uptake has complex kinetics, one component being saturated at about 1–3 μM external serotonin (Lindström *et al.*, 1980) and the other at a serotonin concentration above 25 mM (Hellman *et al.*, 1972d). Serotonin uptake is inhibited by low temperature (Lindström *et al.*, 1980) and imipramine but not by reserpine (Lindström, 1981). Serotonin, incorporated in islet cells, is released

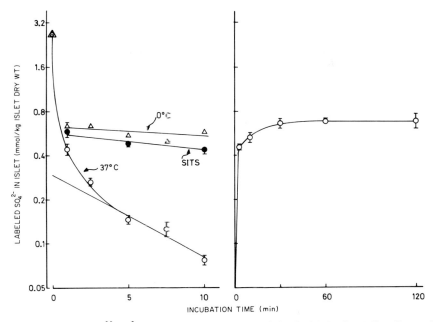

Fig. 2. Fluxes of $^{35}SO_4^{2-}$ in β-cell-rich islets of noninbred *ob/ob* mice. Microdissected islets were incubated in HEPES-buffered (pH 7.4) medium containing Na^+, K^+, Ca^{2+}, Mg^{2+}, Cl^-, $H_2PO_4^-$, and SO_4^{2-} (1.2 mM) at approximately the same concentrations as in Krebs–Ringer buffer. The uptake of $^{35}SO_4^{2-}$ with time is shown on the right. Note the semilogarithmic scale. Extracellular and contaminating $^{35}SO_4^{2-}$ was removed by washing in nonradioactive basal medium for 2 min at 0°C. The efflux of $^{35}SO_4^{2-}$ from islets prelabeled with this ion for 60 min is shown on the left. Efflux was measured in either nonradioactive basal medium at 37°C (open circles) (the regression line calculated from the three last data points has been extrapolated to time zero) or such medium at 0°C (triangles) or such medium containing 1 mM SITS at 37°C (solid circles). Results are mean values ± SEM (bars when larger than symbols) for four to six experiments. Unpublished results of J. Sehlin.

concomitantly with insulin, supporting the view that the former is localized in insulin storage granules (Gylfe, 1978).

VI. SULFONYLUREAS

Studies on the volume distribution of sulfonylurea derivatives indicate that they do not permeate islet cell membranes and that their action may be mediated through membrane binding. Tolbutamide uptake was very close to that of the extracellular space markers sucrose and mannitol when albumin was present in the incubation medium (Hellman *et al.*, 1971g). In the absence of albumin, the tolbutamide uptake was slightly enhanced, but it did not equilibrate in the total water space (Hellman *et al.,* 1973g). This uptake (membrane binding) was saturable and reduced by glibenclamide (Sehlin, 1973). Glibenclamide uptake was considerably greater than that of tolbutamide, whether in the presence (Hellman, 1974) or absence of albumin (Hellman *et al.,* 1973g). However, this uptake was strongly augmented by treatments known to increase the uptake of extracellular space markers without glibenclamide uptake by subcellular particles in islet homogenates being affected. Glibornuride was handled by islets essentially like glibenclamide, the uptake also being inhibited by glibenclamide (Täljedal, 1974). These results suggest that sulfonylureas do not readily enter β cells but bind to their plasma membranes. This idea gains support from the finding that a plasma membrane probe, SITS (Hellman *et al.,* 1973d), inhibits and the addition of cations (Hellman *et al.,* 1976c) augments glibenclamide uptake by islets.

VII. METHYLXANTHINES

Caffeine and theophylline, both potentiators of insulin release, are taken up by rat islets by mediated transport (McDaniel *et al.,* 1977). The half-time for equilibration of either of the methylxanthines was less than 1 min. The transport showed saturation kinetics, and theophylline reduced caffeine uptake and equilibrium concentration. D-Glucose did not clearly affect theophylline uptake. These data suggest that caffeine and theophylline share a common transport site in islet cells (McDaniel *et al.,* 1977).

VIII. THIOL REAGENTS

Evidence has been obtained demonstrating that thiol groups in β-cell plasma membranes are involved in stimulus–secretion coupling (cf. Hellman *et al.,* 1973b).

The uptake of slowly permeable [^{203}Hg] chloromercuribenzene-*p*-sulfonic acid (CMBS) was biphasic with time, one rapid component probably representing surface binding of CMBS and one slower component probably representing permeation into the islet cell plasma membrane (Hellman *et al.,* 1973e). As in erythrocytes (Knauf and Rothstein, 1971), this slow uptake of CMBS in islets was inhibited by SITS (Hellman *et al.,* 1973e) or sulfate ions (Söderberg and Täljedal, 1977). D-Glucose, but not nonsecretagogue analogues, reduced the slow CMBS membrane permeation (Söderberg, 1975), possibly reflecting a change in the configuration of the β-cell membrane associated with D-glucose-induced insulin release.

Iodoacetamide showed a marked accumulation in islets, which was sensitive to dithiothreitol or 5,5'-dithiobis(2-nitrobenzoic acid) (Hellman et al., 1973a). A considerable part of the accumulation may thus be due to the binding of iodoacetamide to thiol groups.

IX. β-CYTOTOXIC AGENTS

Alloxan is thought to react with thiol groups (Patterson et al., 1949) that may be important for β-cell function (see also Chapter 15). The capacity of a number of sugars to protect against the toxic effects of alloxan on islet cells has induced a search for a common transport site. Whereas Cooperstein and Lazarow (1964) and Watkins et al. (1964) did not find any cellular uptake of alloxan in toadfish islets, Hammarström et al. (1966) observed a marked accumulation of alloxan in mouse islets using radioautography. Recently, uptake of radicactively labeled alloxan in rat islets was described (Weaver et al., 1978). This uptake is rapid, temperature-dependent, and confined to alloxan and not any of its degradation products. Among compounds known to protect against alloxan poisoning of islet cells, some (caffeine, 3-O-methyl-D-glucose, and cytochalasin B) reduced the alloxan uptake, but others (D-glucose and D-mannose) augmented the uptake. Thus the existence of a common transport route for alloxan and protective sugars is not clear.

Ninhydrin was also rapidly accumulated by rat islets (McDaniel et al., 1979). D-Glucose or alloxan reduced the ninhydrin uptake. It was suggested that ninhydrin, which is a stable chemical analogue of alloxan, serves as a functional alloxan analogue in studies on alloxan sites in β cells (McDaniel et al., 1979) (see Chapter 5).

X. MARKERS FOR TRANSMEMBRANE pH OR ELECTRICAL POTENTIAL GRADIENTS

Attempts have been made to estimate the intracellular pH of pancreatic β cells by measuring the distribution of 5,5-dimethyloxazolidine-2,4-dione (DMO) in isolated islets from ob/ob mice (Hellman et al., 1972b). The calculated intracellular pH was 7.05, and it was unaffected by D-glucose concentration, diazoxide, epinephrine, and anoxia.

Uptake of the lipophilic TPMP+ cation in ob/ob mouse islets was studied to test its suitability as a probe for β-cell membrane electrical potentials (Sehlin and Täljedal, 1980). Reasonable agreement with data obtained with intracellular electrodes was achieved by correcting for voltage-independent TPMP$^+$ binding. The magnitude of TPMP$^+$-derived potentials was decreased with increasing K$^+$ concentration, was reduced by D-glucose or 2,4-dinitrophenol, but was not affected by 3-O-methyl-D-glucose. These results were reproduced with isolated islet cells from *ob/ob* mice and intact islets from NMRI mice. The effect of D-glucose was abolished by D-mannoheptulose and reduced by Cl$^-$ replacement. The results indicate that TPMP$^+$ may be used as a probe for membrane electrical potentials in intact islets or isolated islet cells and support a role of K$^+$ and Cl$^-$ electrodiffusion mechanisms in β-cell function.

ACKNOWLEDGMENT

The author's original work referred to in this chapter was supported by the Swedish Medical Research Council (12X-04756).

REFERENCES

Ashcroft, S. J. H. (1980). *Diabetologia* **18,** 5–15.
Ashcroft, S. J. H., Bunce, J., Lowry, M., Hansen, S. E., and Hedeskov, C. J. (1978). *Biochem. J.* **174,** 517–526.
Ashcroft, S. J. H., Sugden, M. C., and Williams, I. H. (1980). *In* "Biochemistry and Biophysics of the Pancreatic B-Cell; Hormone and Metabolic Research Supplement No. 10" (W. J. Malaisse and I.-B. Täljedal, eds.), pp. 1–7. Thieme, Stuttgart/New York.
Ashby, J. P., and Speake, R.N. (1975). *Biochem. J.* **150,** 89–96.
Asplund, K., Sehlin, J., and Täljedal, I.-B. (1979). *Biochim. Biophys. Acta* **588,** 232–240.
Asplund, K., Sehlin, J., and Täljedal, I.-B. (1981) (unpublished).
Bander, A., and Schesmer, G. (1970). *Diabetologia* **6,** 36.
Berggren, P. -O., Östensson, C. -G., Petersson, B., and Hellman, B. (1979). *Endocrinology* **105,** 1463–1468.
Berglund, O., and Hellman, B. (1976). *Diabetologia* **12,** 380.
Berglund, O., and Sehlin, J. (1980). *Diabetes* **29,** 151–155.
Berglund, O., Sehlin, J., and Täljedal, I.-B. (1978). *Diabetologia* **15,** 191–195.
Bloom, G. D., Hellman, B., Idahl, L. -A., Lernmark, A., Sehlin, J., and Täljedal, I.-B. (1972). *Biochem. J.* **129,** 241–254.
Boschero, A. C., and Malaisse, W. J. (1979). *Am. J. Physiol.* **236,** E139–E146.
Boschero, A. C., Kawazu, S., Duncan, G., and Malaisse, W. J. (1977). *FEBS Lett.* **83,** 151–154.
Boschero, A. C., Kawazu, S., Sener, A., Herschuelz, A., and Malaisse, W. J. (1979). *Arch. Biochem. Biophys.* **196,** 54–63.
Bukowiecki, L., Trus, M., Matschinsky, F. M., and Freinkel, N. (1979). *Biochim. Biophys. Acta.* **583,** 370–377.
Cegrell, L., Falck, B., and Hellman, B. (1964). *In* "The Structure and Metabolism of the Pancreatic Islets" (S. E. Brolin, B. Hellman, and H. Knutson, eds.), pp. 429–435. Pergamon, Oxford.

Christensen, H. N., Hellman, B., Lernmark, A., Sehlin, J., Tager, H. S., and Täljedal, I.-B. (1971). *Biochim. Biophys. Acta* **241**, 341–348.

Cooperstein, S. J., and Lazarow, A. (1964). *Am. J. Physiol.* **207**, 423–430.

Cooperstein, S. J., and Lazarow, A. (1969). *Am. J. Physiol.* **217**, 1784–1788.

Cooperstein, S. J., and Lazarow, A. (1977). *Am. J. Physiol.* **233**, E19–E27.

Coore, H. G., and Randle, P. J. (1964). *Biochem. J.* **93**, 66–78.

Donatsch, P., Lowe, D. A., Richardson, B. P., and Taylor, P. (1977). *J. Physiol. (London)* **267**, 357–376.

Figlewicz, D. P., Formby, B., Hodgson, A. T., Schmid, F. G., and Grodsky, M. (1979). *In* "Diabetes 1979: Excerpta Medica Intern. Congr. Ser. No. 500" (W. K. Waldhäusl, ed.), pp. 146–153. Excerpta Medica-American Elsevier, Amsterdam/New York.

Formby, B., Capito, K., Egeberg, J., and Hedeskov, C. J. (1976a). *Am. J. Physiol.* **230**, 441–448.

Formby, B., Capito, K., and Hedeskov, C. J. (1976b). *Acta Physiol. Scand.* **96**, 143–144.

Frankel, B. J., Gylfe, E., Hellman, B., Idahl, L. -A., Landström, U., Lövtrup, S., and Sehlin, J. (1978). *Diabetologia* **15**, 187–190.

Freinkel, N., El Younsi, C., Bonnar, J., and Dawson, R. M. (1974). *J. Clin. Invest.* **54**, 1179–1189.

Freinkel, N., El Younsi, C., and Dawson, R. M. C. (1976). *Proc. Natl. Acad Sci. U.S.A.* **73**, 3403–3407.

Freinkel, N., Pedley, K. C., Wooding, P., and Dawson, R. M. C. (1978). *Science* **201**, 1124–1126.

Gagerman, E., Sehlin, J., and Täljedal, I.-B. (1980). *J. Physiol. (London)* **300**, 505–513.

Gagliardino, J. J., Zieher, L. M., Furriza, F. C., Hernández, R. E., and Rodriguez, R. R. (1971). *Horm. Metab. Res.* **3**, 145–150.

Gerich, J. E., Frankel, B. J., Fanska, R., West, L., Forsham, P. H., and Grodsky, G. M. (1974). *Endocrinology* **94**, 1381–1385.

Goetz, F. C., and Cooperstein, S. J. (1962). *Biol. Bull.* **123**, 496.

Grodsky, G. M., Batts, A. A., Bennet, L. L., Vcella, C., McWilliams, N. B., and Smith, D. F. (1963). *Am. J. Physiol.* **205**, 638–644.

Gylfe, E. (1978) *J. Endocrinol.* **78**, 239–248.

Hammarström, L., Hellman, B., and Ullberg, S. (1966). *Diabetologia* **2**, 340–345.

Hellman, B. (1965). *Ann. N.Y. Acad. Sci.* **131**, 541–558.

Hellman, B. (1974). *Pharmacology* **11**, 257–267.

Hellman, B., Sehlin, J., and Täljedal, I.-B. (1971a). *Horm. Metab. Res.* **3**, 219–220.

Hellman, B., Sehlin, J., and Täljedal, I.-B. (1971b). *Biochim. Biophys. Acta* **241**, 147–154.

Hellman, B., Sehlin, J., and Täljedal, I.-B. (1971c). *Diabetologia* **7**, 256–265.

Hellman, B., Sehlin, J., and Täljedal, I.-B. (1971d). *Am. J. Physiol.* **221**, 1795–1801.

Hellman, B., Sehlin, J., and Täljedal, I.-B. (1971e). *Endocrinology* **89**, 1432–1439.

Hellman, B., Sehlin, J., and Täljedal, I.-B. (1971f). *Biochem. J.* **123**, 513–521.

Hellman, B., Sehlin, J., and Täljedal, I.-B. (1971g). *Biochem. Biophys. Res. Commun.* **45**, 1384–1388.

Hellman, B., Sehlin, J., and Täljedal, I.-B. (1972a). *Biochim. Biophys. Acta* **266**, 436–443.

Hellman, B., Sehlin, J., and Täljedal, I.-B. (1972b). *Endocrinology* **90**, 335–337.

Hellman, B., Lernmark, A., Sehlin, J., and Täljedal, I.-B. (1972c). *Metabolism* **21**, 60–66.

Hellman, B., Lernmark, A., Sehlin, J., and Täljedal, I.-B. (1972d). *Biochem. Pharmacol.* **21**, 695–706.

Hellman, B., Idahl, L.-A., Lernmark, A., Sehlin, J., and Täljedal, I.-B. (1973a). *Biochem. J.* **132**, 775–789.

Hellman, B., Idahl, L.-A., Lernmark, A., Sehlin, J., and Täljedal, I.-B. (1973b). *In* "Diabetes: Excerpta Medica Intern. Congr. Ser. No. 312" (W. J. Malaisse and J. Pirart, eds.) pp. 65–78. Excerpta Medica-American Elsevier, Amsterdam/New York.

Hellman, B., Lernmark, A., Sehlin, J., Täljedal, I.-B., and Whistler, R. L. (1973c). *Biochem. Pharmacol.* **22**, 29–35.

Hellman, B., Lernmark, A., Sehlin, J., and Täljedal, I.-B. (1973d). *FEBS Lett.* **34**, 347–349.

Hellman, B., Lernmark, A., Sehlin, J., Söderberg, M., and Täljedal, I.-B. (1973e). *Arch. Biochem. Biophys.* **158**, 435–441.

Hellman, B., Sehlin, J., and Täljedal, I.-B. (1973f). *Pfluegers Arch.* **340**, 51–58.

Hellman, B., Sehlin, J., and Täljedal, I.-B. (1973g). *Diabetologia* **9**, 210–216.

Hellman, B., Idahl, L.-A., Lernmark, A., Sehlin, J., and Täljedal, I.-B. (1974). *Biochem. J.* **138**, 33–45.

Hellman, B., Idahl, L.-A., Sehlin, J., and Täljedal, I.-B. (1975). *Diabetologia* **11**, 495–500.

Hellman, B., Sehlin, J., and Täljedal, I.-B. (1976a). *J. Physiol. (London).* **254**, 639–656.

Hellman, B., Sehlin, J., and Täljedal, I.-B. (1976b). *Science* **194**, 1421–1423.

Hellman, B., Sehlin, J., and Täljedal, I.-B. (1976c). *Horm. Metab. Res.* **8**, 427–429.

Hellman, B., Lenzen, S., Sehlin, J., and Täljedal, I.-B. (1977). *Diabetologia* **13**, 49–53.

Hellman, B., Sehlin, J., and Täljedal, I.-B. (1978). *Pfluegers Arch.* **378**, 93–97.

Hellman, B., Abrahamsson, H., Andersson, T., Berggren, P.-O., Flatt. P., and Gylfe, E. (1979). *In* "Diabetes 1979: Excerpta Medica Intern. Congr. Ser. No. 500" (W. K. Waldhäusl, ed.), pp. 160–165. Excerpta Medica-American Elsevier, Amsterdam/New York.

Hellman, B., Andersson, T., Berggren, P.-O., and Rorsman, P. (1980). *Biochem. Med.* **24**, 143–152.

Henquin, J. C. (1977). *Biochem. Biophys. Res. Commun.* **77**, 551–556.

Henquin, J. C. (1978). *Nature (London)* **271**, 271–273.

Henquin, J. C. (1979a). *J. Physiol. (London)* **296**, 103.

Henquin, J. C. (1979b). *Nature (London)* **280**, 66–68.

Henquin, J. C. (1980). *Biochem. J.* **186**, 541–550.

Henquin, J. C., and Meissner, H. P. (1978). *Biochim. Biophys. Acta* **543**, 455–464.

Henquin, J. C., Meissner, H. P., and Preissler, M. (1979). *Biochim. Biophys. Acta* **587**, 579–592.

Hermansen, K., Christensen, S. E., and Ørskov, H. (1979). *Diabetologia* **16**, 261–266.

Hermansen, K., and Schwartz, T. W. (1979). *Endocrinology* **105**, 1469–1474.

Herschuelz, A., Couturier, E., and Malaisee, W. J. (1980). *Am. J. Physiol.* **238**, E96–E103.

Howell, S. L., and Taylor, K. W. (1968). *Biochem. J.* **108**, 17–24.

Howell, S. L., Montague, W., and Tyhurst, M. (1975). *J. Cell Sci.* **19**, 395–409.

Idahl, L.-A., and Hellman, B. (1968) *Acta Endocrinol.* **59**, 479–486.

Idahl, L.-A., Sehlin, J., and Täljedal, I.-B. (1975). *Nature (London)* **254**, 75–77.

Idahl, L.-A., Lernmark, A., Sehlin, J., and Täljedal, I.-B. (1976). *J. Physiol. (Paris).* **72**, 729–746.

Idahl, L.-A., Lernmark, A., Sehlin, J., and Täljedal, I.-B. (1977). *Biochem. J.* **162**, 9–18.

Idahl, L.-A., Sehlin, J., Täljedal, I.-B., and Tamarit-Rodriguez, J. (1978). *Acta Endocrinol.* **88**, 113–121.

Iversen, J., and Hermansen, K. (1977). *Diabetologia* **13**, 297–303.

Kawazu, S., Boschero, A. C., Delcroix, C., and Malaisse, W. J. (1978). *Pfluegers Arch.* **375**, 197–206.

Kemmler, W., and Löffler, G. (1977). *Diabetologia* **13**, 235–238.

Knauf, P. A., and Rothstein, A. (1971). *J. Gen. Physiol.* **58**, 211–223.

Lacy, P. E., Klein, N. J., and Fink, C. J. (1973). *Endocrinology* **92**, 1458–1468.

Lebowitz, H. E., and Feldman, J. M. (1973). *Fed. Proc. Fed. Am. Soc. Exp. Biol.* **32**, 1797–1802.

Leclercq-Meyer, V., Marchand, J., and Malaisse, W. J. (1973). *Endocrinology* **93**, 1360–1370.

Lernmark, A., Sehlin, J., and Täljedal, I.-B. (1975). *Anal. Biochem.* **63**, 73–79.

Lernmark, A., Nathans, A., and Steiner, D. F. (1976). *J. Cell Biol.* **71**, 606–623.

Lernmark, A., Nielsen, D. A., Parman, A. Ü., Sehlin, J., Steiner, D. F., and Täljedal, I.-B. (1980). *In* "Biochemistry and Biophysics of the Pancreatic B-Cell; Hormone and Metabolic Research Supplement No. 10" (W. J. Malaisse and I.-B. Täljedal, eds.), 55–61. Thieme, Stuttgart/New York.

Levin, D. R., Kasson, B. G., and Dressen, J. F. (1978). *J. Clin. Invest.* **62**, 692–701.

Lin, B. J. (1977) *Diabetologia* **13**, 77–82.

Lindström, P. (1981) *Br. J. Pharmacol.* (in press).

Lindström, P., Sehlin, J., and Täljedal, I.-B. (1980). *Br. J. Pharmacol.* **68**, 773–778.

Löffler, G., and Kemmler, W. (1974). *Hoppe-Seyler's Z. Physiol. Chem.* **355**, 1274.

Ludvigsen, C., McDaniel, M., and Lacy, P. (1979). *Diabetes* **28**, 570–576.

McDaniel, M. L., King, S., Anderson, S., Fink, J., and Lacy, P. E. (1974). *Diabetologia* **10**. 303–308.

McDaniel, M. L., Anderson, S., Fink, J., Roth, C., and Lacy, P. E. (1975). *Endocrinology* **97**, 68–75.

McDaniel, M. L., Weaver, D. C., Roth, C. E., Fink, C. J., Swanson, J. A., Lacy, P. E. (1977). *Endocrinology* **101**, 1701–1708.

McDaniel, M. L., Bry, C. G., Fink, C. J., Homer, R. W., and Lacy, P. E. (1979). *Endocrinology* **105**, 1446–1451.

Mahoney, D., and Feldman, J. M. (1977). *Diabetes* **26**, 257–261.

Malaisse, W. J., Boschero, A. C., Kawazu, S., and Hutton, J. C. (1978a). *Pfluegers Arch.* **373**, 237–242.

Malaisse, W. J., Herschuelz, A., Devis, G., Somers, G., Boschero, A. C., Hutton, J. C., Kawazu, S., Sener, A., Atwater, I. J., Duncan, G., Ribalet, B., and Rojas, E. (1978b). *N.Y. Acad. Sci.* **307**, 562–582.

Malaisse-Lagae, F., and Malaisse, W. J. (1971). *Endocrinology* **88**, 72–80.

Marshall, E. K., Jr., and Davis, D. M. (1914). J. Biol. Chem. **18**, 53–80.

Maske, H. (1957). *Diabetes* **6**, 335–341.

Matschinsky, F. (1972). *In* "Handbook of Physiology" (D. F. Steiner and N. Freinkel, eds.), Vol 1, pp. 200–214. American Physiological Society, Washington, D.C.

Matthews, E. K. (1978). *In* "Secretory Mechanisms: Symposia of the Society for Experimental Biology" (C. R. Hopkins and C. J. Duncan, eds.), pp. 225–249. Cambridge Univ. Press, London and New York.

Meissner, H. P., and Sehlin, J (1981) (unpublished).

Meissner, H. P., Preissler, M., and Henquin, J. C. (1979). *In* "Diabetes 1979: Excerpta Medica Intern. Congr. Ser. No. 500" (W. K. Waldhäusl, ed.), pp. 166–171. Excerpta Medica-American Elsevier, Amsterdam/New York.

Milner, R. D. G., and Hales, C. N. (1970). *In* "The Structure and Metabolism of the Pancreatic Islets" (B. Hellman, S. Falkmer, and I.-B. Täljedal, eds.), pp. 489–493. Pergamon, Oxford.

Neame, K. D. (1968). *In* "Progress in Brain Research" (A. Lajtha and D. H. Ford, eds.), Vol. 29, pp. 185–199. Elsevier, Amsterdam.

Okamoto, K., and Kawaniski, I. (1966). *Endocrinol. Jpn.* **13**, 305–318.

Oxender, D. L., and Christensen, H. N. (1963). *J. Biol. Chem.* **238**, 3686–3699.

Pace, C. S., and Blaustein, M. P. (1979). *Biochim. Biophys. Acta* **585**, 100–106.

Patterson, J. W., Lazarow, A., and Levey, S. (1949). *J. Biol. Chem.* **177**, 197–204.

Pierce, M., and Freinkel, N. (1975). *Biochem. Biophys. Res. Commun.* **63**, 870–874.

Pierce, M., Bukowiecki, L., Asplund K., and Freinkel, N. (1976). *Horm. Metab. Res.* **8**, 358–361.
Pierce, M., Freinkel, N., Dawson, R. M. C., Asplund, K., and Bukowiecki, L. (1978). *Endocrinology* **103**, 971–977.
Scott, D. A. (1934). *Biochem. J.* **28**, 1592–1602.
Sehlin, J. (1972a). *Hormones* **3**, 144–155.
Sehlin, J. (1972b). *Hormones* **3**, 156–166.
Sehlin, J. (1973). *Acta Diabet. Lat.* **10**, 1052–1060.
Sehlin, J. (1976). *Biochem. J.* **156**, 63–69.
Sehlin, J. (1978). *Am. J. Physiol.* **235**, E501–E508.
Sehlin, J. (1980). *In* "Biochemistry and Biophysics of the Pancreatic B-Cell; Hormone and Metabolic Research Supplement No. 10" (W. J. Malaisse and I.-B. Täljedal, eds.), 73–80. Thieme, Stuttgart/New York.
Sehlin, J. (1981). *Upsala J. Med. Sci.* **86**, 177–182.
Sehlin, J., and Täljedal, I.-B. (1974a). *J. Physiol. (London)* **242**, 505–515.
Sehlin, J., and Täljedal, I.-B. (1974b). *FEBS Lett.* **39**, 209–213.
Sehlin, J., and Täljedal, I.-B. (1975). *Nature (London)* **253**, 635–636.
Sehlin, J., and Täljedal, I.-B. (1981). (unpublished).
Söderberg, M. (1975). *Acta Endocrinol.* **79**, 86–94.
Söderberg, M., and Täljedal, I.-B. (1977). *Acta Endocrinol.* **86**, 552–560.
Stein, W. D. (1967). "The Movements of Molecules Across Cell Membranes." Academic Press, New York.
Täljedal, I.-B. (1974). *Hormone Res.* **5**, 211–216.
Watkins, D., Cooperstein, S. J., and Lazarow, A. (1964). *Am. J. Physiol.* **207**, 431–435.
Watkins, D., Cooperstein, S. J., and Lazarow, A. (1970). *Am. J. Physiol.* **219**, 503–509.
Weaver, D. C., McDaniel, M. L., and Lacy, P. (1978). *Endocrinology* **102**, 1847–1855.
Williams, I. H., and Ashcroft, S. J. H. (1978) *FEBS Lett.* **87**, 115–120.
Wollheim, C., Blondel, B., and Sharp, G. W. G. (1976). *Diabetologia* **12**, 287–294.

4

Biosynthesis of Insulin

M. A. PERMUTT

I. INSULIN BIOSYNTHESIS

A. Primary Sequence

Prior to 1950, virtually nothing was known about the transfer of information from the gene to the rest of the cell. Study of the polypeptide hormone insulin has played an important role in the understanding of molecular biology. In the early 1950s, insulin was the first polypeptide whose primary sequence was determined (Ryle *et al.*, 1955). The B chain of insulin, containing 30 amino acids, is joined by two disulfide bridges to the A chain which contains 21 amino acids (Fig. 1). The primary sequence of

75

The Islets of Langerhans
Copyright © 1981 by Academic Press, Inc.
All rights of reproduction in any form reserved.
ISBN 0–12–187820–1

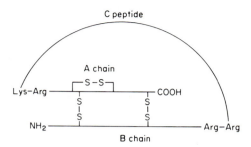

Fig. 1.   Insulin is composed of an A chain (21 amino acids) linked to a B chain (30 amino acids) by disulfide bridges. Cleavage of the single polypeptide chain proinsulin with the removal of two basic amino acids at either end of the connecting peptide (23–31 amino acids) yields insulin.

insulin from diverse species was determined over the next two decades (Smith, 1966). The structure of the B chain (Table I) has been very highly conserved in mammals and birds with the exception of histricomorph rodents (e.g., guinea pig, coypu, chinchilla, casiragua). Fish insulins contain a region at the amino terminus of the B chain which diverges considerably from that of mammalian insulins. The total number of amino acids in the fish B chain is 30, but there is an additional amino acid at the amino terminus, and one less at the carboxyl terminus. The A chain is also highly conserved in mammals and birds, again with the exception of histricomorph rodents. A small core in the middle of the A chain is divergent, but the amino and carboxyl terminii are highly conserved in all species. This conservation of the primary sequence probably accounts for the high level of biological activity of fish insulin in mammals (Yamamoto *et al.*, 1960). It is also interesting to note that the divergent histricomorph rodent insulins have less than 10% of the biological activity of mammalian insulin (Horuk *et al.*, 1979).

B. Site of Synthesis

In 1889, Von Mering and Minkowski (Von Mering *et al.*, 1890) demonstrated that diabetes could be caused by pancreatectomy. Later Banting and Best (1922) discovered that the active principal, insulin, was destroyed by pancreatic enzymes in the extraction process. Today extraction methods have changed little from the original. Fresh or frozen pancreas is extracted with acidified ethanol which solubilizes insulin but inactivates pancreatic proteases. Pancreatic insulin content varies depending on the source, but approximately 1–2 U (40–80 μg)/g of pancreas is obtained (Wrenshall *et al.*, 1952. (The biological activity of crystalline bovine insulin is approximately 25 U/mg.) Fish islets which are well separated from the exocrine portion of the pancreas, contain up to 75 U/g (Bencosme *et al.*, 1965). In mammalian pancreas the site of insulin production is the endocrine islet, which comprises only about 1% of the total pancreatic mass. Ultrastructural (Andersson *et al.*, 1974), immunofluorescent (Howell *et al.*, 1969), and biochemical studies (Howell and Taylor, 1967) have localized insulin in secretion granules within β cells.

C. Biosynthesis

1. Tissues Available for Study

The biosynthesis of insulin has been studied by incubating islet tissue with radioactive amino acids This study has been complicated by lack of availability of pancreatic islet tissue. Whole mammalian pancreas is about 1% islet tissue, and insulin comprises only a fraction of total islet protein. These studies have been facilitated by the isolation of rat and mouse islets from total pancreas by collagenase digestion (Lacy and Kostianovsky, 1967). Human insulinomas (Lazarus *et al.*, 1970) and insulinomas induced in experimental animals by irradiation (Duguid *et al.*, 1976) or exposure to streptozotocin and nicotinamide have also been examined (Itoh and Okamoto, 1977). Fish islets are composed of more than 75% endocrine tissue in most teleost species and have been studied extensively (Rapoport *et al.*, 1974; Humbel, 1963; Grand and Reid, 1968). Neonatal and fetal pancreas have been cultured for brief periods, but no permanent cell line capable of producing insulin has been reported. Hamster insulinoma cells contain a very small amount of insulin (7 ng/mg protein versus 400 μg/mg islet protein in normal islets) and continue insulin production when grown as tumors but not when grown *in vitro* (Rae *et al.*, 1979). The percentage of insulin synthesis in these cells is less than 0.1% and therefore of little use in insulin biosynthesis studies.

2. Synthesis as a Single Polypeptide Chain

Early studies on protein synthesis were performed by Dintzis who incubated reticulocytes with radioactively labeled amino acids for short periods and isolated labeled globin (Dintzis, 1961). In this way it has been determined that proteins are synthesized by the formation of peptide bonds between amino acids in a sequential fashion from the amino to the carboxyl terminus. The time required for synthesis is approximately 0.23 sec per amino acid residue at 37°C, so that globin (approximately 150 amino acids) requires about 37 secs to be synthesized. Using similar methods with

TABLE I

Sequence of Insulin[a]

Amino acid sequence of insulin A chains

	1	2	3	4	5	6	7	8	9	10	11	12	13	14	15	16	17	18	19	20	21	
man[1] NH_2	Gly	Ile	Val	Glu	Gln	Cys	Cys	Thr	Ser	Ile	Cys	Ser	Leu	Tyr	Gln	Leu	Glu	Asn	Tyr	Cys	Asn	COOH
Pig[2]	—	—	—	—	—	—	—	—	—	—	—	—	—	—	—	—	—	—	—	—	—	
Dog[3]	—	—	—	—	—	—	—	—	—	—	—	—	—	—	—	—	—	—	—	—	—	
Rabbit[3]	—	—	—	—	—	—	—	—	—	—	—	—	—	—	—	—	—	—	—	—	—	
Sperm whale[4]	—	—	—	—	—	—	—	—	—	—	—	—	—	—	—	—	—	—	—	—	—	
Fin whale[5]	—	—	—	—	—	—	—	—	—	—	—	—	—	—	—	—	—	—	—	—	—	
Horse[4]	—	—	—	—	—	—	—	—	Gly	Val	—	—	—	—	—	—	—	—	—	—	—	
Elephant[3]	—	—	—	—	—	—	—	—	Gly	Val	—	—	—	—	—	—	—	—	—	—	—	
Cow[6]	—	—	—	—	—	—	—	Ala	—	Val	—	—	—	—	—	—	—	—	—	—	—	
Sheep[2]	—	—	—	—	—	—	—	Ala	Gly	Val	—	—	—	—	—	—	—	—	—	—	—	
Goat[3]	—	—	—	—	—	—	—	Ala	Gly	Val	—	—	—	—	—	—	—	—	—	—	—	
Guinea pig[3,7]	—	—	—	Asp	—	—	—	—	Arg	Thr	—	—	—	His	—	—	Gln	Ser	—	—	—	
Chinchilla[4]	—	—	—	Asp	—	—	—	—	—	Thr	—	—	—	—	—	—	Glu	Ser	—	—	—	
Coypu[7]	—	—	—	Asp	—	—	—	—	Asn	—	—	—	—	Arg	Asn	—	Met	Ser	—	—	—	
Casiragua[8]	—	—	—	—	—	—	—	—	Asn	—	—	—	—	Arg	Asn	—	Leu	Thr	—	—	Asp	
Rat and mouse I and II[3,9-11]	—	—	—	Asp	—	—	—	—	—	—	—	—	—	—	—	—	—	—	—	—	—	
Sei whale[12]	—	—	—	—	—	—	—	Ala	—	Thr	—	—	—	—	—	—	—	—	—	—	—	
Chicken[3]	—	—	—	—	—	—	—	His	Asn	Thr	—	—	—	—	—	—	—	—	—	—	—	
Turkey[13]	—	—	—	—	—	—	—	His	Asn	Thr	—	—	—	—	—	—	—	—	—	—	—	
Duck[14]	—	—	—	—	—	—	—	Glu	Asn	Thr	—	—	—	—	—	—	—	—	—	—	—	
Anglerfish[5]	—	—	—	—	—	—	—	His	Arg	Pro	—	—	—	Phe	Asp	—	Gln	—	—	—	—	
Codfish[16]	—	—	—	Asp	—	—	—	His	Arg	Pro	—	—	—	Phe	Asp	—	Gln	—	—	—	—	
Tuna II[17]	—	—	—	—	—	—	—	His	Lys	Pro	—	—	—	Phe	Asp	—	Gln	—	—	—	—	
Hagfish[15]	—	—	—	—	—	—	—	His	Lys	Arg	—	—	—	—	Asn	—	Gln	—	—	—	—	

Amino acid sequence of insulin B chains

	1	2	3	4	5	6	7	8	9	10	11	12	13	14	15	16	17	18	19	20	21	22	23	24	25	26	27	28	29	30	
man[1] NH_2	Phe	Val	Asn	Gln	His	Leu	Cys	Gly	Ser	His	Leu	Val	Glu	Ala	Leu	Tyr	Leu	Val	Cys	Gly	Glu	Arg	Gly	Phe	Phe	Tyr	Thr	Pro	Lys	Thr	COOH
Elephant[3]	—	—	—	—	—	—	—	—	—	—	—	—	—	—	—	—	—	—	—	—	—	—	—	—	—	—	—	—	—	—	
Horse[4]	—	—	—	—	—	—	—	—	—	—	—	—	—	—	—	—	—	—	—	—	—	—	—	—	—	—	—	—	—	Ala	
Pig[2]	—	—	—	—	—	—	—	—	—	—	—	—	—	—	—	—	—	—	—	—	—	—	—	—	—	—	—	—	—	Ala	
Cow[6]	—	—	—	—	—	—	—	—	—	—	—	—	—	—	—	—	—	—	—	—	—	—	—	—	—	—	—	—	—	Ala	
Sheep[2]	—	—	—	—	—	—	—	—	—	—	—	—	—	—	—	—	—	—	—	—	—	—	—	—	—	—	—	—	—	Ala	
Goat[3]	—	—	—	—	—	—	—	—	—	—	—	—	—	—	—	—	—	—	—	—	—	—	—	—	—	—	—	—	—	Ala	

Dog[1]	—	—	—	—	—	—	—	—	—	—	—	—	—	—	—	—	—	—	—	—	—	Ala
Sperm whale[4]	—	—	—	—	—	—	—	—	—	—	—	—	—	—	—	—	—	—	—	—	—	Ala
Fin whale[5]	—	—	—	—	—	—	—	—	—	—	—	—	—	—	—	—	—	—	—	—	—	Ala
Sei whale[12]	—	—	—	—	—	—	—	—	—	—	—	—	—	—	—	—	—	—	—	—	—	Ala
Rabbit[1]	—	—	—	—	—	—	—	—	—	—	—	—	—	—	—	—	—	—	—	—	—	Ser
Guinea pig[2,7]	—	—	—	—	Ser	Arg	—	—	—	—	—	—	Asn	—	Thr	—	Ser	—	Gln	Asp	Asp	—	Ile	—	Asp
Chinchilla[4]	Ser	Lys	—	—	—	—	—	—	—	—	—	—	—	—	—	—	—	—	—	—	—	Met	Ala
Coypu[7]	Tyr	Ser	—	Arg	—	—	—	—	—	—	—	Gln	Asp	Thr	—	Ser	—	Arg	His	—	Arg	—	Asn	Asp
Casiragua[4]	Tyr	Gly	—	Arg	—	—	—	—	—	—	—	Gln	Asp	Thr	—	Ser	—	Arg	His	—	Arg	—	Ser	Glu
Rat and mouse I[3,9-11]	—	—	Lys	—	—	—	—	—	—	—	—	Pro	—	—	—	—	—	—	—	—	—	—	Ser
Rat and mouse II[3,9-11]	—	—	Lys	—	—	—	—	—	—	—	—	—	—	—	—	—	—	—	—	—	—	Met	Ser
Chicken[1]	Ala	Ala	—	Lys	—	—	—	—	—	—	—	—	—	—	—	—	Ser	—	—	—	—	Met	Ala
Turkey[13]	Ala	Ala	—	—	—	—	—	—	—	—	—	—	—	—	—	—	Ser	—	—	—	—	—	Ala
Duck[14]	Ala	Ala	—	—	—	—	—	—	—	—	—	—	—	—	—	—	Ser	—	—	—	—	—	Thr
Anglerfish[15]	Val	Ala	Pro	Ala	—	—	—	—	Asp	—	—	—	—	Asp	—	Asp	—	Asn	—	—	—	—	—
Codfish[16]	Met	Ala	Pro	Pro	—	—	—	—	Asp	—	—	—	—	Asp	—	Asp	—	Asn	—	—	—	—	—
Tuna II[17]	Val	Ala	Pro	Pro	—	—	—	—	Asp	—	—	—	—	Asp	—	Asp	—	Asn	—	—	—	—	—
Hagfish[18]	Arg	Thr	Thr	Gly	—	Asp	—	Ala	Ile	—	—	—	—	Val	—	—	—	Asp	—	Thr	Lys	Met

[a] Key to references:

1 Nicol and Smith, (1960) *Nature (London)* **187**, 483.

2 Brown, Sanger, and Kitai, (1955). *Biochem. J.* **60**, 556.

3 Smith, (1966) *Am. J. Med.* **40**, 662.

4 Brown, Sanger, and Naughton, (1956) *Arch. Biochem. Biophys.* **65**, 427.

5 Hama, Titani, Sakaki, and Narita, (1964) *J. Biochem. (Tokyo)* **56**, 285.

6 Ryle, Sanger, Smith, and Kitai, (1955) *Biochem. J.* **60**, 541.

7 Smith, (1972) *Diabetes* **21**, Suppl 2, 457.

8 Horuk, Goodwin, O'Connor, Neville, Lazarus, and Stone, (1979) *Nature (London)* **279**, 440.

9 Clark and Steiner, (1969) *Proc. Natl. Acad. Sci. U.S.A.* **62**, 278.

10 Markussen, (1971) *Int. J. Protein Res.* **3**, 149.

11 Bunzli, Glatthaar, Kunz, Mulhaupt, and Humbel, (1972) *Hoppe Seyler's Z. Physiol. Chem.* **353**, 451.

12 Ishihara, Saito, Ito, and Fujino, (1958) *Nature (London)* **181**, 1468.

13 Jentsch (1972) in "Atlas of Protein Sequence and Structure" (Dayhoff, ed.), Vol. 5, National Biomedical Research Foundation, Washington, D.C.

14 Markussen and Sundby, (1973) *Int. J. Pept. Protein Res.* **5**, 37.

15 Neumann, Koldenhof, and Humbel, (1969) *Z. Physiol. Chem.* **350**, 1286.

16 Reid, Grant, and Youngson, (1968) *Biochem. J.* **110**, 289.

17 Neumann and Humbel, (1969) *Int. J. Protein Res.* **1**, 125.

18 Peterson, Steiner, Emdin, and Falkmer (1975) *J. Biol. Chem.* **250**, 5183.

anglerfish islets, Humbel (1965) erroneously concluded that the A and B chains of insulin were synthesized separately. Steiner and Oyer (1967) subsequently demonstrated with human insulinoma slices and isolated rat islets that radioactive amino acids were incorporated into a single polypeptide chain, proinsulin (MW 9000), which was converted into insulin (Fig. 1). The two chains of insulin are synthesized from the amino terminus of the B chain through the so-called connecting peptide (C peptide) to the carboxyl terminus of the A chain as a single polypeptide chain. Porcine proinsulin was the first to be sequenced (Chance *et al.*, 1968). The sequence of the C peptide (Table II) has been more divergent than that of the A or B chain throughout evolution. It has been hypothesized that the main role of the C peptide is to facilitate proper folding of A and B chains prior to cleavage (Steiner *et al.*, 1973). Note that the numbers of amino acids in the A and B chains are highly conserved, while the C peptide varies from 23 to 31 amino acids in different species.

3. Synthesis on Membrane-Bound Polysomes and Conversion of Proinsulin to Insulin

Incubation of isolated rat islets with radioactive amino acids for various periods of time followed by cell fractionation (Permutt and Kipnis, 1972a) or autoradiography (Howell *et al.*, 1969) has revealed that proinsulin is synthesized on membrane-bound polysomes, as are other secretory peptides. Conversion of proinsulin to insulin occurs in membranous vesicles within the cisternae of the rough endoplasmic reticulum or in the Golgi apparatus (Kemmler *et al.*, 1972). At least 95% of proinsulin is cleaved into insulin and C peptide which is stored in secretion granules until both are released into the blood. The primary structures of bovine and porcine proinsulin suggest that enzymes with trypsinlike and carboxypeptidase-B-like activities are required for conversion to insulin, and partially converted forms of bovine proinsulin intermediates have been isolated (Kemmler *et*

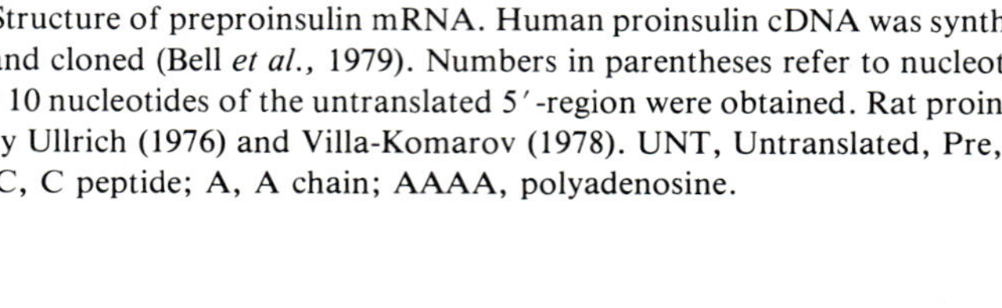

Fig. 2. Structure of preproinsulin mRNA. Human proinsulin cDNA was synthesized from insulinoma and cloned (Bell *et al.*, 1979). Numbers in parentheses refer to nucleotides in each region. Only 10 nucleotides of the untranslated 5′-region were obtained. Rat proinsulin cDNA was cloned by Ullrich (1976) and Villa-Komarov (1978). UNT, Untranslated; Pre, pre region; B, B chain; C, C peptide; A, A chain; AAAA, polyadenosine.

TABLE II

Amino Acid Sequence of Connecting Peptides[a,b]

	NH₂	1	2	3	4	5	6	7	8	9	10	11	12	13	14	15	16	17	18	19	20	21	22	23	24	25	26	27	28	29	30	31	C-OOH
man[1]	NH₂	Glu	Ala	Glu	Asp	Leu	Gln	Val	Gly	Gln	Val	Glu	Leu	Gly	Gly	Gly	Pro	Gly	Ala	Gly	Ser	Leu	Gln	Pro	Leu	Ala	Leu	Glu	Gly	Ser	Leu	Gln	C-OOH
Monkey[2]		—	—	—	—	Pro	—	—	—	—	—	—	—	—	—	—	—	—	—	—	—	—	—	—	—	—	Ala	—	—	—	Pro	Gln	—
Horse[3]		—	—	—	—	Pro	—	—	—	Glu	—	—	—	—	—	—	—	—	—	Gly	—	—	—	Ala	—	—	—	—	—	Pro	Pro	—	—
Pig[4]		—	—	—	Ilu	Pro	Ala	Ala	—	Ala	Leu	—	—	—	—	—	Leu	—	—	x	Gly	—	—	x	—	x	x	—	—	—	Pro	Pro	—
Cow, sheep[5,6]		—	Val	—	Gly	Pro	Leu	Leu	—	Ala	—	—	—	—	—	—	—	—	—	x	Gly	—	x	x	x	x	x	—	—	—	Pro	—	—
Dog[2]		Asp	Val	—	x	x	x	Thr	—	Glu	—	—	—	Ala	Ala	Met	—	—	Glu	—	Gly	—	—	Thr	—	x	Gln	—	—	—	Alu	—	—
Guinea pig[7]		—	Leu	—	—	Pro	—	Leu	Glu	Pro	—	Leu	—	—	—	—	Leu	—	—	—	Asp	—	—	Thr	—	x	—	Val	Val	Ala	Ala	—	—
Rat I[1]		—	Val	—	—	Asp	—	Leu	—	Glu	—	Glu	—	—	—	—	—	—	—	—	Asp	—	—	Thr	—	—	—	Val	Val	Ala	Ala	Arg	—
Rat II[1]		Asp	Val	—	Gln	Pro	Leu	Asn	Gly	Gln	Val	—	His	—	—	—	Val	—	x	x	x	—	x	—	Phe	His	—	Glu	Glu	Tyr	x	—	—
Duck[8]		Asp	Val	—	Gln	Pro	Leu	x	x	x	x	x	—	x	His	—	—	Glu	Val	Glu	x	—	x	—	—	His	—	Val	Glu	Tyr	x	—	—

[a] A hyphen indicates the same amino acid as in man; x indicates a deletion.

[b] Key to references:

1. Oyer, Cho, Peterson, and Steiner (1971) *J. Biol. Chem.* **246**, 1375.
2. Peterson, Nehrlich, Oyer, and Steiner (1972) *J. Biol. Chem.* **247**, 4866.
3. Tager and Steiner (1972) *J. Biol. Chem.* **247**, 7936.
4. Chance, Ellis, and Bromer, (1968) *Science* **161**, 165.
5. Steiner, Cho, Oyer, Terris, Peterson, and Rubenstein, (1971) *J. Biol. Chem.* **246**, 1365.
6. Nolan, Margoliash, Peterson, and Steiner, (1971) *J. Biol. Chem.* **246**, 2780.
7. Smyth, Markussen, and Sundby, (1974) *Nature (London)* **248**, 151.
8. Markussen and Sundby, (1973) *Eur. J. Biochem.* **34**, 401.

al., 1971). Tager *et al.* (1973) have isolated a chymotrypsin-like fragment of rat proinsulin C peptide from whole rat pancreas, suggesting that this occurs naturally in the normal conversion of proinsulin to insulin in the rat. Kallikreins are endopeptidases that generate basal active kinin polypeptides from plasma α-2 globulin substrates or kininogens (Ole-MoiYoi *et al.,* 1979). Kallikrein has been localized to pancreatic β cells within islets with the same distribution as that of insulin in normal human pancreas and in two islet cell tumors. Human pancreatic kallikrein, in concert with carboxypeptidase B, converts bovine proinsulin to a polypeptide with the electrophoretic mobility of insulin. Whether glandular kallikreins play any role in the conversion of proinsulin to insulin is unknown at the present time.

In vivo conversion of proinsulin to insulin is not complete, as evidenced by various intermediates identified in human plasma (De Haën *et al.,* 1978). These comprise only a small percentage of the total immunoreactive insulin in normal subjects and include partially cleaved proinsulins as well as arginyl and diarginyl insulins.

4. Cell-Free Synthesis of Insulin

Studies measuring cell-free synthesis of insulin have been important in understanding the mechanisms of regulation of insulin biosynthesis. Wagel (1965) prepared microsomes from fetal dog pancreas and measured the incorporation of labeled amino acids into insulin. Yip *et al.* (1975) injected islet RNA into frog oocytes and observed labeled peptides bound by antiinsulin serum. The peptides were very heterogeneous in size, ranging in molecular weight from 2000 to 20,000, and no discrete protein was seen.

More recently, RNA has been extracted from fish pancreatic islets (Shields and Blobel, 1977; Permutt *et al.,* 1978), adult and fetal bovine pancreas (Munjaal and Saunders, 1979; Lomedico and Saunders, 1976), isolated rat islets (Chan *et al.,* 1976), and rat and human insulinomas (Duguid and Steiner, 1978; Permutt *et al.,* 1977). Poly-A-rich mRNA was prepared by chromatography on oligo-dT–cellulose and translated in a mRNA-dependent, cell-free, protein-synthesizing system. The estimated molecular weight of the major protein synthesized in these cell-free systems was 12,000. This cell-free product has been called preproinsulin in accordance with other pre forms of secretory proteins, since it contains 23–25 amino acids at the amino terminus of proinsulin.

The amino-terminal extension of secretory proteins, synthesized when the mRNAs are translated in cell-free systems devoid of microsomal membrane, has been postulated to be a sequence extension or signal peptide which plays a role in facilitating movement of the secretory peptide through the membrane (Devillers-Thiery *et al.,* 1975). Shields and Blobel (1977) isolated mRNA from anglerfish and sea raven islets and translated preproinsulin in a cell-free system. Using microsomal membranes isolated from dog pancreas, they cleaved preproinsulin to proinsulin. It was concluded that microsomal membranes and the cleavage process of the pre form of secretory proteins were highly conserved during evolution, since fish preproinsulin could bind to dog microsomal membranes and be correctly processed.

5. Preproinsulin in Intact Cells

Recent studies have suggested that a small amount of preproinsulin is present in intact cells (Permutt *et al.*, 1977; Albert *et al.*, 1979; Patzelt *et al.*, 1978). Catfish islets incubated with labeled amino acids synthesized two peptides (MW 12,000 and 11,000) which were bindable by antiinsulin antibody. They were synthesized before proinsulin and appeared to be "chased" into it. These proteins were shown to contain tryptic peptides of proinsulin. Conversion occurred even when protein synthesis was inhibited by cycloheximide. Rat preproinsulins I and II were observed in isolated rat islets (Patzelt *et al.*, 1978). It thus appears that preproinsulin is a natural precursor of proinsulin in intact islet cells and that conversion may occur as a posttranslational event. Whether some preproinsulin escapes cleavage and accumulates in cytoplasm, as does proinsulin, is unknown at the present time. Nevertheless, even after short incubations, the percentage of preproinsulin is very small and therefore most is converted to proinsulin.

D. Isolation and Characterization of Proinsulin mRNA

1. Isolation of mRNA

Recombinant DNA technology has recently been utilized to isolate individual genes which make up only about one-millionth of the total genome of a mammalian cell. The insulin gene is present in all mammalian cells but is expressed only in pancreatic islet β cells. [Recently (Rosenzweig *et al.*, 1980), a very small amount of insulin was detected by a sensitive radioimmunoassay in every tissue examined. Insulin in these tissues is present at about 40 ng/g, compared to 4 mg/g in islet tissue; i.e., it is 10^5-fold less abundant. Therefore a small amount of insulin gene expression may occur in every cell.] The RNA from pancreatic islets is therefore greatly enriched in proinsulin mRNA. With the use of islet mRNA as a template, cDNA has been synthesized from deoxyribonucleotides with an enzyme known as reverse transcriptase. The cDNA of proinsulin mRNA can be radioactively labeled and used in DNA–RNA hybridization to study expression of the insulin gene.

Proinsulin mRNA has been isolated by techniques used for other eukaryotic messengers. Poly-A-rich mRNA is isolated from total pan-creatic RNA by oligo-dT–cellulose affinity chromatography (Permutt, *et al.*, 1976). Poly-A residues at the 3′-end of mRNA hybridize by hydrogen bonding to the cellulose-bound oligo dT in high-salt buffer, while rRNA and tRNA do not adhere. Cell-free translation of this islet mRNA by wheat germ extracts yielded preproinsulin which comprised between 10 and 23% of the total cell-free product depending on the conditions of cell-free syn-thesis. Blocked methylated 5′-terminal structures have been identified at the 5′-end of many eukaryotic and viral mRNAs, and cap analogues such as 7-methylguanosine inhibit translation of capped mRNA. 7-Methyl-guanosine produced an 80% inhibition of preproinsulin synthesis (Permutt *et al.*, 1978), suggesting the presence of a 7-methylguanosine cap at the 5′-end of preproinsulin mRNA. Proinsulin mRNA was purified by sucrose gradients and elution from agarose urea gels (Permutt *et al.*, 1978). Catfish preproinsulin mRNA was estimated to be of 210,000 molecular weight and to have approximately 650 nucleotides by electrophoresis on denaturing gels. Labeled cDNA of fish preproinsulin mRNA was synthesized and used to monitor purification. Preproinsulin mRNA represented 5% of the total islet mRNA.

2. Cloning cDNA of Proinsulin mRNA

Ullrich *et al.* (1977) obtained total islet poly-A-rich RNA from isolated rat islets and synthesized its cDNA. The single-stranded cDNA was con-verted to double-stranded material and inserted into a circular bacterial plasmid. This recombinant plasmid was used to transform *Escherichia coli*. Sequence analysis of the cloned recombinant DNA showed rat insulin se-quences in the DNA clones. These studies identified 55 nucleotides at the 3′-end of proinsulin mRNA beyond the A chain, which were not trans-lated. The 5′-end was not fully identified at that time.

Villa-Komaroff *et al.* (1978) used recombinant DNA techniques to make rat insulin in bacteria. Proinsulin cDNA was inserted into the bacterial plasmid pBR322 within the coding region for penicillinase. The hybrid plasmid was used to transform *E. coli*. One of the clones expressed a fused protein which bore both insulin and penicillinase antigenic determinants.

RNA has been extracted from human insulinoma, its cDNA synthesized, and cloned in bacteria (Bell *et al.*, 1979). Since there is considerable homol-ogy between rat and human proinsulin (83%), bacterial transformants were screened with rat preproinsulin I cDNA as a probe. The largest cloned cDNA contained 500 base pairs. The primary structure of human proin-sulin mRNA, determined by sequencing the cDNA, agreed precisely with that obtained by previous amino acid sequencing of human proinsulin. The predicted 24-amino-acid sequence of the human prepeptide was very similar to that observed in rat insulin I and the partial sequences obtained from other preproinsulins (Table III). In addition, the nucleotide sequence of 10 bases of 5'-end untranslated messenger and the complete sequence (76 bases of the 3'-end untranslated region) were obtained (Fig. 2, p. 80). When rat and human proinsulin mRNAs were compared, it was observed that the high degree of amino acid sequence homology of the A and B chains extended to the nucleotide sequence. The nucleotide sequence homology of the C peptides was less than that of the pre portions of human and rat proinsulin. The 3'-end untranslated region of human preproinsulin cDNA was 21 residues longer than this region in rat preproinsulin I. Despite the difference in length, there was a 21-nucleotide segment adjacent to the poly-A attachment site that was highly conserved (86%). This suggested that these conserved regions may play an important role in the regulation of transcription, translation, or polyadenylation.

E. Structure of Rat Insulin Genes

Using radioactively labeled cloned cDNA of rat preproinsulin mRNA, two groups have studied rat insulin genes within genomic DNA (Cordell *et al.*, 1979; Lomedico *et al.*, 1979). High-molecular-weight DNA is cut with specific restriction endonucleases (enzymes which cut double-stranded DNA at highly specific sites) and the resulting fragments separated according to size by electrophoresis on agarose gels. The DNA fragments are then transferred out of the gel after denaturation, by a technique called Southern blotting, onto nitrocellulose filters where the DNA is adsorbed (Southern, 1975). The mobilized single-stranded DNA on the filter can then be hybridized with the radioactive cDNA of proinsulin mRNA. The radioactive cDNA probe binds to the insulin gene, and a radioautograph is obtained. In this fashion, the pieces of genomic DNA which contain the insulin gene can be detected. Preparative amounts of high-molecular-weight DNA were digested, resulting DNA fragments separated by preparative electrophoresis, and the fractions hybridizing with the proinsulin cDNA cloned in bacteriophage lambda. Two nonallelic insulin genes were detected in the rat, separated by at least 7000 bases of DNA. There was no obvious similarity in the organization surrounding each gene, although the coding regions of the genes were quite similar.

Further studies on the two nonallelic genes for rat preproinsulins I and II were reported by Lomedico *et al.* (1979). The hybridization patterns using DNA from rat kidney, spleen, or insulinoma were identical to that obtained from liver DNA, suggesting that the insulin gene was not rearranged during development. The noncoding 5'-regions of the genes for rat insulins I and II were very similar, with an intron of 119 base pairs preceding the

TABLE III

Amino Acid Sequence of the Pre Regions of Proinsulin[a,b]

	-24				-20										-10									-1	
MAN[1] NH₂	Met	Ala	Leu	Trp	Met	Arg	Leu	Leu	Pro	Leu	Leu	Ala	Leu	Leu	Ala	Leu	Trp	Gly	Pro	Asp	Pro	Ala	Ala	Ala	Phe
Rat I[2]	—	—	—	—	Ile	—	Phe	—	—	—	—	—	—	—	Ile	—	—	Glu	—	Arg	—	—	Gln	—↓	—
Rat II[2]	—	—	—	—	—	—	Phe	—	—	—	—	—	—	—	Val	—	—	Glu	—	Lys	—	—	Gln	—	—
Bovine[3]	x	x	x	x	x	x	—	x	x	x	x	x	x	x	x	—	x	x	x	x	x	x	x	x↓	x
Anglerfish[4]	x	x	Leu	—	Leu	x	x	Phe	Val	—	—	Val	Val	—	x	Val	—	x	x	x	x	x	—	—↓	Val
Sea raven[5]	x	x	x	x	x	x	x	x	—	—	—	—	—	—	x	—	x	x	x	x	x	x	x↓	x↓	x

(Anglerfish[4] is preceded by Met Met; Sea raven[5] is preceded by Met.)

[a] A hyphen indicates the same amino acid as that in man; x indicates an undetermined residue; ↓ indicates the end of the pre region and the amino terminus of proinsulin.

[b] Key to references:

[1] Bell, Swain, Pictet, and Rutter, (1979) Nature (London) **282**, 525.

[2] Lomedico, Rosenthal, Efstratiadis, Gilbert, Kolodner, and Tizard, (1979) Cell **18**, 545.

[3] Lomedico, Chan, Steiner, and Saunders, (1977) J. Biol. Chem. **252**, 7971.

[4],[5] Shields and Blobel, (1977) Proc. Natl. Acad. Sci. U.S.A. **74**, 2059.

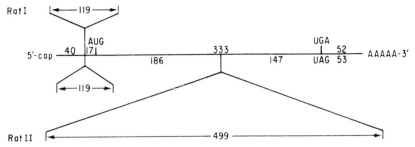

Fig. 3. Structure of rat preproinsulin I and II genes from Lomedico (1979). An intron is present within the portion of the gene coding for the untranslated 5′-portion of preproinsulin I and II mRNAs. An intron of 499 bases appears within the gene coding for the C-peptide region of rat preproinsulin II mRNA. The introns are spliced out of the mature mRNA found in the cytoplasm.

pre region of preproinsulin (Fig. 3). Introns are regions of DNA which are transcribed into mRNA but do not appear in the mature mRNA because they are spliced out (Berget et al., 1977). Another intron of 499 bases was observed within the C-peptide region of the rat insulin II gene but not in the rat insulin I gene. Heteroduplex mapping, or hybridization of single strands of the two genes, revealed that the two sequences of rat insulins I and II diverged immediately after the end of the noncoding 3′-regions. About 500 base pairs upstream from the 5′-capping site of the mRNA are very homologous, however, and probably retain highly conserved base sequences important in the regulation of insulin gene expression. The DNA sequencing data for the first time established the complete amino acid sequence of the pre region of both preproinsulins. This illustrates the importance of recombinant DNA technology in polypeptide hormone studies.

II. REGULATION OF INSULIN BIOSYNTHESIS

A. Potential Sites of Regulation

Very little is known about the regulation of insulin synthesis in whole animals. Hellman (1959) has studied total islet volume during development of the rat. In the newborn, islet volume is 0.14 mm^2 and increases to 3.39 mm^2 in rats 480 days old. Similarly, the number of islets increases from 243 ± 21 in newborn rats to 3320 ± 184 in adult rats. Control of pancreatic insulin reserve, turnover of insulin within β cells, and the effects of aging on the ability of the islets to produce insulin are areas about which little is known. Reaven et al. (1979) showed that β-cell number and islet insulin content doubled in rats from 2 to 18 months, while glucose-stimulated insulin release declined with age. Can insulin be destroyed within the β cell without being released? During starvation, when very little insulin is released from the pancreas, a 50% reduction in pancreatic insulin content was noted. (Malaisse *et al.*, 1967).

A number of potential sites can be identified for the regulation of insulin biosynthesis (Fig. 4): (1) hyperplasia of islet β cells by increased DNA replication, (2) new synthesis of proinsulin mRNA (transcription), (3) splicing out of introns and processing of precursor preproinsulin mRNA to mature mRNA, (4) capping of the 5'-end or polyadenylation of the 3'-end, (5) transport from the nucleus to the cytoplasm (or degradation within the nucleus), and (6) translation and turnover of proinsulin mRNA in the cytoplasm. What little is known of these potential regulatory steps will be discussed below.

B. Regulation of Insulin Biosynthesis by Glucose

Kinash and Haist (1954) reported that, when rats were continuously infused for 6–14 days with glucose, the total amount of islet tissue was greatly increased. In isolated islets incubated in medium containing glucose

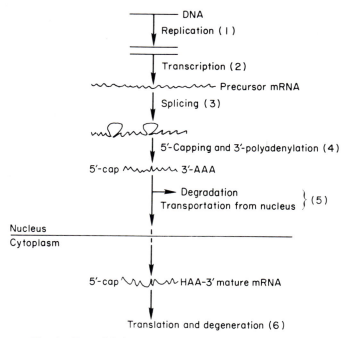

Fig. 4. Potential sites of regulation of insulin biosynthesis.

at 250 mg/dl [³H]leucine incorporation into insulin was approximately 10-fold over that which occurred at 50 mg/dl during a 1-hr incubation (Martin *et al.*, 1963). Morris and Korner (1970a) were the first to report a specific effect of glucose on proinsulin synthesis relative to that of total islet protein. Proinsulin comprised approximately 6% of total islet protein at 5 mM glucose, and 20% at 20 mM glucose.

Studies on the mechanism of glucose stimulation of insulin biosynthesis were begun in 1970. It had been reported that glucose stimulated the incorporation of labeled precursors into RNA by isolated rat islets (Jarrett *et al.*, 1967). Morris and Korner (1970b) used actinomycin D to determine whether RNA synthesis was required for glucose-stimulated insulin biosynthesis. During a 2-hr incubation they noted a 20-fold stimulation of insulin synthesis when glucose was raised from 2 to 20 mM in the absence of actinomycin D, and a 5-fold stimulation in the presence of actinomycin D. Permutt and Kipnis (1972b) reported that the early effects of glucose on insulin biosynthesis (a 1-hr incubation) were independent of new RNA synthesis. At 2 hr, however, the inhibition of RNA synthesis inhibited glucose-stimulated insulin biosynthesis. These data suggested that the early effects of glucose on preexisting mRNA were at a translational level and that there was a delayed effect of glucose on stimulation of new proinsulin mRNA. Cycloheximide was added to islets to block protein synthesis, and the effects of high glucose on the buildup of proinsulin mRNA determined. When the islets were subsequently removed from the cycloheximide, those previously incubated in 16.6 mM glucose synthesized more insulin than those previously incubated in 2.8 mM glucose, in spite of the fact that the glucose concentration during the test period was the same. This effect was blocked by preincubation with actinomycin D. The conclusion was that, while glucose had an immediate effect on the translation of preexisting proinsulin mRNA, it also increased synthesis of new proinsulin mRNA.

Experiments with low doses of cycloheximide, in which ribosome movement along messengers was slowed, were used to estimate the amount of messenger being utilized for total islet protein synthesis and for proinsulin (Permutt, 1974). These experiments further demonstrated that the glucose effect on total islet protein synthesis was not increased by mRNA production. In contrast, increased glucose in the medium increased the total amount of functional proinsulin mRNA, confirming previous studies.

All these studies were only suggestive, however, and an assay for proinsulin mRNA was not available at that time. Itoh *et al.* (1978) incubated isolated rat islets in 3.3 or 36.7 mM glucose for 1 hr and extracted the RNA. This RNA was translated in a cell-free, protein-synthesizing wheat germ system to quantitate proinsulin mRNA. There was no difference in the amount of preproinsulin mRNA in islets incubated for up to 1 hr in low or high glucose. It was concluded that glucose regulated proinsulin synthesis during the first 60 min by enhancing the availability of total insulin mRNA for translation rather than by increasing the amount of proinsulin mRNA.

Glucose stimulation of insulin biosynthesis over a more prolonged period has been studied by Zucker and Logothetopoulos (1975). Rats were infused for 24 hr with glucose sufficient to maintain plasma glucose levels between 350 and 500 mg/dl. Control rats were infused with glucose-free buffer for the same amount of time. After 24 hr of infusion, rat islets were isolated by collagenase digestion and incubated in either 4.5 or 29 mM glucose for 45 min with [^{3}H]leucine. Total islet protein synthesis was increased about fourfold in the glucose-infused animals as compared to controls, whether tested at a low or a high glucose concentration. Glucose infusion over 24 hr had a profound effect on proinsulin and insulin biosynthesis measured during the test period. When control islets were studied, proinsulin and insulin comprised 16% of protein synthesis at low glucose and 30% at high glucose. In contrast, glucose-infused islets synthesized 39% proinsulin and insulin with low glucose in the incubation medium, and 41% with high glucose. The specific effect of increased glucose in the incubation medium on insulin synthesis relative to total islet protein synthesis was eliminated by previously infusing rats with glucose for 24 hr. These data suggest that glucose infusion during the 24 hr prior to the test period maximally induced proinsulin mRNA levels. These studies need to be further evaluated with an assay for proinsulin mRNA.

The effects of glucose on the translation of islet protein synthesis was studied by the isolation of rat islet polyribosomes (Permutt and Kipnis, 1972a). Islets incubated in 16.6 mM glucose were shown to have two- to fourfold increased numbers of ribosomes active in protein synthesis compared to islets incubated in 2.8 mM glucose. Activation of islet polyribosomes occurred in the presence or absence of actinomycin D, thus demonstrating a glucose effect on the overall rate of initiation of islet proteins, which was independent of new RNA synthesis.

C. Regulation of Insulin Biosynthesis by Other Compounds

The effects of compounds other than glucose on insulin biosynthesis have been studied by a number of investigators. Mannose, a potent stimulator of insulin secretion, was also stimulatory for insulin biosynthesis, whereas fructose was not (Lin and Haist, 1969). Glucose- or mannose-stimulated insulin synthesis was inhibited by mannoheptulose. No insulin synthesis occurred in the presence of tolbutamide, ribose, or xylitol, all stimulators of insulin release. While caffeine and dibutyryl cyclic AMP have been shown to be potent stimulators of insulin release, caffeine alone did not have a stimulatory effect on insulin synthesis. Caffeine doubled the synthesis of insulin induced by 4 mM glucose. The effects of sulfonylureas on insulin biosynthesis have variously been reported to be inhibitory or stimulatory (Tanese et al., 1970; Schatz et al., 1978). Schatz et al. (1978) reported the long-term actions of sulfonylureas on insulin biosynthesis. The insulin content was not changed in the glibenclamide group as compared to controls but was reduced about 20% in the tolbutamide group. In vitro no changes were found in insulin biosynthesis after tolbutamide or glibenclamide.

Diazoxide and epinephrine, and the absence of calcium ions, all inhibited insulin release but had no effect on insulin biosynthesis (Lin and Haist, 1973). Serotonin, dopamine, and isoproteronol did not inhibit or stimulate insulin biosynthesis induced by glucose (Lin and Haist, 1973). Methysergide, at a concentration reported to potentiate insulin release, strongly inhibited insulin synthesis (Lin and Haist, 1975). D-Glyceraldehyde, a potent secretagogue of insulin secretion, produced a 10-fold stimulation of insulin synthesis at 1.5 mM without a significant increase in other islet proteins (Jain et al., 1975). Above 1.5 mM glucose, D-glyceraldehyde inhibited insulin synthesis in contrast to glucose.

Alloxan, streptozotocin, and N-nitrosomethylurea have all been reported to inhibit insulin synthesis (Gunnarsson, 1975). Lin et al. (1976) described a more potent inhibitory effect of acetate and fluoride on insulin biosynthesis than on oxidation of glucose in isolated rat pancreatic islets. Cyproheptadine has been reported to be a potent inhibitor of insulin biosynthesis (Hintze et al., 1977). Administration of this drug at 45 mg/kg body weight to rats for 8 days raised plasma glucose concentrations from 136 mg/dl in the control animals to 349 mg/dl. Insulin content was reduced over 90% in drug-treated animals. The total protein content of the pancreas and the DNA content were not altered. When islets were isolated and insulin biosynthesis studied, islets isolated from animals previously treated with cyproheptadine incorporated 7.5 times more radioactivity into proinsulin compared to islets prepared from control rats. Cyproheptadine added directly to the isolated islets at 8×10^{-5} M inhibited leucine incorporation into proinsulin and insulin almost completely, while effects on total protein synthesis were not observed. Cyproheptadine may be an excellent drug for studying the regulation of insulin biosynthesis, since it appears to be quite selective for insulin. It is a serotonin and histamine antagonist used in man, but the recommended human dose is up to 0.5 mg/kg body weight, or approximately 10^2 less than that used in the experimental animals.

D. Defects of Insulin Biosynthesis and Diabetes

Errors in insulin biosynthesis are an obvious potential cause of diabetes, yet very few studies have been reported. In normal and spontaneously diabetic mice (Poffenbarger *et al.,* 1971) no difference in the rate or pattern of incorporation of radioactive amino acids into proinsulin and insulin was noted. Other investigators have reported a reduced rate of insulin biosynthesis in response to glucose in spontaneously diabetic mice (Gunnarsson, 1977). In diabetic sand rats glucose stimulated biosynthesis, and release was greater than in control animals (Wilke *et al.,* 1977).

That a biologically less active insulin is a possible cause of diabetes in man has been considered (Steiner, 1976). Amino acid analysis of insulin isolated from eight pancreases of diabetics did not differ from normal human insulin except in one case in which an excess of lysine and a low value for isoleucine were found (Kimmel and Pollock, 1967). Since the changes were less than molar, it was speculated that the patient was a heterozygote with one normal and one abnormal allele. Negative results were obtained for human insulin from 19 diabetics (Brunfeld *et al.,* 1969).

Gabbay *et al.* (1976) reported a family with a high prevalence of hyperproinsulinemia. The patients were completely asymptomatic and had no abnormalities in carbohydrate tolerance. The plasma immunoreactive insulin in these patients was predominantly proinsulin-like material, as measured by gel filtration chromatography and radioimmunoassay. These authors speculated that this genetic disorder was a defect in the processing of proinsulin to insulin or a structural defect in the proinsulin molecule itself. Since some normal insulin was present, it was again assumed that these patients were heterozygotes.

Tager *et al.* (1979) recently described a structurally abnormal insulin causing human diabetes. The patient had elevated fasting plasma glucose and insulin levels. The proinsulin/insulin ratio was normal, and the plasma did not contain antiinsulin or antiinsulin receptor antibodies. Furthermore, the patient responded normally to exogenously administered insulin and had normal insulin receptors. The patient's insulin had lower than normal activity in stimulating glucose uptake and oxidation in rat adipocytes. The patient's pancreas was removed during exploratory surgery, and enough material was obtained to isolate insulin and partially characterize it chemically. The patient's insulin had impaired ability to displace porcine insulin from human receptors and impaired insulin-mediated glucose transport and oxidation. It was suggested that the abnormal insulin was a mixture of normal insulin and an abnormal variant which contained leucine substituted for phenylalanine at position 24 or 25 of the insulin B chain. The biological activity of the patient's insulin was only 11–12% normal.

The abnormal insulin present in this patient may inhibit binding and action of the normal insulin.

Abnormal human hemoglobin molecules due to point mutations, deletions, insertions, and abnormal crossover have been observed (Konigsberg, 1979). The thalessemias are a group of anemias in which there is insufficient production of either α- or β-globin. The mRNA may be present but contain a premature termination codon. Deletions of genes outside the β-globin gene cause failure of expression of the β-globin. Mutations in the stop codon of β-globin are responsible for hemoglobin variants with extensions at the carboxyl end. No human insulin variant with an extension at the carboxyl end has been noted, however, and may never be found since the carboxyl end of the A chain is critical for biological activity and an extended proinsulin molecule may have no biological activity. It seems reasonable to conclude that mutations in insulin genes are as common as those in globin genes. It remains to be determined how frequently they occur, and what role, if any, they play in diabetes.

REFERENCES

Albert, S., Chyn, R., Goldford, M., and Permutt, A. (1979) *Diabetes* **26**, Suppl. 1, 378.
Andersson, A., Westman, J., and Hellerström, C. (1974) *Diabetologia* **10**, 743–753.
Banting, F. G., and Best, C. H. (1922) *J. Lab. Clin. Med.* **7**, 251–256.
Bell, G. I., Swain, W. F., Pictet, R., Cordell, B., Goodman, H. M., and Rutter, W. J. (1979) *Nature (London)* **282**, 525–527.
Bencosme, S. A., Meyer, J., Bergmar, B. J., and Martinez-Palomo, A. (1965) *Rev. Can. Biol.* **24**, 141–154.
Berget, S. M., Moore, C., and Sharp, P. A. (1977) *Proc. Natl. Acad. Sci. U.S.A.* **74**, 3171–3175.
Brunfeld, T. K., Deckert, T., and Thomsen, J. (1969) *Acta Endocrinol.* **60**, 543–549.
Chan, S. J., Keim, P., and Steiner, D. F. (1976) *Proc. Natl. Acad. Sci. U.S.A.* **73**, 1964–1968.
Chance, R. E., Ellis, R. M., and Bromer, W. W. (1968) *Science* **161**, 165–167.
Cordell, B., Bell, G., Tischer, E., DeNoto, F. M., Ullrich, A., Pictet, R., Rutter, W. J., and Goodman, H. M. (1979) *Cell* **18**, 533–543.
De Haën, C., Little, S. A., May, J. M., and Williams, R. H. (1978) *J. Clin. Invest.* **62**, 727–737.
Devillers-Thiery, A., Kindt, T., Scheele, G., and Blobel, G. (1975) *Proc. Natl. Acad. Sci. U.S.A.* **72**, 5016–5020.
Dintzis, H. M. (1961) *Proc. Natl. Acad. Sci. U.S.A.* **47**, 247–261.
Duguid, J. R., and Steiner, D. F. (1978) *Proc. Natl. Acad. Sci. U.S.A.* **75**, 3249–3253.
Duguid, J. R., Steiner, D. F., and Chick, W. L. (1976) *Proc. Natl. Acad. Sci. U.S.A.* **73**, 3539–3543.
Gabbay, K. H., DeLuca, K., Fisher, J. N., Jr., Mako, M. E., and Rubenstein, A. H. (1976) *New Engl. J. Med.* **294**, 911–945.
Grant, P. T., and Reid, K. B. M. (1968) *Biochem. J.* **106**, 531–541.

Gunnarsson, R. (1975) *Mol. Pharmacol.* **11**, 759–765.

Gunnarsson, R. (1977) *Diabet. Metab.* **3**, 149–153.

Hellman, B. (1959) *Acta Endocrinol.* **32**, 78–91.

Hintz, K. L., Grow, A. V., and Fischer, L. J. (1977) *Biochem. Pharmacol.* **26**, 2021–2027.

Horuk, R., Goodwin, P., O'Connor, K., Neville, R. W. J., Lazarus, N. R., and Stone, D. (1979) *Nature (London)* **279**, 439–440.

Howell, S. L., and Taylor, K. W. (1967) *Biochem. J.* **102**, 922–927.

Howell, S. L., Kostianovsky, M., and Lacy, P. E. (1969) *J. Cell Biol.* **42**, 695–702.

Humbel, R. E. (1963) *Biochem. Biophys. Acta* **74**, 96–104.

Humbel, R. E. (1965) *Proc. Natl. Acad. Sci. U.S.A.* **53**, 583–859.

Itoh, N., and Okamoto, H. (1977) *FEBS Lett.* **80**, 111–114.

Itoh, N., Sei, T., Nose, K., and Okamoto, H. (1978) *FEBS Lett.* **93**, 343–347.

Jain, K., Logothetopoulos, J., and Zucker, P. (1975) *Biochim. Biophys. Acta* **399**, 384–394.

Jarrett, R. J., Keene, H., and Track, N. S. (1967) *Nature (London)* **213**, 634–635.

Kemmler, W., Peterson, J. D., and Steiner, D. F. (1971) *J. Biol. Chem.* **246**, 6786–6791.

Kemmler, W., Peterson, J. D., Rubenstein, A. H., and Steiner, D. F. (1972) *Diabetes* **21**, Suppl. 2, 572–581.

Kimmel, J. R., and Pollock, H. G. (1967) *Diabetes* **16**, 687–694.

Kinash, B., and Haist, R. E. (1954) *Can. J. Biochem. Physiol.* **32**, 428–433.

Konigsberg, W. (1980). *In* "Metabolic Control and Disease" (Bondy and Rosenberg, eds.), pp. 27–72. Saunders, Philadelphia, Pennsylvania.

Lacy, P. E., and Kostianovsky, M. (1967) *Diabetes* **16**, 35–39.

Lazarus, N. R., Tanese, T., Gutman, R., and Recant, L. (1970) *J. Clin. Endocrinol. Metab.* **30**, 273–281.

Lin, B. J., and Haist, R. E. (1969) *Can. J. Physiol. Pharmacol.* **47**, 791–801.

Lin, B. J., and Haist, R. E. (1973) *Endocrinology* **92**, 735–742.

Lin, B. J., and Haist, R. E. (1975) *Endocrinology* **96**, 1247–1253.

Lin, B. J., Henderson, M. J., Levin, B. B., Nagy, B. R., and Nagy, E. M. (1976) *Horm. Metab. Res.* **8**, 353–358.

Lomedico, P. T., and Saunders, G. F. (1976) *Nucleic Acids* **3**, 381–391.

Lomedico, P., Rosenthal, N., Efstratiadis, A., Gilbert, W., Kolodner, R., and Tizard, R. (1979) *Cell* **18**, 545–558.

Malaisse, W. J., Malaisse-Lagae, F., and Wright, P. E. (1967) *Am. J. Physiol.* **213**, 843–848.

Martin, J. M., Gregor, W. H., Lacy, P. E., and Evens, R. G. (1963) *Diabetes* **12**, 538–544.

Morris, G. E., and Korner, A. (1970a) *Biochim. Biophys. Acta* **208**, 404–413.

Morris, G. E., and Korner, A. (1970b) *FEBS Lett.* **10**, 165–168.

Munjaal, R. P., and Saunders, G. F. (1979) *Mol. Cell. Endocrinol.* **15**, 51–60.

Ole-MoiYoi, O., Pinkus, G. S., Spragg, J., and Austen, K. F. (1979) *New Engl. J. Med.* **300**, 1289–1294.

Patzelt, C., Labrecque, A. D., Duguid, J. R., Carroll, R. J., Keim, P. S., Heinrikson, R. L., and Steiner, D. F. (1978) *Proc. Natl. Acad. Sci. U.S.A.* **75**, 1260–1264.

Permutt, M. A., (1974) *J. Biol. Chem.* **248**, 2738–2742.

Permutt, M. A., and Kipnis, D. M. (1972a) *Proc. Natl. Acad. Sci. U.S.A.* **69**, 505–509.

Permutt, M. A., and Kipnis, D. M. (1972b) *J. Biol. Chem.* **247**, 1194–1199.

Permutt, M. A., and Routman, A. (1977) *Biochem. Biophys. Res. Commun.* **78**, 855–862.

Permutt, M. A., Biesbroeck, J., Chyn, R., Boime, I., Szczesna, E., and McWilliams, D., (1976) *Ciba Found. Symp.* **41**, 97–116.

Permutt, M., Biesbroeck, J., and Chyn, R. (1977) *J. Clin. Endocrinol. Metab.* **44**, 536–544.

Permutt, M. A., Boime, I., Chyn, R., and Goldford, M. (1978a) *Biochemistry* **17**, 537–543.

Permutt, M. A., Chyn, R., and Goldford, M. (1978b) *Diabetes* **27**, Suppl. 2, 456.
Poffenbarger, P. L., Chick, W. L., Labine, R. L., Soeldner, S., and Flewelling, J. H. (1971) *Diabetes* **20**, 677–685.
Rae, P. A., Yip, C. C., and Schimmer, B. P. (1979) *Can. J. Physiol. Pharmacol.* **57**, 819–824.
Rapoport, T. A., Prehn, S., Lukowsky, A., and Junghahn, I. (1974) *Acta Biol. Med. Ger.* **33**, 953–961.
Reaven, E. P., Gold, G., and Reaven, G. M. (1979) *J. Clin. Invest.* **64**, 591–599.
Rosenzweig, J. L., Havrankova, J., Lesniak, M. A., Brownstein, M., and Roth, J. (1980) *Proc. Natl. Acad. Sci. U.S.A.* **77**, 572–576.
Ryle, A. P., Sanger, F., Smith, L. F., and Kitai, R. (1955) *Biochem. J.* **60**, 541–556.
Schatz, H., Laube, H., Sieradzki, J. Kamenisch, W., and Pfeiffer, E. F. (1978) *Horm. Metab. Res.* **10**, 23–29.
Shields, D., and Blobel, G. (1977) *Proc. Natl. Acad. Sci. U.S.A.* **74**, 2059–2963.
Smith, L. F. (1966) *Am. J. Med.* **40**, 662–666.
Southern, E. M. (1975) *J. Mol. Biol.* **98**, 503–517.
Steiner, D. F., (1976) *New Engl. J. Med.* **294**, 952–953.
Steiner, D. F., and Oyer, P. B. (1967) *Proc. Natl. Acad. Sci. U.S.A.* **57**, 473–480.
Steiner, D. F., Peterson, J. D., Tager, H., Emdin, S., Ostberg, Y., and Falkmer, S. (1973) *Am. Zool.* **13**, 591–604.
Tager, H. S., Emdin, S. O., Clark, J. L., and Steiner, D. F. (1973) *J. Biol. Chem.* **248**, 3476–3482.
Tager, H., Given, B., Baldwin, D., Mako, M., Markese, J., Rubenstein, A., Olefsky, J., Kobayashi, M., Kolterman, O., and Poucher, R. (1979) *Nature (London)* **281**, 122–125.
Tanese, T., Lazarus, N. R., Devrim, S., and Recant, L. (1970) *J. Clin. Invest.* **49**, 1394–1404.
Ullrich, A., Shin, J., Chirgwin, J., Pictet, R., Tischer, E., Rutter, W. J., and Goodman, H. M. (1977) *Science* **196**, 1313–1319.
Villa-Komaroff, L., Efstratiadis, A., Broome, S., Lomedico, P., Tizard, R., Naber, S. P., Chick, W. L., and Gilbert, W. (1978) *Proc. Natl. Acad. Sci. U.S.A.* **75**, 3727–3731.
Von Mering, J., and Minkowski, O. (1890) *Naunyn-Schmiedebergs Arch. Exp. Pathol. Pharmakol.* **26**, 371–387.
Wagle, S. R. (1965) *Biochim. Biophys. Acta* **107**, 524–530.
Wilke, B., Jahr, H., Schmidt, S., Schäfer, H., Gottschling, D., Fiedler, H., and Zühlke, H. (1977) *Endokrinologie* **69**, 233–238.
Wrenshall, G. A., Bogoch, A., and Ritchie, R. C. (1952) *Diabetes* **1**, 87–107.
Yamamoto, M., Kotaki, A., Okuyama, T., and Satake, K. (1960) *J. Biochem.* **48**, 84–92.
Yip, C. C., Hew, C-L., and Hsu, H. (1975) *Proc. Natl. Acad. Sci. U.S.A.* **72**, 4777–4779.
Zucker, P., and Logothetopoulos, J. (1975) *Diabetes* **24**, 194–200.

5

Interactions of Cell Organelles in Insulin Secretion

MICHAEL L. McDANIEL and PAUL E. LACY

Insulin release from the β cell involves recognition of the stimulus followed by translation of this primary signal via a series of intracellular events, which results in a rapid, controlled release of insulin. This overall secretory process is integrated by the interaction of specific cellular

97

The Islets of Langerhans
Copyright © 1981 by Academic Press, Inc.
All rights of reproduction in any form reserved.
ISBN 0–12–187820–1

organelles, i.e., the plasma membrane, insulin storage granules, and the microtubule–microfilament system. This chapter will focus on the interactions of cell organelles in insulin secretion by describing the role(s) of the plasma membrane in mediating recognition of the stimulus, the storage form of intracellular insulin contained within specialized membrane vesicles or sacs, the directed movement of these insulin storage granules to the plasma membrane via the microtubule–microfilament system, and the membrane fusing of the storage granule and plasma membrane during the emiocytotic discharge of insulin.

I. PLASMA MEMBRANE

A. Stimulus Recognition

1. Glucoreceptor

D-Glucose is the major physiological stimulus for insulin release from the β cell. The molecular mechanism of glucose-induced insulin release, however, remains unclear. Two concepts have been proposed to explain the recognition and initiation of insulin release by glucose: metabolism and the glucoreceptor. These two models have been reviewed recently by Matschinsky *et al.* (1979) and Hedeskov (1980). The metabolism model implies that an alteration in some metabolite of glucose or a complex change in the metabolite pattern initiates insulin release. This model will be discussed further in Chapter 6, and the present discussion will emphasize only approaches in describing recognition via the glucoreceptor mechanism.

A major difficulty in determining the primary event responsible for the initiation of insulin release by D-glucose is the complex interactions of glucose with the β cell. D-Glucose initially interacts with the plasma membrane, rapidly enters the intracellular space via a low-affinity facilitated carrier (see Chapter 3), and subsequently becomes a substrate for metabolism. An experimental approach in attempting to define the primary D-glucose initiation site in the β cell has been to employ chemical probes which demonstrate specificity for the insulin secretory mechanism. The ideal requirements for such a chemical probe would be the induction of insulin release by a reaction at the glucose initiation site and the subsequent formation of a stable chemical bond at this site. In this approach one would anticipate specific steric requirements for recognition between the stimulatory agent or probe and the glucose molecule.

In recent studies, we have evaluated the specificity of alloxan (discussed further in Chapter 15) as a chemical probe to inhibit glucose-induced insulin release in an *in vitro* system employing collagenase-isolated islets.

These studies have shown that a 5-min exposure of isolated rat islets to alloxan (650 μM) results in both stimulation and subsequent inhibition of insulin release (Weaver et al., 1978). The monophasic release of insulin induced by alloxan occurs rapidly 2–3 min following exposure, and similar to glucose-induced insulin release is associated with increased ^{45}Ca uptake. The inhibition of insulin release is completely prevented by the concomitant presence of D-glucose (27.5 mM) during the exposure period (Tomita et al., 1974). The protection by glucose is specific for the D isomer, and no protection is observed in the presence of L-glucose. In addition, when present during the 5-min exposure to alloxan (650 μM), D-glucose protects against the inhibition of insulin release in a dose-dependent manner (Weaver et al., 1978). These findings suggest that the protection provided by D-glucose against alloxan inhibition occurs by a competitive mechanism. Additional studies have examined the specificity of hexose protection by determining the protective ability of the α and β anomers of D-glucose. At low concentrations the α anomer of D-glucose is a more potent protective agent against alloxan inhibition of insulin release than the β anomer (McDaniel et al., 1976). The results with the anomers of D-glucose indicate a close relationship between initiation of insulin release and protection by D-glucose against alloxan inhibition (Rossini et al., 1974; Grodsky et al., 1974).

The competitive interaction between alloxan and D-glucose has suggested that these two molecules may compete for a common initiation site. To determine if common molecular features exist supporting this contention, the structures of D-glucose, alloxan, and their analogues have been compared by computer analysis for molecular similarity. This overall analysis based on x-ray crystallographic data compares structural similarities among these agents, computes the volume required to accommodate them at a common site, and proposes a testable model for their molecular recognition at a glucoreceptor (Weaver et al., 1979). As indicated in Fig. 1, alloxan is a heterocyclic six-membered ring with C-4, N-3, C-2, N-1, and C-6 existing in a common plane. The reactive moiety of the alloxan molecule is a gem-dihydroxy group at C-5 with one of its hydroxyls in the axial position and the other in the equatorial position. An analogue of alloxan, ninhydrin, shares similarities in chemical reactions with alloxan and has been shown both to stimulate insulin release and to inhibit subsequent glucose-induced insulin release (McDaniel et al., 1977). The inhibition of insulin release in vitro by ninhydrin is prevented by D-glucose and D-mannose, as is alloxan inhibition. Molecular analysis of the structure of ninhydrin indicates a similarity to alloxan in the conformation of the gem-dihydroxy group and adjacent carbonyls. Both alloxan and ninhydrin have a slight pucker in the ring that allows their reactive moiety to project out of the principal plane, and both compounds have an electron-dense group at

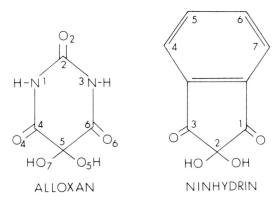

Fig. 1. Chemical formulas of alloxan monohydrate and ninhydrin. From Weaver *et al.*, 1979 with permission.

the opposite end of the molecule. Alloxan has an attached oxygen at C-2 that aligns near the aromatic ring of ninhydrin.

D-Glucose, D-mannose, and their anomers all initiate insulin release and protect against alloxan and ninhydrin. A structural comparison indicates that the slight pucker in the ring of alloxan and ninhydrin allows their reactive moiety, i.e., the gem-dihydroxy group and two adjacent carbonyls, to align with hydroxyls of D-glucose and D-mannose at C-1, C-2, and C-3. The gem-dihydroxy group of both alloxan and ninhydrin has an equatorial and an axial hydroxyl that align at the hexose C-2 with the equatorial hydroxyl of D-glucose and the axial hydroxyl of D-mannose. In addition, the carbonyl group at C-2 of alloxan and the aromatic ring of ninhydrin lie near the CH_2OH group of hexoses. The net result of this comparison is that alloxan and ninhydrin fit almost entirely within the volume demanded by D-glucose, D-mannose, and their anomers. The volume required to accommodate the recognized agents is illustrated in Fig. 2. The steric requirements common to the recognized agents is an oxygen at position 1, either axial or equatorial; a hydroxyl at position 2, either axial or equatorial; an equatorial oxygen at position 3; and an electron-rich region at position 5.

Hershfield and Richards (1976) evaluated the steric and conformational similarities between a series of substituted pyridine derivatives and D-glucose. In this comparison, a variety of substituents (CH_3, F, Br, CN, NH_2, and H) were added to the pyridine nucleus. These pyridine derivatives were observed to bind at both competitive and noncompetitive sites of the glucose transport system of human erythrocytes. In particular, a close steric and conformational homology was shown to exist between the substituted pyridine derivative 2,4-diamino-5-cyano-6-bromopyridine and the D-glu-

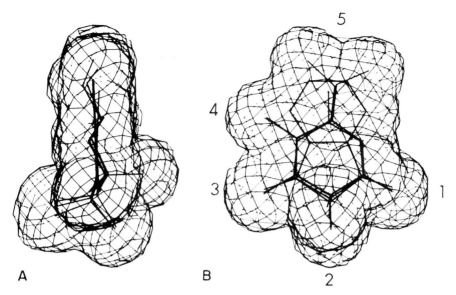

Fig. 2. The receptor-excluded volume in flat (A) and orthogonal projection (B). This volume represents the union of volume required for alloxan, ninhydrin, D-glucose, D-mannose, and their anomers. The darker internal lines represent interatomic bonds. The outer lines represent the molecular volume generated from the Gaussian atom density distribution and contoured to provide a surface representative of the van der Waals radii. (From Weaver *et al.*, 1979 with permission.)

cose molecule. In a subsequent study, Johnson and de Häen (1979) evaluated some of these substituted pyridine derivatives to determine whether the same structure–function relationships were required to produce an insulinotrophic effect in the β cell In the perfused pancreas, these authors demonstrated that the glucose analogue 2,4-diamino-5-cyano-6-bromopyridine caused up to a 20-fold stimulation of insulin release over that caused by glucose alone. An interpretation of this study supports the hypothesis of Hershfield and Richards (1976) that hydrogen-binding possibilities at positions 1, 2, 4, and 5 in relation to the glucose molecule appear necessary for this pyridine derivative to mimic or enhance the effect of glucose on insulin release.

2. Peptide Receptors

A variety of peptide hormones such as glucagon, pancreozymin, secretin, and gastric inhibitory protein (GIP) stimulate insulin release (Rubenstein, 1979). The initial step in the mechanism of hormone-induced insulin release, if it is similar to other systems, presumably involves interactions of these peptides with plasma membrane receptors and subsequent alterations in membrane-related activities such as permeability, ion transport, and adenylate cyclase activity. In islet cells, the hormones glucagon, adrenocorticotrophic hormone, vasoactive intestinal peptide, secretin, and pancreozymin have been shown to stimulate adenylate cyclase activity directly (Sharp, 1979). Interestingly, Capito and Hedeskov (1977) have reported a direct activating effect of D-glucose and two metabolites, phosphoenolpyruvate and pyruvate, on adenylate cyclase activity measured in islet homogenates. This study, however, is at variance with other reports in which no direct effect of glucose on adenylate cyclase activity has been reported (Sharp, 1979).

B. Electrophysiological Studies

In the β cell, glucose stimulation of insulin release is associated with the induction of bursts of electrical activity (Dean and Matthews, 1968, 1970). In the concentration range of 5.5–16.5 mM glucose, a rapid depolarization occurs to a plateau level on which is superimposed spikelike activity or action potentials. This burst of electrical activity ends with spontaneous repolarization of the membrane to the original potential level. These bursts of electrical activity characteristically occur at regular intervals during the course of glucose stimulation.

The association of this electrical activity with insulin release is based on the following observations: (1) The relative duration of the burst of electrical activity is dependent on stimulatory glucose concentrations (Meissner and Schmelz, 1974); (2) the electrical activity in response to square-wave stimulation with glucose proceeds in a biphasic pattern comparable to the pattern of glucose-induced insulin release (Meissner and Atwater, 1976); (3) insulin release from single islets has been shown to be pulsatile, having a periodicity similar to that of bursts of electrical activity (Atwater et al., 1979); and (4) bursts of electrical activity present during glucose stimulation cease after the removal of calcium (Atwater and Beigelman, 1976).

Although glucose stimulation in the β cell affects electrical activity within seconds, the ionic alterations occurring during this phenomena have not been clearly defined (see Chapter 7). It has been shown that physiological concentrations of glucose diminish both potassium efflux (Henquin, 1978) and rubidium permeability (Sehlin and Täljedal, 1975) in islets, and this effect of glucose may be involved in depolarization of the β cell from the resting state to a threshold level from which the burst of electrical activity originates. There is also evidence indicating that voltage-dependent changes in calcium permeability are subsequently involved in initiating the depolarization phase of the electrical activity observed in the β cell (Meissner and Preissler, 1979). In addition, membrane regulation of intracellular calcium by a sodium–calcium exchange mechanism (Donatsch *et al.*, 1977) and ATP-dependent Ca-ATPase activity has been suggested (Formby *et al.*, 1976). A cyclic mechanism explaining the repetitive burst pattern of electrical activity induced by glucose involving changes in membrane permeability and ionic fluxes is an area of current focus.

C. Isolation and Biochemical Characterization of Membrane Fractions

Biochemical approaches in isolating and characterizing functional components of the β-cell membrane directly have been reported. Lernmark *et al.* (1976) have described the isolation of a plasma membrane-enriched fraction from rat islets, using either a continuous or a one-step sucrose gradient separation procedure (Lernmark *et al.*, 1978). In these isolation procedures, ^{125}I-labeled wheat germ agglutinin has been applied as a specific probe for the plasma membrane fraction. With the plasma membrane fraction prepared by a one-step sucrose gradient, both an alkaline phosphatase and a Mg-ATPase activity have been described.

Experiments with fish and mouse islet membranes have been described by Davis and Lazarus (1975). The membranes of both mouse and cod islets were shown to contain a protein phosphokinase. The plasma membranes utilized in this study were identified by enzyme marker activities as well as by electron microscopy. They contained, in addition to protein kinase activity, adenylate cyclase, phosphodiesterase, and ATPase activities.

A procedure for the preparative isolation of a highly enriched islet cell plasma membrane fraction from rat islets has been developed in our laboratory (Naber *et al.*, 1980). This technique utilizes a discontinuous sucrose gradient separation which yields approximately 50–100 μg of plasma membrane obtained from 15–20 rats. This preparation has been characterized by a 10-fold enrichment in 5'-nucleotidase activity and an 11-fold increase in ^{125}I-labeled wheat germ agglutinin binding. Electron microscopic examination of the plasma membrane fraction indicates smooth, membranous vesicles with little contamination by heavier organelles. A high-affinity Ca-ATPase has been identified in this plasma membrane-enriched fraction from islets (McDonald *et al.*, 1980). Two activities have been described, one with a low affinity for calcium (10 μM) and one with a high affinity (0.1 μM). The high-affinity activity is located in the plasma membrane as determined by parallel distributions of 5'-nucleotidase and Ca-ATPase activity among all the subcellular fractions. *In vitro* studies on β-cell membrane fractions represent a direct approach in determining whether insulin secretagogues, i.e., glucose and sulfonylureas, mediate their effects via receptor sites and provide a model for characterizing enzymatic activities responsible for cation movements associated with the insulin secretory process.

II. INSULIN SECRETORY GRANULES

A. Composition and Properties

Insulin storage granules in the β cell have been described ultrastructurally as spherical structures containing a dense core material surrounded by a smooth, membranous sac (Howell and Lacy, 1970). This dense core material is the storage form of insulin, as demonstrated by electron microscopic (Greider *et al.*, 1969) and immunochemical techniques (Misugi *et al.*, 1970). Zinc has been localized in ultramicroscopic sections of β granules (Pihl, 1968), as well as in isolated secretory granules (Coore *et al.*, 1969). These findings suggest that insulin is stored in the mature granule probably as a zinc–insulin complex. Calcium has also been shown to be present in high concentrations in the granule (Herman *et al.*, 1973; Ravazzola *et al.*, 1976). Analysis of the protein content of the storage granule fraction of rat islets by polyacrylamide gel electrophoresis has shown the presence of insulin I and II and also traces of glucagon (Howell and Lacy, 1970). *In vitro* studies characterizing the physical properties of isolated secretory granules from rat islets have indicated that optimal stability is attained at 4°C and pH 6 and that the solubility properties of insulin within the storage granule are similar to those of crystallized insulin (Howell *et al.*, 1969). In addition, agents that stimulate insulin secretion in the intact cell have no effect on the stability of secretory granules from this preparation.

B. Zinc Content and Function

The presence of zinc in the insulin secretory granule has focused attention on the possible roles zinc may play in the biosynthesis, storage, and release of insulin. It has been shown in a cultured islet system that a reduction in extracellular zinc has little effect on proinsulin biosynthesis, the conversion of proinsulin to insulin, or the ability of cells to store newly formed insulin (Howell *et al.*, 1978). Interestingly, this study showed that calcium depletion alone resulted in the formation of large, electron-lucent granules similar to those produced by zinc depletion and suggested that calcium may have an important function in insulin storage.

In vivo studies have correlated zinc content and its localization in secretory granules with the functional state of the islet. In general, the functional state of islets has been correlated with the content of detectable zinc (Maske, 1957; McIsaac, 1955). Zinc deficiency in Chinese hamsters has also been associated with abnormal glucose tolerance (Boquist and Lernmark, 1969); Huber and Gershoff (1973) have reported reduced insulin release in pancreatic slices obtained from zinc-deficient rats compared with those from pair-fed controls. The inhibitory effect of zinc on insulin secretion in the perfused pancreas and in isolated islets has also been reported (Ghafghazi *et al.*, 1979). In both systems, exogenously added zinc inhibited glucose-induced insulin release in a dose-dependent manner. We have demonstrated that insulin release induced by either potassium or L-leucine is also inhibited in a dose-dependent manner by the presence of zinc. The significance of these *in vitro* effects on insulin secretion has not been determined. However, cellular mechanisms responsible for this inhibitory effect of zinc may reflect interactions with calcium, membrane stabilization (Chvapil, 1973), or possibly zinc-induced polymers of tubulin as reported by Larsson *et al.* (1976).

Measurement of the uptake of ^{65}zinc in the intact islet indicates that this is a slow process that continues for hours, reaching 3–5 times the extracellular concentration by 70 min and a 30-fold differential over extracellular concentrations by 24 hr (Ludvigsen *et al.*, 1979). This *in vitro* study indicated that a facilitated mechanism for zinc transport predominated at low zinc concentrations and that a diffusion mechanism of entry predominated at higher zinc concentrations. Zinc uptake at low concentrations (0.5–7 μM) demonstrated saturation kinetics with a K_m and V_m of 1.5 μM and 11 fmol/min per islet, respectively. At higher zinc concentrations, linear relationships between initial rates and zinc concentration were observed. In these studies, zinc uptake at either 2 or 44 μM in short (1–70 min) or long (1–24 hr) incubations was unaffected by concentrations of glucose that stimulated insulin secretion. Comparisons of total zinc content reported per islet (Havu *et al.*, 1977) with that measured by ^{65}zinc incorporation studies suggest that a large pool for zinc is present in excess of that contained in the secretory granule.

The interactions of zinc and insulin have also been examined in relation to a postsecretory event away from the β cell. Arquilla *et al.* (1978) have shown enhanced binding and decreased degradation of insulin with liver plasma membranes either removed from mice pretreated with zinc or treated with zinc *in vitro*. The molecular mechanism and physiological significance of the interaction between zinc and insulin in this system are unknown.

III. MICROTUBULES AND MICROFILAMENTS

A. Physical Description and Orientation

The cytoplasmic structures microtubules and microfilaments have been identified in the β cell and are similar to those described in other types of cells. Microtubules exist as tubular elements 20–25 nm in diameter and are scattered throughout the β-cell cytoplasm (Lacy et al., 1968; Gomez-Acebo and Hermida, 1973). Microfilaments have been described ultrastructurally as subcellular structures of filamentous material located beneath the β-cell plasma membrane. These filaments are 5–7 nm in diameter, are of indefinite length, and extend into the core of the microvilli protruding from the cell surface (Orci et al., 1972; Gabbiani et al., 1974). Microfilaments are believed to consist of actinlike material, based on the binding of heavy meromyosin (Ishikawa et al., 1969) and immunological properties (Gabbiani et al., 1974).

Ultrastructurally, insulin storage granules have been reported to be associated with both cytoplasmic structures. In monolayer cultures of β cells, secretory granules have been observed in ordered columns separated by rows of microtubules (Orci et al., 1973b). Microfilamentous bridges have been described, which connect or associate secretory granules with the plasma membrane (Orci et al., 1979).

Based on the inhibitory effect of colchicine on insulin release from isolated islets, it was proposed that the translocation of secretory granules to the plasma membrane may be interlinked by the microtubule–microfilament system (Lacy et al., 1968). Further biological studies have observed this relationship by examining alterations in insulin secretion following the exposure of isolated islets or the perfused pancreas to a variety of agents which interact with either microtubules or microfilaments. In these studies, vinblastine, vincristine, and colchicine have been most commonly employed to alter the formation of microtubules by disruption, whereas D_2O, hexylene glycol, and ethanol have been used as microtubule-stabilizing agents. The effects of these microtubule-disrupting and stabilizing agents have indirectly indicated that an intact microtubular system is apparently involved in both phases of glucose-induced insulin release. The application and limitations of employing these agents in correlating insulin secretion with microtubule function in the intact cell have been reviewed (Malaisse et al., 1975).

The effect of cytochalasin B, an agent which induces both clumping and aggregation of microfilaments, has been examined for its action on insulin secretion (Orci et al., 1972). This microfilament-sensitive agent markedly potentiates both the first and second phase of glucose-induced insulin release (Lacy et al., 1973; Van Obberghen et al., 1973). Although cytochalasin B also inhibits the facilitated transport of glucose in the islet (McDaniel *et al.*, 1974), the primary site of potentiation of insulin secretion appears to be the microfilaments, since cytochalasin D has no effect on hexose transport but results in a similar marked potentiation of glucose-induced insulin release (McDaniel *et al.*, 1975).

Cinemicrographic studies with monolayer cultures of β cells have been used to support the involvement of microtubules and microfilaments in insulin secretion (Lacy *et al.*, 1975; Somers *et al.*, 1979). In this system, in which the movement of individual secretory granules within a β cell can be continuously monitored, it has been shown that the type of movement of individual granules is unidirectional and occurs at an average rate of 1.5 μm/sec (Lacy *et al.*, 1975). The amount of movement of secretory granules was correlated with insulin secretory activity, since agents which potentiate insulin release resulted in a significant increase in the amount of movement, whereas agents which inhibit insulin release decreased granule movement. In the latter case, the decrease in granule movement produced by the omission of calcium or the presence of D_2O was reversible following either the introduction of calcium or the removal of D_2O from the incubation medium.

B. Quantitative Measurements

1. Tubulin and Microtubules

Microtubules exist in equilibrium with the dimeric subunit tubulin. In a variety of tissues, tubulin polymerization has been shown to be an essential part of microtubule function. Biochemical evidence of the importance of the equilibrium between microtubules and their subunits in the regulation of insulin release has been investigated in islets. In general, the degree of tubulin polymerization is determined by incorporating the binding specificity of [^{3}H] colchicine to the tubulin subunit with isolation techniques which preserve the cellular equilibration between the polymerized and depolymerized forms of tubulin (Pipeleers *et al.*, 1977; Ostlund *et al.*, 1979; Sherline *et al.*, 1974). Using these procedures to quantitate only the tubulin component of this equilibrium, Montague *et al.* (1976)) demonstrated that vinblastine treatment caused an increase in islet tubulin, i.e., shifted the equilibrium in favor of microtubule depolymerization, whereas treatment with D_2O resulted in a decrease in tubulin, i.e., caused an increase in microtubule formation. In this study, long periods of stimulation of insulin by glucose or increased intracellular cyclic AMP (cAMP) levels produced by 3-isobutyl-l-methylxanthine and glucose were also associated with a decrease in tubulin. In a separate study in which the amounts of both polymerized and depolymerized tubulin in islets were measured, Pipe-

leers *et al.* (1976) showed that fasting in rats resulted in a decrease in the
total tubulin pool size and a decrease in the percentage of polymerized
tubulin. Both of these effects were restored by glucose feeding. These
studies indicated that an *in vivo* equilibrium between tubulin and microtubules existed in islets, and that an increase in tubulin polymerization was
associated with the second or sustained phase of insulin secretion.

In the β cell, an increase in glucose concentration initiates insulin release
in a biphasic manner, i.e., a rapid release followed by a return to a basal
rate and then a second sustained phase of secretion. An involvement of the
microtubule–microfilament system in both components of biphasic release
has been proposed based on the decrease in both secretion and intact
microtubules following fasting (Pipeleers *et al.*, 1976), and on the absence
of a first phase and a diminution in the second phase of glucose-induced insulin release from islets maintained in low glucose for 4 days *in vitro* (Lacy
et al., 1976). Studies in our laboratory have examined whether a correlation
exists between the assembly and disassembly of microtubules and the more
rapid events associated with the biphasic pattern of glucose-induced insulin
release (McDaniel *et al.*, 1980). Figure 3 illustrates the biphasic pattern of

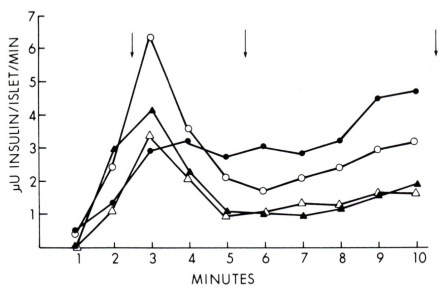

Fig. 3. Biphasic pattern of insulin release in four separate experiments. Isolated islets (100
per chamber) were preincubated for 45 min at 37°C in a glucose-free medium and then
stimulated at 1 min with D-glucose (27.5 m*M*) medium for a duration of 10 min. Arrows represent the sampling time chosen for monitoring both insulin release and microtubule content
from islets in a static incubation system. (From McDaniel *et al.*, 1980 with permission.)

insulin release from perifused islets obtained in four separate experiments. A rapid, consistent first phase was observed occurring between 2 and 3 min, which was followed by a decrease or nadir at approximately 5.5 min. A gradual increase marking the beginning of the second phase was apparent at 10.5 min. Figure 4 shows the microtubule content of islets following glucose stimulation as determined in a static incubation system at given time intervals. At 2.5 min in the presence of 27 mM glucose, insulin release increased threefold and was paralleled by an increase in polymerized tubulin compared to the nonstimulated or basal condition. At this early interval, the percentage of polymerized tubulin increased from 24% under basal conditions to 33% following stimulation. Both insulin release and the amount of polymerized tubulin decreased to basal values at 5.5 min. Although insulin release was enhanced at 10.5 min, the amount of polymerized tubulin remained at a basal level. The changes in polymerized

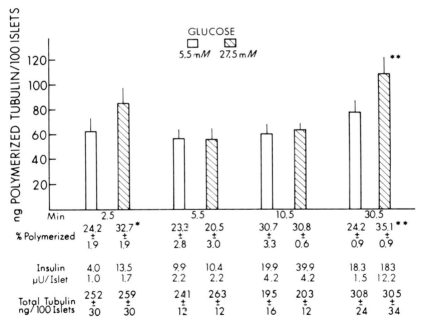

Fig. 4. Microtubule content of islets following glucose stimulation. Isolated islets were preincubated in paired homogenization vessels at 37°C in KRB medium (500 μl) with glucose (5.5 mM) for 30 min. The medium was then changed and replaced with either 5.5 or 27.5 mM glucose for the designated incubation interval. The incubation medium was immediately replaced with microtubule-stabilizing buffer and homogenized. The incubation medium at 30.5 min contained dibutyryl cAMP (2 mM). Five paired experiments were performed at each interval. Values represent the mean ± SEM. *$P < 0.025$; **$P < 0.01$. (From McDaniel et al., 1980 with permission.)

tubulin during the second phase of release were evaluated with glucose and dibutyryl cAMP present in the incubation medium. Under these conditions at 30.5 min, a greatly enhanced rate of release (i.e., 10-fold) was accompanied by an increase in tubulin polymerization from 24 to 35%. These results indicate that the more rapid events associated with the biphasic pattern of insulin release were temporally correlated with changes in polymerized tubulin.

2. Microfilaments

Functional alterations in the microfilamentous component of the cell web have also been studied in relation to the insulin secretory process. Biochemical evidence has been presented indicating that actin filaments specifically bind secretory granules *in vitro* (Ostlund, 1977). This effect has been proposed to relate to a mechanism for the translocation of secretory granules to the plasma membrane surface. In islets, the proportions of actin in the polymerized and depolymerized state have also been measured under insulin-stimulatory conditions, and these results indicate that insulin secretion is accompanied by conversion of G- to F-actin (Howell and Tyhurst, 1980).

C. Regulation

A common or unifying cellular mechanism for regulating functional changes in microtubules and microfilaments in response to secretory activity is not clear. Following glucose stimulation in the β cell, levels of both calcium and cAMP are increased. The essential requirement for calcium in the insulin secretory process has emphasized the importance of defining its effect on these paramenters. However, calcium inhibits microtubule assembly *in vitro* (Fuller and Brinkley, 1976). Recently, the effect of calcium in inhibiting and reversing tubulin polymerization *in vitro* in the presence of a calcium-dependent regulatory (CDR) protein has also been reported (Marcum *et al.*, 1978). A combined effect involving both cAMP and calcium in controlling microtubule function has also been proposed (Gillespie, 1975). Ostlund (1977) has compared the similarities of insulin secretion in the β cell to muscle contraction and proposed that a contractile force for granule movement in the β cell may be mediated by microfilamentous contraction resulting from activation of an actomyosin ATPase activity. Obviously, the control mechanism for the assembly and disassembly of microtubules and the involvement and regulation of microfilaments in this process represent a continued challenge in the area of hormone secretion.

IV. EMIOCYTOSIS

A. Ultrastructural Studies

Emiocytosis is a mechanism for the release or discharge of stored insulin contained in the secretory granule from the β cell into the extracellular space. In the β cell this process involves the movement of secretory granules to the cell surface via the microtubule–microfilament system. Fusion subsequently occurs between the membrane of the secretory vesicle and the plasma membrane, followed by ejection of the insulin granule into the extracellular space. In this overall process, energy is required, and there is also a requirement for extracellular calcium (Grodsky, 1972). Experimental approaches in describing both granule movement by cinemicrographic techniques and the involvement of the cytoskeletal components, microtubules and microfilaments, in the process of insulin release have been discussed.

Evidence for interaction of the insulin storage granule with the β-cell plasma membrane during the emiocytotic event has been obtained with different experimental approaches. Initial observations, from which the emiocytotic process was proposed to occur in the β-cell, came from electron microscopic studies following insulin stimulation by glucose and other secretogogues *in vivo* (Lacy *et al.*, 1959; Williamson *et al.*, 1961). In the fetal rat pancreas, Orci *et al.* (1968) observed intact secretory granules, devoid of their membranous sacs, in the extracellular space following incubation in the presence of high concentrations of potassium. Howell *et al.* (1969) had shown previously that isolated secretory granules were stabilized in a potassium-rich medium. Scanning electron microscopic techniques have also been used to correlate insulin secretory activity with the appearance of cytoplasmic projections on the β-cell membrane (Lacy, 1970), and freeze-etch microscopy has been used to detect prominent modifications of the plasma membrane with exocytotic activity (Orci *et al.*, 1973a).

B. Role of Calcium in Emiocytosis

Studies directed toward the molecular mechanism of membrane fusion during emiocytosis, and the role calcium may play in this process, have been reported. Secretory vesicles isolated from pancreatic islets have been shown to fuse in the presence of calcium (Dahl and Gratzl, 1976). Intervesicular fusion of secretory vesicles and interaction with the plasma membrane have been observed in glucose-stimulated β cells (Berger *et al.*, 1975; Dahl *et al.*, 1976). This type of exocytotic process involving both intervesicular fusion and vesicular fusion with the plasma membrane has been shown to exist in the mast cell (Douglas, 1974). *In vitro* fusion of secretory vesicles isolated from rat liver was found to be calcium-specific and to exhibit properties similar to those of the exocytotic process occurring in a variety of secretory cells (Gratzl and Dahl, 1978). Cochrane and Douglas (1974) have shown that isolated peritoneal mast cells from the rat extrude secretory granules when exposed to the stimulus 48/80 or the ionophores A23187 and X537A. These results are consistent in this system with the interpretation that calcium influx mediates the exocytotic process.

Fusion of the granule membrane with the plasma membrane during this process should result in an increase in the surface area of the β-cell membrane unless recycling mechanisms are operative. Orci *et al.* (1973c) have reported studies indicating that membrane recycling parallels the extrusion of insulin from the β cell.

C. Insulin Release by Subcellular Fractions of Islets

An *in vitro* insulin-secreting system has been reported by Lazarus *et al.* (1976) and Davis and Lazarus (1977). This system consists of plasma membranes isolated from the cod principal islet incubated with insulin granules isolated from either mouse or rabbit pancreatic islets. In this *in vitro* system, when glucose (17 mM), ATP (5 μM), and Ca^{2+} (2 μM) are present concomitantly, all the insulin contained within the granules is rapidly released into the medium. In this model, it has also been found that the phosphorylated intermediates glucose 6-phosphate and phosphoenolpyruvate cause insulin release in the presence of ATP and calcium. These authors propose that secretion in this system is initiated by glucose interacting with its receptor on the plasma membrane and that following this event continued insulin release is controlled by phosphorylated intermediates of glucose operating via a membrane-bound protein kinase.

V. CONCLUDING COMMENTS

It is apparent that the interaction of cell organelles during the insulin release process underlies a series of specialized, complex biological processes. Stimulus recognition for insulin release involves interactions with the β-cell plasma membrane, most likely via receptor-mediated mechanisms. Alterations in electrical activity at the β-cell membrane following stimulation occurs rapidly, with concomitant changes in ionic fluxes involving both calcium and potassium. Although confronted with limitations in the quantity of islet tissue available for experimentation, approaches in subcellular isolation procedures are emerging which will allow biochemical characterization of plasma membrane receptors and transport systems possibly involved in the gating of ions across the cell membrane. The significant role of calcium and cAMP in the insulin secretory process focuses on many aspects of interactions of cellular organelles in the β cell, i.e., the cytoskeleton, granule movement, and membrane fusion. The translocation of insulin storage granules to the cell surface involves specific interactions of components of the cytoskeleton in the β cell. At this point, the biochemical mechanism for the generation of a motive or contractile force for granule movement involving microtubules and microfilaments and the possible role of calcium and cAMP in this process remains speculative. Characterization of regulatory mechanisms in the β cell involving protein phosphorylations dependent on either cAMP or calcium and calcium-dependent regulatory protein(s) represents an important area in understanding interactions of cell organelles. Delineation of the specific role of calcium in fusion of the secretory membrane with the plasma membrane is also required for describing the emiocytotic discharge of insulin. Further elucidation of the molecular mechanisms of the interactions of cell organelles in the β cell will provide the necessary basis for understanding the physiological control of hormone secretion.

REFERENCES

Arquilla, E. R., Packer, S., Tarmas, W., and Miyamoto, S. (1978). *Endocrinology* **103**, 1440–1449.

Atwater, I., and Beigelman, P. M. (1976). *J. Physiol. (London)* **258**, 13–14P.

Atwater, I., Rojas, E., and Scott, A. (1979). *J. Physiol. (London)* **291**, 57P.

Berger, W., Dahl, G., and Meissner, H. P. (1975). *Cytobiologie* **12**, 119–139.

Boquist, L., and Lernmark, A. (1969). *Acta Pathol. Microbiol. Scand.* **76**, 215–228.

Capito, K., and Hedeskov, C. J. (1977). *Biochem. J.* **162**, 569–573.

Chvapil, M. (1973). *Life Sci.* **13**, 1041–1049.

Cochrane, D. E., and Douglas, W. W. (1974). *Proc. Natl. Acad. Sci. U.S.A.* **71**, 408–412.

Coore, H. G., Hellman, B., Pihl, E., and Täljedal, I. B. (1969). *Biochem. J.* **111**, 107–113.

Dahl, G., and Gratzl, M. (1976). *Cytobiologie* **12**, 344–355.

Dahl, G., Berger, W., and Meissner, H. P. (1976). *J. Physiol. (Paris)* **72**, 703–709.

Davis, B., and Lazarus, N. R. (1975). *J. Membr. Biol.* **20**, 301–318.

Davis, B., and Lazarus, N. R. (1977). *J. Physiol. (London)* **271**, 273–288.

Dean, P. M., and Matthews, E. K. (1968). *Nature (London)* **219**, 389–390.

Dean, P. M., and Matthews, E. K. (1970). *J. Physiol. (London)* **210**, 255–264.

Donatsch, P., Lowe, D. A., Richardson, B. P., and Taylor, P. (1977). *J. Physiol. (London)* **267**, 357–376.

Douglas, W. (1974). *Biochem. Soc. Symp.* **39**, 1–28.

Formby, B., Capito, K., Egeberg, J., and Hedeskov, C. J. (1976). *Am. J. Physiol.* **230**, 441–448.

Fuller, G. M., and Brinkley, B. R. (1976). *J. Supramol. Struct.* **5**, 497–514.

Gabbiani, G., Malaisse-Lagae, F., Blondel, B., and Orci, L. (1974). *Endocrinology* **95**, 1630–1635.
Ghafghazi, T., Ludvigsen, C. W., McDaniel, M. L., and Lacy, P. E. (1979). *IRCS Medi. Sci. Pharmacol.* **7**, 122.
Gillespie, E. (1975). *Ann. N.Y. Acad. Sci.* **253**, 771–779.
Gomez-Acebo, J., and Hermida, G. O. (1973). *J. Anat.* **114**, 421–437.
Gratzel, M., and Dahl, G. (1978). *J. Membr. Biol.* **40**, 343–364.
Greider, M. H., Howell, S. L., and Lacy, P. E. (1969). *J. Cell Biol.* **41**, 162–166.
Grodsky, G. M. (1972). *Diabetes* **21**, Suppl. 2, 584–593.
Grodsky, G. M., Fanska, R., West, L., and Manning, M. (1974). *Science* **186**, 536–538.
Havu, N., Lundgren, G., and Falkmer, S. (1977). *Acta Endocrinol.* **86**, 570–577.
Hedeskov, C. J. (1980). *Physiol. Rev.* **60**, 442–509.
Henquin, J. C. (1978). Nature (London) **271**, 271–273.
Herman, L., Sato, T., and Hales, C. N. (1973). *J. Ultrastruct. Res.* **42**, 298–311.
Hershfield, R., and Richards, F. M. (1976). *J. Biol. Chem.* **251**, 5141–5148.
Howell, S. L., and Lacy, P. E. (1970). *In* "Memoirs of the Society for Endocrinology: Subcellular Organization and Function in Endocrine Tissues" (H. Heller and K. Lederis, eds.). No. 19, pp. 469–480. The syndics of the Cambridge University Press, London.
Howell, S. L., and Tyhurst, M. (1980). *Sixth Intern. Congr. Endocrinol. Prog. Abstr., Australia* p. 456.
Howell, S. L., Tyhurst, M., Duvefelt, H., Anderson, A., and Hellerström, C. (1978). *Cell Tissue Res.* **188**, 107–118.
Howell, S. L., Young, D. A., and Lacy, P. E. (1969). *J. Cell Biol.* **41**, 167–176.
Huber, A. M., and Gershoff, S. N. (1973). *J. Nutr.* **103**, 1739–1744.
Ishikawa, H., Bischoff, R., and Holtzer, H. (1969). *J. Cell Biol.* **43**, 312–328.
Johnson, D. G., and de Häen, C. (1979). *Mol. Pharmacol.* **15**, 287–293.
Lacy, P. E. (1970). *Diabetes* **19**, 895–905.
Lacy, P. E., Cardeza, A. F., and Wilson, W. D. (1959). *Diabetes* **8**, 36–44.
Lacy, P. E., Howell, S. L., Young, D. A., and Fink, C. J. (1968). *Nature (London)* **219**, 1177–1179.
Lacy, P. E., Klein, N. J., and Fink, C. J. (1973). *Endocrinology* **92**, 1458–1468.
Lacy, P. E., Finke, E. H., and Codilla, R. C. (1975). *Lab. Invest.* **33**, 570–576.
Lacy, P. E., Finke, E. H., Conant, S., and Naber, S. (1976). *Diabetes* **25**, 484–493.
Larsson, H., Wallin, M., and Edström, A. (1976). *Exp. Cell Res.* **100**, 104–110.
Lazarus, N. R., Davis, B., and O'Connor, K. J. (1976). *J. Physiol. (Paris)* **72**, 787–794.
Lernmark, Å., Nathans, A., and Steiner, D. F. (1976). *J. Cell Biol.* **71**, 606–623.
Lernmark, Å., Nielsen, D. A., and Steiner, D. F. (1978). *J. Supramol. Struct.* **9**, 327–336.
Ludvigsen, C., McDaniel, M. L., and Lacy, P. E. (1979). *Diabetes* **28**, 570–576.
McDaniel, M. L., King, S., Anderson, S., Fink, J., and Lacy, P. E. (1974). *Diabetologia* **10**, 303–308.
McDaniel, M., Roth, C., Fink, J., Fyfe, G., and Lacy, P. E. (1975). *Biochem. Biophys. Res. Commun.* **66**, 1089–1096.
McDaniel, M. L., Roth, C. E., Fink, J., and Lacy, P. E. (1976). *Endocrinology* **99**, 535–540.
McDaniel, M. L., Roth, C. E., Fink, C. J., Swanson, J. A., and Lacy, P. E. (1977). *Diabetologia* **13**, 603–606.
McDaniel, M. L., Bry, C. G., Homer, R. W., Fink, C. J., Ban, D., and Lacy, P. E. (1980). *Metabolism* **29**, 762–766.
McDonald, J. M., Pershadsingh, H. A., Bry, C. G., McDaniel, M. L., and Lacy, P. E. (1980). *Fed. Proc. Fed. Am. Soc. Exp. Biol.* **39**, 380.
McIsaac, R. J. (1955). *Endocrinology* **57**, 571–579.

Malaisse, W. J., Malaisse-Lagae, F., Van Obberghen, E., Somers, G., Devis, G., Ravazzola, M., and Orci, L. (1975). *Ann. N.Y. Acad. Sci.* **253**, 630–652.

Marcum, J. M., Dedman, J. R., Brinkley, B. R., and Means, A. R. (1978). *Proc. Natl. Acad. Sci. U.S.A.* **75**, 3771–3775.

Maske, H. (1957). *Diabetes* **6**, 335–341.

Matschinsky, F. M., Pagliara, A. A., Zawalich, W. S., and Trus, M. D. (1979). *In* "Endocrinology" (L. J. DeGroot *et al.*, eds.), Vol. II, pp. 935–949. Grune & Stratton, New York.

Meissner, H. P., and Atwater, I. J. (1976). *Horm. Metab. Res.* **8**, 11–16.

Meissner, H. P., and Preissler, M. (1979). *Adv. Exp. Med. Biol.* **119**, 97–107.

Meissner, H. P., and Schmelz, H. (1974). *Pfluegers Arch.* **351**, 195–206.

Misugi, K., Howell, S. L., Greider, M. H., Lacy, P. E., and Sorenson, G. D. (1979). *Arch. Pathol.* **89**, 97–102

Montague, W., Howell, S. L., and Green, I. C. (1976). *Horm. Metab. Res.* **8**, 166–169.

Naber, S. P., McDonald, J. M., Jarett, L., McDaniel, M. L., Ludvigsen, C. W., and Lacy, P. E. (1980) *Diabetologia* **19**, 439–444.

Orci, L., Stauffacher, W., Beaven, D., Lambert, A. E., Renold, A. E., and Rouiller, C. (1968). *Acta Diabetol. Lat.* **6**, 271.

Orci, L., Gabbay, K. H., and Malaisse, W. J. (1972). *Science* **175**, 1128–1130.

Orci, L., Amherdt, M., Malaisse-Lagae, F., Rouiller, C., and Renold, A. E. (1973a). *Science* **179**, 82–83.

Orci, L., Like, A. A., Amherdt, M., Blondel, B., Kanazawa, Y., Marliss, E. R., Lambert, A. E., Wollheim, C. B., and Renold, A. E. (1973b). *J. Ultrastruct. Res.* **43**, 270–297.

Orci, L., Malaisse-Lagae, F., Ravazzola, M., Amherdt, M., and Renold, A. E. (1973c). *Science* **181**, 561–562.

Orci, L., Amherdt, M., Roth, J., and Perrelet, A. (1979). *Diabetologia* **16**, 135–138.

Ostlund, R. E. (1977). *Diabetes* **26**, 245–252.

Ostlund, R. E., Leung, J. T., and Hajek, S. V. (1979). *Anal. Biochem.* **96**, 155–164.

Pihl, E. (1968). *Acta Pathol. Microbiol. Scand.* **74**, 145–160.

Pipeleers, D. G., Pipeleers-Marichal, M. A., and Kipnis, D. M. (1976). *Science* **191**, 88–89.

Pipeleers, D. G., Pipeleers-Marichal, M. A., Sherline, P., and Kipnis, D. M. (1977). *J. Cell Biol.* **74**, 341–350.

Ravazzola, M., Malaisse-Lagae, F., Amherdt, M., Perrelet, A., Malaisse, W. J., and Orci, L. (1976). *J. Cell Sci* **27**, 107–117.

Rossini, A. A., Berger, M., Shadden, J., and Cahill, G. F. (1974). *Science* **183**, 424.

Rubenstein, A. H. (1979). *In* "Endocrinology" (L. J. DeGroot, ed.), Vol. 2, pp. 951–957. Grune & Stratton, New York.

Sehlin, J., and Täljedal, I. B. (1975). *Nature (London)* **253**, 635–636.

Sharp, G. W. G. (1979). *Diabetologia* **16**, 287–296.

Sherline, P., Bodwin, C. K., and Kipnis, D. M. (1974). *Anal. Biochem.* **62**, 400–407.

Somers, P., Blondel, B., Orci, L., and Malaisse, W. J. (1979). *Endocrinology* **104**, 255–264.

Tomita, T., Lacy, P. E., Matschinsky, F. M., and McDaniel, M. L. (1974). *Diabetes* **23**, 517–524.

Van Obberghen, E., Somers, P., Devis, G., Malaisse-Lagae, F., and Malaisse, W. J. (1973). *J. Clin. Invest.* **52**, 1041–1051.

Weaver, D. C., McDaniel, M. L., Naber, S. P., Barry, C. D., and Lacy, P. E. (1978). *Diabetes* **27**, 1205–1214.

Weaver, D. C., Barry, C. D., McDaniel, M. L., Marshall, G. R., and Lacy, P. E. (1979). *Mol. Pharmacol.* **16**, 361–368.

Williamson, J. R., Lacy, P. E., and Grisham, J. W. (1961). *Diabetes* **10**, 460–469.

6

Metabolic Controls of Insulin Secretion

S. J. H. ASHCROFT

I. INTRODUCTION

The hypothesis that the stimulation of insulin release by glucose involves metabolism of the sugar by the β cell dates from the earliest *in vitro* studies

117

The Islets of Langerhans
Copyright © 1981 by Academic Press, Inc.
All rights of reproduction in any form reserved.
ISBN 0-12-187820-1

on insulin release by Coore and Randle (1964) using rabbit pancreas pieces, and by Grodsky *et al.* (1963) using a perfused rat pancreas preparation. The essential findings were that insulin release was stimulated by glucose and mannose, which are readily metabolized by mammalian tissues, but not by sugars such as 2-deoxyglucose, 3-*O*-methylglucose, and galactose. It was also observed that mannoheptulose was a potent inhibitor of glucose- or mannose-stimulated insulin release, and, in studies with liver slices, Coore and Randle found that mannoheptulose blocked glucose metabolism at the level of phosphorylation. It was realized that, if sugar metabolism mediated in some way the insulin-releasing action of glucose, then varying blood glucose concentrations could be transduced by the β cell into varying rates of glucose metabolism, hence insulin release. The β-cell glucose sensor was therefore the enzyme catalyzing the rate-limiting step for the entry of glucose into β-cell metabolism. Such a model was first described explicitly by Randle *et al* (1968) as the "substrate site hypothesis," a mechanism essentially distinct from the alternative "regulator site hypothesis"; in the latter the glucose sensor mechanism is envisaged as a glucoreceptor, presumably a protein located in the β-cell membrane, to which glucose and other sugars directly bind, thereby eliciting an undefined series of events leading to insulin release. The two models are illustrated in Fig. 1.

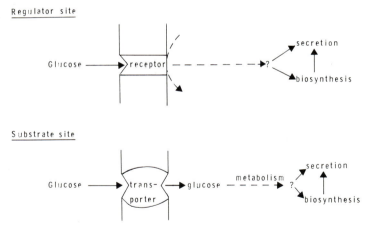

Fig. 1. β-Cell glucose sensor mechanisms. In the regulator site model (top) glucose binds to a glucoreceptor and induces a conformational change that triggers the series of events leading to insulin secretion. In the substrate site model (bottom) the metabolism of glucose within the β cell causes changes in the concentration of one or more metabolites or cofactors that act as triggers for the release of insulin; the glucose sensor in this model is the enzyme or transporter participating in the rate-limiting step for the metabolism of glucose to the trigger metabolite(s). The models as drawn include the view that the same *initial* events are involved in the recognition of glucose as a signal for both insulin release and insulin biosynthesis.

With the advent of methods for the isolation of viable pancreatic islets (Hellerstrom, 1964; Moskaleski, 1965; Keen *et al.,* 1965) suitable for *in vitro* metabolic studies, it became possible to subject these ideas to experimental testing. Special attention has been given to carbohydrate metabolism in view of the physiological importance of glucose as a stimulator of insulin release. However, the stimulation of insulin release by other metabolites, e.g., amino acids, raises the question as to whether a substrate site hypothesis also applies to such agents. In this chapter the major emphasis will be to review to what extent current evidence supports a metabolic basis for the recognition of sugars and other fuels as stimulants of insulin release. The question may then be posed as to the mechanisms whereby metabolic events are linked to the exocytotic process. A primary role for a rise in cytosolic free Ca^{2+} as the event most closely linked to the release process is strongly supported by available data, as discussed in Chapter 7, hence consideration is given to the way in which the metabolism of nutrients may be coupled to movements of Ca^{2+} and other ions.

II. GENERAL CONSIDERATIONS

Insulin release and biosynthesis are energy-requiring processes. Moreover, the integrity of the β cell depends on energy-dependent functions such as maintenance of the intracellular ionic milieu. Hence investigation of the role of the metabolism of nutrients in insulin release is complicated by the fuel functions of metabolites, which may be distinct from other possible trigger functions. That these functions are indeed distinct is indicated by the following observations suggesting that the β cell is not critically dependent on exogenous nutrients for maintenance of ATP content. (1) In islets incubated without exogenous substrate the rate of oxygen uptake is constant for at least 3 hr at approximately 80% of that found in the presence of 20 mM glucose (Hellerstrom, 1967), and ATP content shows only a modest fall (Ashcroft *et al.,* 1973). (2) ATP content and adenylate energy charge are maximal in the presence of glucose concentrations insufficient to elicit insulin release (Ashcroft *et al.,* 1973; Malaisse *et al.,* 1979a). (3) Measurements of $^{14}CO_2$ evolution from islets prelabeled with [^{14}C]palmitate indicate that endogenous lipid fuels may constitute a major energy reserve (Malaisse *et al.,* 1979b).

The substrate site hypothesis possesses predictive power not shared by the regulator site model. In the latter, the properties of insulin secretory responses, such as concentration dependence and specificity, are ascribable to properties of the postulated receptor molecule. On the other hand, the substrate site hypothesis requires the existence of parallels between metabolic fluxes and insulin release—and the model can be disproved if a dissociation between these parameters can be demonstrated. It also must be stressed that, no matter how many such parallels are established, they will not suffice to prove the model; at any time one unequivocal example of dissociation may disprove the hypothesis. It is thus true and not just an engaging paradox that the substrate site hypothesis cannot be proved and the regulator site hypothesis cannot be disproved. A second conceptual difference between the models also exists. Based on the regulator site model it should be possible to construct a defined map of the specificity requirement for sugars to stimulate in terms of the actual minimum molecular structure necessary for stimulation (see Chapter 5). Such a defined structure should be of general application to sugars, since the glucoreceptor is a defined entity with a fixed recognition site. In the substrate site hypothesis, however, the glucoreceptor is *not* a fixed entity, and such a defined structure need not exist. This follows from the fact that specificity is the result of a combination of successive discriminatory steps, namely, transport, phosphorylation, and subsequent metabolism of the sugar. Thus sugars which fail to enter the β cell are nonstimulatory, but so too are sugars which enter but are not phosphorylated. Moreover, a more complex pattern of inhibition is predicted by the substrate site hypothesis. Thus the effects on insulin release of sugars whose initial metabolic transformations differ may be blocked by quite different inhibitors. To give a specific example, mannoheptulose inhibits glucose metabolism at the level of phosphorylation but does not inhibit the metabolism of glyceraldehyde. The finding that mannoheptulose inhibits glucose-stimulated insulin release but not that stimulated by glyceraldehyde has thus a ready explanation in the substrate site hypothesis. In the regulator site model these observations require the unattractive postulate of a receptor for glyceraldehyde distinct from that for glucose.

Finally, the phenomenon of potentiation requires comment. It has been found that a number of potential metabolites, ineffective alone as stimulants of insulin release, are nevertheless able to stimulate secretion in the presence of nonstimulatory concentrations of glucose or another primary stimulant (Ashcroft *et al.,* 1972b): fructose is an example which has received particular attention. A possible explanation of this behavior based on the regulator site model envisages cooperative interactions of subunits of the receptor. The substrate site model, however, seeks to explain such behavior on the basis that the metabolism of the potentiator alone fails to attain the rate necessary for stimulation, but that the sum of the flux from the potentiator and from a substimulatory concentration of glucose is sufficient to elicit release. Accurate quantitation of metabolic fluxes is essential to substantiate this view.

III. INSULIN SECRETORY RESPONSES TO POTENTIAL
β-CELL METABOLIC SUBSTRATES

Table I lists potential β-cell metabolic substrates that have been reported to elicit insulin release. Stimulation has been described with hexoses, hexosamines, pentoses, a tetrose, trioses, glycolytic products, amino acids, 2-oxoacids, and purine ribonucleosides. To what extent the β-cell metabolism of these agents may underlie the stimulation of release will be considered for each of these classes in turn. The major metabolic pathways that may be involved are outlined in Fig. 2.

TABLE I

Metabolic Substrates Stimulating Insulin Release

Class	Substrate[a]	Comment
Hexoses	Glucose	α Anomer more effective than β anomer
	Mannose	α Anomer more effective than β anomer
	Fructose	Potentiator only
Hexosamines	N-Acetylglucosamine	
	N-Propionylglucosamine	
	N-Dichloroacetylglucosamine	
	Glucosamine	Also inhibits glucose-stimulated release
Other sugars	Erythrose	
	Glyceraldehyde	
	Dihydroxyacetone	
Glycolytic	Pyruvate	Potentiator only
products	Lactate	Potentiator only
Amino acids	Leucine	
	Arginine	Potentiator only?
	Lysine	May be species differences
	Phenylalanine	May be species differences
	Tryptophan	May be species differences
2-Oxoacids	4-Methyl-2-oxopentanoate	
	3-Methyl-2-oxopentanoate	
	2-Oxopentanoate	
Purine ribo-	Inosine	
nucleosides	Guanosine	Inhibition at micromolar concentrations
	Adenosine	Inhibition at micromolar concentrations

[a] Sugars are the D stereoisomer and amino acids are the L stereoisomer.

Extracellular

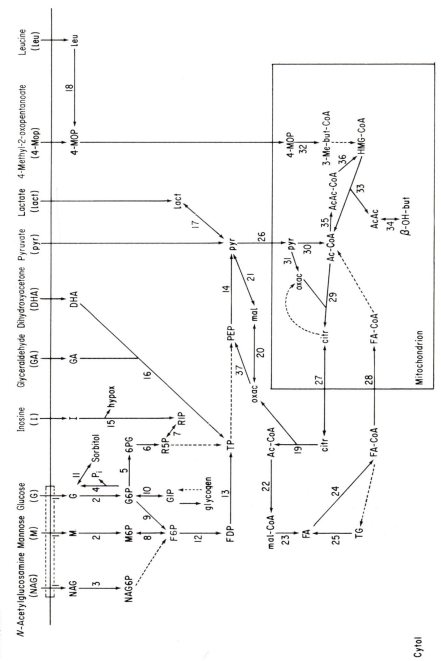

Cytol

A. Hexoses

1. Specificity

Insulin release from isolated islets is stimulated by glucose and mannose (Ashcroft *et al.*, 1972b), and for both sugars the α anomer is more potent that the β anomer (Niki *et al*, 1974, 1979). Galactose, despite some claims (Landgraf *et al.*, 1971), is generally accepted as ineffective (Hellman *et al.*, 1974a; Ashcroft and Lowry, 1979). Allose, altrose, gulose, idose, and talose do not stimulate insulin release (Ashcroft and Lowry, 1979). Fructose is ineffective alone at concentrations up to 50 mM but elicits insulin release if a low concentration of glucose or other primary stimulant is also present (Ashcroft *et al.*, 1972b, 1973, Curry, 1974). Ineffective as stimulants are 3-*O*-methyglucose, 2-deoxyglucose, L-glucose, 1,5-anhydroglucitol, and goldthioglucose (Ashcroft *et al.*, 1972b, 1973; Hellman *et al.*, 1974a). Glucose is metabolized by islets, as evidenced by $^{14}CO_2$ output from [^{14}C]glucose (Ashcroft *et al.*, 1970), ^3H_2O output from [5-^{3}H]glucose (Ashcroft *et al.*, 1972a), lactate output (Ashcroft and Lowry, 1979), maintenance of ATP content (Ashcroft *et al.*, 1973), and stimulation of respiration (Hellerstrom, 1967). Mannose is also well metabolized, as shown by measurements of output of $^{14}CO_2$ (Ashcroft *et al*, 1970), ^3H_2O (Zawalich *et al.*, 1979), and lactate (Ashcroft and Lowry, 1979) and maintenance of ATP content (Ashcroft *et al* 1973). Fructose is metabolized, but at rates considerably lower than glucose or mannose, never exceeding the value of about 50 pmol/hr per islet attained with threshold concentrations of glucose or mannose (Zawalich *et al.*, 1979). Assuming additive glycolytic

Fig. 2. Pathways of the metabolism of metabolic substrates stimulating insulin release. The reactions numbered are as follows; those marked with an asterisk have been directly demonstrated in pancreatic islets (see text for references). Dotted arrows indicate pathways not given in detail. * 1, Glucose transporter; * 2, glucokinase; 3, * *N*-acetylglucosamine kinase; * 4, glucose 6-phosphatase; * 5, glucose-6-phosphate dehydrogenase; * 6, 6-phosphogluconate dehydrogenase; 7, phosphoribomutase; 8, phosphomannose isomerase; * 9, phosphoglucose isomerase; 10, phosphoglucomutase; * 11, aldose reductase; * 12, phosphofructokinase; 13, aldolase; * 14, pyruvate kinase; * 15, nucleoside phosphorylase; 16, triokinase; * 17, lactate dehydrogenase; * 18, leucine aminotransferase; 19, ATP-citrate lyase; * 20, malate dehydrogenase; * 21, malic enzyme; 22, acetyl-CoA carboxylase; 23, fatty acid synthetase; 24, fatty acid thiokinase; 25, triglyceride lipase; 26, pyruvate transporter (mitochondrial); 27, citrate transporter (mitochondrial); 28, carnitine acyltransferase; * 29, citrate synthase; 30, pyruvate dehydrogenase; * 31, pyruvate carboxylase; 32, branched-chain 2-oxoacid dehydrogenase; 33, hydroxymethylglutaryl-CoA cleavage enzyme; * 34, β-hydroxybutyrate dehydrogenase; 35, thiolase; 36, hydroxymethylglutaryl-CoA synthase; 37, * PEP carboxykinase. In addition to those defined on the diagram the following nonstandard abbreviations are used: TP, triose phosphate; FA, fatty acid; FA-CoA, fatty acyl-CoA; 3-Me-but-CoA, 3-methylbutyryl-CoA; AcAc, acetoacetate; β-OH-but, β-hydroxybutyrate; HMG-CoA, 3-hydroxymethylglutaryl CoA; hypox, hypoxanthine; mal, malate; citr, citrate; oxac, oxaloacetate.

rates, however, the combination of low glucose and fructose gave a summated metabolic flux that was correlated with insulin release values in the same way as that between corresponding sets of metabolism and release data obtained from glucose alone (Zawalich *et al.*, 1979). No appreciable metabolism by islets of allose, altrose, gulose, idose, galactose, talose, or L-glucose is found; this conclusion is based on measurements of lactate output (Ashcroft & Lowry, 1979), $^{14}CO_2$ evolution (Macdonald *et al.*, 1975), and ATP content (Ashcroft *et al.*, 1973).

Conflicting results have been reported with 3-O-methylglucose. Matschinsky and Ellerman (1973) claimed to have observed increased lactate formation without concomitant insulin release in the presence of 3-O-methylglucose. However, other workers reported 3-O-methylglucose to be without effect on islet glycolysis (Ashcroft, 1976; Hellman *et al.*, 1974a). Since Matschinsky's group later was unable to reproduce the stimulatory effect of 3-O-methylglucose on islet glycolysis (Zawalich *et al.*, 1977a), it is probable that 3-O-methylglucose, although entering islets via the glucose transporter (Hellman *et al.*, 1973b), is not appreciably metabolized. Effects of 3-O-methylglucose on acylglucosamine metabolism are discussed further below.

The greater efficacy of α-D-glucose compared with β-D-glucose as a stimulator of insulin release has prompted the search for a metabolic counterpart. Idahl *et al.* (1976) found no evidence for preferential utilization of α-D-glucose using ^3H_2O production as an index of glycolysis. Moreover, no difference between the anomers was observed when the glucose 6-phosphate content was measured in islets exposed to a sudden increment in glucose concentration. The conclusion that recognition of glucose involved more than metabolism via glucose 6-phosphate provided considerable support for the regulator site model. However, this problem was further studied by Malaisse *et al.* (1976a). It was demonstrated that islet phosphoglucose isomerase was stereospecific for α-D-glucose 6-phosphate and that the concentration of glucose 6-phosphate was lower and that of later glycolytic intermediates (fructose 6-phosphate, fructose 1,6-disphosphate, and triose phosphates) higher in islets exposed to the α anomer of D-glucose. The rate of conversion of the α anomer to lactate and CO_2 was also higher than that of β-D-glucose. It was concluded that the more marked insulinotropic effect of α- as distinct from β-D-glucose was entirely compatible with the substrate site hypothesis. However, the question still remains unsettled at the present time in view of a recent report (Niki *et al.*, 1979) that the effect of mannose on insulin release also shows a preference for the α anomer, whereas, at least in other tissues, phosphomannose isomerase shows no such anomeric preference. Further studies on islet metabolism of mannose are required to resolve this issue.

2. Concentration Dependence

The curve relating rates of insulin release to glucose concentration is sigmoidal, with a threshold value at 4 mM, a half-maximum (K_m) value at 8 mM, and maximal release occurring at about 15 mM (Malaisse *et al.,* 1967a; Ashcroft *et al.,* 1972b; Ashcroft, 1976). For mannose, values of threshold, K_m, and maximally stimulating concentrations are 10, 15, and 20 mM, respectively (Zawalich *et al.,* 1977b). Measurements of utilization rates of both these sugars, using ^3H_2O output, have shown concentration dependencies in most studies similar to that seen for release (Ashcroft *et al.,* 1972a; Zawalich *et al.,* 1977b). Conflicting data from Zawalich and Matschinsky (1977), who reported that islet glucose utilization changed little and lactate output not at all on raising the extracellular glucose from 4 to 10 mM, are at variance with other studies including several from the same laboratory (Zawalich *et al.,* 1977b; Zawalich, 1979).

3. Effects of Inhibitors

Insulin release stimulated by glucose or mannose is inhibited by mannoheptulose, 2-deoxyglucose, glucosamine, and iodacetate. The first of these has proved to be of the greatest utility, since the other agents possess multiple actions that make it difficult to draw unequivocal conclusions. Thus, although 2-deoxyglucose is generally regarded as exerting its main effect on the conversion of glucose 6-phosphate or mannose 6-phosphate to fructose 6-phosphate, it also inhibits the metabolism of *N*-acetylglucosamine (Zawalich *et al.,* 1979) which is likely to bypass the above step. Nevertheless, in all situations in which hexose metabolism is inhibited by 2-deoxyglucose, a corresponding reduction in the rate of insulin release has been observed. The rate of metabolism of 2-deoxyglucose by islets is very low. The effects of glucosamine are discussed below. The use of iodacetate as a tool for probing glucoreceptor models has generated much confusion. Matschinsky and Ellerman (1973) reported that iodacetate could be used to dissociate islet glucose metabolism from glucose-stimulated insulin release, i.e., inhibition of glycolysis but not of insulin secretion. This finding is at variance with a number of other studies (Georg *et al.,* 1971; Hellman *et al.,* 1974b). Moreover, it could not be confirmed in a subsequent report from the same laboratory (Zawalich *et al.,* 1977a). The problem appears to be twofold: first, iodacetate is by no means specific for triosephosphate dehydrogenase, and, second, iodacetate possesses intrinsic insulin-releasing ability (Hellman *et al.,* 1973a). Detailed studies on iodacetate (Sener *et al.,* 1978a) have shown that, when the facilitating effect of iodacetate on insulin release is taken into account, there is an expected coincidence between the inhibition of metabolic and secretory events. Sener *et al.* conclude that iodoacetate was not an adequate tool for dissociating the metabolic and secretory functions of glucose.

Mannoheptulose inhibits islet glucose and mannose metabolism (Ashcroft *et al.,* 1970; Zawalich *et al.,* 1978). The effect is reversible and correlates closely with the effects of mannoheptulose on insulin release stimulated by these sugars. Neither the metabolism nor the insulin-releasing activity of other metabolites is inhibited by mannoheptulose (Zawalich, 1979).

The inhibitory action of mannoheptulose on islet glucose (and mannose) metabolism is ascribed to the inhibition of phosphorylation of the sugars (Ashcroft and Randle, 1970).

4. Metabolic Pathways

Glucose enters the β cell rapidly by a system of facilitated diffusion. Both the V_{max} and the K_m of the transporter are considerably greater than the V_{max} and K_m for glucose utilization (Hellman *et al.,* 1973b). Thus transport of glucose is non-rate-limiting, and intraislet glucose concentrations are essentially the same as extracellular concentrations (Matschinsky and Ellerman, 1968). The consequence of non-rate-limiting glucose transport is that glucose utilization is relatively insensitive to inhibitors of sugar transport, e.g., phloridzin (Ashcroft and Nino, 1978). The prediction of the substrate site hypothesis that glucose-stimulated insulin release therefore should also be relatively insensitive to transport inhibitors has been tested. Thus 3-*O*-methylglucose competes with glucose for entry but does not inhibit glucose utilization or glucose-stimulated insulin release (Hellman *et al.,* 1973b; Ashcroft *et al.,* 1980). Caffeine, which also inhibits glucose transport into islets (McDaniel *et al.,* 1977), does not inhibit glycolytic flux or glucose-stimulated insulin release (Ashcroft *et al.,* 1980). Both phloretin and phloridzin inhibit islet glucose transport without inhibiting glucose utilization (Hellman *et al.,* 1972; Ashcroft and Nino, 1978). Results of studies on the effects of phloretin on glucose-stimulated insulin release are complex: Low concentrations of phloretin that did not inhibit islet glucose utilization, glucose oxidation, or ATP content produced a 50% inhibition of glucose-stimulated insulin release (Ashcroft and Nino, 1978). This observation suggests a dissociation of release and metabolism, supporting the regulator site model. However, caution is necessary in interpretation, since phloretin may have other sites of action. In islets leucine-stimulated release was also inhibited by this concentration of phloretin (Ashcroft and Nino, 1978), and phloretin also has a marked effect on anion permeability of lipid bilayers.

Phosphorylation of glucose and mannose is the rate-limiting step for their utilization by pancreatic islets. Hence according to the substrate site hypothesis this step constitutes the glucose sensor. Extracts of rat or mouse islets contain glucose-phosphorylating activity with the kinetic properties of hexokinase; clearly such an activity, with a K_m for glucose of $10^{-4} M$, cannot account for the observed kinetics of glucose utilization. However, evidence has been obtained suggesting the presence of a second glucose-phosphorylating enzyme (Ashcroft and Randle, 1970). The activity has a K_m for glucose of approximately 10 mM and is not inhibited by glucose 6-phosphate. These properties are similar to those of liver glucokinase with which the islet enzyme has been tentatively identified. It must be pointed out that such a conclusion remains preliminary pending separation of the "glucokinase" from the hexokinase; this has not yet been achieved. The presence of glucose-6-phosphatase has been reported in mouse islets, but it has not been found in rat or hamster islets (Täljedal, 1969; Ashcroft and Randle, 1972). Mouse islet glucose-6-phosphatase has a K_m for glucose 6-phosphate of 1 mM and is inhibited by glucose. Its theoretical contribution to net glucose phosphorylation has been calculated (Ashcroft and Randle, 1969), but from experiments aimed at measurement of glucose formation from mannose in intact mouse islets it was concluded that glucose-6-phosphatase was not a significant factor in control of the net rate of glucose 6-phosphate formation (Ashcroft and Randle, 1968). The properties of the glucokinase account at least qualitatively for the K_m for glucose and sensitivity to mannoheptulose of glucose- (and mannose-) stimulated insulin release, but purification and characterization of this enzyme are still required.

Islets are enzymatically equipped for the synthesis and degradation of glycogen, but the activities are considerably lower than those found in liver (Brolin and Berne, 1970). The islet glycogen store is dependent on the glucose concentration to which the islets have been exposed, either *in vivo* or *in vitro*. Thus in one study islets isolated from rats contained no detectable glycogen but, after maintenance of the islets with 83.3 mM glucose for 20 hr, up to 63 mmol glucose residue/kg dry wt (73 pmol/islet) was found (Malaisse *et al.*, 1977). Even this value is about 25-fold lower than that of liver. In lean mice, fresh islets contained 4 mmol/kg dry wt (Hellman and Idahl, 1970), and rat islets in this study contained about 1 mmol glucose residues/kg; obese hyperglycemic mice had an islet glycogen content of 10 mmol/kg dry wt, which was increased to 30 mmol/kg dry wt in islets isolated after elevation of blood sugar by an intraperitoneal injection. Up to 90% of the islet glycogen store of these mice is mobilized during incubation of islets in the absence of glucose or of oxygen for 45 min (Hellman and Idahl, 1970). Rates of glycogen synthesis are slow, amounting to less than 0.2% of the rate of glucose utilization (Hedeskov and Capito, 1974). Thus in normal situations glycogen synthesis is not a major route of islet glucose metabolism. Moreover, in islets from obese hyperglycemic mice, the measured glycogen store can support the observed rate of oxygen uptake in the absence of exogenous substrate for about 15 min, whereas oxygen uptake is constant for up to 150 min (Hellerstrom, 1967). Glycogen does not therefore represent a major endogenous energy store.

The significance of the metabolism of glucose via the pentose cycle has been controversial. In four studies (Snyder *et al.*, 1969; Ashcroft *et al.*, 1972a, Hedeskov and Capito 1975a; Malaisse *et al.*, 1976b) the fractional contribution of the pentose cycle flux to the generation of triose phosphate was found to be less than 3% at 16.7 mM extracellular glucose. The net flux of substrate through the pentose cycle was not increased when the glucose concentration was raised from 2.8 to 16.7 mM. The net flux is calculated to be 5–7 pmol glucose 6-phosphate per islet per hour irrespective of the extracellular glucose concentration. This conclusion has been challenged by Verspohl *et al.* (1979) who claim that insulin released by the islets into the medium inhibits the pentose cycle flux. When measurements of the pentose cycle flux were conducted in the presence of antiinsulin serum to bind such secreted insulin, the rate of glucose oxidation via the pentose cycle was calculated to increase about sevenfold on raising the glucose concentration from 5.6 to 15.7 mM. However, the usually observed dependence of the glucose utilization rate on glucose concentration was also modified by the addition of antiinsulin serum; rates of glucose utilization were identical at 5.6 mM glucose with or without antiinsulin serum (754 and 765 pmol/3 hr per 10 islets), but whereas in the absence of antiinsulin serum the glucose utilization rate was increased sixfold at 16.7 mM glucose, in the presence of antiinsulin serum there was no significant increase at 16.7 mM glucose (Verspohl *et al.*, 1979).

The activities of glucose-6-phosphate and 6-phosphogluconate dehydrogenases in islet homogenates are very much greater than the measured pentose cycle fluxes (Ashcroft and Randle, 1970), and it is suggested that flux is controlled by the concentration of NADP$^+$ and NADPH. It should be emphasized that this view is diametrically opposed to that of Verspohl *et al.* (1979) who envisaged that flux through the cycle controls NADPH and NADP$^+$ rather than vice versa. In the context of this disagreement, it is relevant to note that the islet has other enzymes capable of generating NADPH (Ashcroft and Randle, 1970; Ashcroft and Christie 1979).

The sorbitol pathway has been studied in rat islets (Malaisse *et al.*, 1974). Although exogenous sorbitol is oxidized by islets, it was concluded that the metabolism of glucose via the sorbitol pathway did not contribute to any significant extent to the formation of triose phosphates.

The studies described thus far indicate that glycolysis represents the major pathway for glucose utilization in quantitative terms, and also in terms of significance for control by glucose of insulin secretion. About 95% of the net uptake of glucose is accounted for by the formation of triose phosphates, and more than 90% of the triose phosphates are formed via the glycolytic pathway. The pathway has been most conveniently quantitated by measurements of rates of ^3H_2O formation from [5-^{3}H]glucose or -mannose (Ashcroft et al., 1972a; Zawalich et al., 1977b). This parameter demonstrates parallels with the effects of hexoses on insulin release as described above. Interestingly, islets do not display the Pasteur effect (Hellman et al., 1975), although the allosteric properties of phosphofructokinase are similar to those found in other tissues (Sener and Malaisse, 1978). Measurements of maximally extractable activities of glycolytic enzymes are consistent with phosphofructokinase representing the rate-limiting step for glycolysis (Sener and Malaisse, 1978); however, more rigorous approaches, e.g., measurement of mass-action ratios, are necessary to substantiate this conclusion. Islets release pyruvate; in rat islets the rate is 12 pmol/hr per islet and is relatively independent of the extracellular glucose concentration (5.6–27.8 mM) (Sener and Malaisse, 1978). Lactate output is considerably greater and is highly dependent on medium glucose concentration, rising from 16 pmol/hr per islet in the absence of glucose to 120 pmol/hr per islet at 16.7 mM glucose, the latter value representing about 50% of the glucose utilized (Sener and Malaisse, 1978). In another study, however, only 20% of glucose uptake was accounted for by lactate formation (Reese et al., 1973); it was also shown that [1-^{14}C]glucose gave rise to [3-^{14}C]lactate, indicating that lactate formation from pyruvate occurred directly without prior metabolism of the pyruvate via the Krebs cycle.

Although rates of lactate formation and glucose utilization estimated as ^3H_2O production usually vary at least qualitatively in the same way, this is not invariably true. A striking example is a recent study in which mannoheptulose reduced glucose utilization at 27.5 mM glucose from 129 to 40 pmol/hr per islet without alteration in the lactate output (Zawalich et al., 1977a).

The metabolism of lactate and pyruvate via the Krebs cycle is considered below. Other minor pathways for glucose metabolism exist in islets. The incorporation of glucose carbon into triacylglycerol and phospholipids of islets from obese hyperglycemic mice amounted to less than 1–2% of the rate of glucose utilization (Berne, 1975); there is no evidence that these pathways are involved in the control of insulin secretion. The incorporation of radioactivity from [^{14}C]glucose into islet amino acids has also been demonstrated (Gylfe and Sehlin, 1976; Gylfe and Hellman, 1974). Most radioactivity was found in aspartate, followed by glutamate and γ-aminobutyrate. A high concentration of glucose enhanced incorporation into

S. J. H. Ashcroft

glutamate but not aspartate or γ-aminobutyrate. The results provided no evidence that these metabolic pathways were involved in glucose-stimulated insulin release.

5. Conclusions

The ability of hexoses to stimulate insulin release correlates with their rate of metabolism via glycolysis in islets with regard to specificity, concentration dependence, and effects of inhibitors. Islets possess a high K_m glucose-phosphorylating activity, possibly identical to liver glucokinase, that may constitute the glucose sensor.

B. Hexosamines

1. Specificity

Insulin release from rat islets is stimulated by N-acetyl-D-glucosamine (NAG) but not by N-acetyl-D-mannosamine (Ashcroft et al., 1976; Ashcroft, 1980). Glucosamine elicits release, albeit weakly, but inhibits release stimulated by glucose (Coore and Randle (1964); Zawalich et al., 1979). The effects of other acylglucosamines have been studied in the presence of caffeine and a low glucose concentration: N-Propionyl-D-glucosamine stimulated insulin release, but with a further increase in the length of the acyl side chain insulin-releasing ability was diminished. However, N-dichloroacetyl-D-glucosamine was a highly potent insulin secretagogue both in vitro and in vivo (Ashcroft and Crossley, 1975; Ashcroft et al., 1976).

Islets metabolize NAG as evidenced by (1) maintenance of the ATP content of mouse islets (Ashcroft et al., 1973), (2) formation of $^{14}CO_2$ from [1-^{14}C]NAG in rat islets (Williams and Ashcroft, 1978), and (3) formation of ^3H_2O from [1-^{3}H]NAG in rat islets (Zawalich et al., 1979). Glucosamine is also metabolized by rat or mouse islets (Zawalich et al., 1979).

2. Concentration Dependence

Curves relating rates of NAG oxidation and NAG-stimulated insulin release to NAG concentration were similar, half-maximum values being obtained at 12–15 mM NAG (Williams and Ashcroft, 1978). The weaker stimulatory action of glucosamine on insulin release was correlated with its slower rate of metabolism (Zawalich et al., 1979).

3. Effects of Inhibitors

Insulin release stimulated by NAG is inhibited by phloretin and by caffeine (Williams and Ashcroft, 1978), by 3-O-methylglucose (Ashcroft et al., 1980), by 2-deoxyglucose, and by iodoacetate but not by mannoheptulose (Zawalich *et al.*, 1979; Ashcroft *et al.*, 1978). This pattern is clearly different from glucose-induced insulin release; therefore study of NAG metabolism has permitted a rather stringent test of the substrate site hypothesis. The prediction of the latter that NAG metabolism should be blocked by phloretin, caffeine, 3-*O*-methylglucose, 2-deoxyglucose, and iodoacetate but not by mannoheptulose has been confirmed (Williams and Ashcroft, 1978; Ashcroft *et al.*, 1980). For glucosamine, insulin-releasing ability and metabolism are both inhibited by 2-deoxyglucose and iodo-acetate but not by mannoheptulose (Zawalich *et al.*, 1979).

4. Metabolic Pathways

Only NAG will be considered here. Phosphorylation of NAG is catalyzed by a specific NAG kinase with the following properties: It does not phosphorylate *N*-acetylmannosamine; increasing the acyl side-chain length of *N*-acylglucosamines is accompanied by an increase in K_m; it is not inhibited by mannoheptulose (Ashcroft, 1976). These properties are consistent with observed properties of insulin release elicited by NAG. However, the K_m for NAG of islet NAG kinase is 20 μM, whereas the concentration of NAG required for half-maximal rates of insulin release or NAG metabolism is about 20 mM. Moreover, the maximally extractable activity of NAG kinase in rat islets is considerably higher than observed rates of NAG utilization. These observations suggest that, in contrast to glucose metabolism, NAG metabolism has transport rather than phosphorylation as the rate-limiting step. Since a specific carrier for NAG is unlikely, it also seems feasible that the NAG enters via the glucose transporter. This possibility is supported by the following findings. First, in contrast to glucose, NAG metabolism is markedly inhibited by low concentrations of the glucose transport inhibitor phloretin (Williams and Ashcroft, 1978). Second, caffeine, which also inhibits islet sugar transport (McDaniel *et al.*, 1977), markedly inhibits NAG oxidation (Williams and Ashcroft, 1978). This action underlies the paradoxical inhibitory action of methylxanthines on NAG-stimulated release of insulin; the effect is envisaged as a direct action of the methyl-xanthines per se, since it is not reproduced by dibutyryl cyclic AMP (Williams and Ashcroft, 1978; Ashcroft *et al.*, 1980). Third, results with 3-*O*-methylglucose provide convincing support. 3-*O*-Methylglucose is transported into islets by the glucose transporter but is not metabolized and does not stimulate insulin release; nor, since glucose transport is non-rate-limiting, does 3-*O*-methylglucose inhibit glucose utilization or glucose-stimulated insulin release. However, competition between 3-*O*-methylglu-cose and NAG would be expected to inhibit NAG metabolism, hence, based on the substrate site hypothesis, NAG-stimulated insulin release; these predictions have been verified (Ashcroft *et al.*, 1980).

The subsequent metabolism of NAG phosphate is not known in detail. It is assumed to enter the glycolytic pathway via fructose 6-phosphate; approximately 4% of the NAG utilized is incorporated into glycoprotein, presumably via UDP NAG (Williams, 1979).

5. Conclusions

As for glucose, a metabolic basis for the stimulation of insulin release by NAG is supported by available evidence. Unlike that for glucose metabolism, the rate-limiting step for metabolism of NAG by islets is transport into the cell; hence this step serves the discriminatory function of a "NAG receptor."

C. Pentoses, Tetroses, and Trioses

1. Specificity

Stimulatory effects of certain pentose sugars on insulin release (Kuzuya et al., 1966; Montague and Taylor, 1968) have not been confirmed by other workers (Ashcroft et al., 1972a; Malaisse et al., 1967a) and will not be considered here. In one study, the insulinotropic action of erythrose was reported (Sener et al., 1977). It was found that erythrose stimulated insulin release in the absence of glucose and lowered the K_m but did not affect the V_{max} for glucose-stimulated insulin release. This insulinotropic action was paralleled by an increased glycolytic flux. Stimulation of insulin release by glyceraldehyde and by dihydroxyacetone has been studied in more detail. Stimulation occurs in vivo (Ashcroft and Crossley, 1975) as well as in vitro (Ashcroft et al., 1973; Hellman et al., 1974b; Jain et al., 1975; Zawalich et al., 1978). The secretory response to D-glyceraldehyde is biphasic in time and is potentiated by theophylline, arginine, or cytochalasin B; L-glyceraldehyde does not initiate secretion but potentiates the effects of glucose or D-glyceraldehyde; dihydroxyacetone elicits insulin release, but the maximal rate is only one-third to one-half that observed with glyceraldehyde (Hellman et al., 1974b; Jain et al., 1975). D-Glyceraldehyde is well metabolized by islets, as evidenced by $^{14}CO_2$ evolution from [U-^{14}C]glyceraldehyde (Ashcroft et al., 1973; Hellman et al., 1974b) or ^3H_2O production from [2-^{3}H]glyceraldehyde (Zawalich et al., 1978). Dihydroxyacetone metabolism has not been measured directly but has been inferred from isotope dilution studies with [U-^{14}C]glucose (Hellman et al., 1974b). In quantitative terms a threshold usage rate of 35 pmol/hr per islet has to be reached before glyceraldehyde stimulates insulin release; thus glyceraldehyde is about three times as efficient as glucose as regards triose equivalents required to initiate insulin release (Zawalich et al., 1978).

2. Concentration Dependence

At low concentrations (2–4 mM) glyceraldehyde is a more potent secretagogue than glucose (Jain *et al.*, 1975). The curve relating insulin release rate to glyceraldehyde concentration is sigmoidal, with a K_m of 2.5–4 mM (Hellman *et al.*, 1974b; Zawalich *et al.*, 1978). The K_m for glyceraldehyde utilization is similar to that for release (Zawalich *et al.*, 1978).

3. Effects of Inhibitors

The metabolism of glyceraldehyde is unaffected by mannoheptulose nor does the latter inhibit glyceraldehyde- or dihydroxyacetone-stimulated insulin release (Ashcroft *et al.*, 1973; Hellman *et al.*, 1974b). Neither 2-deoxyglucose nor glucosamine inhibits glyceraldehyde metabolism or glyceraldehyde-stimulated release (Zawalich *et al.*, 1978).

4. Metabolic Pathways

It is assumed that glyceraldehyde and dihydroxyacetone enter glycolysis at the level of triose phosphate, via triokinase. However, no studies on the latter enzyme have been reported. Increasing the glyceraldehyde concentration to about 5 mM leads to a progressive decrease in mouse islet ATP content (Ashcroft *et al.*, 1973); a possible explanation is that the ability of triokinase to phosphorylate glyceraldehyde exceeds the ability of the islet to utilize for ATP formation the triose phosphate formed. A parallel fall in the rate of glyceraldehyde-induced insulin release at high glyceraldehyde concentrations has been observed (see above).

5. Conclusions

Studies with trioses support the substrate site hypothesis. In particular the failure of mannoheptulose to inhibit glyceraldehyde metabolism and glyceraldehyde-stimulated insulin release is not readily incorporated into a regulator site model.

D. Lactate and Pyruvate

1. Specificity

In the absence of glucose or in the presence of maximally stimulating glucose concentrations, neither L-lactate nor pyruvate at concentrations up to 30 mM augmented the rate of insulin release; however, at intermediate glucose concentrations (5.6–11 1 mM) both agents enhanced the secretory response (Sener *et al.*, 1978b; Malaisse *et al.*, 1979b). Pyruvate also enhanced insulin release in the presence of fructose, leucine, or 4-methyl-2-oxopentanoate (Sener *et al.* 1978b), whereas lactate increased release in the presence of fructose but not 4-methyl-2-oxopentanoate (Malaisse *et al.,* 1979b).

2. Concentration Dependence

The magnitude of the shift to the left of the sigmoidal curve relating the rate of insulin release to glucose concentration is such that a 30 mM concentration of pyruvate or L-lactate is equivalent to 2 or 2.8 mM glucose, respectively (Malaisse *et al.,* 1979b). On a molar basis the insulinotropic ability of nutrients is D-glucose > > L-lactate > pyruvate = DL-lactate > D-lactate. However, measurements of $^{14}CO_2$ output show that the oxidation of L-lactate, which increases with lactate concentration over the range 1–30 mM, is considerably less than that of pyruvate; oxidation of the latter is comparable to that of glucose (Sener *et al.,* 1978b). There is thus a discrepancy between the relative abilities of glucose, L-lactate, and pyruvate to elicit insulin release and to be oxidized by islets. In particular the high rate of oxidation of pyruvate compared to its feeble insulinotropic activity has been noted in several studies (Jain *et al.,* 1978; Sener *et al.,* 1978b; Hedeskov *et al.,* 1972). One explanation would be that the major signal for insulin release arises from glucose metabolism prior to the formation of pyruvate, and the modest potentiatory effects of lactate and pyruvate accounted for by their metabolism via pyruvate carboxylase (Ashcroft and Randle, 1970) and phosphoenolpyruvate (PEP) carboxykinase (Hedeskov and Capito, 1980) to intermediates higher in the glycolytic sequence. However, an alternative explanation is possible. When allowance is made for the effects of intracellular conversion of lactate and pyruvate and the relative sparing effect of exogenous nutrients on the utilization of endogenous fuels, a close correlation is found among the abilities of glucose, lactate, and pyruvate to generate reducing equivalents and to stimulate insulin release (Malaisse *et al.,* 1979b). Thus a role for mitochondrial oxidation of pyruvate in nutrient-induced insulin release has been suggested (Sener *et al.,* 1978b). These findings have been challenged. When islets from *ob/ob* mice were used, the opposite conclusion was reached, namely, that glucose but not pyruvate decreased metabolism of endogenous fuels; hence there is a dissociation between net gain of reducing equivalent and insulinotropic capacity of pyruvate and glucose (Lenzen and Panten, 1980).

3. Effects of Inhibitors

The oxidation of pyruvate by rat islets is inhibited by anoxia, antimycin A, KCN, and iodoacetate (Sener *et al.,* 1978b). Effects on pyruvate-potentiated insulin release have not been reported but would not be easily interpretable in view of the requirement for glucose and the known fall in ATP content with anoxia or respiratory poisons (Ashcroft *et al.,* 1973).

Pyruvate oxidation is also inhibited by cyanocinnamic acid, an inhibitor of mitochondrial pyruvate transport; rates of pyruvate oxidation at 5 mM pyruvate were decreased to 25% by 1 mM cyanocinnamic acid (S. J. H. Ashcroft and M. Lowry, unpublished). Inhibition of pyruvate oxidation by mannoheptulose has also been reported (Hedeskov *et al.,* 1972); no explanation of the mechanism has to my knowledge been put forward.

4. Metabolic Pathways

Lactate is rapidly taken up by islets, but the total rate of lactate oxidation and conversion into pyruvate, 0.1 nmol/hr per islet, is well below the activity of lactate dehydrogenase in islet homogenates (14.6 nmol/hr per islet) (Sener and Malaisse 1978). Uptake of exogenous pyruvate is also rapid and appears to be saturable, with a K_m of 8–9 mM (Sener *et al.,* 1978b). The inhibition of pyruvate oxidation by cyanocinnamate (above) suggests that entry of pyruvate into the mitochondria occurs via a pyruvate transporter. The intramitochondrial oxidation of pyruvate within the mitochondrion accounts for a major fraction of the generation of ATP from glucose. However, there is little information available on metabolic events of the Krebs cycle in islets. In recent studies in this laboratory J. Merritt has measured the activity of Krebs cycle enzymes in a mitochondrial fraction from rat islets. The results are shown in Table II. The lowest activity is that of NAD-isocitrate dehydrogenase; estimates of maximum citrate cycle flux from measurements of oxygen uptake suggest that the cycle operates at well below maximum capacity in the intact islet. As in rat heart mitochondria, however, NADP-isocitrate dehydrogenase is also present, at higher maximal activity than NAD-isocitrate dehydrogenase. Operation of the Krebs cycle therefore may be capable of sustaining a high rate of reduction of NADP as well as NAD. Kinetic data for some Krebs cycle enzymes are also included in Table II. There are no available data on islet mitochondrial metabolite levels to permit conclusions concerning possible regulatory sites in the cycle.

5. Conclusions

Interpretation of the potentiatory effects of pyruvate and lactate on insulin release in terms of their metabolism requires consideration of their effects on the metabolism of endogenous nutrients. In some but not all studies, the effects of these agents on net production of reducing power are correlated with their effects on insulin release.

E. Amino Acids and 2-Oxoacids

1. Specificity

In the absence of glucose, insulin release is stimulated by leucine (Ashcroft *et al.,* 1973; Milner and Hales, 1967). Other amino acids, with

TABLE II

Activities and Properties of Mitochondrial Enzymes in Rat Islets[a]

Enzyme	Maximal activity at 30°C (pmol/min per islet)	Kinetic properties	
		Substrate	K_m (μM)
Citrate synthase	67	Acetyl-CoA	10
		Oxalacetate	4
NAD$^+$-isocitrate dehydrogenase	3	—	—
NADP$^+$-isocitrate dehydrogenase	33	Isocitrate	10
		NADP$^+$	15
2-Oxoglutarate dehydrogenase	93	NAD$^+$	19
		CoA	9
Succinate dehydrogenase	143	—	—
Fumarase	195	Malate	84
Malate dehydrogenase	1030	Oxalacetate	22
		NADH	150

[a] A mitochondrial fraction was obtained from rat islets as described by Ashcroft and Christie (1979). The recovery was assessed by comparison of citrate synthase activity in the fraction with that in the whole homogenates. Enzyme activities were measured spectrophotometrically by methods described in "Methods in Enzymology" (S. P. Colowick and N. O. Kaplan, eds.), Academic Press; the activities given have been converted for recovery.

the possible exception of arginine, are ineffective. For arginine conflicting results have been reported: Thus arginine stimulated insulin release from perfused rat pancreas in the absence of glucose in one study (Gerich et al., 1974) but failed to do so in another (Pagliara et al., 1974). Since arginine is only feebly metabolized by pancreatic islets (Hellman et al., 1971), it is of importance to resolve this point to further understanding of the mechanisms involved. Discussion of the mechanism of action of leucine is centered around whether the metabolism of leucine within the β cell plays a role in its insulinogenic activity, i.e., the substrate site hypothesis. In particular the effects of nonmetabolizable analogues and of potential metabolites, especially the corresponding 2-oxoacid, have been investigated.

In the presence of low concentrations of glucose, insulin release is augmented by several amino acids. In humans (Floyd et al., 1966) and rats (Malaisse and Malaisse-Lagae, 1968) lysine, arginine, phenylalanine, and tryptophan are effective. There is insufficient information available on the metabolism of these amino acids, in particular their possible effects on the metabolism of endogenous nutrients, to permit conclusions as to the mechanism involved. The present account will therefore be confined to the action of leucine and 2-oxoacids. Of the latter, DL-3-methyl-2-oxopentanoate, 4-methyl-2-oxopentanoate, and 2-oxopentanoate have been reported to elicit insulin release and to be metabolized by isolated islets (Hutton *et al.*, 1979a,b; Lenzen and Panten, 1980). Leucine is also well metabolized by islets, as evidenced by maintenance of the ATP content (Ashcroft *et al.*, 1973) or as $^{14}CO_2$ evolution (Hellman *et al.*, 1971). The stimulation of insulin release by the nonmetabolizable leucine analogue 2-aminobicyclo [2.2.1] heptane-2-carboxylic acid [(−)BCH] was suggested to indicate that leucine metabolism was not involved in insulin secretion (Christensen *et al.*, 1971). However, it has become apparent that (−)BCH does in fact elicit metabolic changes in islets including effects on nicotinamide adenine dinucleotide fluorescence (Panten *et al.*, 1972), on glutanate dehydrogenase activity (Sener and Malaisse, 1980) and on glucose oxidation (Gylfe, 1974); therefore, the effects of (−)BCH on insulin release do not rule out a role for leucine metabolism in leucine-stimulated insulin release.

2. *Concentration Dependence*

Most data are available on the effects of 4-methyl-2-oxopentanoate (Hutton *et al.*, 1979a,b), and it is generally assumed that the mechanism of stimulation of insulin release by this metabolic product of leucine is the same as that of leucine itself. Insulin release is stimulated by 4-methyl-2-oxopentanoate at concentrations greater than 4 m*M*, a maximal response occurring in the presence of 25–50 m*M* 4-methyl-2-oxopentanoate. Rates of islet respiration, acetoacetate production, and 4-methyl-2-oxopentanoate utilization, oxidation, and amination were a hyperbolic function of the 4-methyl-2-oxopentanoate concentration with maximal responses at 25 m*M*. Responses of ATP content, ATP/ADP ratio, and energy change were also hyperbolic but were maximally increased by 1 m*M* 4-methyl-2-oxopentanoate. The $NADPH/NADP^+$ ratios were correlated with rates of insulin release and metabolic fluxes with a maximum at 25 m*M* 4-methyl-2-oxopentanoate; a maximum value for the $NADH/NAD^+$ ratio was achieved at 10 m*M* 4-methyl-2-oxopentanoate. These studies and also those of Lenzen and Panten (1980) are consistent with the view that metabolism of 2-oxoacids is involved in their stimulatory effect on insulin release.

3. *Effects of Inhibitors*

The oxidation of 4-methyl-2-oxopentanoate by rat islets is inhibited by rotenone, a respiratory chain inhibitor, by uncoupling agents, by the K^+ ionophore valinomycin, and by the mitochondrial F_0-F_1 ATPase inhibitor oligomycin (Hutton *et al.*, 1979a); parallel changes in the insulin secretory response also occur (Hutton *et al.*, 1980), although they may be primarily a consequence of decreased islet ATP content (Ashcroft *et al.*, 1973). However, parallel inhibition of 4-methyl-2-oxopentanoate oxidation and insulin release by hydroxycyanocinnamate, an inhibitor of 2-oxoacid transport, has also been reported (Hutton *et al.*, 1979a). In the absence of Ca^{2+}, stimulation of insulin release and oxidation of 4-methyl-2-oxopentanoate are impaired, but oxidation of the nonstimulatory 3-methyl-2-oxobutyrate is unaffected (Lenzen and Panten, 1980).

4. Metabolic Pathways

The probable metabolic pathway for metabolism of leucine is shown in Fig. 2. Studies (Hutton *et al.*, 1979a) with labeled 4-methyl-2-oxopentanoate have shown that incorporation by islets occurs into CO_2, H_2O, acetoacetate, L-leucine, and to a lesser extent protein and lipids. Carbon atoms C-2, C-3, and C-4 of the acetoacetate produced are derived from the 4-methyl-2-oxopentanoate, but carboxy group carbon is derived from CO_2. The acetoacetate produced is not utilized further. Amination proceeds via a branched-chain aminotransferase. Of considerable importance is the observation that the same amounts of $^{14}CO_2$ are released from [1-^{14}C]3-methylbutyrate, which does not stimulate insulin release, as from [2-^{14}C]4-methyl-2-oxopentanoate (Holze and Panten, 1979). Since both compounds are oxidized via 3-methylbutyryl–coenzyme A, the oxidative decarboxylation of 4-methyl-2-oxopentanoate is implicated in its insulin-releasing activity. This might suggest a role for the mitochondrial $NADH/NAD^+$ ratio as a metabolic coupling factor. However, the studies of Hutton *et al.* (1979b) referred to earlier, although they measured whole tissue concentrations of pyridine nucleotides, seemed to discount the $NADH/NAD^+$ ratio as being of importance in the stimulus–secretion coupling mechanism and pointed instead to a role for the $NADPH/NADP^+$ ratio. The mechanism whereby 4-methyl-2-oxopentanoate increases the $NADPH/NADP^+$ ratio is not clear, especially in view of the demonstration that under anoxic conditions, in which 4-methyl-2-oxopentanoate oxidation (and insulin release) is blocked, the 4-methyl-2-oxopenanoate-induced rise in the islet $NADPH/NADP^+$ ratio is not inhibited (Hutton *et al.*, 1979b). With leucine itself, increases in the $NADPH/NADP^+$ ratio have also been demonstrated, and the effects of the thiol oxidants diamide and *tert*-butylhydroperoxide were to oppose leucine-induced increases in both insulin release and the $NADPH/NADP^+$ ratio. (Ammon *et al.*, 1979).

5. Conclusions

There is considerable evidence that 4-methyl-2-oxopentanoate, and by inference leucine, stimulate insulin release by a mechanism that involves their metabolism. Data so far indicate that the major metabolic flux occurs via the pathway delineated in other tissues. Evidence suggests that metabolites after the oxidative decarboxylation step are not important in stimulus–secretion coupling. However, it is not clear how the increased reduction of NADP is elicited; a role for allosteric activation of glutamate dehydrogenase has been suggested. The mode of stimulation of insulin release by other amino acids such as arginine remains obscure.

F. Purine Ribonucleosides

1. Specificity

In mouse islets insulin release is stimulated by inosine, guanosine, and adenosine, and maximal secretory responses are close to those seen with glucose (Jain and Logothetopoulos, 1978). Free purine bases had no effect on insulin release (Jain and Logothetopoulos, 1978) nor did hypoxanthine or free ribose (Capito and Hedeskov, 1976). Measurement of $^{14}CO_2$ evolution (Jain and Logothetopoulos, 1978) showed that inosine and guanosine were well-metabolized by mouse islets, and the ability of islets to metabolize inosine was further established by measurements of islet lactate output and the amount of ATP, glucose 5-phosphate, and fructose 1,6-diphosphate plus triose phosphates (Capito and Hedeskov, 1976). For rat islets, however, conflicting reports have been published. Thus Jain and Logothetopoulos (1978) found no stimulation of insulin release with inosine, guanosine, or adenosine. Campbell and Taylor (1977), however, showed stimulation of insulin release from rat islets (but not from rabbit islets) by inosine. Nevertheless, where both metabolic and secretory parameters have been measured, parallellism has generally been observed; in particular, in the studies of Jain and Logothetopoulos (1978) mouse islets oxidized adenosine five times faster and inosine three times faster than rat islets.

2. Concentration Dependence

Near-maximal secretory responses to purine nucleosides were reached at 2.5–5 mM (Jain and Logothetopoulos 1978). Dose dependencies of metabolic parameters have not yet been systematically investigated. It is noteworthy that, at micromolar concentrations, adenosine and guanosine markedly inhibit insulin secretory responses to glucose and other stimuli in rat islets (Ismail et al., 1977; Ismail and Montague, 1977). These effects are suggested to be by the direct action of adenosine and guanosine on the cyclic AMP and cyclic GMP systems.

3. Effects of Inhibitors

The stimulation of insulin release by inosine is not inhibited by man-noheptulose (Capito and Hedeskov, 1976). p-Nitrobenzylthioguanosine, an inhibitor of nucleoside transport, inhibited purine ribonucleoside-induced insulin release; formycin B, an inhibitor of purine nucleoside phos-phorylase, inhibited the effects of inosine and adenosine; coformycin, an inhibitor of adenosine deaminase, inhibited only adenosine-induced insulin release (Jain and Logothetopoulos, 1978). Coformycin also inhibited ox-idation of $[U{-}^{14}C]$adenosine but not of inosine; the oxidation of inosine was reduced by formycin B and almost abolished by p-nitrobenzylthio-guanosine.

4. Metabolic Pathways

An outline of the probable metabolic pathway involved in the metabolism of inosine is given in Fig 2. The presence of purine nucleoside phosphorylase in mouse islets has been demonstrated and evidence pro-vided that the ribose-1-phosphate moiety is further metabolized through the pentose cycle (Capito and Hedeskov, 1976). Campbell and Taylor (1977) showed that rabbit islets, in which inosine failed to stimulate insulin release, had much lower nucleoside phosphorylase activity than rat islets, which in their experiments could be stimulated by inosine to release insulin.

5. Conclusions

The ability of inosine and other ribonucleosides to elicit insulin release is correlated with their ability to be metabolized by pancreatic islets.

IV. EXPERIMENTAL MANIPULATIONS

The substrate site hypothesis has been further explored by measuring metabolic parameters under conditions in which secretory responses have been modified. Here are considered studies on islets from fasting animals, on glucose-loaded islets, and on islets during development.

A. Fasting

A diminished insulin secretory response to glucose during starvation has been noted in several species (Cahill et al., 1966; Vance et al., 1968; Malaisse et al., 1967b). There is, however, evidence that this effect may not be confined to the response to glucose; thus diminished secretion in response to leucine and high K^+ (Ashcroft, 1976; Hedeskov and Capito,

1975b), tolbutamide (Ashcroft, 1976), and inosine (Capito and Hedeskov, 1976) has also been observed and the tendency of caffeine to restore secretory responses to normal may indicate an effect on the adenylate cyclase system. Direct support for this possibility has been provided by the demonstration of long-term effects of glucose on islet adenylate cyclase activity (Howell et al., 1973). In other studies (Levy et al., 1976), however, starvation specifically decreased glucose-stimulated insulin release, responses to leucine, tolbutamide, and glyceraldehyde being unaffected by fasting. Evidence from several studies suggests a metabolic basis for the impairment by starvation of the insulin response to glucose and to inosine. In homogenates of islets from fasted rats, the rates of glucose and fructose 6-phosphate phosphorylation were diminished; a preferential effect on the high K_m enzyme for glucose phosphorylation was observed (Malaisse et al., 1976c). Hedeskov and Capito (1974) found that islet glucose utilization and lactate output were decreased in islets from starved mice. These authors suggested that the V_{max} of glucokinase was unchanged but that its effective K_m in the whole islet was increased by starvation. On the other hand, Malaisse et al. (1976c) concluded that in rat islets the effect of starvation was on the V_{max} and not on the K_m of glucokinase. Despite these differences it is clear that the decrease in glucose utilization in islets from starved animals may account, at least in part, for the reduced secretory responses to glucose (Levy et al., 1976).

It has also been found that islet inosine metabolism, as measured by lactate output, is markedly depressed by starvation, in parallel with inosine-stimulated insulin release (Capito and Hedeskov, 1976). Inosine produced a higher content of fructose 1,6-diphosphate plus triose phosphate during starvation than that seen in islets from fed mice; this change is opposite that seen with glucose. No effect of starvation on islet nucleotide phosphorylase activity could be detected (Capito and Hedeskov, 1976).

B. Glucose Loading

If glycolysis from exogenous glucose underlies the stimulatory action of glucose on insulin release, then it should also be possible to elicit insulin release by breakdown of endogenous glycogen. However, normal islet glycogen stores are low and contribute little if at all to glycolytic flux. Malaisse et al. (1977) preincubated rat islets for 20 hr in the presence of high (83.3 mM) glucose; this procedure greatly elevated the islet content of glycogen. When such islets were subsequently incubated in the absence of glucose, theophylline elicited a marked stimulation of glycogenolysis and glycolysis, which was accompanied by a dramatic stimulation of insulin release. These findings further support the substrate site hypothesis.

C. Development

In a number of species glucose is a poor stimulus of insulin release during the late fetal and immediate neonatal periods (Grasso *et al.,* 1968; Asplund, 1972; Milner, 1969) (see also Chapter 2). Attempts to implicate the cyclic AMP system in this phenomenon have not been conclusive (Grill *et al.,* 1975). Therefore a metabolic basis has been sought. It has been found that in contrast to glucose, glyceraldehyde is a potent stimulator of insulin release in islets isolated from neonatal rats (Agren *et al.,* 1976). Therefore any metabolic defect is likely to occur at a step during or prior to triose phosphate formation. Glucose phosphorylation is an obvious candidate, and evidence has been found that glucokinase activity may be lower in neonatal rat islets (Andersson *et al.,* 1975). Moreover, the induction of sensitivity to glucose by culture of neonatal islets parallels the appearance of glucokinase (Agren *et al.,* 1975). The introduction of tissue culture techniques and the long-term effects of glucose, hormones, and other factors on secretory responses of cultured islets affords the possibility of further definition of the regulatory components of the stimulus–response systems.

V. METABOLITES AND COFACTORS OF POSSIBLE IMPORTANCE IN STIMULUS–SECRETION COUPLING

Insulin secretion is dependent on an adequate supply of ATP, and in situations where islet ATP production is impaired secretory responses show a parallel decline (Ashcroft *et al.,* 1973). However, as discussed earlier, stimulation of the release of insulin by exogenous fuels cannot be attributed solely to the generation of ATP, and changes in the concentration of metabolites or cofactors as a consequence of metabolic transformation of stimulatory nutrients are envisaged to play a key role in stimulus–secretion coupling. Studies on the way in which the metabolism of glucose and other metabolized secretagogues may be linked to the rise in intracellular Ca^{2+} concentration, the event believed to be of prime importance in triggering exocytosis, have thus far produced evidence relating to two possible control events. The first of these concerns the hypothesis that the extent of reduction of nicotinamide adenine dinucleotides within the β cell may be of critical importance in regulating Ca^{2+} flux into the β-cell cytosol. Electrophysiological data and measurements of K^+ or Rb^+ fluxes (Henquin, 1977, 1978; Matthews and Sakamoto, 1975; Meissner, 1976) have indicated that Ca^{2+} influx occurs via a voltage-dependent Ca^{2+} channel opened by a decrease in membrane permeability to K^+. The latter could conceivably be regulated by the redox state of sulfhydryl groups in membrane proteins

(Hellman et al., 1978) linked directly, or via an intermediary redox couple such as the glutathione system (Ammon et al., 1977), to a nicotinamide adenine dinucleotide redox system. The second possibility explored is that islet mitochondrial Ca^{2+} uptake may play a role in the regulation of cytosolic free Ca^{2+} concentration.

A. Nicotinamide Adenine Dinucleotides

Evidence for an involvement of the extent of reduction of nicotinamide adenine dinucleotides in stimulus–secretion coupling has come from several lines of experimentation. Microfluorimetry of intact pancreatic islets has demonstrated increases in the fluorescence of islet nicotinamide adenine dinucleotides in response to various stimulants including glucose, leucine, and 2-oxoacids (Panten et al., 1973, 1974). Measurements of the nicotinamide adenine dinucleotide content in islets exposed to stimulants such as glucose, pyruvate, leucine, and 4-methyl-2-oxopentanoate (Malaisse et al., 1979a,c; Sener et al., 1978b; Hutton et al., 1979b; Ammon et al., 1979) or to inhibitors such as menadione, NH_4^+, and methylene blue (Malaisse et al., 1978a,b; Sener et al., 1978c; Ammon and Vespohl, 1979) show correlations between rates of insulin release and the whole-tissue concentrations of reduced nicotinamide adenine dinucleotides. For 4-methyl-2-oxopentanoate-induced insulin release, as discussed above, the $NADPH/NADP^+$ ratio was correlated more closely with insulin release than the $NADH/NAD^+$ ratio. A limitation of the above studies is that they do not give information on the changes in any particular cellular compartment, whereas it is known that the mitochondrial and cytosolic $NADPH/NADP^+$ and $NADH/NAD^+$ ratios may differ by several orders of magnitude. So far only one study attempted to overcome this problem of compartmentation. With a method originally applied to liver (Veech et al., 1969), the islet cytosolic $NADPH/NADP^+$ ratio was estimated (Ashcroft and Christie, 1979). It was found that this ratio was increased from 16 to 26 when the extracellular glucose concentration was increased from 2 to 20 mM. The observed cytosolic $NADPH/NADP^+$ ratios were considerably greater than the whole-tissue ratios of 1.3–2.7 reported by Malaisse et al. (1978b), underlining the importance of the problem of compartmentation.

B. Phosphoenolpyruvate

In addition to influx into the cell, it is likely that the uptake and release of Ca^{2+} by intracellular organelles is important in controlling the Ca^{2+} concentration of the β-cell cytosol. A mitochondrial fraction from rat islets was shown to accummulate $^{45}Ca^{2+}$ in the presence of respiratory substrate and a permeant anion (Sugden and Ashcroft, 1978). Uptake was enhanced by ATP and inhibited by respiratory chain inhibitors, by uncoupling agents, or by ruthenium red. Evidence was also obtained for an inhibitory effect of methylxanthines on mitochondrial Ca^{2+} uptake. That such a system may be modulated by glucose metabolism was suggested by the finding that Ca^{2+} uptake was inhibited by certain glycolytic intermediates, including fructose 1,6-diphosphate and PEP. The effect of PEP was observed at physiological concentrations of this intermediate. The possible importance of this action of PEP was indicated by the finding that the islet content of PEP was increased by glucose or by glyceraldehyde; mannoheptulose prevented the glucose-induced rise in PEP but not that evoked by glyceraldehyde (Sugden and Ashcroft, 1977). Thus it was suggested (Sugden and Ashcroft, 1978) that PEP may influence the magnitude, duration, and intracellular location of the increase in cytosolic Ca^{2+} in response to glucose or glyceraldehyde, via inhibition of mitochondrial Ca^{2+} uptake. Studies on the intracellular distribution of Ca^{2+} in glucose-stimulated islets have provided some support for this concept (Hahn *et al.*, 1979).

The following working hypothesis has been proposed (Ashcroft, 1980) on the basis of these observations. An increased glucose concentration leads to an increase in glucose metabolism, generating an increase in islet PEP and the $NADPH/NADP^+$ ratio. The latter change decreases membrane K^+ permeability, and the consequent depolarization causes Ca^{2+} influx through voltage-dependent Ca^{2+} channels. An increase in cytosolic Ca^{2+} concentration ensues, which leads to exocytosis; PEP, by restraining the uptake of Ca^{2+} into mitochondria, helps to maintain the elevated Ca^{2+} concentration. It is possible that the regulation of mitochondrial Ca^{2+} uptake may also be involved in the response to stimulants other than glucose and glyceraldehyde, but there is no relevant evidence.

VI. CONCLUSIONS

The concept that the ability of glucose to stimulate insulin release is dependent upon its metabolism within the β cell, the substrate site hypothesis, has been subjected to extensive investigation. In general the results of the studies reviewed here have provided convincing support for the model. There are no clear-cut examples of dissociation of metabolic flux from secretory ability and many instances of verification of rather strong predictions of the substrate site hypothesis. Although outside the scope of this chapter, there is also good evidence of the applicability of the model to glucose-stimulated insulin biosynthesis (Ashcroft *et al.*, 1978) (see

Chapter 4). In addition, available data point to a metabolic basis for the recognition of leucine as a stimulant for insulin release. However, the effects of other amino acids such as arginine are not so readily explicable. Nor can one conclude that the substrate site model represents the sole mechanism for recognition of sugars, particularly in view of the studies of Davis and Lazarus (1976). Major gaps in our knowledge of the control of insulin secretion include a lack of quantitative information on the energetics of β-cell processes involved in exocytosis and precise identification of the components of the discharge system. As in many other biochemical processes, further progress will demand a deeper understanding of events within and across cellular membranes.

REFERENCES

Agren, A., Brolin, S. E., and Hellerstrom, C. (1975). *Diabetologia* **11**, 329.
Agren, A., Andersson A., and Hellerstrom, C. (1976). *FEBS Lett.* **71**, 185.
Ammon, H. P. T., and Verspohl, E. J. (1979). *Diabetologia* **17**, 41.
Ammon, H. P. T., Akhtar, M. S., Niklas, H., and Hegner, D. (1977). *Mol. Pharmacol.* **13**, 598.
Ammon, H. P. T., Hoppe, E., Akhtar, M. S., and Niklas, H. (1979) *Diabetes* **28**, 593.
Andersson, A., Grill, V., Asplund, K., Berne, C., Agren, A., and Hellerstrom, C. (1975). *In* "Early Diabetes in Early Life" (R. Camerini-Davalos and H. S. Cole, eds.), pp. 49–56. Academic Press, New York.
Ashcroft, S. J. H. (1976) *Ciba Symp.* **41**, 117.
Ashcroft, S. J. H. (1980) *Diabetologia* **18**, 5.
Ashcroft, S. J. H., and Christie, M. R. (1959). *Biochem. J.* **184**, 697.
Ashcroft, S. J. H., and Crossley, J. R. (1975). *Diabetologia* **11**, 279.
Ashcroft, S. J. H., and Lowry, M. (1979). *Diabetologia* **17**, 165.
Ashcroft, S. J. H., and Nino S. (1978). *Biochim. Biophys. Acta* **538**, 334.
Ashcroft, S. J. H., and Randle, P. J. (1968). *Nature (London)* **219**, 857.
Ashcroft, S. J. H., and Randle, P. J. (1969). *Acta Diabetol. Lat.* **6**, Suppl. 1, 538.
Ashcroft, S. J. H., and Randle, P. J. (1970). Biochem. J. **119**, 5.
Ashcroft, S. J. H., Hedeskov C. J , and Randle, P. J. (1970). *Biochem. J.* **118**, 143.
Ashcroft, S. J. H., Weerasinghe. L. C. C., Bassett, J. M., and Randle, P. J. (1972a). *Biochem. J.* **126**, 525.
Ashcroft, S. J. H., Bassett, J. M., and Randle, P. J. (1972b). *Diabetes* **21**, Suppl 2, 538.
Ashcroft, S. J. H., Weerasinghe, L. C. C., and Randle, P. J. (1973), *Biochem, J.* **132**, 223.
Ashcroft, S. J. H., Crossley, J. R , and Crossley, P. C. (1976). *Biochem. J.* **154**, 701.
Ashcroft, S. J. H., Bunce, J., Lowry, M., Hansen, S. E., and Hedeskov, C. J. (1978) *Biochem. J.* **174**, 517.
Ashcroft, S. J. H., Sugden, M. C., and Williams, I. H. (1980). *Horm. Metab. Res. Suppl. Ser.* **10**, 1.
Asplund, K. (1972). *Diabetologia* **8**, 13.
Berne, C. (1975). *Biochem. J.* **152**, 667.
Brolin, S. E., and Berne, C. (1970). *In* "The Structure and Metabolism of the Pancreatic Islets" (S. Falkmer, B. Hellman, and I.-B. Täljedal, eds.), pp. 245–252. Pergamon, Oxford.

Cahill, J. F., Herrera, M. G., Morgan, A. P., Soeldner, J. S., Steinke, J., Levy, P. L., Reichard, G. H., and Kipnis, D. M. (1966). *J. Clin. Invest.* **45**, 1751.

Campbell, I. L., and Taylor, K. W. (1977). *Biochem. J.* **168**, 591.

Capito, K., and Hedeskov, C. J. (1976). *Biochem. J.* **158**, 335.

Christensen, N. H., Hellman, B., Lernmark, A., Sehlin, J., Tager, H. S., and Taljedal, I-B (1971). *Biochim. Biophys. Acta* **241**, 341.

Coore H. G., and Randle, P. J. (1964). *Biochem. J.* **93**, 66.

Curry, D. L. (1974). *Am. J. Physiol.* **226**, 1073.

Davis, B., and Lazarus, N. (1976). *J. Physiol. (London)* **256**, 709.

Floyd, J. C., Fajans, S. S., Conn, J. W., Knopf, R. F., and Rull, J. (1966). *J. Clin. Invest.* **45**, 1487.

Georg, R. H., Sussman, K. E., Leitner, J. W., and Kirsch, K. M. (1971). *Endocrinology* **89**, 169.

Gerich, J. E., Charles, M. A., and Grodsky, G. M. (1974). *J. Clin. Invest.* **54**, 833.

Grasso, S., Saporito, N., Messina, A., and Reitano, G. (1968). *Lancet* **2**, 755.

Grill, V., Asplund, K., Hellerstrom, C., and Cerasi, E. (1975). *Diabetes* **24**, 746.

Grodsky, G. M., Batts, A. A., Bennett, L. L., Vcella, C., McWilliams, N. B., and Smith, D. F. (1963). *Am. J. Physiol.* **205**, 638.

Gylfe, E. (1974). *Biochim. Biophys. Acta* **343**, 584.

Gylfe, E., and Hellman, B. (1974) *Endocrinology* **94**, 1150.

Gylfe, E., and Sehlin, J. (1976). *Horm. Metab. Res.* **8**, 7.

Hahn, H. J., Gylfe, E., and Hellman, B. (1979). *FEBS Lett.* **103**, 348.

Hedeskov, C. J., and Capito, K. (1974). *Biochem. J.* **140**, 423.

Hedeskov, C. J., and Capito, K. (1975a). *Biochem. J.* **152**, 571.

Hedeskov, C. J., and Capito, K. (1975b). *Horm. Metab. Res.* **7**, 1.

Hedeskov, C. J., and Capito, K. (1980). *Horm. Metab. Res. Suppl. Ser.* **10**, 8.

Hedeskov, C. J., Hertz, L., and Nissen, C. (1972). *Biochim. Biophys. Acta* **261**, 388.

Hellerstrom, C. (1964). *Acta Endocrinol.* **45**, 122.

Hellerstrom, C. (1967). *Endocrinology* **81**, 105.

Hellman, B., and Idahl, L.-A. (1970). *In* "The Structure and Metabolism of the Pancreatic Islets" (S. Falkmer, B. Hellman, and Täljedal, I.-B. eds.), pp. 253–262. Pergamon, Oxford.

Hellman, B., Sehlin, J., and Täljedal, I.-B. (1971). *Biochem. J.* **123**, 513.

Hellman, B., Lernmark, A., Sehlin, J., and Täljedal, I.-B. (1972). *Metabolism* **21**, 60.

Hellman, B., Idahl, L.-A., Lernmark, A., Sehlin, J., and Täljedal, I.-B. (1973a). *Biochem. J.* **132**, 775.

Hellman, B., Sehlin, J., and Täljedal, I.-B. (1973b). *Pfluegers Arch.* **340**, 51.

Hellman, B., Idahl, L.-A., Lernmark, A., Sehlin, J., and Täljedal, I.-B. (1974a). *Biochem. J.* **138**, 33.

Hellman, B., Idahl, L-A., Sehlin, J., and Täljedal, I.-B. (1974b). *Arch. Biochem. Biophys.* **162**, 448.

Hellman, B., Idahl, L.-A., Sehlin, J., and Täljedal, I.-B. (1975). *Diabetologia* **11**, 495.

Hellman, B., Lernmark, A., Sehlin, J., Soderberg, M., and Täljedal, I.-B. (1978). *Endocrinology* **99**, 1398.

Henquin, J. C. (1977). *Biochem. Biophys. Res. Commun.* **77**, 551.

Henquin, J. C. (1978). *Nature (London)* **271**, 271.

Holze, S., and Panten, U. (1979). *Biochim. Biophys. Acta* **588**, 211.

Howell, S. L., Green, I. C., and Montague, W. (1973). *Biochem. J.* **136**, 343.

Hutton, J. C., Sener, A., and Malaisse, W. J. (1979a). *Biochem. J.* **184**, 291.

Hutton, J. C., Sener, A., and Malaisse, W. J. (1979b). *Biochem. J.* **184**, 303.

Hutton, J. C., Sener, A., Herchuelz, A., Atwater, I., Kawazu, S., Boschero, A. C., Somers, C., Devis, G., and Malaisse, W. J. (1980). *Endocrinology* **106**, 203.

Idahl, L.-A., Rahemtulla, F., Sehlin, J., and Täljedal, I.-B. (1976). *Diabetes* **25**, 450.

Ismail, N. A., and Montague, W. M (1977). *Biochim. Biophys. Acta* **498**, 325.

Ismail, N. A., El Denshary, E. S. M., and Montague, W. M. (1977). *Biochem. J.* **164**, 409.

Jain, K., and Logothetopoulos, J. (1978). *Biochem. J.* **170**, 461.

Jain, K. Logothetopoulos, J., and Zucker, P. (1975). *Biochim. Biophys, Acta* **399**, 384.

Keen, H., Sells, R., and Jarrett, R. J. (1965). *Diabetologia* **1**, 28.

Kuzuya, T., Kanagawa, Y., and Kosaka, K. (1966). *Metab. Clin. Exp.* **15**, 1149.

Landgraf, R., Kotler-Brajtburg, J., and Matschinsky, F. M. (1971). *Proc. Natl. Acad. Sci. U.S.A.* **68**, 536.

Lenzen, S., and Panten, U. (1980). *Biochem. J.* **186**, 135.

Levy, J., Herchuelz, A., Sener, A., and Malaisse, W. J. (1976). *Metabolism* **25**, 583.

McDaniel, M. L., Weaver, D. C., Roth, C. E., Fink, C. J., Swanson, C. J., and Lacy, P. E. (1977). *Endocrinology* **101**, 1701.

Macdonald, M. J., Ball, D. H., Patel, T. N., Lauris, U., and Steinke, J. (1975). *Biochim. Biophys. Acta* **385**, 188.

Malaisse, W. J., and Malaisse-Lagae F. (1968). *J. Lab. Clin. Med.* **72**, 438.

Malaisse, W. J., Malaisse-Lagae, F., and Wright, P. H. (1967a). *Endocrinology* **80**, 99.

Malaisse W. J., Malaisse-Lagae, F., and Wright, P. H. (1967b). *Am J. Physiol.* **213**, 843.

Malaisse, W. J., Sener, A., and Mahy, M. (1974). *Eur. J. Biochem.* **47**, 365.

Malaisse, W. J., Sener, A., Koser, M., and Herchuelz, A. (1976a). *J. Biol. Chem.* **251**, 5936.

Malaisse, W. J., Sener, A., Levy, J., and Herchuelz, A. (1976b). *Acta Diabetol. Lat.* **13**, 202.

Malaisse, W. J., Sener, A., and Levy, J. (1976c). *J. Biol. Chem.* **251**, 1731.

Malaisse, W. J., Sener, A., Koser, M., Rawazzola, M., and Malaisse-Lagae, F. (1977). *Biochem. J.* **164**, 647.

Malaisse, W. J., Sener, A., Boschero, A. C., Kawazu, S., Devis, G., and Somers, G. (1978a). *Eur. J. Biochem.* **87**, 111.

Malaisse, W. J., Hutton, J. C., Kawazu, S., and Sener A. (1978b). *Eur. J. Biochem.* **87**, 121.

Malaisse, W. J., Sener, A., Herchuelz, A., and Hutton, J. C. (1979a). *Metabolism* **28**, 373.

Malaisse, W. J., Kawazu, S., Herchuelz, A., Hutton, J. C., Somers, G., Devis, G., and Sener, A. (1979b). *Arch. Biochem. Biophys.* **194**, 49.

Malaisse, W. J., Hutton, J. C., Kawazu, S., Herchuelz, A., Valverde, I., and Sener, A. (1979c). *Diabetologia,* **16**, 331.

Matschinsky F. M., and Ellermann, J. E. (1968). *J. Biol. Chem.* **243**, 2730.

Matschinsky, F. M., and Ellerman, J. (1973). *Biochem. Biophys. Res. Commun.* **50**, 193.

Matthews, E. K., and Sakamoto, Y. (1975). *J. Physiol. (London)* **246**, 439.

Meissner, H. P. (1976). *J. Physiol.* **72**, 757.

Milner, R. D. G. (1969). *J. Endocrinol.* **44**, 267.

Milner, R. D. G., and Hales, C. N. (1967). *Diabetologia* **3**, 47.

Montague, W., and Taylor, K. W. (1968) *Biochem. J.* **109**, 333.

Moskalewski, S. (1965). *Gen. Comp. Endocrinol.* **5**, 342.

Niki, A., Niki, H., Miwa, I., and Okuda, J. (1974). *Science* **186**, 150.

Niki, A., Niki, H., and Miwa, I (1979). *Endocrinology* **105**, 1051.

Pagliara, A. S., Stillings, S. N., Hover B., Martin, D. M., and Matschinsky, F. M. (1974). *J. Clin Invest.* **54**, 819.

Panten, U., v. Kriegstein, E., Poser, W., Schonborn, J., and Hasselblatt, A. (1972). *FEBS Lett.* **20**, 225.

Panten, U., Christians, J., Kriegstein, E. V., Poser, W., and Hasselblatt, A. (1974). *Diabetologia* **10**, 149.

Randle, P. J., Ashcroft, S. J. H., and Gill, J. R. (1968). *In* "Carbohydrate Metabolism and Its Disorders" (F. Dickens, P. J. Randle, and W. J. Whelan, eds.), Vol. 1, pp. 427–447. Academic Press, New York.

Reese, A. C., Landau, B. R., Craig, J. W., Gin, G., and Rodman, H. M. (1973). *Metabolism* **22**, 467.

Sener, A., and Malaisse, W. J. (1978). *Diabete et metab. (Paris)* **4**, 127.

Sener, A., and Malaisse, W. J. (1980). *Nature (London)* **288**, 187.

Sener, A., Devis, G., Somers, G., and Malaisse, W. J. (1977). *Diabetologia* **13**, 125.

Sener, A., Pipeleers, D. G., Levy, J., and Malaisse, W. J. (1978a). *Metabolism* **27**, 1505.

Sener, A., Kawazu, S., Hutton, J. C., Boschero, A. C., Devis, G., Somers, G., Herchuelz, A., and Malaisse, W. J. (1978b). *Biochem. J.* **176**, 217.

Sener, A., Hutton, J. C., Kawazu, S., Boschero, A. C., Somers, G., Devis, G., Herchuelz, H., and Malaisse, W. J. (1978c). *J. Clin. Invest.* **62**, 868.

Snyder, P. J., Kashket, S., and O'Sullivan, N. B. (1969). *Am. J. Physiol.* **219**, 876.

Sugden, M. C., and Ashcroft, S. J. H. (1977). *Diabetologia* **13**, 481.

Sugden, M. C., and Ashcroft, S. J. H. (1978). *Diabetologia* **15**, 173.

Täljedal, I.-B. (1969). *Biochem. J.* **114**, 387.

Vance, J. E., Buchanan, K. D., and Williams, R. H. (1968). *J. Lab. Clin. Med.* **72**, 290.

Veech, R. L., Eggleston, L. V., and Drebs, H. A. (1969). *Biochem. J.* **115**, 609.

Verspohl, E. J., Handel, M., and Ammon, H. P. T. (1979). *Endocrinology* **105**, 1269.

Williams, I. H. (1979). D. Phil. Thesis, Univ. of Oxford, Oxford.

Williams, I. H., and Ashcroft, S. J. H. (1978). *FEBS Lett.* **87**, 115.

Zawalich (1979). *Diabetes* **28**, 252.

Zawalich, W. S., and Matschinsky, F. M. (1977). *Endocrinology* **100**, 1.

Zawalich, W. S., Pagliara, A. S., and Matschinsky, F. M. (1977a). *Endocrinology* **100**, 1276.

Zawalich, W. S. Rognstad, R., Pagliara, A. S., and Matschinsky, F. M. (1977b). *J. Biol. Chem.* **252**, 8519.

Zawalich, W. S., Dye, E. S., Rognstad, R., and Matschinsky, F. M. (1978). *Endocrinology* **103**, 2027.

Zawalich, W. S., Dye, E. S., and Matschinsky, F. M. (1979). *Biochem. J.* **180**, 145.

7

Inorganic Ions in Insulin Secretion

W. J. MALAISSE, A. HERCHUELZ,
and A. SENER

I. INTRODUCTION

The sequence of cytophysiological events leading to the release of insulin by the pancreatic B cell in response to stimulation by appropriate secretagogues includes three major steps.

149

The Islets of Langerhans
Copyright © 1981 by Academic Press, Inc.
All rights of reproduction in any form reserved.
ISBN 0–12–187820–1

The first step consists of the recognition of insulinotropic agents by the B cell. The modality of such a recognition process differs from one insulin-releasing agent to another. It is currently thought that hormones and neurotransmitters such as catecholamines, cholinergic agents, and polypeptidic hormones which participate in either enteroinsular axis or intraislet paracrine processes bind to specific membrane receptors in islet cells, and that their stimulatory or inhibitory effects upon insulin release are initiated by such a binding phenomenon (Goldfine *et al.,* 1972; Verspohl and Ammon, 1980). In the case of nutrient secretagogues, e.g., glucose and leucine, there is increasing evidence implying that the metabolism of these nutrients is an essential component of their recognition by islet cells (Ashcroft, 1980; Malaisse *et al.,* 1979b) (see Chapter 6). Yet, with other secretagogues, e.g., hypo- or hyperglycemic sulfonamides and the tumor promoter phorboldiester, an interference with some biophysical property of the B-cell membrane may represent the initial event in the secretory sequence (Couturier and Malaisse, 1980; Malaisse *et al.,* 1980b).

The second step in such a sequence consists of the coupling of the recognition process to activation of the effector system responsible for the exocytosis of secretory granules. Here emphasis is currently given to the role of intracellular Ca^{2+} as an apparent trigger for insulin release (Malaisse *et al.,* 1978b). It is obvious that, because of the variety of processes involved in the recognition of insulinotropic agents, an equally variable series of coupling factors may participate in the control of Ca^{2+} movements in islet cells. If the assumption is made that the accumulation of Ca^{2+} in the cytosol of the B cell, or in its ectoplasmic compartment, indeed triggers insulin release, all coupling factors should somehow either alter the transport of Ca^{2+} across the plasma membrane and/or the membrane of intracellular organelles in the B cell or, otherwise, affect the binding of Ca^{2+} to molecular structures in contact with the cytosol.

The last step in the secretory sequence can be viewed as motile events responsible for the translocation of secretory granules and their extrusion from the B cell by exocytosis. A microtubule–microfilament system is here thought to play a key role in controlling the access of secretory granules to the exocytotic sites (Malaisse and Orci, 1979) (see Chapter 5).

Each of these three major steps in the secretory sequence may be affected by or closely dependent on the movements and concentrations of ions. Since the pilot studies of Grodsky and Bennett (1966) and those of Milner and Hales (1967), the participation of ions in the insulin secretory sequence continues to be the subject of so many investigations that it is almost beyond our capacity to provide a balanced overview of this field of research. Let us therefore use the excuse of limitations in space to justify the bias of this chapter, which is restricted to selected topics on the general theme of ions and insulin release.

II. PARTICIPATION OF IONS IN THE RECOGNITION OF INSULINOTROPIC AGENTS

The ionic environment of the B cell may affect the recognition of insulinotropic agents in several ways. First, certain ions may influence the binding of the secretagogue to the plasma membrane or its transport across such a membrane. For instance, the accumulation of glibenclamide in pancreatic islets is affected by the concentration of Na^+ and divalent cations in the incubation medium (Hellman et al., 1976). Second, in the case of nutrient secretagogues, the ionic environment may feed back on the rate of nutrient utilization. Indeed, in the B cell, as in other tissues, a significant fraction of the energy generated by the metabolism of nutrients may be used, at the intervention of specific ATPases, to maintain appropriate ionic gradients across membrane system(s). Third, a change in the extracellular or intracellular concentration of ions may affect the activity of certain enzymes involved in the recognition of secretagogues.

A few examples of such interferences will be considered here.

A. Islet Function and the HCO_3^- Ion

Henquin and Lambert (1976) first reported that a sufficient concentration of HCO_3^- was required for glucose to exert its normal insulinotropic action. In a more recent work, we observed that the absence of extracellular HCO_3^- markedly reduced the rate of O_2 consumption, whether in the presence or absence of an exogenous nutrient (Hutton and Malaisse, 1980). This phenomenon may be related to the presence in islet cells of a HCO_3^--sensitive ATPase (Sener et al., 1979) (Fig. 1). Since nutrient secretagogues invariably augment the rate of both O_2 consumption and CO_2 production by the islets (Hellerström, 1967; Hellerström and Gunnarsson, 1970), it is tempting to consider that changes in the CO_2 and/or HCO_3^- generation rate may play a role in the fine control of catabolic events in this fuel sensor organ.

B. Glucose Metabolism and Insulin Release in K^+-Deprived Islets

It is well established that changes in the extracellular concentration of Na^+, H^+, or Ca^{2+} affect the metabolism of glucose in isolated islets (Hellman et al., 1974a; Hutton et al., 1980; Malaisse et al., 1978c). Such metabolic effects are currently considered examples of feedback control mechanisms in the regulation of fuel utilization (Malaisse et al., 1980c). Indeed, if the metabolism of glucose plays a key role in causing the remodeling of ionic fluxes eventually leading to insulin release, changes in the ionic environment may in turn affect glucose metabolism so that, under normal

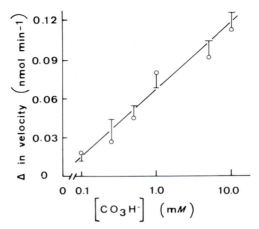

Fig. 1. Effect of HCO_3^- on ATPase activity in islet homogenates. The increase in velocity (nmoles per minute per islet) attributable to HCO_3^- is shown as a function of the HCO_3^- concentration (logarithmic scale).

conditions, the catabolic flux eventually and precisely matches the energy demand of stimulated islet cells.

With this perspective, we have recently explored the situation found in K^+-deprived islets in order to evaluate the role of K^+–Na^+-activated ATPase in the ATP turnover of islet cells (Sener *et al.*, 1980). The results of this study suggest that such an ATPase accounts for approximately 10% of the basal energy expenditure in isolated islets. The latter value is in good agreement with a 1:2 stoichiometry for ATP–K^+ active inflow into the islet cells (Malaisse *et al.*, 1980c).

From the functional standpoint, although the prevalent short-term effect of K^+ deprivation is to augment basal or glucose-stimulated insulin release (Herchuelz and Malaisse, 1980b; Somers *et al.*, 1980a, inhibition of glucose-stimulated proinsulin biosynthesis and insulin secretion was evident in long-term experiments (Sener and Malaisse, 1980). A comparison of the time course and reversibility of the inhibitory action of K^+ deprivation and glucose deprivation, respectively, upon insulin release led us to propose that the accumulation of K^+ evoked by nutrient secretagogues in islet cells may somehow participate in their "memory," i.e., their enhanced capacity to release insulin after a prior period of exposure to glucose (Grill and Cerasi, 1978).

C. Participation of Calmodulin in Insulin Release

It is well established that glucose increases the calcium content of islet cells as judged from chemical (Malaisse *et al.*, 1978b), radioisotopic

(Malaisse-Lagae and Malaisse, 1971), or ultrastructural criteria (Ravazzola et al., 1976; Schäfer and Klöppel, 1974). Most other secretagogues examined for such a purpose also affect the handling of calcium in islet cells. It is assumed, but remains to be proved, that the accumulation of calcium in islet cells coincides with an increased cytosolic concentration of ionized Ca^{2+}. It was recently reported that islets contained a calcium-dependent regulatory protein known as calmodulin (Sugden et al., 1979; Valverde et al., 1979). This finding has suggested that the accumulation of Ca^{2+} in islet cells may in turn affect enzyme systems susceptible to regulation by calmodulin. Much work remains to be performed to scrutinize, in the islets, the effect of calmodulin upon such enzymes as cyclic AMP and cyclic GMP phosphodiesterases, Ca^{2+}-activated ATPase, and protein kinases, in order to assess the role of calmodulin in insulin release.

So far, it has been found that calmodulin binds to a subcellular particulate fraction derived from the islets and activates adenylate cyclase in the same fraction (Valverde et al. 1979). Both the binding and activation phenomena are modulated by the concentration of ionized Ca^{2+} in the 10^{-7}–$10^{-4}M$ range. These data provide a possible explanation for the capacity of several insulin secretagogues, known to cause Ca^{2+} accumulation in islet cells, to increase the production or content of cyclic AMP in these cells (Hellman et al., 1974b). The K_m of adenylate cyclase for calmodulin (Fig. 2) is close to 0.1 μM (Valverde et al., 1981), a concentration far below the actual concentration of calmodulin in islet cells (ca. 50 μM). These findings are in good agreement with the view that the cytosolic concentration of Ca^{2+}, rather than that of calmodulin, represents the rate-limiting factor in the activation of adenylate cyclase by the Ca^{2+}-dependent regulatory protein.

Cyclic AMP is known to enhance insulin release evoked by a variety of secretagogues (Malaisse et al., 1967). This effect is apparently due, in part at least, to an intracellular redistribution of Ca^{2+} leading to the cytosolic accumulation of this cation (Brisson et al., 1972; Sehlin, 1976; Sugden and Ashcroft, 1978). The interaction among Ca^{2+}, calmodulin, adenylate cyclase, and cyclic AMP is thus well suited to provide amplification of the secretory response to a given stimulus (Fig. 3).

In a recent work, we have used two presumed specific antagonists of calmodulin to further investigate the validity of the model depicted in Fig. 3. Although these drugs (e.g., trifluoperazine) indeed suppressed the calmodulin-induced increment in adenylate cyclase activity in the islet subcellular fraction, side effects on glucose oxidation, calcium influx, and basal adenylate cyclase activity were observed, so that no definite information on the role of calmodulin in insulin release could be obtained from these experiments (Valverde et al., 1981).

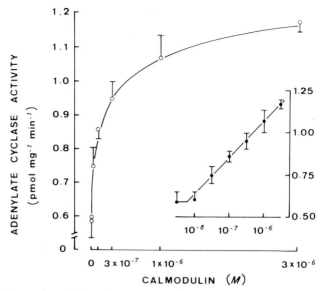

Fig. 2. Dose–action relationship for the effect of exogenous calmodulin on adenylate cyclase activity in an islet subcellular fraction. In the inset, the same data are ranged on a logarithmic scale.

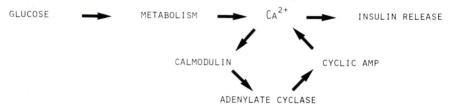

Fig. 3. Schematic model of the interaction among Ca^{2+}, calmodulin, adenylate cyclase, and cyclic AMP in the process of glucose-induced insulin release.

III. PARTICIPATION OF IONS IN THE COUPLING OF STIMULATION TO RELEASE

In considering the ionic aspects of B-cell function, the most complex problem involves the participation of ions in the coupling of the recognition step to the activation of the effector system. For the sake of clarity, we will consider this problem mainly in the framework of the process of glucose-induced insulin release. In introducing such a topic, we will first describe the bioelectrical events recorded in the B cell when stimulated by glucose.

A. Bioelectrical Events in the B Cell

It has been known for more than 12 yr that pancreatic B cells exhibit electrical activity in response to glucose and various other secretagogues (Dean and Matthews, 1968). It has been shown that electrical activity can be correlated with the release of insulin and that changes in membrane potential played a significant role in the mechanisms by which glucose stimulates the release of insulin Hence considerable work has been devoted to study the ionic basis of the glucose-induced potential changes in the pancreatic B cell.

In the absence of any secretagogue, the B cell displays a stable membrane potential of about -45 to -60 mV (Meissner and Preissler, 1979). When the cell is suddenly exposed to an insulinotropic glucose concentration, a slow depolarization of about 15 mV develops within 45–105 sec depending on the glucose concentration used. When the membrane reaches a threshold potential, a further, rapid 10 mV depolarization is observed, which brings the membrane to a plateau potential on which spike activity is superimposed (Fig. 4). After about 30 sec of firing, spike activity stops and the membrane repolarizes to a level slightly more negative than the threshold potential. The electrical activity then proceeds in bursts con-

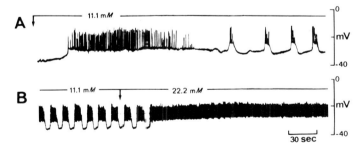

Fig. 4. Membrane potential recordings from two pancreatic B cells showing glucose-induced electrical activity. (A) Phasic response to a sudden increase in glucose concentration from 0 to 11.1 mM in the perifusion solution. Glucose was introduced into the chamber at the time indicated by the arrow. (B) Oscillatory response in the presence of 11.1 mM glucose and continuous spike activity in the presence of 22.2 mM glucose. The glucose concentration in the perifusion solution was switched at the time indicated by the arrow; the solution in the chamber was equilibrated within 5 sec. The vertical axis at the right gives intracellular potential with respect to the potential of the perifusion solution in the chamber. This illustration was kindly provided by Dr. Illani Atwater (Norwich).

sisting of regular sequences of depolarization, spike activity, and repolarization. The bursts which immediately follow the aforementioned initial train of spike activity are short-lived, but their duration progressively increases with time. The threshold, the plateau, and the repolarization potentials are independent of the glucose concentration. Instead, increasing concentrations of glucose affect the duration of spike activity and, at high glucose concentrations, the burst pattern is replaced by a continuous spike activity.

Several lines of evidence suggest that the initial depolarization from the resting to the threshold potential may result from a decrease in the membrane's permeability to potassium. First, glucose depolarization is associated with an increased resistance of the B-cell membrane (Atwater et al., 1978), a finding which suggests that the initial depolarization is not attributable to any major increase in cationic permeability. In agreement with the latter view, the depolarizing effect of glucose is not affected in the absence of extracellular Na^+ or in the presence of cobalt, a selective blocker of calcium entry into the B cell (Meissner and Preissler, 1979). Second, the islet cell membrane potential is K^+-dependent (Meissner et al., 1978). Third, glucose reduces $^{42}K^+$ or $^{86}Rb^+$ efflux from isolated islets, an effect which displays the same dose–action relationship as the glucose-induced initial depolarization (see following section). Last, drugs which decrease islet cell K^+ permeability (e.g., quinine and 9-aminoacridine) depolarize (Meissner and Preissler, 1979), while valinomycin, which increases K^+ permeability, hyperpolarizes the B-cell membrane (Henquin and Meissner, 1978). While this evidence convincingly supports the participation of K^+ in the initial depolarizing effect of glucose, it does not rule out that changes in the handling of other ions may be involved in the sugar depolarizing action. In this respect, it was demonstrated that glucose increased chloride (Sehlin, 1978) and phosphate efflux (Freinkel et al., 1974) from isolated islets, suggesting that these increased permeabilities did indeed participate in the glucose-induced B-cell depolarization.

The fast depolarization from the threshold to the plateau potential has been attributed to the inflow of Ca^{2+} into the B cell (Meissner and Preissler, 1979). It is indeed suppressed under experimental conditions known to impair the entry of Ca^{2+} into the B cell, while the amplitude and the rate of depolarization are increased at a high extracellular Ca^{2+} concentration.

As already mentioned, the bioelectrical (Meissner and Atwater, 1976) and possibly the secretory (Malaisse et al., 1980c) response to glucose appears as a discontinuous or rhythmic phenomenon, except at very high concentrations of glucose. This observation raises the question as to the factor(s) responsible for repolarization at the end of each burst of spikes.

It has been proposed that the repolarization may be due to a calcium-induced activation of potassium permeability (Atwater *et al.*, 1979a,b). Thus glucose in causing Ca^{2+} accumulation in the B cell leads to the latter activation. In good agreement with such a view, both tetraethylammonium and 9-aminoacridine were found to inhibit the repolarization phase (Henquin *et al.*, 1979; Meissner and Preissler, 1979). The repolarization phase of the slow waves may also be brought about partially by the activity of an electrogenic Na^+-K^+- pump (Atwater and Meissner, 1975). It then remains to be explained why, at high glucose concentrations, the spike activity is continuous. To our knowledge there is as yet no satisfactory explanation for the latter phenomenon. It is simply hypothesized that, at high concentrations of glucose, the decrease in potassium permeability is so great as to suppress the effect of factors tending to increase K^+ permeability or activate the electrogenic Na^+ pump (Matthews and O'Connor, 1979).

Matthews and O'Connor (1979) recently reported on a computer simulation of the electrical activity induced by glucose in the B cell. This model illustrates how the ionic mechanisms deduced from experimental observations can account for the electrical patterns produced by B cells in the presence of glucose. Among other features, this model was able to reproduce the oscillation in B-cell transmembrane potential with superimposed bursts of electrical activity. At this point, however, it should be noted that oscillation in metabolic events could conceivably also represent a pacemaker for oscillation in ionic fluxes (Malaisse *et al.*, 1980c).

B. Regulation of K^+ Conductance

The glucose-induced decrease in K^+ conductance apparently represents an essential step of the stimulus–secretion coupling process (Sehlin and Täljedal, 1974). It is indeed responsible for the slow phase of depolarization, hence for the subsequent gating of voltage-dependent Ca^{2+} channels. Incidentally, changes in the fluxes of other ions, such as an increased efflux of Cl^- (Sehlin, 1978), may also participate in the phenomenon of depolarization.

Because of its essential role, the decrease in K^+ conductance was the object of several recent studies based mainly on the use of $^{86}Rb^+$ as a tracer for the movements of $^{39}K^+$ (Boschero and Malaisse, 1979; Carpinelli and Malaisse, 1980a,c,d; Henquin, 1978, 1979, 1980; Malaisse *et al.*, 1978a). The validity for such a procedure was fully assessed by the comparison of data obtained with $^{86}Rb^+$ and $^{42}K^+$ (Boschero *et al.*, 1977; Malaisse *et al.*, 1978a). However, considerable caution should be exerted in ascribing changes in $^{86}Rb^+$ fractional outflow rate from perifused islets solely to alteration in the plasma membrane conductance for K^+. Indeed, radioisotopic data may well reflect, to a limited extent, redistribution of the tracer ion between distinct subcellular compartments, such as the cytosol and mitochondria (Carpinelli and Malaisse, 1980c,d). With this reservation in mind, there seems little doubt that the decrease in K^+ conductance is tightly coupled to the metabolism of nutrient secretagogues in islet cells (Boschero and Malaisse, 1979). Emphasis is currently given to the apparent role of reducing equivalents (e.g., NADH and NADPH) in the control of K^+ conductance (Henquin, 1980; Malaisse *et al.*, 1978d; Sener *et al.*, 1978). A contributive role of changes in the generation rate of ATP and H^+ in the regulation of K^+ conductance should, however, not be ruled out (Carpinelli and Malaisse, 1980c,d). Incidentally, there is some indication that the effect of glucose on K^+ conductance may indeed be a dual or discontinuous phenomenon (Carpinelli and Malaisse, 1980a).

C. Effects of Glucose on Ca^{2+} Movements in the Islets

The influence of glucose on Ca^{2+} movements in islet cells was recently and extensively reviewed by Herchuelz and Malaisse (1981). The major effects of glucose apparently consist of both a stimulation of Ca^{2+} entry into and an inhibition of Ca^{2+} outflow from the islet cells. These two effects are closely dependent on the integrity of glucose metabolism in the islet cells but display vastly different dose–action relationships at increasing concentrations of glucose (Herchuelz and Malaisse, 1980a), as well as vastly different time courses in reponse to a square-wave increase in the sugar concentration (Malaisse *et al.*, 1981).

The stimulant action of glucose on Ca^{2+} inflow into the islet cells is inferred, *inter alia,* from the secondary rise in $^{45}Ca^{2+}$ outflow occurring a few minutes after the administration of glucose to perifused prelabeled islets. This increase, which can be dissociated from the release of insulin (Herchuelz and Malaisse, 1978), does not occur in the absence of extracellular Ca^{2+}, hence may reflect a phenomenon of exchange between influent $^{40}Ca^{2+}$ and effluent $^{45}Ca^{2+}$ (Herchuelz *et al.*, 1980a). The secondary rise in $^{45}Ca^{2+}$ efflux is delayed relative to the glucose-induced decreases in $^{86}Rb^+$ outflow (Fig. 5) and thus may well be a consequence of the membrane depolarization and subsequent gating of voltage-dependent Ca^{2+} channels (Malaisse *et al.*, 1981). It was also reported that various agents known to affect K^+ conductance (e.g., quinine or tetraethylammonium) and/or to cause depolarization mimic, to a given extent, the effect of glucose upon Ca^{2+} fluxes in the islets (Herchuelz *et al.*, 1980c,d, 1981).

The glucose-induced decrease in Ca^{2+} fractional outflow rate was attributed to inhibition of Na^+–Ca^{2+} countertransport (Herchuelz *et al.,* 1980b), possibly as a result of an increase in the H^+ generation rate (Carpinelli *et al., 1980). The latter view is supported by the finding that H^+ in-

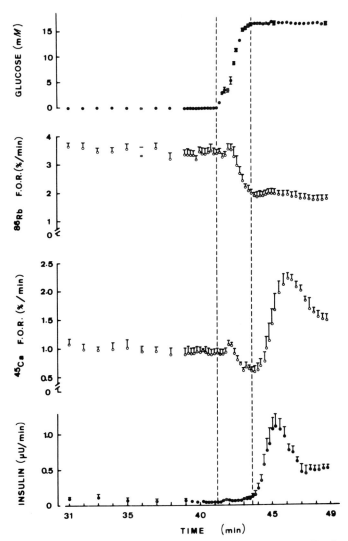

Fig. 5. Timing of the changes in glucose concentration, $^{86}Rb^+$ and $^{45}Ca^{2+}$ fractional outflow rates (F.O.R.), and insulin release in perifused islets.

deed inhibits Na^+-Ca^{2+} countertransport as mediated, in an artificial system, by either the antibiotic ionophore A23187 (Malaisse *et al.,* 1980a) or native ionophores extracted from the islet cells (Anjaneyulu *et al.,* 1980). It is also consistent with the observations that (1) the dose–action relationships for the glucose-induced increment in H^+ net output and decrease in

$^{45}Ca^{2+}$ outflow, respectively, display a comparable hyperbolic pattern (Malaisse *et al.*, 1979a), and (2) the decrease in $^{45}Ca^{2+}$ outflow rate temporally coincides with an increase in the output of lactic and pyruvic acids from the islets (Malaisse *et al.*, 1981).

A last possible effect of glucose on Ca^{2+} handling by islet cells would be to mobilize this cation from intracellular organelles, such as mitochondria and secretory granules. Wollheim and his colleagues (Kikuchi *et al.*, 1979; Wollheim *et al.*, 1978) believe that the first phase of insulin release is mainly caused by such an intracellular translocation which, however, remains to be factually documented.

We have purposedly restricted these considerations to current concepts concerning Ca^{2+} handling by islet cells. There are, however, several relevant findings and views that have not been discussed. Among them, we may mention the idea that the effect of glucose in facilitating Ca^{2+} influx into islet cells may, to a limited extent, be independent of the decrease in K^+ conductance (Boschero *et al.*, 1979). An alternative possibility is that glucose increases the fluidity of the plasma membrane (Table I; Deleers *et al.*, 1981) and, by doing, so, facilitates the transport of calcium, as mediated by native ionophores, in a manner comparable to that found in liposomes (Deleers and Malaisse, 1980).

Another less common view is that Ca^{2+} may somehow exert inhibitory effects in the B cell (Hellman, 1977). It has also been observed that, when tetracycline is used as a probe to investigate the interaction of calcium with the B-cell membrane, glucose reduces the intensity of the calcium-dependent tetracycline fluorescence (Täljedal, 1978, 1979).

D. Quantification of Ca^{2+} Movements

The quantification of Ca^{2+} movements in the islets was recently made possible from the analysis of $^{45}Ca^{2+}$ efflux from prelabeled islets (Herchuelz *et al.*, 1979). This model indicates that glucose (16.7 mM) increases the inflow–outflow rate of Ca^{2+} transport across the cell membrane from a basal value of 120 ± 25 to 275 ± 27 fmol/min per islet (Table II). Based on a mean diameter for the islet cell of 10 μm and a mean intracellular volume of 2.5 nl/islet, the glucose-induced increment in Ca^{2+} inflow represents close to 10 pmol/cm^2 per minute. According to Meissner and Preissler (1979), with 16.7 mM glucose, the plateau phase of electrical activity occupies 74% of the total time with close to 2.5 spikes/sec of active phase, i.e., about 110 spikes/min. Our data thus imply that each spike corresponds to approximately 0.1 pmol/cm^2 of entering Ca^{2+}. The latter value is identical to that calculated by Matthews *et al.* (1975) using a postulated membrane capacitance of 1 μF/cm^2 and an observed action potential of

TABLE I

Glucose-Induced Decrease in Membrane Viscosity[a]

Glucose (mM)	Paired decrease in viscosity		P	n
	Millipoises	Percentage of basal		
Nil	0	0	—	10
5.6	67.1 ± 20.4	3.42 ± 1.12	< 0.02	10
11.1	192.2 ± 46.8	8.76 ± 1.91	< 0.02	5
16.7	300.9 ± 49.5	15.31 ± 2.74	< 0.001	10

[a] The membrane viscosity was measured under steady-state conditions of exposure to increasing concentrations of glucose, the value reached at 37°C being derived from records obtained at increasing temperatures. Mean values (±SEM) for the paired decrease in viscosity below basal value (no glucose) are expressed in both absolute (millipoises) and relative (percentage) terms and are shown together with their statistical significance (P) and the number of individual observations (n). The basal viscosity averaged 2010 ± 120 mP.

TABLE II

Effect of Glucose upon Ionic Fluxes in Islets

Ionic parameter	No glucose	Glucose, 16.7 mM
K^+ total pool (pmol/islet)	161 ± 11	312 ± 38
K^+ inflow-outflow (pmol/min per islet)	14.3 ± 1.6	13.8 ± 1.6
K^+ fractional outflow rate (percentage/min)	8.88 ± 0.34	4.23 ± 0.74
Na^+ total pool (pmol/islet)	157 ± 7	119 ± 7
Na^+ cytosolic pool (percentage of total)	72.3 ± 5.5	75.5 ± 5.4
Na^+ vacuolar pool (percentage of total)	27.7 ± 2.6	24.5 ± 2.3
Na^+ inflow-outflow (pmol/min per islet)	28.4 ± 3.3	40.6 ± 5.0
Na^+ fractional outflow rate (percentage/min)	18.3 ± 1.3	29.8 ± 2.0
Na^+ intracellular translocation (pmol/min per islet)	1.7 ± 0.3	1.5 ± 0.2
H^+ net outflow rate (pmol/min per islet)[c]	1.10 ± 0.18	2.35 ± 0.33
Ca^{2+} total pool (pmol/islet)	6.61 ± 1.51	24.94 ± 1.67
Ca^{2+} cytosolic pool (pmol/islet)	2.58 ± 0.51	9.54 ± 0.93
Ca^{2+} vacuolar pool (pmol/islet)	4.03 ± 1.08	15.41 ± 1.11
Ca^{2+} inflow-outflow (pmol/min per islet)	0.12 ± 0.03	0.27 ± 0.03
Ca^{2+} fractional outflow rate (percentage/min)	4.62 ± 0.36	2.93 ± 0.29
Ca^{2+} intracellular translocation (pmol/min per islet)	0.03 ± 0.01	0.09 ± 0.01

[a] The net output of H^+ was measured in a bicarbonate-free medium.

20mV and assuming that Ca^{2-} was the main ion carrying depolarizing current.

Another implication of our model is that the inflow rate of Na^+ required to cause Na^+-Ca^{2+} countertransport, assuming a 3:1 stoichiometry as is indeed observed with islet native ionophores (Anjaneyulu et al., 1980), does not exceed 1.1 pmol/min per islet, i.e., about 2.6% of the total influx of

Na$^+$. The glucose-induced inhibition of Ca^{2+} outflow, if attributable to the substitution of H$^+$ for Ca^{2+}, implies an increase in H$^+$ output of 0.33 pmol/min per islet (Herchuelz et al., 1979), a value compatible with the observed glucose-induced increment in the net output of H$^+$ from the islets (i.e., 1.25 pmol/min per islet; see Malaisse et al., 1979a).

E. Phosphate "Flush"

Freinkel and co-workers first reported that glucose caused a transient increase in inorganic phosphate release from the islets (Freinkel et al., 1974) (see also Chapter 3). Such a phosphate flush is triggered by D-glucose but not L-glucose and by the α rather than the β anomer of D-glucose (Pierce and Freinkel, 1975). It can also be elicited by D-mannose (Freinkel et al., 1974) and D-glyceraldehyde (Freinkel, 1979) but not by D-galactose or D-fructose. Mannoheptulose (Freinkel et al., 1976) and 2-deoxyglucose (Larson et al., 1979) block the glucose-mediated phosphate flush. Leucine and one of its nonmetabolizable analogues, 2-aminobicyclo[2.2.1]heptane-2-carboxylic acid (BCH), both elicit a phosphate flush (Freinkel et al., 1976). The dose–response relationship of the glucose-induced phosphate flush (Fig. 6) is shifted somewhat to the left in comparison with data for glucose-induced insulin release (Pierce et al., 1976). Activation of the phosphate flush by glucose is significantly altered by fasting (Asplund and Freinkel, 1978). The phosphate flush can be dissociated (e.g., by Ni^{2+}) from the augmented release of ^{45}Ca^{2+} and insulin evoked by glucose (Bukowiecki and Freinkel, 1976). Virtually all the released radioactivity consists of [^{32}P]orthophosphate (Bukowiecki et al., 1979). Histochemical and microprobe examinations of B cells show the accumulation of inorganic phosphate adjacent to the plasmalemma and nucleolus, which is lost during stimulation by glucose (Freinkel et al., 1978).

Freinkel (1979) considers that the phosphate flush reflects an early event in the sequence of stimulus–secretion coupling, such as the recognition of nutrient stimuli at the cell surface. We rather believe that the phosphate flush is secondary to metabolic events evoked by nutrient secretagogues, such as an increase in both O$_2$ uptake and the production rate of NAD(P)H and ATP (Carpinelli and Malaisse, 1980b). The time course for the phosphate flush virtually coincides with that of the first phase of insulin release and thus is delayed relative to the glucose-induced decrease in both ^{86}Rb$^+$ and ^{45}Ca^{2+} fractional outflow rates (Malaisse et al., 1981).

F. Islet Function and the Na$^+$ Ion

It is well established that the accumulation of Na$^+$ in islet cells, due to either facilitation of Na$^+$ influx by veratridine or inactivation of the

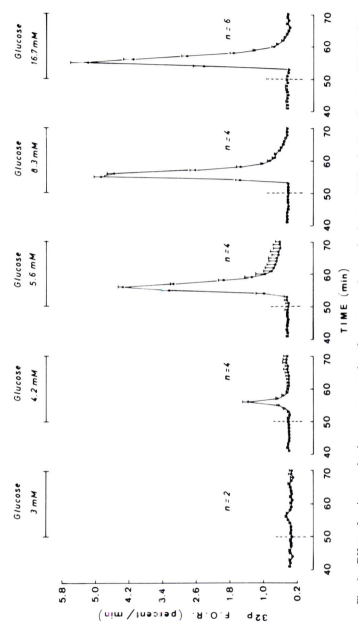

Fig. 6. Effect of an increase in glucose concentration (from zero to the stated value) on ^{32}P fractional outflow rate (F.O.R.) from perifused islets.

K^+–Na^+-dependent ATPase results in the stimulation of insulin release (Donatsch *et al.,* 1977; Lowe *et al.,* 1976; Somers *et al.,* 1980). The latter effect is mainly due to a mobilization of Ca^{2+} from intracellular organelles (Herchuelz and Malaisse, 1980b).

The question should be raised therefore whether an accumulation of intracellular Na^+ participates in the normal process of glucose-induced insulin release. Two independent series of observations suggest that such is not the case.

First, the influence of Na^+ accumulation in islet cells on the efflux of $^{45}Ca^{2+}$ differs in some respects from that evoked by glucose (Herchuelz and Malaisse, 1980b). For instance, when the islets are exposed to a K^+-free perifusate, the enhanced rate of $^{45}Ca^{2+}$ outflow is significantly decreased upon the administration of glucose.

Second, the data so far available do not support the idea that glucose increases the steady-state content of Na^+ in islet cells. According to Kalkhoff and Siegesmund (1979), and as judged by energy-dispersive x-ray diffraction analysis, glucose decreases the Na^+ content of islet cells. Likewise, Kawazu *et al.* (1978) reported that the steady-state content of $^{22}Na^+$ was decreased in islets stimulated by glucose. In the latter study, however, data were obtained suggesting that such a decreased content represented the balance between an increased rate of Na^+ inflow into islet cells and an even more marked increase in the fractional outflow rate of Na^+ from islet cells (Table II). The latter phenomenon did not appear to be attributable to any increase in the activity of the ouabain-sensitive Na^+–K^+-activated ATPase (Kawazu *et al.,* 1978). Nevertheless, we have already mentioned that the repolarization ending each burst of spikes in islets exposed to intermediate concentrations of glucose may be attributable, in part at least, to the activation of such an electrogenic Na^+ pump (Atwater and Meissner, 1975).

Maybe one of the most important roles of Na^+ in islet cells, from the perspective of insulin secretion, consists of the coupling of Ca^{2+} outward transport across the cell membrane with the inward transport of Na^+ by the process known as Na^+–Ca^{2+} countertransport (Herchuelz *et al.,* 1980b).

IV. PARTICIPATION OF IONS IN THE MECHANICAL EVENTS LEADING TO INSULIN RELEASE

The accumulation of Ca^{2+} at a critical site of the B cell may represent the trigger for insulin release. The modality by which Ca^{2+} provokes the exocytosis of secretory granules will be considered first. The participation of other ions in the exocytotic process will then be discussed.

A. Calcium as the Trigger for Insulin Release

We are aware of at least two proposals concerning the mechanism by which the presumed accumulation of ionized Ca^{2+} in the cytosol of the B cell may eventually cause the release of secretory granules.

The first hypothesis, put forward by Matthews (1970), postulates that secretory granules reach the cell membrane by a stochastic or diffusional process. One function of divalent cations, such as calcium, would be to cause a collapse of the potential energy barrier to granule–membrane interaction. According to Dean (1973), islet granules have a surface charge density of about 42 esu/mm², and Ca^{2+} in the 1–50 mM range decreases such a surface charge density. Estimations of the time required for a granule to cover a given distance in the stochastic model (Matthews, 1970) and of the localized increase in Ca^{2+} concentration due to Ca^{2+} entry during the action potential (Dean, 1973) appear quantitatively compatible with this hypothesis.

In the second hypothesis, first postulated by Lacy et al. (1968) and Orci et al. (1972), secretory granules are thought to move toward the plasma membrane along oriented microtubular pathways (Pipeleers et al., 1976), and the microfilamentous cell web, to which the microtubules may be anchored, acts as a sphincter both in controlling and facilitating the access of secretory granules to the plasma membrane. In this model, Ca^{2+} may act by causing contraction of the microfilaments (Somers et al., 1979). We have reviewed on several occasions the findings in support of such a model (Malaisse et al., 1975; Malaisse and Orci, 1979). As far as the role of Ca^{2+} is concerned, it was shown that the ionophore A23187 indeed stimulated contractile-like movements at the boundary of islet cells examined by time-lapse cinematography (Somers et al., 1979).

The two hypotheses under consideration here are not necessarily exclusive of one another. Matthews (1970) calculated the time required (t seconds) for the displacement (x centimeters) of a granule from the diffusion law of Einstein, in which $x^2 = 2Dt$ with, for spherical particles, $D = kT/6\pi\eta r$ where k is the Boltzmann constant, T the absolute temperature, η the cytoplasmic viscosity (taken as 0.06 P), and r the particle radius (taken as a 0.1 μm). We observed that the distance covered by saltatory movements of secretory granules in a monolayer culture of endocrine pancreatic cells yielded a Poisson-like distribution and occurred at a mean speed of 0.8–0.9 μm/sec (Somers et al., 1979). From the above-mentioned equations, the mean speed for the stochastic process of granule translocation would amount to 0.87 μm/sec. The similarity between the observed and calculated values indicates that the back-and-forth saltatory movements of secretory granules along oriented microtubular pathways occur at a speed compatible with the diffusional concept, thus raising the question whether saltation of secretory granules in islet cells represents an ATP-requiring process.

B. Chemosmotic Hypothesis for Exocytosis

We have so far emphasized the role of calcium as a trigger for insulin release. Other ions, however, may participate in the mechanical events responsible for exocytosis of secretory granules.

The ultimate event in the secretory sequence consists of the fusion and fission of membranes at the exocytotic site. Recently, Pollard and colleagues (Brown *et al.,* 1978; Pazoles and Pollard, 1978; Pollard *et al.,* 1977) proposed a chemosmotic hypothesis for the release of epinephrine, parathyroid hormone, and serotonin from intact cells or isolated secretory vesicles. According to this hypothesis, when secretory granules form a fusion complex with the plasma membrane, an anion transport site, presumably derived from the granule-limiting membrane, spans the membrane separating the intragranular space and the extracellular medium, so that the downhill transport of ions (Cl^-, OH^-) into the granule eventually leads to fission of the membrane by osmotic lysis. We have recently shown (Somers *et al.,* 1980b) that this hypothesis may be extended to the process of insulin release, which is inhibited (1) when a sufficient amount of extracellular Cl^- is replaced by an impermeant anion (e.g., isethionate), (2) when the osmolarity of the extracellular medium is sufficiently increased (e.g., by the addition of sucrose) to prevent osmotic lysis, and (3) when an anion transport-blocking agent (e.g., probenecid) is used to prevent the downhill transport of Cl^- and OH^-.

The chemosmotic hypothesis also implies that, when secretory granules move in the close vicinity of one another, no fission of membrane occurs as long as one of the granules does not establish contact with the plasma membrane. This is in good agreement with current morphological observations (Orci and Perrelet, 1977). Thus, although exposure of the B cell to glucose may somehow favor the close apposition and binesis of secretory granules (Gabbay *et al.,* 1975), fission between adjacent granules is usually observed only when one of them is already in direct communication with the extracellular space (Fig. 7). Since insulin granules in the B cell are often disposed in parallel rows along oriented microtubular pathways, this anatomical organization, taken in conjunction with the chemosmotic mechanism, may account for the fusion and fission of several secretory granules at the same exocytotic site (Fig. 7), a phenomenon known as chain release (Orci and Malaisse, 1980).

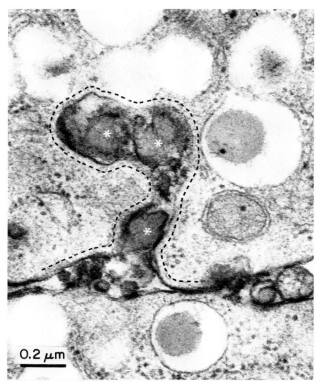

Fig. 7. Insulin-containing cells from isolated islets of Langerhans were stimulated with glucose (16.7 mM). The islets were fixed with 2% cacodylate-buffered glutaraldehyde containing 1% alcian blue to stain the cell coat, dehydrated in ethanol, and embedded in Epon. The dense staining of the plasma membrane coat reveals a profound invagination of the surface (outlined by dotted lines) containing three granule cores (asterisks) exposed to the extracellular space, hence blackened by the stain at their periphery. This image results from the fusion of several secretory granule membranes one with another and with the plasma membrane, allowing several granule cores to be discharged through a single exocytotic stoma. ×62,000. Bar = 0.2 μm. This illustration was kindly provided by Dr. Lelio Orci (Geneva).

V. CONCLUSION

This far from exhaustive review of the participation of ions in the process of insulin release emphasizes the view that ions act on or participate in a great variety of discrete events, each of which represents a single step in the insulin secretory sequence. Because of such a multiple involvement, the ionic aspects of insulin secretion will, in coming years, undoubtedly remain a subject for further fruitful investigations. Indeed, this chapter, through its numerous weaknesses, calls for less speculative and more illuminating contributions.

REFERENCES

Anjaneyulu, K., Anjaneyulu, R., and Malaisse, W. J. (1980). *J. Inorg. Biochem.* **13**, 178–188.
Ashcroft, S. J. H. (1980). *Diabetologia* **18**, 5–15.
Asplund, K., and Freinkel, N. (1978). *Acta Endocrinol.* **88**, 545–555.
Atwater, I., and Meissner, H. P. (1975). *J. Physiol. (London)* **247**, 56–57.
Atwater, I., Ribalet, B., and Rojas, E. (1978). *J. Physiol. (London)* **278**, 117–139.
Atwater, I., Dawson, C. M., Ribalet, B., and Rojas, E. (1979a). *J. Physiol. (London)* **288**, 575–588.
Atwater, I., Ribalet, B., and Rojas, E. (1979b). *J. Physiol. (London)* **288**, 561–574.
Boschero, A. C., and Malaisse, W. J. (1979). *Am. J. Physiol.* **236**, E139–E146.
Boschero, A. C., Kawazu, S., Duncan, G., and Malaisse, W. J. (1977). *FEBS Lett.* **83**, 151–154.
Boschero, A. C., Kawazu, S., Sener, A., Herchuelz, A., and Malaisse, W. J. (1979). *Arch. Biochem. Biophys.* **196**, 54–63.
Brisson, G. R., Malaisse-Lagae, F., and Malaisse, W. J. (1972). *J. Clin. Invest.* **51**, 232–241.
Brown, E. M., Pazoles, C. J., Creutz, C. E., Aurbach, G. D., and Pollard, H. B. (1978). *Proc. Natl. Acad. Sci. U.S.A.* **75**, 876–880.
Bukowiecki, L., and Freinkel, N. (1976). *Biochim. Biophys, Acta* **436**, 190–198.
Bukowiecki, L., Trus, M., Matschinsky, F. M., and Freinkel, N. (1979). *Biochim. Biophys. Acta* **583**, 370–377.
Carpinelli, A. R., and Malaisse, W. J. (1980a). *Mol. Cell. Endocrinol.* **17**, 103–110.
Carpinelli, A. R., and Malaisse, W. J. (1980b). *Diabetologia.* **19**, 458–464.
Carpinelli, A. R., and Malaisse, W. J. (1980c). *Diab. Metab.* **6**, 193–198.
Carpinelli, A. R., and Malaisse, W. J. (1980d). *J. Endocrinol. Invest.* **4**, 365–370.
Carpinelli, A. R., Sener, A., Herchuelz, A., and Malaisse, W. J. (1980). *Metabolism* **29**, 540–545.
Couturier, E., and Malaisse, W. J. (1980). *Diabetologia* **19**, 335–340.
Dean, P. M. (1973). *Diabetologia* **9**, 111–114.
Dean, P. M., and Matthews, E. K. (1968). *Nature (London)* **219**, 389–390.
Deleers, M., and Malaisse, W. J. (1980). *Biochem. Biophys. Res. Commun.* **95**, 650–657.
Deleers, M., Ruysschaert, J. M., and Malaisse, W. J. (1981). *Biochem. Biophys. Res. Commun.* **98**, 255–260.
Donatsch, P., Lowe, D. A., Richardson, B. P., and Taylor, P. (1977). *J. Physiol. (London)* **267**, 357–376.
Freinkel, N. (1979). *In* "Treatment of Early Diabetes" (R. A. Camerini-Davalos and B. Hanover, eds.), pp. 71–77. Plenum, New York.
Freinkel, N., El Younsi, C., Bonnar, J., and Dawson, R. M. C. (1974). *J. Clin. Invest.* **54**, 1179–1189.
Freinkel, N., El Younsi, C., and Dawson, R. M. C. (1976). *Proc. Natl. Acad. Sci. U.S.A.* **73**, 3403–3407.
Freinkel, N., Pedley, K. C., Wooding, P., and Dawson, R. M. C. (1978). *Science* **201**, 1124–1126.
Gabbay, K. H., Korff, J., and Schneeberger, E. E. (1975). *Science* **187**, 177–179.
Goldfine, I. D., Roth, J., and Birnbaumer, L. (1972). *J. Biol. Chem.* **247**, 1211–1218.

Grill, V., and Cerasi, E. (1978). *J. Clin. Invest.* **61**, 1034-1043.

Grodsky, G. M., and Bennett, L. L. (1966). *Diabetes* **15**, 910-913.

Hellerström, C. (1967). *Endocrinology* **81**, 105-112.

Hellerström, C., and Gunnarsson R. (1970). *Acta Diabetol. Lat.* **7**, Suppl. 1, 127-151.

Hellman, B. (1977). *In* "Diabetes Research Today" (E. Lindenlaub, ed.), pp. 207-222. Schattauer, Stuttgart.

Hellman, B., Idahl, L. -Å., Lernmark, A., Sehlin, J., and Täljedal, I. B. (1974a). *Biochem. J.* **138**, 33-45.

Hellman, B., Idahl, L. -Å., Sehlin, J., and Täljedal, I. B. (1974b). *Proc. Natl. Acad. Sci. U.S.A.* **71**, 3405-3409.

Hellman, B., Sehlin, J., and Täljedal, I. B. (1976). *Horm. Metab. Res.* **8**, 427-429.

Henquin, J. C. (1978). *Nature (London)* **271**, 271-273.

Henquin, J. C. (1979). *Nature (London)* **280**, 66-68.

Henquin, J. C. (1980). *Biochem. J.* **186**, 541-550.

Henquin, J. C., and Lambert, A. E. (1976). *Am J. Physiol.* **231**, 713-721.

Henquin, J. C., and Meissner, H. P. (1978). *Biochim. Biophys. Acta* **543**, 455-464.

Henquin, J. C., Meissner, H. P , and Preissler, M. (1979). *Biochim. Biophys. Acta* **587**, 579-592.

Herchuelz, A., and Malaisse, W. J. (1978). *J. Physiol. (London)* **283**, 409-424.

Herchuelz, A., and Malaisse, W. J. (1980a). *Am. J. Physiol.* **238**, E87-E95.

Herchuelz, A., and Malaisse, W. J. (1980b). *J. Physiol. (London)* **302**, 263-280.

Herchuelz, A., and Malaisse, W. J. (1981). *In* "Calcium in Normal and Pathological Biological Systems" (L. J. Anghileri, ed.) CRC Press, Boca Raton (in press).

Herchuelz, A., Delcroix, C., and Malaisse, W. J. (1979). *Biochem. Med.* **22**, 156-164.

Herchuelz, A., Couturier, E., and Malaisse, W. J. (1980a). *Am. J. Physiol.* **238**, E96-E103.

Herchuelz, A., Sener, A., and Malaisse, W. J. (1980b). *J. Membr. Biol.* **57**, 1-12.

Herchuelz, A., Thonnart, N., Carpinelli, A., and Sener, A., Malaisse, W. J. (1980c). *J. Exp. Pharmacol. Ther.* **215**, 213-220.

Herchuelz, A., Thonnart, N., Sener, A., and Malaisse, W. J. (1980d). *Endocrinology* **107**, 491-497.

Herchuelz, A., Lebrun, P., Carpinelli, A., Thonnart, N., Sener, A., and Malaisse, W. J. (1981). *Biochim. Biophys. Acta* **640**, 16-30.

Hutton, J. C., and Malaisse, W. J. (1980). *Diabetologia* **18**, 395-405.

Hutton, J. C., Sener, A., Herchuelz, A., Valverde, I., Boschero, A. C., and Malaisse, W. J. (1980). *Horm. Metab. Res.* **12**, 294-298.

Kalkhoff, R. K., and Siegesmund, K. (1979). *Diabetes* **28**, 394.

Kawazu, S., Boschero, A. C., Delcroix, C., and Malaisse, W. J. (1978). *Pfluegers Arch.* **375**, 197-206.

Kikuchi, M., Wollheim, C. B., Siege. E. G., Renold, A. E., and Sharp, G. W. G. (1979). *Endocrinology* **105**, 1013-1019.

Lacy, P. E., Howell, S. L., Young, D. A., and Fink, C. J. (1968). *Nature (London)* **219**, 1177-1179.

Larson, B. A., Williams, T. L., Showers, M. D., and Vanderlaan, W. P. (1979). *Diabetologia* **17**, 117-120.

Lowe, D.A., Richardson, B. P., Taylor, P., and Donatsch, P. (1976). *Nature (London)* **260**, 337-338.

Malaisse, W. J., and Orci, L. (1979). *Methods and Achievements in Exp. Pathol.* **9**, 112-136.

Malaisse, W. J., Malaisse-Lagae, F., and Mayhew, D. A. (1967). *J. Clin. Invest.* **46**, 1724-1734.

Malaisse, W. J., Malaisse-Lagae, F., Van Obberghen, E., Somers, G., Devis, G., Ravazzola, M., and Orci, L. (1975). *Ann. N.Y. Acad. Sci.* **253**, 630–652.

Malaisse, W. J., Boschero, A. C., Kawazu, S., and Hutton, J. C. (1978a). *Pfluegers Arch.* **373**, 237–242.

Malaisse, W. J., Herchuelz, A., Devis, G., Somers, G., Boschero, A. C., Hutton, J. C., Kawazu, S., Sener, A., Atwater, I., Duncan, G., Ribalet, B., and Rojas, E. (1978b). *Ann. N.Y. Acad. Sci.* **307**, 562–582.

Malaisse, W. J., Hutton, J. C., Sener, A., Levy, J., Herchuelz, A., Devis, G., and Somers, G. (1978c). *J. Membr. Biol.* **38**, 193–208.

Malaisse, W. J., Sener, A., Boschero, A. C., Kawazu, S., Devis, G., and Somers, G. (1978d). *Eur. J. Biochem.* **87**, 111–120.

Malaisse, W. J., Hutton, J. C., Kawazu, S., Herchuelz, A., Valverde, I., and Sener, A. (1979a). *Diabetologia* **16**, 331–341.

Malaisse, W. J., Sener, A., Herchuelz, A., and Hutton, J. C. (1979b). *Metabolism* **28**, 373–386.

Malaisse, W. J., Anjaneyulu, K., Anjaneyulu, R., and Couturier, E. (1980a). *Mol. Cell. Biochem.* **30**, 67–70.

Malaisse, W. J., Sener, A., Herchuelz, A., Carpinelli, A. R., Poloczek, P., Winand, J., and Castagna, M. (1980b). *Cancer Res.* **40**, 3827–3831.

Malaisse, W. J., Sener, A., Herchuelz, A., Valverde, I., Hutton, J. C., Atwater, I., and Leclercq-Meyer, V. (1980c). *Horm. Metab. Res. Suppl.* **10**, 61–66.

Malaisse, W. J., Carpinelli, A. R., and Sener, A. (1981). *Metabolism* (in press).

Malaisse-Lagae, F., and Malaisse, W. J. (1971). *Endocrinology* **88**, 72–80.

Matthews, E. K. (1970). *Acta Diabetol. Lat.* **7**, Suppl. 1, 83–89.

Matthews, E. K., and O'Connor, M. D. L. (1979). *J. Exp. Biol.* **81**, 75–91.

Matthews, E. K., Dean, P. M., and Sakamoto, Y. (1975). In "Insulin II" (A. Hasselblatt and Y. von Bruckhausen, eds.), pp. 157–173. Springer-Verlag, Berlin and New York.

Meissner, H. P., and Atwater, I. J. (1976). *Horm. Metab. Res.* **8**, 11–16.

Meissner, H. P., and Preissler, M. (1979). In "Treatment of Early Diabetes" (R. A. Camerini-Davalos and B. Hanover, eds.), pp. 97–107. Plenum, New York.

Meissner, H. P., Henquin, J. C., and Preissler, M. (1978). *FEBS Lett.* **94**, 87–89.

Milner, R. D. G., and Hales, C. N. (1967). *Diabetologia* **3**, 47–49.

Orci, L., and Malaisse, W. J. (1980). *Diabetes* **29**, 943–944.

Orci, L., and Perrelet, A. (1977). In "The Diabetic Pancreas" (B. W. Volk and K. F. Wellman, eds.), pp. 171–210. Plenum, New York.

Orci, L., Gabbay, K. H., and Malaisse, W. J. (1972). *Science* **175**, 1128–1130.

Pazoles, C. J., and Pollard, H. B. (1978). *J. Biol. Chem.* **253**, 3962–3969.

Pierce, M., and Freinkel, N. (1975). *Biochem. Biophys. Res. Commun.* **63**, 870–874.

Pierce, M., Bukowiecki, L., Asplund, K., and Freinkel, N. (1976). *Horm. Metab. Res.* **8**, 358–361.

Pipeleers, D. G., Pipeleers-Marichal, M. A., and Kipnis, D. M. (1976). *Science* **191**, 88–90.

Pollard, H. B., Tack-Goldman, K., Pazoles, C. J., Creutz, C. E., and Shulman, N. R. (1977). *Proc. Natl. Acad. Sci. U.S.A.* **74**, 5295–5299.

Ravazzola, M., Malaisse-Lagae, F., Amherdt, M., Perrelet, A., Malaisse, W. J., and Orci, L. (1976). *J. Cell Sci.* **27**, 107–117.

Schäfer, H. J., and Klöppel, G. (1974). *Virchows Arch. A* **362**, 231–245.

Sehlin, J. (1976). *Biochem. J.* **156**, 63–69.

Sehlin, J. (1978). *Am. J. Physiol.* **235**, E501–E508.

Sehlin, J., and Täljedal, I. B. (1974). *J. Physiol. (London)* **242**, 505–515.

Sener, A., and Malaisse, W. J. (1980). *Endocrinology* **106**, 778–785.

Sener, A., Hutton, J. C., Kawazu, S., Boschero, A. C., Somers, G., Devis, G., Herchuelz, A., and Malaisse, W. J. (1978). *J. Clin. Invest.* **62,** 868–878.

Sener, A., Valverde, I., and Malaisse, W. J. (1979). *FEBS Lett.* **105,** 40–42.

Sener, A., Kawazu, S., and Malaisse, W. J. (1980). *Biochem. J.* **186,** 183–190.

Somers, G., Blondel, B., Orci, L., and Malaisse, W. J. (1979). *Endocrinology* **104,** 255–264.

Somers, G., Devis, G., and Malaisse, W. J. (1980a). *Pfluegers Arch.* **385,** 217–222.

Somers, G., Sener, A., Devis, G., and Malaisse, W. J. (1980b). *Pfluegers Arch.* **388,** 249–253.

Sugden, M. C., and Ashcroft, S. J. E. (1978). *Diabetologia* **15,** 173–180.

Sugden, M. C., Christie, M. R., and Ashcroft, S. J. H. (1979). *FEBS Lett.* **105,** 95–100.

Täljedal, I. B. (1978). *J. Cell. Biol.* **76,** 652–674.

Täljedal, I. B. (1979). *Biochem. J.* **178,** 187–193.

Valverde, I., Vandermeers, A., Anjaneyulu, R., and Malaisse, W. J. (1979). *Science* **206,** 225–227.

Valverde, I., Sener, A., Lebrun, P., Herchuelz, A., and Malaisse, W. J. (1981). *Endocrinology* **108,** 1305–1312.

Verspohl, E. J., and Ammon, H. P. T. (1980). *J. Clin. Invest,* **65,** 1230–1237.

Wollheim, C. B., Kikuchi, M., Renold, A. E., and Sharp, G. W. G. (1978). *J. Clin. Invest.* **62,** 451–458.

8

Interrelationships between Prostaglandins and Biogenic Amines during Modulation of Beta-Cell Function

R. P. ROBERTSON

I. INTRODUCTION

A common theme running through the many pathophysiological phenomena found in diabetics is the failure of cells to recognize and respond to glucose signals appropriately. For example, non-insulin-dependent diabetics with fasting hyperglycemia do not have first-phase or acute insulin responses to intravenous glucose (1) but have preserved responses to secretogogues such as secretin (2), isoproterenol (3), amino acids (4), and

The Islets of Langerhans
Copyright © 1981 by Academic Press, Inc.
All rights of reproduction in any form reserved.
ISBN 0–12–187820–1

glucagon (5). Similarly, insulin-dependent diabetics fail to secrete glucagon appropriately during hypoglycemia but have normal responses following arginine stimulation (6). This general trend has also been observed in extra-pancreatic tissues. This can be readily appreciated if one recalls that in diabetic subjects there is subnormal suppression of growth hormone by glucose (7) and an increased threshold for the sense of taste for the glucose molecule (8). For these reasons, it seems appropriate and potentially pro-ductive to focus investigative energy on the question of why the beta cell in-adequately responds to glucose signals. An obvious place to search for the answers is within the pancreatic islet itself, because the islet contains two resident classes of inhibitors of glucose-induced insulin secretion. These are the prostaglandins and biogenic amines (9,10). The information that follows is presented on the premise that a better understanding of the behavior of endogenous substances that negatively modulate beta-cell func-tion will provide fresh insights into pathogenetic mechanisms that con-tribute to the syndrome of diabetes mellitus.

In this chapter, three goals will be pursued. First, a description will be presented of the effects of prostaglandins and biogenic amines on insulin secretion. Second, an examination will be made of functional interrelation-ships between prostaglandins and biogenic amines in their role as negative modulators of beta-cell function. Third, once the interrelationships of these two pharmacological families have been presented, speculation will be offered regarding the implications of the actions of these molecules for the pathogenesis and treatment of diabetes mellitus.

II. ACTIONS OF PROSTAGLANDINS AND BIOGENIC AMINES ON INSULIN SECRETION

A. Prostaglandin Pharmacology

Prostaglandins are less familiar than biogenic amines to most investi-gators interested in beta-cell function. Consequently, a brief description of prostaglandin pharmacology and physiology at this point should prove helpful. Contrary to the implication of their name, these fatty acids are not localized to a specific gland. Rather, all tissues and presumably all cells synthesize a variety of prostaglandins. The three major groups of these substances currently receiving the most attention (Fig. 1) are the "classical" prostaglandins (represented in the figure by PGE), thrombox-ane A_2, and prostacyclin (PGI_2). The synthesis of these molecules begins with plasma membrane phospholipid from which is cleaved arachidonic acid. This step is enzymatically governed by phospholipase A_2 (Fig. 2) and

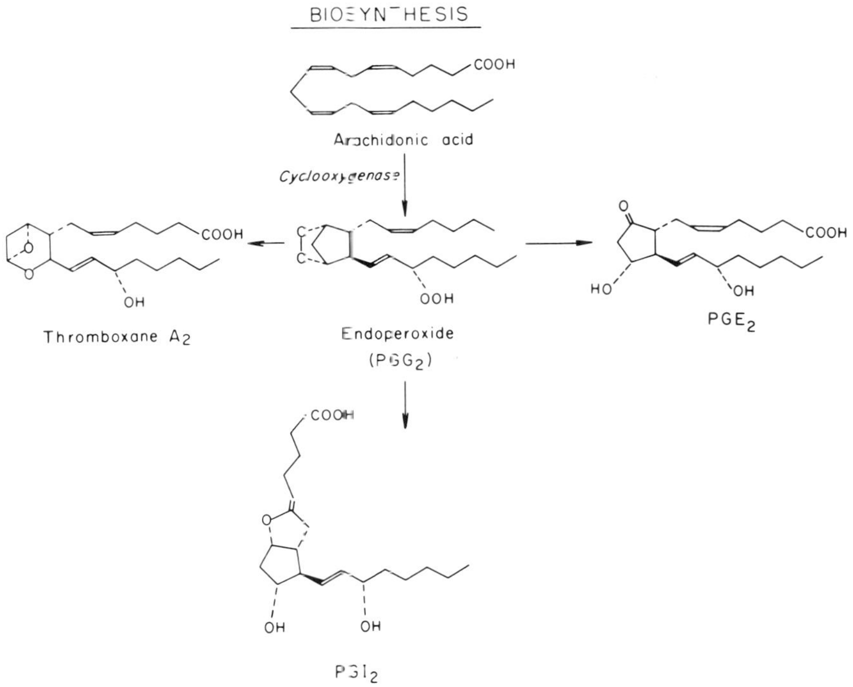

Fig. 1. Molecular structures of the major prostaglandins and their precursors. PGI$_2$ is prostacyclin; the classical prostaglandins are represented here by PGE$_2$. The key intermediates for these three pathways are endoperoxides, represented here by PGG$_2$.

blocked by corticosteroids. Following the cleavage of arachidonic acid, the enzyme cyclooxygenase promotes the formation of cyclic endoperoxides. It is at this step that several clinically well-known antiinflammatory drugs exert a blocking effect. For example, acetylsalicylic acid and indomethacin prevent the formation of endoperoxide and, consequently, the classical prostaglandins, thromboxane A$_2$, and prostacyclin. Once the endoperoxides are formed, three subsequent pathways are possible, thereby making endoperoxides the key intermediates for synthesis. Whether one, two, or all three of these pathways are used depends upon the tissue being examined and the metabolic forces in its environment. Consequently, it is pointless to speculate about which prostaglandin is the most or least important. Rather, specific physiological and pathophysiological questions must be asked about specific tissues under specific conditions.

Although the physiological and the pathophysiological properties of prostaglandins are too numerous to develop fully in this chapter, at least three fundamental considerations should be kept in mind. First, it is essen-

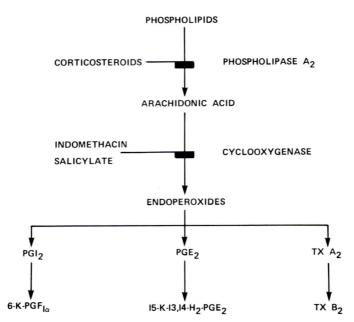

Fig. 2. Pathways for the biosynthesis and degradation of prostaglandins. The classical prostaglandins are represented here by PGE_2. Corticosteroids block the phospholipase-mediated step from phospholipids to arachidonic acid. Nonsteroidal antiinflammatory agents block the cyclooxygenase-mediated step from arachidonic acid to endoperoxides. The three metabolites shown (6-K-$PGF_{1\alpha}$; 15-K-13,14-H_2-PGE_2; and TX B_2) are the ones formed first.

tial not to think of prostaglandins as hormones, because a hormone is a substance that is synthesized by a specific tissue, released into the circulation, and delivered to a distant target organ to exert a specific metabolic action. Since prostaglandins are made in all tissues, it is unlikely that a given tissue is dependent upon prostaglandin synthesis by another tissue. However, this is not to say that in certain pathophysiological states excessive amounts of prostaglandins cannot enter the circulation, travel to distant sites, and cause adverse effects. However, such phenomena must not be confused with hormonal action. A second important consideration about prostaglandins is their rapid half-lives. For example, it has been estimated that under physiological conditions the half-life is under 30 sec for thromboxane A_2 and is less than several minutes for prostacyclin. Both these compounds undergo spontaneous degradation. Although more chemically stable, PGE is quickly and extensively degraded by both the lung and the liver. Circulating PGE is approximately 90% degraded in a single pass through either of these organs. Third, one should not expect prostaglandins to perform the same general type of function in different tissues. For example, PGE stimulates some types of smooth muscle (gut, uterus) but relaxes others (arterial). Again, while PGE usually stimulates adenylate cyclase, in a few tissues it does not. A recent issue is whether PGE and prostacyclin utilize the same cellular receptor. While this appears to be the case in some tissues (11), the contrary has been found in other tissues (12,13). Consequently, once again we are left with the conclusion that an attempt to generalize too much about prostaglandins will only lead to confusion about their roles in physiology and pathophysiology. The more prudent approach is to focus on specific issues in specific tissues. Perhaps the one generalization that will stand the test of time is that prostaglandins appear to be intracellular modulators of on-going biochemical activity rather than primary effectors. Viewed in this context, their multiple actions, some of which may appear to be paradoxical, can be more easily understood.

B. Prostaglandins and Beta-Cell Function

Given the caveats mentioned about prostaglandins thus far, it should not be surprising that in the past there has been a good deal of confusion regarding the action of these agents on the beta cell. It now seems clear that prostaglandins of the E series are the most important ones with regard to the regulation of insulin secretion. Virtually all the data obtained *in vivo* indicate that PGE inhibits insulin release (14). While some *in vitro* data substantiate these findings (15), others do not (16,17). However, in instances where PGE has been observed to stimulate insulin secretion, it appears that activation of PGE-sensitive adenylate cyclase may also have occurred (16). Since the generation of cyclic AMP augments insulin secretion, experiments in which PGE has been shown to have stimulatory effects on beta-cell function seem to reflect more its ability to simulate adenylate cyclase than its direct effect on insulin secretion. An example of the inhibitory effect of PGE on glucose-induced insulin release is shown in Fig. 3. These data indicate that an intravenous infusion of PGE_2 in normal human subjects results in partial inhibition of the acute insulin response to intravenous glucose. It has been observed that PGE in relatively larger doses lowers basal insulin levels during similar studies on dogs (18). Studies have also been published describing the use of analogues of PGE in both humans (19) and animals *in vivo* (20). In all instances these substances inhibited glucose-induced insulin secretion. PGE_1 and PGE_2 have the same effect on beta-cell function (21). It has also been demonstrated that the infusion of PGA_1 inhibits insulin secretion; however, unlike PGE, the PGA effect appears to be mediated by reflex sympathetic stimulation rather than direct inhibition of beta-cell function (22). Thus far, the few publications

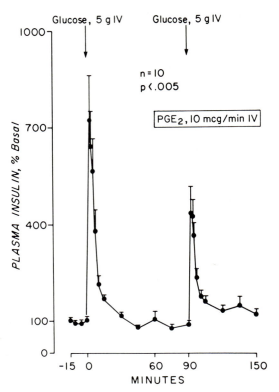

Fig. 3. The inhibitory effect of an intravenous infusion of PGE_2 in humans on the acute insulin response to intravenous glucose pulses.

dealing with prostacyclin and thromboxanes have failed to demonstrate effects on islet function (23).

An understanding of the effects of PGE on insulin secretion has also been approached through studies on inhibitors of prostaglandin synthesis. Here the results have consistently demonstrated that a variety of different inhibitors augment glucose-induced insulin secretion with one exception (24–28), namely, indomethacin. However, it must be remembered that indomethacin has many pharmacological actions in addition to inhibiting the synthesis of PGE. This drug can also inhibit the degradation of PGE (29), inhibit cyclic AMP-dependent protein kinase (30), and inhibit translocation of calcium across cell membranes (31). All three of these effects tend to decrease insulin secretion. Since PGE consistently inhibits insulin secretion *in vivo* and since all other inhibitors of prostaglandin synthesis stimulate insulin secretion, the weight of the evidence seems to indicate that the inhibitory effect of indomethacin on beta-cell function is an event unrelated to the inhibition of PGE synthesis.

III. BIOGENIC AMINES AND BETA-CELL FUNCTION

It has been appreciated for a much longer period of time that biogenic amines have inhibitory effects on insulin secretion. Two catecholamines—epinephrine and norepinephrine—and serotonin are the amines that have been the most extensively studied. Epinephrine and norepinephrine consistently inhibit glucose-induced insulin section *in vitro* (32) and *in vivo* (33). This inhibitory effect is ascribed to alpha-adrenergic receptor stimulation, because alpha-adrenergic antagonists block it (34). Like PGE, the alpha-adrenergic property of the catecholamines appears to be relatively glucose-specific, since nonglucose secretogogues such as secretin are not prevented by catecholamines from stimulating insulin secretion (35). In humans and primates, an additional observation has been made with epinephrine, which relates to basal secretion of insulin (Fig. 4). Immediately following the onset of epinephrine infusion (36), there is a decrement in circulating insulin to approximately 50% of the basal level. Within a short period of time (approximately 10–20 min), the nadir is reached. Thereafter, a recovery phase occurs during which circulating insulin again reaches basal levels and then surpasses them. This recovery phase can be blocked by propranolol, a beta-adrenergic antagonist; consequently, the initial decline in

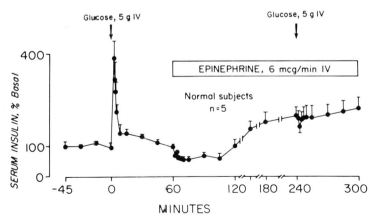

Fig. 4. Epinephrine inhibition of the acute insulin response to intravenous glucose pulses. This catecholamine also causes a decrement in basal insulin levels during the first $\frac{1}{2}$ hr of its infusion in humans.

basal levels has been ascribed to the alpha-adrenergic properties of epinephrine (36).

Although many investigations have been performed with serotonin, interpretation of the data is more difficult than with the catecholamines. One reason for this is that very few studies have been performed *in vivo* with serotonin itself. Most *in vivo* studies have utilized antagonists of serotonin and frequently have resulted in contradictory results. Much of the confusion may arise from the fact that some of the serotonin antagonists that have been used are mixed antagonists, hence they also bind to nonserotonin receptor sites. An example of this is cyproheptadine which is a potent antagonist of both serotonin and histamine. Given that the effects of histamine on beta-cell function have not been completely elucidated, it is difficult to interpret experiments with this drug. In general, the consensus appears to be that serotonin inhibits insulin secretion. Demonstration of this phenomenon can be seen in Fig. 5. In this study, in which adrenergic influences were removed by combined alpha- and beta-adrenergic block-

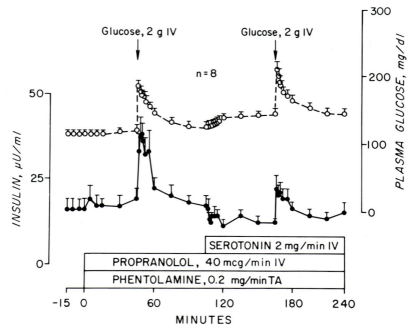

Fig. 5. The inhibitory effect of serotonin infused into the thoracic aorta (to avoid immediate pulmonic degradation) in dogs on the acute insulin response to intravenous glucose pulses. The animals were pretreated with propranolol and phentolamine to provide combined alpha- and beta-adrenergic blockage. Open circles, plasma glucose; solid circles, plasma insulin.

age, serotonin caused a partial inhibition of glucose-induced insulin secretion (37). It cannot be said whether this inhibitory effect is specific for glucose, since the ability of serotonin to inhibit the effects of nonglucose secretogogues has not been fully examined.

IV. INTERRELATIONSHIPS BETWEEN PROSTAGLANDINS AND BIOGENIC AMINES

Since it has been established that PGE, catecholamines, and serotonin inhibit glucose-induced insulin secretion, a search can be made for interrelationships among the actions of these molecules. That this is more than simply an intellectual exercise becomes apparent when one considers that all three of these substances are synthesized by the pancreatic islet and that gap junctions exist between various cells within the islet. Thus the stage is set for these substances to be potential local messengers between islet cells. For example, it is conceivable that PGE or biogenic amines produced by one cell might migrate to the beta cell to exert a negative modulatory influence on insulin secretion. A scheme illustrating all the possible interactions is given in Fig. 6. In this scheme the common result is the inhibition of insulin secretion. The question is whether any of these agents depend on another to exert this effect.

Soon after it was established that PGE infusions *in vivo* inhibited glucose-induced insulin secretion, it was ascertained whether this effect was dependent on or independent of the adrenergic nervous system. One reason this was particularly pressing was that the PGE infusion in some of the studies caused hypotension. This could have caused catecholamine release which theoretically then could have been responsible for the inhibition of beta-cell function. In several instances the approach was to treat

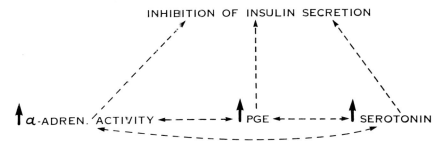

Fig. 6. Theoretical schema of the interrelationships among alpha-adrenergic agonists, PGE, and serotonin as inhibitors of insulin secretion. This schema illustrates all possible interrelationships.

simultaneously with alpha-adrenergic antagonists and PGE. In all such cases, ranging from rodents to man (18,38,39), PGE continued to exert its inhibitory effect on insulin secretion despite the presence of alpha-adrenergic antagonists. Thus it has been concluded that the inhibitory effect of PGE is independent of endogenous catecholamines. Some time later it was demonstrated in another series of experiments (37) that methysergide, a serotonin antagonist, reversed the inhibitory effect of PGE on insulin secretion in the dog (Fig. 7). During these experiments, methysergide was studied at various doses and it was found to be equipotent in antagonizing serotonin and PGE during different degrees of inhibition of beta-cell function. The most direct interpretation of these studies is that endogenous serotonin plays a role in mediating the inhibitory effect of PGE on beta-cell function in the dog. The alternate hypothesis that methysergide is an antagonist of both a serotonin receptor and a PGE receptor is not as attractive, since the PGE and serotonin molecules are structurally dissimilar. Therefore one reaches the tentative conclusion that PGE action is not mediated by endogenous alpha-adrenergic forces but that it may be dependent on endogenous serotonin action.

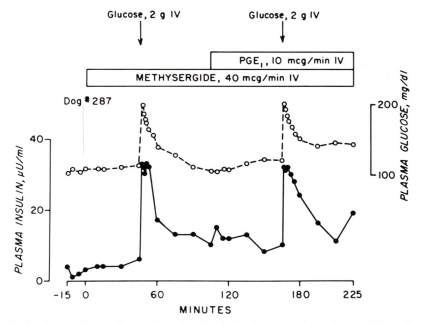

Fig. 7.   Reversal by methysergide of the ability of an intravenous infusion of PGE₁ in dogs to inhibit glucose-induced acute insulin responses. Open circles, plasma glucose; solid circles, plasma insulin.

Quite recently, it has been examined whether inhibitors of endogenous prostaglandin synthesis can alter the ability of epinephrine to inhibit glucose-induced insulin secretion (Fig. 8). While the effect of epinephrine on basal insulin secretion did not appear to be affected, a striking restoration of glucose-induced insulin secretion despite epinephrine infusion was observed (40). This experiment was conducted using two structurally dissimilar inhibitors of PGE synthesis, namely, sodium salicylate and indomethacin. Both these drugs have been demonstrated to decrease PGE synthesis in cultures of neonatal rat pancreatic islets (41). Additionally, almost a decade ago it was demonstrated that methysergide, a serotonin antagonist, could antagonize the inhibitory effect of alpha-adrenergic activity on insulin secretion *in vitro* (42). More recently, unpublished data have been collected in our laboratory indicating the same to be true in the intact, anesthetized dog. Therefore an intriguing possibility concerning the interrelationships between prostaglandins and biogenic amines arises. The experiments using epinephrine and inhibitors of endogenous prostaglandin synthesis suggest that the inhibitory effect of catecholamines on glucose-induced insulin secretion (which previously had been attributed to stimulation of the alpha-adrenergic receptor) may be at least in part mediated by endogenous prostaglandins. In this regard it is important to emphasize again that prostaglandins are synthesized by isolated pancreatic islets and by cultures of neonatal rat pancreatic islets and that catecholamines are stimulators of prostaglandin synthesis. These findings combined with the observations that methysergide can block PGE and catecholamine action on the beta-cell support the notion that alpha-adrenergic effects might be mediated by PGE. However, in none of these studies was the inhibitory effect of epinephrine completely reversed. One must therefore allow for the possibility that epinephrine exerts an inhibitory effect on beta-cell function independent of PGE and serotonin.

These experiments allow us to modify the hypothetical schema as illustrated in Fig. 9. It suggests that (1) alpha-adrenergic effects are at least partially mediated by PGE, (2) PGE is mediated by serotonin and not alpha-adrenergic activity, and (3) serotonin effects are independent of PGE and catecholamines. This schema is further supported by experiments in which an inhibitor of endogenous prostaglandin synthesis failed to prevent serotonin from inhibiting glucose-induced insulin secretion in the dog (37). Additionally, it should be recalled that the inhibitory effect of serotonin on glucose-stimulated insulin secretion was not reversed by combined alpha- and beta-adrenergic blockage in the dog (37). One obvious difficulty with this hypothesis is that its construction has required the use of various species. For example, the key observation that inhibitors of prostaglandin synthesis can partially reverse the inhibitory effects of catecholamines was

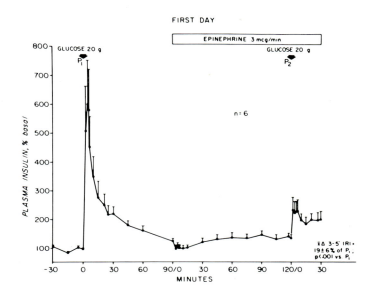

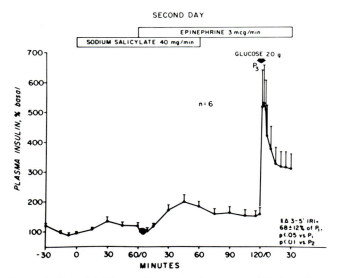

Fig. 8. Reversal of the inhibitory effect of an intravenous infusion of epinephrine in humans on glucose-induced acute insulin responses.

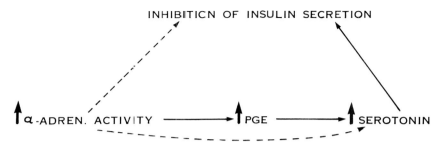

Fig. 9. Alteration of the theoretical schema shown in Fig. 6 to indicate that the inhibitory effect of PGE may be operating through the release of endogenous serotonin in the pancreatic islet. The inhibitory effect of alpha-adrenergic agonists can be at least partially attributed to the release of endogenous PGE. The possibility is left open that alpha-adrenergic agonists may have inhibitory effects on insulin secretion, which are independent of the PGE-serotonin pathway.

made in humans but has not yet been reproduced in other species. Another difficulty is that there are no reliable PGE antagonists that can be used in humans. Instead, one must rely on nonspecific inhibitors of endogenous prostaglandin synthesis. Consequently, much more work is needed in this area before the schema illustrated in Fig. 9 can be accepted with confidence.

V. IMPLICATIONS FOR THE PATHOGENESIS AND TREATMENT OF DIABETES MELLITUS

Turning from the realm of hypotheses about the interplay between prostaglandins and biogenic amines, we will now consider the effects of drugs which antagonize the action or synthesis of these substances when given to subjects with diabetes mellitus. Phentolamine, an alpha-adrenergic antagonist, was the first drug demonstrated to cause partial restoration of glucose-induced acute insulin responses (43). Even though the magnitude of the restoration was quite small, it was intriguing because circulating levels of plasma catecholamines are elevated in some diabetic subjects (43). This is particularly true in subjects under stress and with ketoacidosis. More recently, intravenous infusions of sodium salicylate, an inhibitor of prostaglandin synthesis *in vivo* in humans (44) and in cultures of neonatal rat pancreatic islets (41), were found to result in a much more striking restoration of glucose-induced acute insulin responses (45) in diabetics (Fig. 10). Moreover, there was a fourfold augmentation of second-phase insulin release. These phenomena were accompanied by marked improvement in glucose disappearance rates, which suggests that the augmented insulin

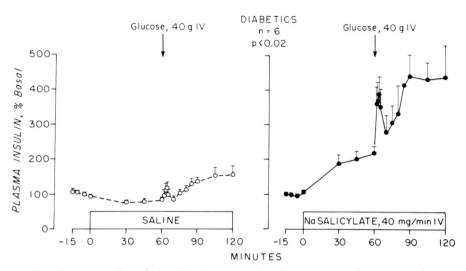

Fig. 10. Restoration of virtually absent acute insulin responses to intravenous glucose pulses given to adult-onset diabetics through treatment with an intravenous infusion of sodium salicylate. Sodium salicylate elevates basal insulin levels, partially restores the acute insulin response, and causes a marked increase in second-phase insulin secretion.

secretion was biologically meaningful. The notion that endogenous prostaglandins may be involved in the pathogenesis of diabetes mellitus is also supported by data suggesting that either PGE or thromboxanes may be overproduced by platelets from diabetic subjects (46,47). In this context, it is interesting that tolbutamide and chlorpropamide, oral hypoglycemic agents, have been shown to inhibit synthesis of PGE in the toad bladder (48). Although this phenomenon has not been reproduced in pancreatic islets, it is intriguing to speculate that the elusive mechanism of the chronic action of these drugs might be related to the inhibition of intraislet prostaglandin synthesis. Finally, it has been reported that methysergide improves oral glucose tolerance in diabetic subjects but not in normal subjects (49). This observation is consistent with the notion that serotonin is an endogenous inhibitor of glucose-induced insulin secretion that may mediate PGE effects on the beta cell.

If one takes pause for a moment and steps away from all the individual experiments, one finds reason for optimism as regards therapy for diabetics. Whether or not endogenous prostaglandins and biogenic amines are operative during abnormal insulin secretion in diabetics and whether or not these two classes of pharmacological compounds work in concert, it is clear that abnormal glucose recognition by the islet in hyperglycemic, non-insulin-dependent diabetics can be improved. It has now been demonstrated that drugs are capable of at least partially restoring virtually absent glucose-induced acute insulin secretion. This indicates that the pathogenetic mechanisms responsible for defective glucose recognition are reversible. The clear challenge is to design drug therapy that will allow the pancreas in diabetics to better recognize and respond to glucose signals. However, a fundamental, as yet unrealized, goal needs to be achieved before this kind of rational drug therapy can be approached effectively. It is essential to isolate in viable form the different cells residing within the islet so that each can be examined as a separate unit to better understand the regulation of its secretory mechanisms. It will be essential to determine what type of cell surface or intracellular receptors are present and to ascertain whether these include receptors for PGE, alpha-adrenergic agonists, and serotonin.

REFERENCES

1. Brunzell, J. D., Robertson, R. P., Lerner, R. L., Hazzard, W. R., Ensinck, J. W., Bierman, E. L., and Porte, D., Jr. (1976). *J. Clin. Endocrinol. Metab.* **42**, 222–229.
2. Lerner, R. L. (1979). *J. Clin. Endocrinol. Metab.* **48**, 462–466.
3. Robertson, R. P., and Porte, D., Jr. (1973). *J. Clin. Invest.* **52**, 870–876.
4. Palmer, J. P., Benson, J. W., Walter, R. M., and Ensinck, J. W. (1976). *J. Clin. Invest.* **58**, 565–570.
5. Crockford, P. M., Hazzard, W. R., and Williams, R. H. (1969). *Diabetes* **18**, 216–244.
6. Gerich, J. E., Langlois M., Noacco, C., et al. (1976) *J. Clin. Invest.* **58**, 320–325.
7. Sacca, L., Sherwin, R., Hendler, R., et al. (1979). *J. Clin. Invest.* **63**, 849–857.
8. Porte, D., Jr., Robertson, R. P., Halter, J. B., et al. (1977). *Int. Symp. Food Intake and chemical Senses.* pp. 331–342. Univ. of Tokyo Press, Tokyo.
9. Hamamdzic, M., and Malik, K. U. (1977). *Am. J. Physiol.* **232**, 201–209.
10. Lundquist, L., Ekholm, R., and Ericson, L. E. (1971). *Diabetologia* **7**, 414–422.
11. Siegl, A. M., Smith, J. B., and Silver, M. J. (1979). *J. Clin. Invest.* **63**, 215–220.
12. Oien, H. G., Babiarz, E. M., Sodeman, D. D., Ham, E. A., and Kuehl, F. A., Jr. (1979). *Prostaglandins* **17**, 525–542.
13. Robertson, R. P., Westcott, K. R. Storm, D. R., and Rice, M. R. (1980). *Am. J. Physiol.* **239**, E75–80.
14. Robertson, R. P. (1979). *Diabetes* **28**, 943–948.
15. Burr, I. M., and Sharp, R. (1977). *Endocrinology* **94**, 835–39.
16. Johnson, D. G., Fugimoto, W. Y., and Williams, R. H. (1973). *Diabetes* **22**, 658–63.
17. Pek, S., Tai, Tong-Yuan, and Elster, A. (1978). *Diabetes* **27**, 801–809.
18. Robertson, R. P., Gavareski, D. J., Porte, D., Jr., and Bierman, E. L. (1974). *J. Clin. Invest.* **54**, 310–15.
19. Konturek, S. J., Mikos, E. M., Krol, R., Wierzicki, Z., and Dobraznska, M. (1978). *Prostaglandins* **15**, 591–602.
20. Dodi, G., Santoro, M. D., and Jaffe. B. M. (1978). *Surgery,* **83**, 206–13.
21. Robertson, R. P. (1974). *Prostaglandins* **6**, 501–508.
22. Sacca, L., Rengo, F. Chaircello, M., and Condorelli, M. (1973). *Endocrinology* **92**, 31–34.

23. Akpan, J. O., Hurley, M. C., Pek, S., and Lunds, W. E. M. (1979). *Can. J. Biochem.* **57**, 540–547.
24. Field, J. B., Boyle, C., and Remer, A. (1978). *Lancet,* **1**, 1191–94.
25. Micossi, P., Pontiroli, A. E., Baron, S. H., Tamayo, R. C., Lengel, F., Bevilacqua, M., Raggi, U., Norbiato, G., and Foa, P. O. (1978). *Diabetes* **27**, 1196–1204.
26. Chen, M., and Robertson, R. P. (1979). *Prostaglandins* **18**, 557–567.
27. Syvalahti, E. K. G. (1974) *Int. J. Clin. Pharmacol.* **10**, 111–16.
28. Widstrom, A. (1977). *Horm. Metab. Res.* **9**, 172–75.
29. Flower, F. J. (1974). *Pharmacol. Rev.* **26**, 33–67.
30. Kantor, H. D., and Hampton, M. (1978). *Nature (London)* **276**, 841–42.
31. Radomirov, R., and Petkov, V. (1977). *C. R. Acad. Bulg. Sci.* **30**, 775–77.
32. Porte, D., Jr., Graber, A. L., Kuzuya, T., and Williams, R. H. (1966). *J. Clin. Invest.* **45**, 228.
33. Porte, D., Jr., and Robertson, R. P. (1973). *Fed. Proc. Fed. Am. Soc. Expo. Biol.* **32**, 1792–1796.
34. Porte, D., Jr. (1967). *J. Clin. Invest.* **46**, 86–94.
35. Lerner, R. L., and Porte, D., Jr. (1972) *J. Clin. Invest.* **51**, 2205–2210.
36. Robertson, R. P., and Porte, D., Jr. (1973). *Diabetes* **22**, 1–8.
37. Robertson, R. P., and Guest, R. J. (1978). *J. Clin. Invest.* **63**, 1014–19.
38. Sacca, L., Perez, G., Rengo, F., Pascucci, I., and Condorelli, R. (1975). *Acta Endocrinol.* **79**, 266–74.
39. Giugliano, D. Torella, R., Sgambato, S., and D'Onofrio, F. (1979). *J. Clin. Endocrinol. Metab.* **48**, 302–08.
40. Metz, S. A., and Robertson, R. P. (1980). *Am. J. Physiol.* **239**, E490–500.
41. Metz, S. A., Robertson, R. P., and Fugimoto, W. (1981). *Diabetes* (in press).
42. Feldman, J. M., Quickel, K. E., and Lebovitz, H. E. (1972) *Diabetes* **21**, 779–88.
43. Robertson, R. P., Halter, J. B., and Porte, D., Jr. (1977). *J. Clin. Invest.* **57**, 791–795.
44. Hamberg, M. (1972). *Biochem. Biophys. Res. Commun.* **49**, 720–726.
45. Robertson, R. P., and Chen, M. (1977). *J. Clin. Invest.* **60**, 747–753.
46. Halushka, P. V., Lurie, D., and Colwell, J. A. (1977). *N. Engl. J. Med.* **297**, 306–10.
47. Ziboh, V. A., Maruta, H., Lord, J. T., Cagle, W. D., and Lucky, W. (1978). *Clin. Res.* **26**, 430A.
48. Zusman, R. M., Keiser, H. R., and Handler, J. S. (1977). *Fed. Proc. Fed. Am. Soc. Exp. Biol.* **36**, 2728–29.
49. Quickel, K. E., Jr., Feldman, J., and Lebovitz, H. E. (1971). *J. Clin. Endocrinol. Metab.* **33**, 877–81.

9

Biosynthesis of Glucagon and Somatostatin

B. D. NOE, D. J. FLETCHER, AND G. E. BAUER

I. INTRODUCTION

The discovery by Steiner and associates (Steiner and Oyer, 1967; Steiner *et al.*, 1967) that insulin is synthesized via proinsulin (see Chapter 4) stimulated many studies designed to ascertain whether other peptide hormones are also synthesized by way of precursors. As a result, precursor–product mechanisms have been found to exist for the synthesis of a number of peptide hormones including glucagon and somatostatin (see below). Of all the known precursor–product relationships, the most thoroughly

The Islets of Langerhans
Copyright © 1981 by Academic Press, Inc.
All rights of reproduction in any form reserved.
ISBN 0–12–187820–1

studied are proinsulin–insulin and proparathyroid hormone–parathyroid hormone (PTH). As a result of efforts to determine if larger precursors of proinsulin and pro-PTH exist, it was demonstrated that, when mRNA isolated from islets (Yip *et al.*, 1975; Chan *et al.*, 1976; Shields and Blobel, 1977) or parathyroid glands (Kemper *et al.*, 1974; Habener *et al.*, 1978) is translated in *in vitro* cell-free protein synthesis systems, the products synthesized are larger than the proinsulin and pro-PTH peptides which can be extracted from intact tissue. The extension peptides are found at the N-terminus of the prohormones, and the amino acid sequences of the extensions found in several species have been determined. Subsequently, "pre-prohormones" for glucagon and somatostatin, as well as those for insulin and PTH, have been found.

It has been known for some time that newly synthesized polypeptides destined for export from the cell cross the membranes and enter the cisternae of the endoplasmic reticulum (ER). This occurs either concomitantly with or shortly after their synthesis. Milstein *et al.* (1972), Blobel and Dobberstein (1975a,b), and Devillers-Thiery *et al.* (1975) have performed a number of experiments demonstrating that immunoglobulins in murine myeloma cells and zymogens in the exocrine pancreas have an N-terminal extension which is cleaved from the precursor either during or shortly after transport across the ER membranes. Partial sequence analyses of the extension peptides of prezymogens (Devillers-Thiery *et al.*, 1975), preproinsulin (Chan *et al.*, 1976; Shields and Blobel, 1977), pre-pro-PTH (Habener *et al.*, 1978), and a growing number of other prepropolypeptides have shown that all have regions of marked hydrophobicity.

The results from these studies have confirmed the "signal hypothesis" proposed by Blobel and Sabatini (1971). The hydrophobic N-terminal sequence presumably serves as a lipid-soluble "signal" which can initiate binding of ribosomes to ER membranes and facilitate movement of the growing polypeptide chain into the ER cisternae. The explanation for the inability to find significant quantities of pre-propolypeptides in intact tissue is that, in most tissues, the signal peptide is rapidly cleaved from the growing polypeptide chain by an enzyme called signal peptidase located on the inner aspect of ER cisternal membranes. Thus, in most studies using intact tissue, the predominant form of precursor found is the prohormone rather than the pre-prohormone.

Confirmation of the signal hypothesis has also generated information regarding the minimum allowable size of polypeptides destined for export from the cell. Blobel and Dobberstein (1975a) have calculated that, for a peptide having a signal of 20 amino acids which is fully extended into the ER cisternal space, it would take a chain of at least 78 amino acids to span the distance from the cleft between the large and small ribosomal subunits and the N-terminus of the peptide. The signal peptides sequenced to date range in size from 16 to 25 amino acid residues. This suggests that all polypeptides destined for export from the cell have to be at least 74 amino acids in length prior to signal cleavage. Thus small peptide hormones such as glucagon (29 amino acids) and somatostatin (14 amino acids) might be expected to be synthesized as larger precursors. It is therefore perhaps not surprising that pre-prohormones for glucagon and somatostatin have been identified. In this chapter, we review the information available regarding the mechanisms of glucagon and somatostatin biosynthesis, as well as proteolytic processing of prohormones to yield cleavage intermediates and peptide hormone products.

II. GLUCAGON BIOSYNTHESIS

A. Evidence for the Existence of a Glucagon Precursor

1. Large Glucagon Immunoreactive Peptides from Pancreas, Gut, Plasma, and Glucagon-Producing Tumors

One indication that glucagon may be synthesized via a precursor is the identification of peptides, from a number of sources, which are larger than glucagon but show glucagon immunoreactivity in glucagon radioimmunoassays (RIAs). Rigopoulou et al. (1970) first reported the existence of "large glucagon immunoreactivity" (LGI) peptides. They were found in gel filtration eluates of extracts of pancreases from dog, duck, cow, rat, and human. The LGI peptides detected varied in molecular size, but all were larger than 6 kilodaltons (kd). Preincubation with 8 M urea, 6 M guanidine hydrochloride, and 0.1 M mercaptoethanol failed to alter the gel filtration elution volume of canine LGI peptides, indicating the absence of noncovalent interactions or disulfide bonding between them.

Since this initial paper, numerous other reports of LGI peptides from the pancreas, gut, plasma, and glucagon-secreting tumors have appeared in the literature. A representative list of such contributions is given in Table I. The range in molecular size reported for these LGI peptides is from 4.5 to 160 kd. The nature of the very large glucagon immunoreactive components and their role in glucagon production, if any, has not yet been determined. As will be discussed later in this chapter, it is highly unlikely that any of these components having a molecular size greater than 18 kd serves as a biosynthetic precursor of glucagon.

TABLE I
Investigations in Which Large Glucagon Immunoreactive Peptides Have Been Identified[a]

Source and reference	Size of LGI peptide (kd)	Species
Pancreas		
Rigopoulou et al. (1970)	>6	Dog, duck, rat, cow, human
Krug and Mialhe (1971)	6	Duck
Noe and Bauer (1971, 1975)	12, 9, 4.9	Anglerfish
Hellerström et al. (1972, 1974)	18, 9	Guinea pig
Tager and Steiner (1973)	4.5	Cow, pig
O'Connor et al. (1973, 1976a)	9, 8.2	Rat, pigeon, ox, dog, rat, turkey
Tung (1973), Tung et al. (1976)	69, 9	Pigeon
Trakatellis et al. (1975)	9.1	Anglerfish
Srikant et al. (1977)	9	Dog
Tager and Markese (1979)	12, 9, 8	Rabbit
Patzelt et al. (1979)	19, 18, 13, 4.5	Rat
Lund et al. (1980)		Anglerfish (cell-free products)
Shields et al. (1981)		Anglerfish (cell-free products)
Gut		
Krug and Mialhe (1971)	6	Duck
Villanueva et al. (1976)	>40	Human
Sundby et al. (1976)	11.6	Pig
Jacobsen et al. (1977)	12, 4.5	Pig
Bhathena et al. (1977)		
(salivary gland)	29	Rat, mouse, guinea pig, human
Srikant et al. (1977)	65, 9	Dog
Chisholm et al. (1978)	9–10	Cat
Conlon et al. (1979)	12, 8, 5	Dog
Tager and Markese (1979)	12, 8	Rabbit
Plasma		
Valverde et al. (1974)	>150	Human
Weir et al. (1975)	160	Human
Jaspan and Rubenstein (1976)	>40, 9	Human
Jaspan et al. (1976)	>40, 9	Human
Kuku et al. (1976)	9	Human
Boden and Owen (1977)	79, 9	Human
Holst et al. (1978)	~9–10	Pig
Palmer et al. (1978)	~10–20, 9	Human
Glucagonomas		
Berger et al. (1980)	>9	Human
Holst and Bang Pederson (1975)	—	Human
Valverde et al (1976)	60, 9	Human
Danforth et al. (1976)	9	Human
Weir et al. (1977)	9	Human
Holst (1978)	—	Human
von Schenck et al. (1979)	~9	Human

[a] Representative list.

2. Chemical Characterization of Glucagon-Containing Peptides Larger Than Glucagon

Several glucagon immunoreactive peptides larger than glucagon have been partially (by amino acid composition or biological activity) or completely (by amino acid sequence) characterized. In 1973, Tager and Steiner published the complete amino acid sequence of a 4.5-kd peptide isolated from a commercial preparation of bovine-porcine glucagon. This peptide consisted of glucagon extended from its C-terminus by eight amino acids. Three of the eight additional amino acids were basic amino acids, and two of these three (lysine and arginine) were positioned at the N-terminus of the extending peptide, a fact which is significant with regard to proteolytic processing of the peptide (Section V). Tager and Steiner also found in the crystalline glucagon preparation several other peptides ranging in molecular size from 3.7 to 9 kd. In view of the sequence of the 4.5-kd peptide, it seems probable that each of the peptides detected is a fragment of a glucagon precursor.

Other investigators have achieved partial characterization of "big glucagons" isolated from several different sources: bovine pancreas (O'Connor and Lazarus, 1976a), pigeon islets (Tung et al., 1976), anglerfish islets (Trakatellis et al., 1975), and porcine gut (Sundby et al., 1976; Jacobsen et al., 1977). Partial sequence analysis data are available only for the porcine gut glucagon-like immunoreactive peptide which has an approximate molecular size of 11.6 kd and has been called glicentin or GLI-1. The sequence of the 11 amino acids at the C-terminal end of GLI-1 consists of the C-terminal three amino acids of pancreatic glucagon plus an eight amino acid extension (Jacobsen et al., 1977). This extension has a sequence identical to that of the C-terminus of the 4.5-kd peptide characterized by Tager and Steiner except for an inverted amino acid pair near the center of the peptide. The sequence of the N-terminal tridecapeptide of GLI-1 has also been determined and found not to contain any sequence present in glucagon (Sundby et al., 1976). These results suggest that GLI-1 may closely resemble pancreatic LGI peptide.

Additional evidence for the similarities between GLI-1 and pancreatic LGI is available. Using immunochemical techniques in conjunction with limited enzymatic digestion, Tager and Markese (1979) have demonstrated that glucagon-immunoreactive peptides which can be extracted from both the gut and pancreas of rabbits are virtually identical. It was shown that 12-kd or 8- to 9-kd immunoreactive peptides from either tissue source had extensions of the same length attached to both the C- and N-termini of glucagon. These results not only provide additional evidence for the existence of a glucagon precursor but also suggest that similar, if not identical, prohormones are present in gut and pancreatic islets. Further support for this latter possibility comes from the work of Ravazzola *et al.* (1979). Using an antiserum against GLI-1 which does not react with glucagon, these investigators localized GLI-1 by immunohistochemical means in the same cells of gut *and* pancreas containing pancreatic glucagon. Taken together, the results from these studies indicate that the cells of the gut and pancreas are ontogenetically related and that their secretory product(s) may be synthesized by similar precursors. The major difference between the cells is in the size of the products stored. In the intestine, the 12-kd and 8- to 9-kd peptides predominate, whereas the 3.5-kd form (glucagon) is the predominant peptide in the pancreas. This difference appears to be related to differential posttranslational proteolytic processing of the two precursors.

B. Studies on Glucagon Biosynthesis

In addition to chemical evidence for the existence of precursor–product relationships, it is necessary to demonstrate precursor-to-product transformation in metabolic studies performed either *in vivo* or *in vitro*. This is usually accomplished by incorporating radioactively labeled amino acids into the peptides of interest using pulse or pulse-chase incubations. A biosynthetic precursor should be larger than its product, it should become labeled more rapidly than the product, and metabolic transfer of label from precursor to product should occur during prolonged pulse or chase incubations. Investigations of glucagon biosynthesis have been performed in several species.

1. Studies Employing Fish Islets

In several species of fish, the pancreatic islet tissue is partially or completely separated anatomically from the exocrine pancreatic tissue. One can obtain from a single anglerfish (*Lophius americanus*) as much as 200–250 mg of zymogen-free islet tissue using simple dissection. In 1952, Audy and Kerly demonstrated glucagon-like biological activity in extracts of anglerfish islets. This was the first evidence that glucagon-producing cells might be present in this tissue. In a more recent immunohistochemical study, Johnson *et al.* (1976) showed that 90–95% of the volume of anglerfish islets was comprised of insulin-, somatostatin-, and glucagon-containing cells. Morphometric analyses yielded insulin/somatostatin/glucagon ratios of 9:6:4 for these cells. Thus the content of glucagon and somatostatin is high relative to that found in most other species.

The first successful attempts to obtain metabolic evidence for the existence of a glucagon precursor were made using anglerfish islet tissue. Noe and Bauer (1970, 1971) demonstrated the incorporation of [³H]tryptophan

(tryptophan is not found in proinsulin but is a component of glucagon) initially into a glucagon immunoreactive peptide having a molecular size of about 12 kd. Cycloheximide blocked the synthesis of this peptide, indicating ribosomal participation in its synthesis. Prolonged incubation or gentle trypsin treatment of the 12-kd component resulted in the generation of a ^{3}H-labeled component having the molecular size, electrophoretic mobility, and immunological characteristics of pancreatic glucagon. It was therefore suggested that the 12-kd peptide might serve as a biosynthetic precursor of glucagon (Noe and Bauer, 1971). In subsequent studies using pulse-chase incubations, it was possible to demonstrate that the conversion process apparently occurs in a stepwise fashion involving at least three cleavage steps. Cleavage intermediates of approximately 9 and 4.9 kd (Noe and Bauer, 1975; Noe, 1977) have been identified. Figure 1 shows the results obtained in a typical pulse-chase incubation. The 4.9-kd peptide was found to be highly basic (Noe, 1977) and is possibly similar to the proglucagon fragment isolated and characterized by Tager and Steiner (1973). Efforts to isolate and characterize the 4.9-, 9-, and 12-kd glucagon-containing peptides from anglerfish islet are currently in progress.

Preliminary studies on glucagon biosynthesis have also been performed using catfish pancreatic islets which are partially separated anatomically from exocrine tissue. The results showed that radiolabeled tryptophan was incorporated into peptides with sizes corresponding to those of the 12-, 9-, and 4.9-kd glucagon-containing peptides from anglerfish islets. It was possible to demonstrate that glucagon immunoreactivity was associated with the 9- and 4.9-kd peptides from catfish islets (Fletcher *et al.*, 1978).

2. Studies Employing Avian Islets

Several species of birds have islets in which alpha cells predominate. Knowledge of this situation led to the use of pigeon pancreatic islets in studies on glucagon biosynthesis. Tung and Zerega (1971) reported the incorporation of [^{3}H]tryptophan into two glucagon immunoreactive components from pigeon islets. One of these components had the molecular size of glucagon, whereas the other eluted near the void volume on BioGel P-10 gel filtration. Trypsin treatment of the larger component yielded a product having the approximate molecular size of glucagon. Although time-course incubations were not performed and no evidence for metabolic transfer of radioactivity from the larger to the smaller glucagon-related component was presented, these authors suggested that the larger molecule may serve as a biosynthetic precursor of glucagon. In a subsequent paper, Tung (1973) described a 69-kd polypeptide from pigeon islets, which could be labeled with [^{3}H]tryptophan. Tryptic hydrolysates of this component contained peptides having the molecular size and migration pattern on thin-

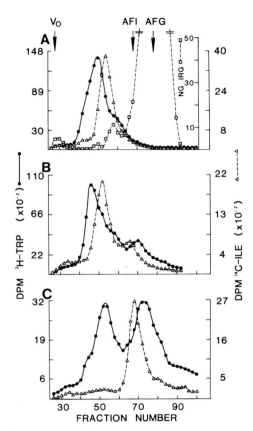

Fig. 1. Pulse-chase incubation of 200-mg anglerfish islet tissue using [³H]tryptophan and [¹⁴C]isoleucine. After 20 min of incubation in the presence of isotopes, the tissue was washed thoroughly in isotope-free medium containing 200 μg/ml unlabeled amino acids. Prior to the initiation of chase incubation in the wash medium, one-quarter of the tissue was removed and homogenized, and an acid ethanol extract of the resulting TCA precipitate was made. The final extract was adjusted to the equivalent of 1 M acetic acid and filtered on a 1.6 × 92 cm column of BioGel P-10 in 1 M acetic acid (A). After 1 hr (B), 3 hr (not shown), and 6 hr (C) of chase incubation, one-fourth of the remaining tissue was removed for extraction. Each extract was filtered on the same P-10 column. The distribution of immunoreactive glucagon (IRG) after filtration of an extract of 1.4 g of unlabeled tissue on this column is shown in (A). Anglerfish [¹⁴C]insulin (AFI) and a 4.9-kd [³H]glucagon immunoreactive peptide appear and accumulate during the chase incubation. Conversion of 12-kd proglucagon apparently progresses through 9- and 4.9-kd intermediates and proceeds very slowly to 3.5-kd glucagon (C). AFG, Anglerfish glucagon. (Reproduced from *Endocrinology* **97**, 870 with permission of J. B. Lippincott Co.)

layer chromatography of tryptic products of porcine glucagon. Since the 69-kd component retained its size after treatment with dissociative agents, the author proposed that it may serve as a glucagon precursor. Tung (1974) also reported the presence of 9- and 6-kd tryptophan-containing glucagon immunoreactive components in extracts of pigeon islets, which might serve as cleavage intermediates in precursor-to-product conversion.

O'Connor and Lazarus (1976a,b) also employed isolated pigeon islets for studies on glucagon biosynthesis. They identified large (20-kd) and small (~ 3.5-kd) glucagon immunoreactive components into which small amounts of [³H]trytophan could be incorporated after an incubation of 3.5 hr or longer. Although pulse-chase incubations were performed, no transfer of radioactivity from the large to the small component and no change in the ratio of glucagon immunoreactivity between them was found. These authors concluded that the 20-kd component did not serve as a biosynthetic precursor of pigeon glucagon.

3. Studies Employing Guinea Pig Islets

The first reports of studies using mammalian islets to study glucagon biosynthesis were published by Hellerström and co-workers. Their initial report described the incorporation of [³H]tryptophan into an 18-kd peptide in isolated islets from guinea pig (Hellerström et al., 1972). The 18-kd peptide was stable in 8 M urea and eluted from gel filtration columns irrigated with NH_4HCO_3 at pH 8.8 in a region where glucagon immunoreactivity could be detected. No evidence suggesting a role for the 18-kd peptide in glucagon biosynthesis was obtained. Accumulation of ³H radioactivity in glucagon was not observed even after islet culture in the presence of isotope for a period of 6 days.

In a subsequent publication, Hellerström et al. (1974) demonstrated that the material which eluted in the 18-kd region at alkaline pH appeared as a 9-kd peptide when eluted in 3 M acetic acid. These authors suggested that the 9-kd component elutes as a dimer at alkaline pH. Prolonged culture of guinea pig islets from 6 to 14 days resulted in the appearance of [³H]tryptophan labeled material eluting near the glucagon marker region. Even though no direct evidence for a precursor–product relationship between the 9-kd peptide and glucagon was obtained in these studies, it is possible (as the authors suggested) that in the guinea pig precursor conversion occurs at an extremely slow rate.

4. Studies Employing Rat or Mouse Pancreas or Islets

O'Connor et al. (1973) were the first to use rats in studies on glucagon biosynthesis. Using the isolated perfused pancreas, these investigators observed the initial incorporation of [³H]tryptophan into a 9-kd peptide having glucagon immunoreactivity. Prolonged incubation resulted in the incorporation of ³H label into a peptide which coeluted with glucagon on gel filtration and comigrated with glucagon when subjected to electrophoresis. Immunobinding was employed to demonstrate that the 3.5-kd labeled component was newly synthesized glucagon. However, no evidence for metabolic transfer of radioactivity from the 9-kd to the 3.5-kd component was obtained.

Petersen *et al.* (1975) described the labeling of a 16-kd glucagon immunoreactive peptide in islets from EMC-virus-infected mice. Labeling of a peptide having the size of glucagon, if observed, was not discussed. Again, no evidence that the larger glucagon-related peptide might serve as a glucagon precursor was presented. Similar results were obtained by Östenson *et al.* (1980) using isolated mouse islets.

The most compelling evidence for the existence of a precursor–product relationship generated from studies on glucagon biosynthesis using mammalian islets was published by Patzelt *et al.* (1979). In this elegant series of experiments, the radioactive peptides generated from incubations of isolated rat islets were analyzed by sodium dodecyl sulfate (SDS) polyacrylamide gel electrophoresis (PAGE). Glucagon immunoreactive peptides were identified by immunoprecipitation from gel slice eluates. Peptides having molecular sizes of 19, 18, 13, 4.5, and 3.5 kd were shown to possess glucagon-like immunological determinants. The 3.5-kd component was identified as glucagon. Peptide mapping of the enzymatic cleavage products of the 19- and 18-kd components proved that both contained structural segments identical with cleavage products of glucagon. Differential labeling combined with enzyme digestion was used to demonstrate that both N- and C-terminal extensions of the glucagon molecule were present in the LGI peptides and that the extensions were linked to glucagon by pairs of basic amino acids.

Patzelt *et al.* (1979) also employed pulse-chase incubations to examine the kinetics of glucagon biosynthesis in isolated rat islets. The first of the larger glucagon-containing peptides to appear as a labeled product in extracts was the 18-kd component. This component was subsequently subjected to a posttranslational modification which increased its molecular size to 19 kd. To determine whether this modification was a form of glycosylation of the 18-kd peptide, the 19-kd component was tested for affinity for a variety of plant lectins. It showed no affinity for the lectins tested, and radioactively labeled sugars did not become incorporated. Moreover, incubation in the presence of tunicamycin, a known inhibitor of glycosylation of proteins, failed to inhibit its formation. Thus the nature of the posttranslational modification of the 18-kd component remains to be determined.

Prolonged chase incubation (30–180 min) resulted in conversion of the 19-kd form to smaller intermediates and glucagon. Glucagon-containing intermediates of 13- and 4.5-kd were identified. A third intermediate of 10 kd was shown by peptide mapping to lack any of the structural components of glucagon but contained peptides present in the 18-kd precursor. The kinetics of label transfer from the 18-kd peptide through the various intermediates to glucagon were consistent with the existence of a precursor–product relationship. On the basis of these results, the authors have identified the 18-kd peptide as rat proglucagon.

5. Studies Employing Human Islets

Only one report of studies on glucagon biosynthesis using human pancreatic islets has appeared in the literature. Noe et al. (1975) demonstrated the incorporation of [³H]tryptophan into a glucagon-containing peptide of approximately 10 kd in addition to 3.5-kd human glucagon. Limited trypsin treatment of the 10-kd peptide yielded ³H-labeled peptides having glucagon immunoreactivity and the electrophoretic mobility of human glucagon and monodesamido glucagon. Labeled peptides larger than 10 kd which possessed glucagon-like immunoreactivity were also observed but not characterized in these studies. The presence of these larger glucagon-related peptides which become labeled with [³H]tryptophan during in vitro incubations is consistent with the existence of a precursor–product relationship in human glucagon biosynthesis. However, since no evidence of metabolic transfer of radioactivity from larger to smaller peptides was obtained, further investigation will be necessary to provide conclusive proof.

6. Summary of Results from Studies on Glucagon Biosynthesis

Metabolic transfer of radioactivity from larger glucagon-containing peptides through cleavage intermediates to glucagon was demonstrated using continuous-pulse or pulse-chase incubations in studies with anglerfish islets (Noe and Bauer, 1971, 1975; Noe, 1977) and rat islets (Patzelt et al., 1979). These results provide strong evidence for the existence of a precursor–product relationship in glucagon biosynthesis. It is not clear why it has been difficult to obtain similar results with many of the other experimental systems employed. The difficulties may in part be related to the peripheral disposition of the alpha cells in the islets of many mammals and the traumatization of these cells during islet isolation. Alternatively, some stimulus to normal synthesis and processing may be lacking in the various in vitro systems employed. The apparent difference in size between rat (18 kd) and anglerfish (12 kd) proglucagon is also somewhat puzzling. Obtaining a better understanding of the relationship between these two glucagon precursors must await determination of the primary structures of both.

C. Proposed Model for the Structure of Proglucagon

Although the complete amino acid sequence is not yet available for any of the putative proglucagons, sufficient evidence has been generated to allow formulation of a model for the structure of proglucagon. Such a model is shown in Fig. 2B. Figure 2A shows a model of the well-known structure of proinsulin for reference. The proglucagon model is adapted from models proposed by Tager and Markese (1979) and Patzelt *et al.* (1979) for mammalian proglucagons and porcine gut GLI-1 by Jacobsen *et al.* (1977). In islets of anglerfish and rabbit and in intestine from pig and

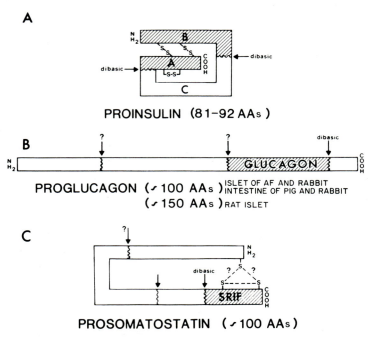

PROINSULIN (81–92 AAs)

PROGLUCAGON (∼100 AAs) ISLET OF AF AND RABBIT INTESTINE OF PIG AND RABBIT
(∼150 AAs) RAT ISLET

PROSOMATOSTATIN (∼100 AAs)

Fig. 2. Models for the structure of proinsulin (A), proglucagon (B), and prosomatostatin (C). The model for proinsulin is based on the known structures of proinsulins from various species (see Chapter 4). The model for proglucagon is adapted and modified from the models proposed by Jacobsen *et al.* (1977), Tager and Markese (1979), and Patzelt *et al.* (1979). Its structure is based on results from studies using anglerfish (AF), rabbit, and rat islets and rabbit and/or porcine intestine (see text). The model for prosomatostatin is based primarily on results from studies using intact anglerfish islets, analyses of cell-free translation products of mRNA from anglerfish islets (Shields, 1980a,b), and precursor sequences deduced from cloned cDNAs (Hobart *et al.,* 1980). Dibasic refers to sites in the respective precursors where it has been demonstrated that pairs of basic residues are positioned (i.e., cleavage sites for proteolytic processing); ?→ , possible location of additional cleavage sites; S-S, sites of intrachain disulfide bonds; S-?-S, possible location of additional intrachain disulfide bonds.

rabbit, the candidate prohormone appears to have a molecular size of
~ 12 kd and to consist of about 100 amino acids. The exception is found in
rat islets where proglucagon is 18 kd in molecular size. The difference in
the rat peptide appears to be the result of an additional extension of the
N-terminus of the peptide found in other species. With the exception of the
anglerfish prohormone, where the primary structure is not yet known, all
proglucagons have an octapeptide extension of the C-terminus of glucagon.
The first two amino acids in this extension are basic amino acids which provide a cleavage site similar to that found in many prohormones. Results
from enzyme cleavage studies suggest that the N-terminal extension is also
joined to glucagon by a pair of basic amino acid residues (Tager and
Markese, 1979). In Fig. 2 the arrows with question marks (Fig. 2B) indicate
potential cleavage sites in proglucagon. Their locations were determined on
the basis of the sizes of glucagon immunoreactive peptides, found in tissue
extracts, which may be cleavage products of proglucagon.

III. SOMATOSTATIN BIOSYNTHESIS

Since its initial isolation from ovine hypothalami and determination of
its primary structure (Burgus *et al.*, 1973), somatotropin release-inhibiting
factor (SRIF), or somatostatin, has been identified in various regions of the
central nervous system, the gastrointestinal mucosa, several endocrine
organs, and the blood (Parsons *et al.*, 1976; Luft *et al.*, 1978; Harris *et al.*,
1978). The highest concentration of SRIF activity, aside from that in the
brain, has been reported in the islets of Langerhans (Falkmer *et al.*, 1977).
SRIF has been localized in pancreatic D cells by immunofluorescent and
immunocytochemical techniques (Luft *et al.*, 1974). Following the development of SRIF radioimmunoassays, numerous investigators have demonstrated that SRIF is released in response to secretagogues from endocrine
cells in diverse tissues (see Chapter 11). However, few studies have directly
addressed the question of the mechanism of SRIF biosynthesis.

A. Evidence for the Existence of a Somatostatin Precursor

1. Large SRIF Immunoreactive Peptides from Various Sources

Studies on the molecular size heterogeneity of SRIF immunoreactive
peptides in tissue extracts have shown the presence of peptides larger than
authentic (tetradecapeptide) SRIF. These observations support the concept
that SRIF, like other small biologically active peptides, may be synthesized
by way of a precursor peptide (Table II). Of particular significance are
reports demonstrating that these larger peptides (a) can be cleaved by selec-

TABLE II
**Investigations in Which Large Somatostatin Immunoreactive
Peptides Have Been Identified**

Reference	Agent tested	Size of large SRIF (kd)	Source
A. Processing of large SRIF immunoreactive peptides to SRIF was demonstrated or is implicit in structure			
Conlon et al. (1978)	Trypsin	3.5	Pancreas (dog)
Esch et al.	—	2.7, 3.1	Hypothalamus (sheep)
Lauber et al. (1979)	Trypsin, endogenous protease(s)	15, 10, 6	Hypothalamus (mouse)
Hobart et al. (1980)	—	13.3, 14.1	Islet (anglerfish)
Millar (1978)	Aminopeptidase, carboxypeptidase B	5, ~3.5	Hypothalamus (sheep)
Noe et al. (1978)	Endogenous protease(s)	8–15	Islet (anglerfish)
Noe et al. (1979a)	Trypsin	8–15	Islet (anglerfish)
Oyama et al. (1980a)	—	3.1	Islet (catfish)
Patzelt et al. (1980)	Endogenous protease(s)	12.5	Islet (rat)
Pradayrol et al. (1978)	—	~2.4	Small Intestine (pig)
Pradayrol et al. (1980)	—	3.1	Small intestine (pig)
Schally et al. (1980)	—	3.1	Hypothalamus (pig)
Spiess and Vale (1980)	Trypsin	12	Hypothalamus (rat)
Zingg and Patel (1979, 1980)	Hypothalamic extract	25, 4	Hypothalamus (rat)
B. Demonstration of large SRIF-like peptide stability using dissociative or reducing agents			
Boyd et al. (1978)	Urea	<5	Hypothalamus (pig)
Conlon et al. (1978)	Urea, guanidine	12, 3.5	Pancreas (dog)
Conlon et al. (1981)	SDS, guanidine, DTT	12.5, 3.0	Pancreatic tumor (human)
Ensinck et al. (1978)	Urea	160, ~12, ~3.5	Pancreas (rat), hypothalamus (rat)
Lauber et al. (1979)	Urea, dithiothreitol	15, 10, 6	Hypothalamus (mouse)
Noe et al. (1979a)	Urea, guanidine, mercaptoethanol	15 (labeled), 8–10 (unlabeled)	Islet (anglerfish)
Patel and Reichlin (1978)	Urea	<5	Stomach, cortex, hypothalamus, islets (rat)
Spiess and Vale (1978)	Guanidine, mercaptoethanol	8.5–10, 6–7.5, 3.5–5	Pancreas (pigeon)
Spiess and Vale (1980)	Urea, guanidine, mercaptoethanol, SDS	12, 4	Hypothalamus (rat)
Weir et al. (1976)	Urea	<5	Pancreas (chicken)
C. Detection of large SRIF immunoreactive peptides which were not characterized			
Arimura et al. (1975)	—	>5	Stomach, pancreas (rat)
Harris et al. (1978)	—	150	Plasma (dog)
Larsson et al. (1977)	—	5, <5	Somatostatinoma (human)

TABLE II (cont.)

Reference	Agent tested	Size of large SRIF (kd)	Source
McIntosh et al. (1978)	—	> 5	Pancreas, stomach (human)
Chayvialle et al. (1978)	—	< 5	Stomach, duodenum (human)
Rorstad et al. (1977)	—	< 5, 3–4	Median eminence, anterior hypophysis, amygdala, cerebral cortex (rat)

tive proteolysis to yield a peptide with the molecular size (1.6 kd) and immunological or biological activity of authentic SRIF (Table IIA) or (b) possess dibasic residues (cleavage sites) as part of their primary structures (Table IIA). These larger peptides, and intermediate derivative forms, are definite candidates for precursors in the biosynthesis of SRIF. Other larger peptides with SRIF-like immunological activities, shown to retain their size following treatments that disrupt noncovalent and/or disulfide linkages (Table IIB), must also be considered possible precursors or intermediates in SRIF biosynthesis. Determination of the possible role of the remaining large molecular species with SRIF-like activity, which are listed in Table IIC, must await further investigation.

A marked similarity in the molecular size of SRIF-like peptides identified from diverse sources is observed. Aside from peptides of ~ 150 kd which probably represent SRIF bound loosely to other proteins (as identified in plasma by Harris et al., 1978), the larger SRIF-like peptides were reported to be 1.6, 3.5, 6, 8–10 and 12–15 kd in molecular size. As will be discussed in Section III, C, the available evidence indicates that prosomatostatin is in the range of 12 kd to 16 kd in size. Support for this view has been obtained recently from studies on mouse hypothalamus. In the studies of Lauber et al. (1979), the largest SRIF-immunoreactive peptide observed in extracts of mouse hypothalami had an apparent molecular size of 15 kd. Since the extracts were subjected to fairly rigorous dissociative conditions, the estimated size of this peptide can be considered reasonably accurate. Upon incubation of the 15-kd material with endogenous proteolytic enzymes derived from tissue extracts, the peptide was converted to smaller SRIF-immunoreactive peptides of 10, 6, and 1.6 kd. Although supporting the possible existence of a 15-kd prosomatostatin, these studies do not provide proof that the larger peptides are obligatory intermediates in the biosynthesis of SRIF.

2. Chemical Characterization of Somatostatin-Containing Peptides Larger Than SRIF

Limited proteolysis was used to characterize the chemical structure of a possible intermediate in SRIF biosynthesis by Millar (1978). A urea-stable, 5-kd peptide with SRIF-like immunoreactivity was partially purified from extracts of ovine hypothalami, treated with aminopeptidase or carboxypeptidase B, and refiltered on a Sephadex G-25 column. Aminopeptidase treatment markedly reduced SRIF-like immunoreactivity and cleaved the 5-kd molecule into several smaller peptides, but carboxypeptidase B treatment increased the SRIF-like immunoreactivity of the 5-kd peptide (presumably by unfolding a C-terminal extension). The author concluded that a short N-terminal extension and a longer C-terminal extension are probably present in the 5-kd SRIF-containing peptide. Of all the SRIF-containing peptides which have been sequenced, however, none have C-terminal extensions.

A SRIF-related peptide with a molecular size of about 3.1 kd has been purified from the pig small intestine (Pradayrol *et al.,* 1980). Amino acid sequence analysis has shown that the peptide consists of somatostatin with a 14-amino-acid N-terminal extension. Subsequently, octacosapeptides having amino acid sequences identical to this gut peptide have been found in ovine (Esch *et al.,* 1980) and porcine (Schally *et al.,* 1980) hypothalamic extracts. This peptide, which has up to 10 times the bioactivity of somatostatin-14 (Brazeau *et al.,* 1981), is now referred to as somatostatin-28. A pair of basic amino acids links the N-terminal extension to tetradecapeptide somatostatin in somatostatin-28. This fact, in combination with results from studies of somatostatin biosynthesis (see below), suggests that somatostatin-28 may be a cleavage intermediate in the processing of prosomatostatin to somatostatin.

Finally, another SRIF-related peptide isolated from catfish islets has 22 amino acids but differs significantly in primary structure from somatostatin-28. It was found to have signficant SRIF-like bioactivity, however (Oyama *et al.,* 1980a). The relationship of this peptide to tetradecapeptide somatostatin and its potential role in the biosynthesis of this unusual form of somatostatin found in the catfish remain to be determined.

B. Studies on Somatostatin Biosynthesis

1. Studies Employing Anglerfish Islet

The first successful studies on SRIF biosynthesis employed the principal islet of the anglerfish (*L. americanus*) (Noe *et al.,* 1976). The fortuitous aggregation of islet tissue into this macroscopic organ and the high concentration of SRIF-containing D cells (Johnson *et al.*, 1976) promote the active incorporation of radioactively labeled amino acids into SRIF-like peptides in an *in vitro* system.

In initial attempts to demonstrate the biosynthesis of somatostatin in this tissue, it was assumed that the primary structure of SRIF in the anglerfish islet was similar or identical to the ovine and porcine hypothalamic hormone. Therefore it was reasoned that, by incubating anglerfish islets in the presence of radioactive amino acids known to be constituents of SRIF, labeling of anglerfish islet SRIF would be observed. Tritiated tryptophan and reduced [^{35}S]cystine (cysteine) were selected as amino acid precursors. Tryptophan labels glucagon-related peptides (Section II,B), and cysteine labels insulin-related peptides (Noe, 1971; Fletcher *et al.*, 1981). It was anticipated that both isotopes would be incorporated into newly synthesized SRIF-related peptides. Two additional factors had to be considered before conducting these studies: (1) In earlier studies on glucagon biosynthesis, labeling of trichloroacetic acid (TCA)-precipitable acid ethanol-soluble peptides having the gel filtration elution position expected for SRIF was not observed (Fig. 1). Presumably, significant losses of SRIF occurred as a result of incomplete precipitation by TCA. (2) The molecular size of SRIF (1.6 kd) was insufficiently large to ensure its separation during BioGel P-10 gel filtration from free (unincorporated) labeled amino acids. These problems were avoided by extracting islet peptides directly in 2 *M* acetic acid and then removing unincorporated labeled amino acids by gel filtration on a BioGel P-2 column. The desalted extract then was applied to a BioGel P-10 column (fractionation range, 20–1.5 kd) to effect separation of the peptides of interest. After incubation under a variety of conditions with [^{3}H]tryptophan and reduced [^{35}S]cystine, samples of islet tissue extracts were analyzed for incorporated ^{3}H and ^{35}S radioactivity and SRIF-like immunoactivity by RIA.

Extracts of tissue incubated for short periods (up to 1 hr) contained [^{3}H]proglucagon and [^{35}S]proinsulin, whereas no labeling of insulin (6 kd), glucagon (3.5 kd), or SRIF (1.6 kd) occurred. After incubations of 2–6 hr, however, labeling of insulin, proglucagon conversion intermediates, and SRIF-like peptides increased progressively. As predicted, a peptide having the molecular size of SRIF was doubly labeled with ^{3}H (tryptophan residues) and ^{35}S (cysteine residues), whereas glucagon and insulin were labeled only with ^{3}H and ^{35}S. respectively. When subjected to inverted alkaline PAGE, anglerfish SRIF-like peptide migrated toward the cathode with a rate identical to that of a mammalian hypothalamic SRIF standard (Noe *et al.*, 1976, 1978, 1979a). In addition, the peptide isolated by PAGE showed SRIF-like immunoreactivity by RIA. Further evidence that [^{3}H]tryptophan and [^{35}S]cysteine residues were present in the anglerfish SRIF-like peptide was obtained by binding the doubly labeled 1.6-kd material on an affinity chromatography column to which anti-SRIF antibody had been complexed. These results demonstrated that [^{3}H]tryptophan and [^{35}S]cysteine were incorporated into anglerfish somatostatin.

Recent work has confirmed the original assumption that anglerfish islet SRIF is similar to ovine hypothalamic SRIF. The amino acid sequence and biological activity of SRIF from anglerfish islet were found to be identical to those of synthetic SRIF (Noe *et al.*, 1979b). Indeed, the amino acid sequences of tetradecapeptide somatostatin from a number of sources have been found to be identical: ovine (Burgus *et al.*, 1973) and porcine (Schally *et al.*, 1976) hypothalamic, pigeon pancreatic (Spiess *et al.*, 1979), porcine intestinal (Pradayrol *et al.*, 1980), anglerfish islet (Noe *et al.*, 1979b), and rat pancreatic SRIF (Benoit *et al.*, 1980). These findings suggest that the frequency of mutation in the gene coding for this peptide is remarkably low.

Results from pulse-chase incubations of anglerfish islets demonstrated the metabolic transfer of radioactivity from SRIF immunoreactive peptides in the 8- to 15-kd size range to somatostatin during the chase incubations (Fig. 3). The molecular size of the labeled large SRIF immunoreactive peptides was not altered by treatment with 6 *M* guanidine HCl, 8 *M* urea plus 5% thioglycolic acid, or boiling (5 min) in 8 *M* guanidine HCl plus 5% mercaptoethanol. However, when radioactively labeled material from the 8- to 15-kd region of gel filtration eluates was exposed to cell-free extracts of unlabeled islet tissue containing lysed secretory granules or subjected to limited trypsin treatment, a labeled peptide with the molecular size, electrophoretic mobility, and immunoreactivity of SRIF was generated. These results suggested that SRIF was covalently bound within a larger peptide. Based on this conclusion and the results from pulse-chase incubations, the authors suggested that a precursor peptide eluting in the 8-to 15-kd portion of gel filtration eluates participated in the biosynthesis of somatostatin (Noe *et al.*, 1979a).

It should be noted that labeled SRIF immunoreactive peptides larger than 15 kd were also identified in anglerfish islet extracts. These larger peptides, unlike the putative precursors, were readily cleaved to smaller peptides when treated with dissociative agents. Therefore, none of this material is thought to be involved in the biosynthesis of anglerfish islet peptides.

2. Studies Employing Rat Brain or Pancreas

Attempts to demonstrate the biosynthesis of somatostatin in mammalian tissues (e.g., hypothalamus and islets of Langerhans) have met with limited success, largely because of the presence of relatively low concentrations of SRIF-containing cells in these tissues. Even in pancreatic islets isolated

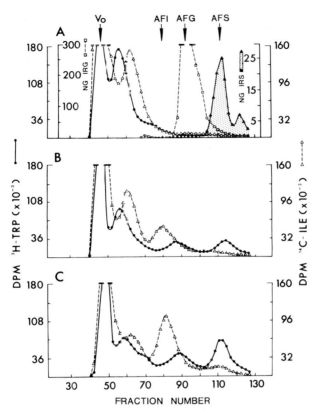

Fig. 3. Pulse-chase incubation of 200-mg anglerfish islet tissue using [³H]tryptophan and [¹⁴C]isoleucine. After a 30-min pulse incubation in the presence of isotopes, the tissue was washed thoroughly in isotope-free medium containing 50 μg/ml unlabeled amino acids and 100 μg/ml cycloheximide. Prior to postincubation, one-third of the tissue was removed for homogenization and extraction in 2 M acetic acid. The desalted extract was subjected to gel filtration in 2 M acetic acid on a 1.6 × 95 cm column of BioGel P-10 (A). Unlike the extraction of TCA precipitates with acid ethanol (Fig. 1), direct extraction in acetic acid results in the retention of SRIF in the extract. One-third of the tissue was removed for extraction and gel filtration after 2 hr (B) and 4 hr (C) of chase incubation in the presence of wash medium. AFI, AFG, and AFS indicate the elution positions of the major peaks of insulin, glucagon, and SRIF immunoreactivity, respectively. In addition to the accumulation of labeled insulin and glucagon resulting from the processing of their respective precursors, [³H]SRIF accumulates during chase incubations performed under conditions in which protein synthesis is inhibited. (IRG, Immunoreactive glucagon; IRS, immunoreactive somatostatin. Reproduced from *Diabetes* **28**, 726, 1979, with permission of the American Diabetes Assoc., Inc.)

from the rat, only about 5% of the tissue is comprised of D cells (Luft *et al.*, 1978), and in most laboratories only 200–300 islets (about 3 mg of tissue wet wt) can be obtained under ideal conditions from a rat pancreas.

In the studies of Ensinck *et al.* (1978), slices of anterior or posterior hypothalamus, pancreas, or isolated pancreatic islets were incubated in an *in vitro* system containing [³H]phenylalanine for periods up to 8 hr. Acetic acid extracts of tissue homogenates or media were neutralized and filtered through an anti-SRIF affinity column. The radioactive material retained by the immunoadsorbant ([³H]SLI) then was gel-filtered on Sephadex G-50 columns. The predominant [³H]SLI material in all tissue and media extracts eluted at the void volume (V_0) of the columns, with the media yielding two- to fourfold more [³H]SLI than the tissues at all incubation time periods (2–6 hr). With increasing duration of incubation, [³H]SLI eluting at the V_0 increased, and material having the molecular size of SRIF appeared after 4 and 6 hr of incubation. After 6 M urea treatment of the [³H]SLI which eluted at the V_0, it was refiltered on a Sephadex G-100 column. Its molecular size was estimated to be 160 kd. Incubation of hypothalamic slices in the presence of cycloheximide significantly reduced the total [³H]SLI but not labeled material in the SRIF fraction. No evidence for a precursor–product relationship between the large SLI material and SRIF was generated in these studies.

Additional evidence for the biosynthesis of SRIF by mammalian pancreatic islets was obtained by Zühlke *et al.* (1978). Islets were isolated from rats by collagenase digestion and incubated in medium containing [³H]phenylalanine for 5 hr. After homogenizing the washed islets, aliquots of the tissue extract were incubated overnight in the presence of anti-SRIF serum with or without the addition of unlabeled SRIF. Any reduction in the binding of ³H label by added (unlabeled) SRIF was considered to represent displacement by newly synthesized SRIF or SRIF immunoreactive peptides. Whereas the study provided evidence for the presence of newly synthesized [³H]SRIF-related material in the incubated islets, no data on the kinetics of labeling were provided (i.e., only one incubation time period was tested), nor was there any estimate of the molecular size of the SRIF-like peptide(s).

The most convincing evidence in support of a precursor–product relationship in somatostatin biosynthesis in mammals has been obtained by Patzelt *et al.* (1980). Using isolated rat islets, it was possible to demonstrate that a polypeptide of 12.5 kd becomes labeled initially during pulse incubations, then progressively loses its radioactivity during chase incubations. Newly synthesized somatostatin accumulated during chase incubations. Since all of the tryptic peptides of somatostatin were found after trypsin treatment of the 12.5-kd protein (indicating there is no extension of the

C-terminal tryptic fragment of SRIF), it was concluded that tetradecapeptide SRIF is located at the COOH-terminus of the putative precursor. Further studies on SRIF biosynthesis in mammalian tissues are required, however, because (a) the 12.5-kd protein could not be precipitated with antisera to SRIF, (b) direct evidence for metabolic transfer of label from precursor to product during chase incubation was not obtained, and (c) no cleavage intermediates were identified in the studies of Patzelt et al.

3. Summary of Results from Studies on Stomatostatin Biosynthesis

The results from studies performed using anglerfish islet leave little doubt that somatostatin, like insulin and glucagon, is synthesized by way of a biosynthetic precursor. The data from this work, and results from recent studies in which the products from cell-free translation of mRNA from anglerfish islet were analyzed extensively (Shields, 1980a,b) and the sequences of several preprosomatostatins which were determined using recombinant DNA methodology (Hobart et al., 1980; Goodman et al., 1980), indicate that prosomatostatin in anglerfish islets has a molecular size of 12–16 kd (Section IV). Although proteolytic processing of prosomatostatin yields somatostatin, further investigation will be necessary to identify any intermediates which may be generated during cleavage.

C. Proposed Model for the Structure of Prosomatostatin

A model for the structure of anglerfish prosomatostatin is presented in Fig. 2C. The recent work of Shields (1980a,b) and Hobart et al. (1980) provides convincing evidence that anglerfish prosomatostatin has a molecular size of 12–16 kd and that SRIF is located at the C-terminus of the precursor (Section IV). Therefore the model depicts a peptide consisting of ∼100 amino acids with C-terminal somatostatin.

An additional feature incorporated into the model is the presence of intrachain disulfide bonds which facilitate approximation of the C-terminus (somatostatin) to the midregion or N-terminal portion of the prohormone. The number and exact placement of these cross-links have not yet been determined. The rationale for proposing the existence of these intrachain disulfide bonds derives from several types of experimental evidence. The first is that treatment of the large SRIF immunoreactive peptides obtained from several different tissue sources with a reducing agent (dithiothreitol or mercaptoethanol) results in dissociation of the larger peptides to smaller immunoreactive components (Spiess and Vale, 1978; Conlon et al., 1978; Noe et al., 1979a). These observations are consistent with the existence, in the tissues of origin, of prosomatostatin molecules that have undergone proteolytic processing at one or more sites (e.g., at the proposed sites of dibasic residues in Fig. 2C) but in which the cleaved chains are still held together by disulfide bonds. The various chains would then be dissociated upon exposure to reducing agents, but only those cleavage products retaining the C-terminal end would possess somatostatin immunoreactivity. Experiments performed recently in our laboratory to test this hypothesis have yielded data in its support. Results from earlier work had shown that newly labeled 8- to 15-kd precursors from anglerfish islets were not dissociated into smaller components by treatment with dissociative or reducing agents (Noe *et al.,* 1979a). Labeled anglerfish islet precursor pool peptides (previously treated with 8 *M* urea and 6 *M* guanidine HCl) were subjected to very limited tryptic digestion, and one-half of the tryptic digest analyzed by gel filtration. Only minimal accumulation of labeled or SRIF immunoreactive material appeared in the SRIF-containing portion of the eluate. The remaining one-half of the tryptic digest was incubated with dithiothreitol prior to filtration. A marked accumulation of both ^{3}H radioactivity and SRIF immunoreactivity appearing at the elution position of SRIF was observed, suggesting that reduction was required, in addition to proteolysis, in the processing of prosomatostatin (B.D. Noe, unpublished).

Finally, the positioning of the dibasic residues in the prosomatostatin model (Fig. 2C) is based on numerous reports in the literature describing SRIF immunoreactive peptides smaller than 15 kd but larger than 1.6 kd (Table II). The only placement of dibasic residues which is firmly established at the time of this writing is the one located at the N-terminus of SRIF. Its positioning is based on the structure of somatostatin-28 described by Pradayrol *et al.* (1980), Schally *et al.* (1980), and Esch *et al.* (1980) and the results of Hobart *et al.* (1980).

IV. DISCOVERY OF PREPROGLUCAGONS AND PREPROSOMATOSTATINS

As indicated in Section I, it is probable that most, if not all, peptides destined for export from their cells of origin (or for incorporation into lysosomes or peroxisomes) are synthesized as pre-pro forms to facilitate penetration of the membranes of the ER. Accordingly, preprohormones have been identified for several peptide hormones including insulin (see Chapter 4). It is thus reasonable to assume that preprohormones for glucagon and somatostatin should exist as well.

Results from two laboratories working independently have recently confirmed the existence of several forms of anglerfish preproglucagon. After cell-free translation of poly A (messenger) RNA from anglerfish islets, glucagon-containing products were precipitated using specific antisera. Lund *et al.* (1980) identified a protein of 14.5 kd as preproglucagon. The addition of microsomal membranes to the translation mixtures resulted in the processing of the 14.5-kd protein to a 12.5-kd glucagon-immuno-reactive peptide which became cotranslationally segregated within micro-somes (proglucagon). Shields *et al.* (1981), using highly resolutive SDS gels, were able to identify two preproglucagon molecules of approximately 14 kd and a third having a molecular size of 16 kd. In addition, these workers made the intriguing observation that during cotranslational processing of these preprohormones in the presence of microsomal membranes, the 16-kd component was processed to a slightly smaller polypeptide whereas the 14-kd components were processed to larger (15 kd) polypeptides. Further work will be necessary to determine the nature of this additive mode of processing and the primary structures of these various preproglucagons from the same tissue source.

Preprosomatostatins have also recently been identified and character-ized. Shields (1980a) used immunoprecipitation, limited proteolysis, and peptide mapping of cell-free translation products of anglerfish islet mRNA to demonstrate clearly that an 18-kd polypeptide is a preprosomatostatin. The results from peptide mapping studies placed tetradecapeptide SRIF at the immediate C-terminus of the preprohormone and showed that an arginine–lysine sequence linked the N-terminus of SRIF to the remainder of the peptide. Subsequently, Shields (1980b) was able to demonstrate the presence of a second distinct (19 kd) preprosomatostatin molecule. Good-man *et al.* (1980a), also using anglerfish islet message, obtained similar results with the estimated sizes of the two immunoprecipitable prepro-somatostatins being 16 kd and 14 kd. The differences in size estimates of the preprosomatostatins identified in these two laboratories are most likely due to the use of different SDS gel systems. A 15-kd polypeptide has also been identified as a preprosomatostatin by immunoprecipitation of cell-free translation products of poly A containing RNA from rat or mouse hypothalami (Joseph-Bravo *et al.*, 1980).

Hobart *et al.* (1980) and Goodman *et al.* (1980b) have independently cloned, in bacteria, DNAs complementary to mRNAs coding for preproso-matostatins in anglerfish islet. The cloned cDNAs have been sequenced, and from these data the complete amino acid sequences of the preprosoma-tostatins were deduced. Hobart *et al.* have described the sequence of two distinct preprosomatostatins (I = 13.3 kd and II = 14.1 kd). "Preproso-matostatin I" has 121 amino acids with tetradecapeptide SRIF at its COOH-terminus. "Preprosomatostatin II" is 125 amino acids in length and has a COOH-terminal tetradecapeptide similar to SRIF but has amino acid substitutions at positions 7 and 10. The single preprosomatostatin described by Goodman *et al.* (1980b) is similar in size to preprosomato-statin I of Hobart *et al.* (119 amino acids vs 121) and has SRIF at its C-terminus, but it differs in sequence at 19 positions of the prohormone segment. The results of these studies correlate well with, and confirm the results from, work on SRIF biosynthesis using intact anglerfish islet (Noe *et al.*, 1976, 1978, 1979a,b; Fletcher *et al.*, 1980) and cell-free translation of islet mRNA (Shields, 1980a,b; Goodman *et al.*, 1980a). The accumulated data support the proposed structure of prosomatostatin shown in Fig. 2C. Preprosomatostatin consists of prosomatostatin extended from its N-terminus by a signal sequence of ~ 20 amino acids.

The results from the cell-free translation experiments and cDNA se-quencing demonstrate convincingly that the extremely large glucagon (LGI) or SRIF immunoreactive (LSI) peptides found in plasma or tissues of various organisms (Tables I and II) are not synthetic products of islet or hypothalamic tissue. It is improbable that any insulin-, glucagon- or SRIF-containing peptides > 18 kd are synthesized in or released from islets or other tissues. A possible exception to this is in the rat islet where preproglucagon may be as large as 21 kd (Patzelt *et al.*, 1979). It is therefore probable that LGI and LSI peptides with molecular sizes > 20 kd represent smaller glucagon- and somatostatin-containing peptides bound noncovalently to larger components.

V. CONVERSION OF ISLET PROHORMONES AT THE SUBCELLULAR LEVEL

Investigation of the subcellular conversion of glucagon or somatostatin precursors has been almost exclusively limited to studies using the angler-fish islet (Noe *et al.*, 1977a,b; Fletcher *et al.*, 1980, 1981). The advantages of the anglerfish islet for the investigation of glucagon and somatostatin biosynthesis in intact tissue also make this system extremely favorable for investigation at the subcellular level. The only other studies on the subcellular conversion of proglucagon have been conducted with guinea pig islets. Hellerström *et al.* (1974) reported the presence of a tryptophan-labeled, 9-kd peptide in A_2-cell (A-cell) secretory granules isolated from guinea pig islets. However, conversion to 3.5-kd glucagon was not detected. In a related study using electron microscopic autoradiography, Howell *et al.* (1974) demonstrated the transfer of radiolabel from rough ER through the Golgi complex to secretory granules of guinea pig A_2 cells. There have been no reports of studies on somatostatin biosynthesis at the subcellular level in any islet system other than the anglerfish islet.

Noe *et al.* (1977a) developed a fractionation procedure which yielded seven subcellular fractions. Two of these were secretory granule fractions and one consisted of microsomes. By assaying the distribution of nucleic acids and immunoreactive hormones and by electron microscopic examination of the fractions, it was determined that the microsome and granule fractions were highly purified. Further characterization of the microsome and granule fractions (Fletcher *et al.*, 1980, 1981) showed that these fractions contained 76% of the total cellular immunoreactive insulin, 80% of the immunoreactive glucagon, and 86% of the immunoreactive somatostatin. When the seven fractions were assessed for the distribution of specific enzyme markers for cellular components, it was shown that the secretory granule fractions contained only 10% of the total β-N-acetylglucosaminidase activity (a lysosome marker) and 8% of the 5'-nucleotidase activity (a plasma membrane marker). These results indicated that the secretory granules and, to a lesser degree, the microsomes obtained from anglerfish islet tissue were suitable for the study of islet prohormone conversion at the subcellular level.

The results from initial studies by Noe *et al.* (1977b) showed that both proglucagon and proinsulin were synthesized in the microsomes and then transported to the secretory granules. This was demonstrated by the selective radiolabeling of the two prohormones and gel filtration analysis of extracts to determine the content of precursor and product peptides. These authors also found that conversion of both prohormones began in the microsome fraction and continued in the granules. The detection of converting activity in the microsomes was somewhat surprising, since only limited converting activity had been observed in microsomal fractions in studies using other species (Sorenson *et al.*, 1970; Creutzfeldt *et al.*, 1973; Sun *et al.*, 1973). The appearance of radiolabeled glucagon and insulin in the microsome fraction indicated that the processing of both prohormones to their respective products began in the ER–Golgi complex.

Investigation of the subcellular conversion of anglerfish proglucagon and proinsulin was continued by Fletcher *et al.*, (1981), who also examined conversion of a somatostatin precursor to somatostatin at the subcellular level (Fletcher *et al.*, 1980). Figure 4A shows the gel filtration profile of an extract of secretory granules isolated from tissue incubated in the presence of [³H]tryptophan and [¹⁴C]isoleucine and then postincubated for 7 hr. Granules extracted at the beginning of the postincubation contained only minute amounts of radiolabeled hormones. The gel filtration pattern shown in Fig. 4A was virtually identical to that observed when microsomes were anlayzed under similar conditions and is very similar to that observed for whole tissue (Fig. 3C). This was the first demonstration of the conversion of a somatostatin precursor to somatostatin by subcellular components of islet tissue. Furthermore, the conversion products resulting

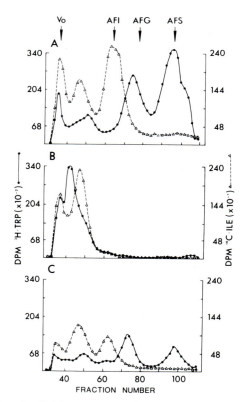

Fig. 4. Conversion of radiolabeled prohormones to hormones by secretory granules. (A) Secretory granules were isolated from anglerfish islets incubated 3 hr in the presence of [³H]tryptophan and [¹⁴C]isoleucine. After suspension in 0.02 *M* sodium acetate buffer, pH 5.2, granules were postincubated 7 hr at 30°C and then extracted with 2 *M* acetic acid. The extract was filtered on a 1.6 × 90 cm column of BioGel P-10 in 2 *M* acetic acid. (B) Filtration pattern of a 2 *M* acetic acid extract of a mixture of lysed secretory granules prepared from unlabeled tissue and labeled 8- to 15-kd precursor pool peptides prepared separately. The mixture was suspended in 0.02 *M* sodium acetate buffer, pH 5.2. No conversion of prohormones is evident. (C) A mixture identical to that described in (B) was allowed to postincubate 6 hr at 30°C prior to extraction and gel filtration. AFI, AFG, and AFS indicate the elution positions of the predominant peaks of immunoreactive insulin, glucagon, and SRIF, respectively. The results from the conversion of exogenous labeled prohormones by lysed secretory granules (C) are indistinguishable from those obtained upon postincubation of intact secretory granules containing endogenous labeled precursors (A). (Reproduced from Fletcher *et al.*, in press, *J. Cell Biol.*, with permission of the Rockefeller University Press.)

from the endogenous conversion of precursor peptides were found to have the same respective electrophoretic mobilities as somatostatin, glucagon, and insulin from intact tissue.

By calculating the percentage of conversion of proinsulin to insulin and the percentage of accumulation of glucagon and somatostatin (since the somatostatin and glucagon precursors cannot be identified by gel filtration alone), the conversion rates for each prohormone were assessed. The rate of conversion (or product accumulation) for each prohormone in the secretory granules was very similar to that observed in whole tissue. For all three converting activities, the pH optimum for conversion *in vitro* was in the range from pH 4.5 to 5.5, which was similar to the pH optimum for proinsulin conversion in rat islets (Sorenson *et al.*, 1972). Disruption of the granules prior to postincubation did not affect conversion of any of the precursor peptides. Electron microscopic examination of granules subjected to repeated freeze-thawing or osmotic shock revealed that ~95% of the granules were lysed, but conversion rates in lysed granules were similar to those in control. This indicated that integrity of the granule membrane was not essential for converting activity. Sorenson *et al.* (1972) also found that lysis of secretory granules from rat islets did not significantly reduce the conversion of proinsulin.

In addition to endogenous converting activities, both granules and microsomes (unlabeled) converted exogenously radiolabeled prohormones to their respective products. Figure 4B and C illustrates conversion of exogenously labeled precursors by a granule preparation. The lysed granule-prohormone mixture was either extracted immediately (Fig. 4B) or allowed to postincubate for 6 hr (Fig. 4C). The conversion products have the elution positions of insulin, glucagon, and somatostatin, respectively.

In another series of conversion experiments using exogenously labeled precursors, the membranous and soluble components of granules were examined for converting activity. After separation of the two components by repeated freeze-thawing and high-speed centrifugation, membranes and the resulting supernates were postincubated in the presence of radiolabeled prohormones. Both the membranous and soluble components of the granules were found to have significant converting activity for all 3 prohormones. The conversion of all 3 prohormones by both membranes and supernates was significantly inhibited in the presence of leupeptin, an arginine-containing peptide aldehyde that inhibits serine and thiol proteinases (Umezawa and Aoyagi, 1977). HPLC and electrophoretic analyses of conversion products which accumulated in either the membranous or soluble component of the granule preparation demonstrated that the converting activities represented actual cleavage of the prohormones and not a nonspecific degradation of the precursor peptides.

These data indicated that the converting activities present in the membranes and supernates were very similar in terms of specificity and mode of action. A reasonable interpretation of these results is that the converting enzyme(s) is loosely associated with the granule membranes and that some of the enzyme becomes dislodged or detached upon granule lysis. Since integrity of the granule membrane is not required for converting activity, the enzyme could function while suspended in the supernate.

Further characterization of the converting enzyme(s) was accomplished by investigating the effects of various proteinase inhibitors on converting activity in postincubated secretory granules. Significant inhibition of all three converting activities was observed when lysed granules were incubated in the presence of leupeptin or antipain, another arginine-containing peptide aldehyde (Umezawa and Aoyagi, 1977), or in the presence of *p*-chloromercuribenzoate (PCMB) or dithiodipyridine (DDP), both of which are thiol proteinase inhibitors. Inhibition by these four compounds was not due to a detectable conformational alteration of the precursor peptides, since the gel filtration elution positions of the prohormones were unchanged. There was no significant reduction of conversion in the presence of serine proteinase inhibitors, such as diisopropyl fluorophosphate and *p*-nitrophenyl-*p'*-guanidinobenzoate, or EDTA, a metal ion chelator. Chloroquine and *N*-*p*-tosyl-L-lysine-chloromethyl ketone HCl, both inhibitors of cathepsin B (Wibo and Poole, 1974; Barrett, 1977), also failed to inhibit conversion significantly.

Based on the proteinase inhibitor data, the converting enzyme(s) appears to be a thiol proteinase. The primary evidence in support of this conclusion is that conversion was inhibited by PCMB and DDP and the demonstration that the inhibition by both agents was reversed in the presence of a reducing agent. The finding that conversion *in vitro* was optimal in the pH 4.5 to pH 5.5 range also supports this conclusion, since most thiol proteinases have maximum enzymatic activity at acidic pH values (Barrett, 1977). Kemmler *et al.* (1973) reported that the conversion of rat proinsulin in a crude secretory granule preparation was inhibited by PCMB, which suggests the involvement of a thiol proteinase in rat islet also. Inhibition of the anglerfish converting enzyme(s) by leupeptin and antipain suggests a specificity for arginine residues since these two peptides contain an arginine aldehyde essential for inhibition (Umezawa and Aoyagi, 1977). However, when the granules were assayed for the presence of enzymatic activity using the fluorescent substrate Z-Gly-Gly-Arg-amino-methylcoumarin, very little activity was detected (D. J. Fletcher and J. P. Quigley, unpublished).

Various enzymes with a specificity for basic residues have been proposed as converting enzymes for proinsulin (and other islet prohormones). These include trypsin-like enzymes (Kemmler *et al.,* 1973; Zühlke *et al.,* 1977), cathepsin B (Ansorge *et al.,* 1977; Puri *et al.,* 1978), kallikrein-kininase (ole-Moi Yoi *et al.,* 1979), and plasminogen activator (Virgi *et al.,* 1980). Inhibitors which could block the activity of each of these enzymes (Wibo and Poole, 1974; Pisano, 1975; Danø and Reich, 1975; Barrett, 1977) were tested in the anglerfish islet secretory granule system with no significant effect on conversion of the three major prohormones (Fletcher *et al.,* 1980, 1981). It is thus proposed that the converting enzyme(s) in the anglerfish islet is a unique intracellular proteinase with the characteristics of a thiol proteinase and a possible specificity for arginine residues.

A further indication that the anglerfish converting enzyme is distinct from other enzymes previously characterized comes from the results of conversion experiments in which increasing amounts of anglerfish islet prohormones or porcine proinsulin were added to lysed granules and labeled precursors (Fig. 5). While the presence of 600 μg/ml porcine proinsulin in the incubation mixture resulted in a small amount of inhibition ($\sim$ 10–20%) of all three converting activities, the degree of inhibition attained was significantly lower than that caused by the same concentration of a crude preparation of unlabeled anglerfish prohormones. The addition of 300 μg/ml porcine proinsulin to an equal amount of unlabeled precursor preparation resulted in no significant change in the degree of inhibition caused by 300 μg/ml anglerfish islet precursors alone. The recognition or binding site(s) of the artificial substrate tested (porcine proinsulin) is apparently significantly different from those on anglerfish islet prohormones. These findings suggest that the anglerfish converting enzyme(s) is species-specific, i.e., that it is a unique islet proteinase which mediates islet prohormone conversion. Since conversion can be detected in isolated microsomes, it is possible that the converting enzyme(s) is synthesized along with the preprohormones in the rough ER, inserted into ER membrane, and transported along with the prohormones through the Golgi to secretory granules as a membrane-associated protein. Additional answers to questions regarding the synthesis and control of converting enzyme activity and the intracellular site of the initiation of conversion must await further investigation.

VI. CURRENT DIRECTIONS IN RESEARCH ON ISLET HORMONE BIOSYNTHESIS

A number of questions regarding the production of islet hormones remain to be answered experimentally. This is especially true for glucagon and somatostatin biosynthesis. A great deal of information regarding the biosynthesis of insulin and the structure of insulin precursor(s) is available (see Chapter 4). Research addressing the mechanisms of somatostatin

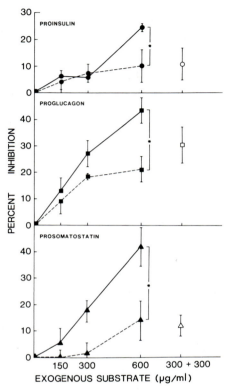

Fig. 5. Comparison of the effects of an "artificial" substrate (porcine proinsulin) and "natural" substrate (8- to 15-kd peptides from gel filtration pools of anglerfish islet extracts) on conversion of the three major islet prohormones. Varying amounts of porcine proinsulin (dashed lines) and unlabeled 8- to 15-kd peptides (solid lines) were added to incubation mixtures identical to those described in Fig. 4B and C. After postincubation, the accumulation of insulin, glucagon, and SRIF in extracts was monitored by gel filtration. Data are expressed as percentage of inhibition and were generated by comparing amounts of labeled products accumulated in the presence of exogenous substrate with the amounts accumulated in control incubations having no exogenous substrate. Bovine serum albumin at 600 μg/ml had no effect on converting activity. The results show that 600 μg/ml of natural substrate inhibited the conversion of all three precursors between 25 and 45%. However, porcine proinsulin at the same concentration was significantly less effective ($P \leq$ 0.05,*) in inhibiting precursor conversion (see text for discussion). Open symbols: Addition of 300 μg/ml each of natural and artificial substrate. (From Fletcher *et al.*, 1980, 1981; reproduced with the permission of the American Diabetes Association and the Rockefeller University Press.)

biosynthesis has proceeded at an amazingly rapid rate, culminating in the use of recombinant DNA technology to determine the amino acid sequences of several preprosomatostatins. However, even though most of the available evidence suggests that a precursor–product mechanism is involved in glucagon biosynthesis as well, the putative prohormone has not yet been isolated and sequenced. Moreover, only the sequences of preprosomatostatins from anglerfish islet are known at the present time with different sequences having been published for the same polypeptide by two laboratories. This emphasizes the need for additional work to characterize not only the anglerfish polypeptides, but pre- and prosomatostatins from other species as well. Thus the isolation and characterization of proglucagon and prosomatostatin from various sources are the focus of work proceeding in several laboratories. It would be of great interest to compare the primary structures of the prohormones from various tissues and species. For example, comparison of the structure of the 18-kd proglucagon from rat islet with that of the 12-kd form from anglerfish islet (or proglucagons from other sources) should contribute to a better understanding of the evolution of biosynthetic precursors. Also, once the complete primary structure of the prohormones is known, it will be possible to examine the non-glucagon- and non-somatostatin-containing portions of the peptides for the sequence(s) of other known biologically active peptides. It is possible that the "nonhormonal" portions of the precursors of glucagon and SRIF are comprised of peptides not usually considered products of islet tissue. Such a situation would not be without precedent. The classic example of a propeptide which yields several biologically active products after differential proteolysis is pro-ACTH endorphin (Mains et al., 1977).

Another area which bears further investigation relates to the transport of newly synthesized peptides across the membranes and into the cisternae of the ER. Signal peptides containing pre-pro forms of proinsulin, proglucagon and prosomatostatin have been identified. Elucidation of the primary structures of the signal peptides for each of the pre-pro peptides from islets should provide further insight into the mechanism of transport of proteins through intracellular membranes. Knowing the nature of the cleavage site for the signal peptides should also provide a valuable addition to information which could be used for further investigation of the nature and regulation of signal peptidase.

A better definition of the intracellular sites and control of proteolytic processing of prohormones is needed as well. Several enzymes identified in or isolated from islets or whole pancreas have been suggested as candidates for proinsulin-converting enzyme(s). However, further investigation is required since definitive evidence is lacking in each case. Isolation and characterization of an authentic cleavage enzyme(s) would provide an in-

valuable tool for additional study of the nature and regulation of the proteolytic processing of each islet prohormone. Questions such as the following remain to be answered: (1) Can the same enzyme(s) accurately cleave
each prohormone? (2) What are the control mechanisms regulating the conversion process? (3) How is the converting enzyme(s) synthesized, sequestered, and transported within the cell?

Finally, very little is known about regulation of the biosynthetic process
in general. The signals and effectors involved in modulating gene regulation, transcription, and translation are, for the most part, not understood.
Fortunately, many of the experimental tools which will allow investigation
of these types of processes in eukaryotic cells are currently being developed. Therefore prospects for the expansion of knowledge in this area appear to be promising. Work performed during the next decade should provide many exciting and important additions to the information available on
islet hormone biosynthesis.

ACKNOWLEDGMENTS

The authors wish to thank Sandra Lemmon, Ann Hunter, Gail Debo, and Carolyn
Williams for their able technical assistance, and Margaret Pierce for help in preparation of the
manuscript. The work described in this chapter which was performed in the authors'
laboratories was supported by research grants from the National Science Foundation
(GB43456) and the National Institutes of Health (NIH) (AM-16921, AM19890, and
AM19223). During a portion of the course of these investigations, Dr. Noe was supported by a
Research Career Development Award from NIH (AM-00142) and Dr. Fletcher was supported
by a National Research Service Award from NIH (F32 AM05662).

REFERENCES

Ansorge, S., Kirschke, H., and Freidrich, K. (1977). *Acta Biol. Med. Ger.* **36**, 1723–1727.
Arimura, A., Sato, H., Dupont, A., Nishi, N., and Schally, A. V. (1975). *Science* **189**,
    1007–1009.
Audy, G., and Kerly, M. (1952). *Biochem. J.* **52**, 70–74.
Barrett, A. J. (1977). *In* "Proteinases in Mammalian Cells and Tissues" (A. J. Barrett, ed.),
    pp. 181–208. North-Holland Publ., Amsterdam.
Benoit, R., Böhlen, P., Brazeau, P., Ling, N., and Ginillemin, R. (1980). *Endocrinology*
    107, 2127–2129.
Berger, M., Teuscher, A., Halban, P., Trimble, E., Studer, P. P., Wollheim, C. B., Zimmer-
    mann-Telschow, H., and Muller, W. A. (1980). *Horm. Metab. Res.* **12**, 144–150.
Bhathena, S. J., Smith, S. S., Voyles, N. R., Penhos, J. C., and Recant, L. (1977). *Bio-
    chem. Biophys. Res. Commun.* **74**, 1574–1581.
Blobel, G., and Dobberstein, B. (1975a). *J. Cell Biol.* **67**, 835–851.
Blobel, G., and Dobberstein, B. (1975b). *J. Cell Biol.* **67**, 852–862.

Blobel, G., and Sabatini, D. (1971). In "Biomembranes" (L. A. Manson, ed.), pp. 193–195. Plenum, New York.

Boden, G., and Owen, O. E. (1977). N. Engl. J. Med. 296, 534–538.

Boyd III, A. E., Sanchez-Franco, F., Spencer, E., Patel, Y. C., Jackson, I. M. D., and Reichlin, S. (1978). Endocrinology 103, 1075–1083.

Brazeau, P., Ling, N., Esch, F., Böhlen, P., Benoit, R., and Guillemin, R. (1981). Regul. Pept. 1, 255–264.

Burgus, R., Ling, N., Butcher, M., and Guillemin, R. (1973). Proc. Natl. Acad. Sci. U.S.A. 70, 684–688.

Chan, S. J., Keim, P., and Steiner, D. F. (1976). Proc. Natl. Acad. Sci. U.S.A. 73, 1964–1968.

Chayvialle, J. A. P., Descos, F., Bernard, C., Martin, A., Barbe, C., and Partensky, C. (1978). Gastroenterology 75, 13–19.

Chisholm, D. J., Alford, F. P., Harewood, M. S., Findlay, D. M., and Gray, B. N. (1978). Metabolism 27, 261–273.

Conlon, J. M., Zyznar, E., Vale, W., and Unger, R. H. (1978). FEBS Lett. 94, 327–330.

Conlon, J. M., Murphy, R. F., and Buchanan, K. D. (1978). Biochim. Biophys. Acta 577, 229–240.

Conlon, J. M., McCarthy, D., Krejs, G. and Unger, R. H. (1981). J. Clin. Endocrinol. Metab. 52, 66–73.

Creutzfeldt, C., Track, N. S., and Creutzfeldt, W. (1973). Eur. J. Clin. Invest. 3, 371–384.

Danforth, D. N., Triche, T., Doppman, J. L., Bezly, R. M., Perrino, P. V., and Recant, L. (1976). N. Engl. J. Med. 295, 242–245.

Danø, K., and Reich, E. (1975). In "Proteases and Biological Control: Cold Spring Harbor Conferences on Cell Proliferation" (E. Reich, D. B. Rifkin, and E. Shaw, eds.), Vol. 2, pp. 357–366. Cold Spring Harbor Laboratory, New York.

Devillers-Thiery, A., Kindt, T., Scheele, G., and Blobel, G. (1975). Proc. Natl. Acad. Sci. U.S.A. 72, 5016–5020.

Dupont, A., and Alvarado-Urbina, G (1976). Life Sci. 19, 1431–1433.

Ensinck, J. W., Laschansky, E. C., Kanter, R. A., Fujimoto, W. Y., Koerker, D. J., and Goodner, C. J. (1978). Metabolism 27, 1207–1210.

Esch, F., Böhlen, P., Ling, N., Benoit, R., Brazeau, P., and Guillemin, R. (1980). Proc. Natl. Acad. Sci. U.S.A. 77, 6827–6831.

Falkmer, S., Elde, R. P., Hellerström, C., Petersson, B., Efendíc, S., Fohlman, J., and Siljevall, J. B. (1977). Arch. Histol. Jpn. 40, Suppl., 99–117.

Fletcher, D. J., Noe, B. D., and Hunt, E. L. (1978). Gen. Comp. Endocrinol. 35, 121–126.

Fletcher, D. J., Noe, B. D., Bauer, G. E., and Quigley, J. P. (1980). Diabetes 29, 593–599.

Fletcher, D. J., Bauer, G. E., Quigley, J. P., and Noe, B. D. (1981). J. Cell Biol. (in press).

Goodman, R. H., Jacobs, J. W., Chin, W. W., Lund, P. K., Dee, P.C. and Habener, J. F. (1980b). Proc. Natl. Acad Sci. U.S.A. 77, 5869–5873.

Goodman, R. H., Lund, P. K., Jacobs, J. W., and Habener J. F. (1980a). J. Biol Chem. 255, 5649–6552.

Habener, J. F., Rosenblatt, M., Kemper, B., Kronenberg, H. M., Rich, A., and Potts, J. T., Jr. (1978). Proc. Natl. Acad. Sci. U.S.A. 75, 2616–2620.

Harris, V., Conlon, J. M., Srikant, C. B., McCorkel, K., Schusdziarra, V., Ipp, E., and Unger, R. H. (1978). Clin. Chim. Acta 87, 275–283.

Hellerström, C., Howell, S. L., Edwards, J. C., and Andersson, A. (1972). FEBS Lett. 27, 97–101.

Hellerström, C., Howell, S. L., Edwards, J. C., Andersson, A., and Östenson, C.-G. (1974). Biochem. J. 140, 13–23.

Hobart, P., Crawford, R., Shen, L., Pictet, R., and Rutter, W. J. (1980). Nature (London) 288, 137–141.

Holst, J. J. (1978). *In* "Gut Hormones" (S. R. Bloom, ed.), p. 599. Churchill, London.

Holst, J. J., and Bang Pederson, N. (1975). *Acta Endocrinol.* **80**, Suppl. 199, 379.

Holst, J. J., Kreutzfeldt, M., Holm, G., Jensen, E., Poulsen, J. S. D., Sparsø B., and Schmidt, A. (1978). *Diab Metab.* **4**, 75–79.

Howell, S. L., Hellerström, C., and Tyhurst, M. (1974) *Horm. Metab. Res.* **6**, 267–271.

Jacobsen, H., Demandt, A., Moody, A. J., and Sundby, F. (1977). *Biochim. Biophys. Acta* **493**, 452–459.

Jaspan, J. B., and Rubenstein, A. H. (1976). *Diabetes* **26**, 887–902.

Jaspan, J. B., Kuku, S. F., Locker, J. D., Huen, A. H.-J., Emanouel, D. S., Katz, A. I., and Rubenstein, A. H. (1976). *Metabolism* **25**, Suppl. 1, 1397–1401.

Johnson, D. E., Torrence, J. L., Elde, R. P., Bauer, G. E., Noe B. D., and Fletcher, D. J. (1976) *Am J. Anat.* **147**, 119–124

Joseph-Bravo, P., Charli, J. L., Sherman, T., Boyer, H., Bolivar, F., and McKelvy, J. F. (1980). *Biochem. Biophy. Res. Commun.* **94**, 1004–1012.

Kemmler, W., Steiner, D. F., and Borg, J. (1973). *J. Biol. Chem.* **248**, 4544–4551.

Kemper, B., Habener, J. F., Mulligan R. C., Potts, Jr., J. T., and Rich, A. (1974). *Proc. Natl. Acad. Sci. U.S.A.* **71**, 3731–3735.

Krug, E., and Mialhe, P. (1971). *Horm. Metab. Res.* **3**, 24–27.

Kuku, S. F., Zeidler, A., Emmanouel, D. S., Katz, A. I., Rubenstein, A. H., Levin, N. W., and Tello, A. (1976). *J. Clin. Endocrinol. Metab.* **42**, 173–176.

Larsson, L.-I., Holst, J. J., Kuhl, C., Lundqvist, G., Hirsch, M. A., Ingemanson, S., Lindkaer Jensen, S., Rehfeld, J. F., and Schwartz, T. W. (1977). Lancet **1**, 666–668.

Lauber, M., Camier, M., and Cohen, P. (1979). *Proc. Natl. Acad. Sci. U.S.A.* **76**, 6004–6008.

Luft, R., Efendíc, S., Hökfelt, T., Johansson, O., and Arimura, A. (1974). *Med. Biol.* **52**, 428–430.

Luft, R., Efendíc, S., and Hökfelt, T. (1978). *Diabetologia* **14**, 1–13.

Lund, P. K., Goodman, R. H., Jacobs, J. W., and Habener, J. F. (1980). *Diabetes* **29**, 583–586.

McIntosh, C., Arnold, R., Bothe, E., Becker, H., Köbberling, J., and Creutzfeldt, W. (1978). *Gut* **19**, 655–663.

Mains, R. E., Eipper, B. A., and Ling, N. (1977). *Proc. Natl. Acad. Sci. U.S.A.* **74**, 3014–3018.

Millar, R. P. (1978). *J. Endocrinol.* **77**, 429–430.

Milstein, C., Brownlee, G. G., Harrison, T. M., and Mathews, M. B. (1972). *Nature New Biol.* **239**, 117–120.

Noe, B. D. (1971). Ph.D. Thesis, Univ. of Minnesota.

Noe, B. D. (1977). *In* "Glucagon: Its Role in Physiology and Clinical Medicine" (P. P. Foá, J. S. Bajaj, and N. L. Foá, eds.), pp. 31–50. Springer-Verlag, Berlin and New York, New York.

Noe, B. D., and Bauer, G. E. (1970). *Biol. Bull.* **139**, 431 (Abstr.).

Noe, B. D., and Bauer, G. E. (1971). *Endocrinology* **89**, 642–651.

Noe, B. D., and Bauer, G. E. (1975) *Endocrinology* **97**, 868–877.

Noe, B. D., Bauer, G. E., Steffes, M. W., Sutherland, D. E. R., and Najarian, J. S. (1975). *Horm. Metab. Res.* **7**, 314–322.

Noe, B. D., Weir, G. C., and Bauer, G. E. (1976) *Biol. Bull.* **151**, 422–423 (Abstr.).

Noe, B. D., Baste, C. A., and Bauer, G. E. (1977a). *J. Cell Biol.* **74**, 578–588.

Noe, B. D., Baste, C. A., and Bauer, G. E. (1977b). *J. Cell Biol.* **74**, 589–604.

Noe, B. D., Fletcher, D. J., Bauer, G. E., Weir, G. C., and Patel, Y. (1978). *Endocrinology* **102**, 1675–1685.

Noe, B. D., Fletcher, D. J., and Spiess, J. (1979a). *Diabetes* **28**, 724–730.

Noe, B. D., Spies, J., Rivier, J., and Vale, W. (1979b). *Endocrinology* **105**, 1410–1415.
O'Connor, K. J., and Lazarus, N. R. (1976a). *Biochem. J.* **156**, 265–277.
O'Connor, K. J., and Lazarus, N. R. (1976b). *Biochem. J.* **156**, 279–288.
O'Connor, K. J., Gay, K., and Lazarus, N. R. (1973). *Biochem. J.* **134**, 473–480.
ole-Moi Yoi, O., Seldin, D. C., Spragg, J., Pinkus, G. S., and Austen, K. F. (1979). *Proc. Natl. Acad. Sci. U.S.A.* **76**, 3612–3616.
Östenson, C. G., Andersson, A., Eriksson, U., and Hellerström, C. (1980). *Diabete Metab. (Paris)* **6**, 141–149.
Oyama, H., Bradshaw, R. A., Bates, O. J., and Permutt, A. (1980a). *J. Biol. Chem.* **255**, 2251–2254.
Oyama, H., O'Connell, K., and Permutt, A. (1980b). *Endocrinology* **107**, 845–847.
Palmer, J. P., Werner, P. L., Benson, J. W., and Ensinck, J. W. (1978). *J. Clin. Invest.* **61**, 763–769.
Parsons, J. A., Erlandsen, S. L., Hegre, O. D., McEvoy, R. C., and Elde, R. P. (1976). *J. Histochem. Cytochem.* **24**, 877–882.
Patel, Y. C., and Reichlin, S. (1978). *Endocrinology* **102**, 523–530.
Patzelt, C., Tager, H. S., Carroll, R. J., and Steiner, D. F. (1979). *Nature (London)* **282**, 260–282.
Patzelt, C., Tager, H. S., Carroll, R. J., and Steiner, D. F. (1980). *Proc. Natl. Acad. Sci. U.S.A.* **77**, 2410–2414.
Petersen, K.-G., Heilmeyer, P., and Kerp, L. (1975). *Diabetologia* **11**, 21–25.
Pisano, J. J. (1975). In "Proteases and Biological Control: Cold Spring Harbor Conferences on Cell Proliferation." (E. Reich, D. B. Rifkin, and E. Shaw, eds.), pp. 199–222. Cold Spring Harbor Laboratory, New York.
Pradayrol, L., Chayvialle, J. A., Carlquist, M., and Mutt, V. (1978). *Biochem. Biophys. Res. Commun.* **85**, 701–708.
Pradayrol, L., Jörnvall, H., Mutt, V., and Ribet, A. (1980). *FEBS Lett.* **109**, 55–58.
Puri, R. B., Anjaneyulu, K., Kidwai, J. R., and Rao, V. K. M. (1978). *Acta Diabet. Lat.* **15**, 243–250.
Ravazzola, M., Spierstein, M., Moody, A. J., Jacobsen, H., and Orci, L. (1979). *Endocrinology* **105**, 499–508.
Rigopoulou, D., Valverde, I., Marco, J., Faloona, G., and Unger, R. H. (1970). *J. Biol. Chem.* **245**, 496–501.
Rorstad, O., Epelbaum, J., Brazeau, P., and Martin, J. B. (1977). *Clin. Res.* **25**, 684A.
Schally, A. V., Dupont, A., Arimura, A., Redding, T. W., Nishi, N., Linthicum, G. L., and Schlesinger, D. H. (1976). *Biochemistry* **15**, 509–514.
Schally, A. V., Huang, W.-Y., Chang, R. C. C., Arimura, A., Redding, T. W., Millar, R. P., Hunkapiller, M. W., and Hood, L. E. (1980). *Proc. Natl. Acad. Sci. U.S.A.* **77**, 4489–4493.
Shields, D. (1980b). *J. Biol. Chem.* **255**, 11625–11628.
Shields, D., and Blobel, G. (1977). *Proc. Natl. Acad. Sci. U.S.A.* **74**, 2059–2063.
Shields, D., Warren, T. G., Roth, S. E., and Brenner, M. J. (1981). *Nature (London)* **289**, 511–514.
Sorenson, R. L., Steffes, M. W., and Lindall, A. W. (1970). *Endocrinology* **86**, 88–96.
Sorenson, R. L., Shank, R. D., and Lindall, A. W. (1972). *Proc. Soc. Exp. Biol. Med.* **139**, 652–655.
Spiess, J., and Vale, W. (1978). *Metabolism* **27**, 1175–1178.
Spiess, J., Rivier, J. E., Rodkey, J A., Bennett, C. D., and Vale, W. (1979). *Proc. Natl. Acad. Sci. U.S.A.* **76**, 2974–2978.
Spiess, J., and Vale, W. (1980). *Biochemistry* **19**, 2861–2866.

Strikant, C. B., McCorkle, K., and Unger, R. H. (1977). *J. Biol. Chem.* **252**, 1847–1851.

Steiner, D. F. and Oyer, P. E. (1967). *Proc. Natl. Acad. Sci. U.S.A.* **57**, 473–480.

Steiner, D. F., Cunningham, D., Spigelman, L., and Aten, B. (1967). *Science* **157**, 697–700.

Sun, A. M., Lin, B. J., and Haist, R. E. (1973). *Can. J. Physiol. Pharmacol.* **51**, 175–182.

Sundby, F., Jacobsen, H., and Moody, A. J. (1976). *Horm. Metab. Res.* **8**, 366–371.

Tager, H. S., and Markese, J. (1979). *J. Biol. Chem.* **254**, 2229–2233.

Tager, H. S., and Steiner, D. F. (1973). *Proc. Natl. Acad. Sci. U.S.A.* **70**, 2321–2325.

Trakatellis, A. C., Tada, K., Yamaji, K., and Gardiki-Kouidou, P. (1975). *Biochemistry* **14**, 1508–1512.

Tung, A. K. (1973). *Horm. Metab. Res.* **5**, 416–424.

Tung, A. K. (1974). *Can J. Biochem.* **52**, 1081–1086.

Tung, A. K., and Zerega, F. (1971). *Biochem. Biophys. Res. Commun.* **45**, 387–395.

Tung, A. K., Rosenzweig, S. A., and Foá, P. P. (1976). *Proc. Soc. Exp. Biol. Med.* **153**, 344–349.

Umezawa, H., and Aoyagi, T. (1977). *In* "Proteinases in Mammalian Cells and Tissues" (A. J. Barrett, ed.), pp. 637–662. North-Holland Publ. Amsterdam.

Valverde, I., Villanueva, M. L., Lozano, I., and Marco, J. (1974). *J. Clin. Endocrinol. Metab.* **39**, 1090–1098.

Valverde, I., Lemon, H. M., Kessinger, A., and Unger, R. H. (1976). *J. Clin. Endocrinol. Metab.* **42**, 804–808.

Villanueva, M. L., Hedo, J. A., and Marco, J. (1976). *Diabetologia* **12**, 613–616.

Virji, M. A. G., Vassalli, J.-D., Estensen, R. D., and Reich, E. (1980). *Proc. Natl. Acad. Sci. U.S.A.* **77**, 875–879.

von Schenck, H., Thorell, J., Berg, J., Bojs, G., Dymling, J. F., Hallengren, B., Ljungberg, O., and Tibblin, S. (1979). *Acta Med. Scand.* **205**, 155–162.

Weir, G. C., Knowlton, S. D., and Martin, D. B. (1975). *J. Clin. Endocrinol. Metab.* **40**, 296–302.

Weir, G. C., Horton, E. S., Aoki, T. T., Slovik, D., Jaspan, J., and Rubenstein, A. H. (1977). *J. Clin. Invest.* **59**, 325–330.

Weir, G. C., Goltsos, P. C., Steinberg, E. P., and Patel, Y. C. (1976). *Diabetologia* **12**, 129–132.

Wibo, M., and Poole, B. (1974). *J. Cell Biol.* **63**, 430–440.

Yip, C. C., Hew, C.-L., and Hsu, H. (1975). *Proc. Natl. Acad. Sci. U.S.A.* **72**, 4777–4779.

Zingg, H. H., and Patel, Y. C. (1979). *Biochem. Biophys. Res. Commun.* **90**, 466–472.

Zingg, H. H., and Patel, Y. C. (1980). *Biochem. Biophys. Res. Commun.* **93**, 1274–1279.

Zülke, H., Kohnert, K.-D., Jahr, H., Schmidt, S., Kirschke, H., and Steiner, D. F. (1977). *Acta. Biol. Med. Ger.* **36**, 1695–1703.

Zülke, H., Ziegler, M., Jahr, H., Titze, R., and Schmidt, S. (1978). *Acta Biol. Med. Ger.* **37**, 1915–1918.

10

Secretion of Glucagon

M. ITOH, G. REACH, B. FURMAN, and J. GERICH

I. INTRODUCTION

Methodological Approaches to the Study of Glucagon Secretion

Numerous experimental methods have been used to study the physiology, biochemistry, and pathology of pancreatic islet A cells. *In vivo* studies have provided much insight into how various physiological and pathological conditions may alter circulating glucagon levels and thus the concentration of glucagon to which target tissues are exposed. However, such studies cannot quantitate glucagon release nor provide direct assessment of A-cell function to the same degree that *in vitro* studies can; examination of

225

The Islets of Langerhans
Copyright © 1981 by Academic Press, Inc.
All rights of reproduction in any form reserved.
ISBN 0-12-187820-1

A-cell calcium fluxes, cyclic nucleotide concentrations, and substrate utilization are precluded during *in vivo* studies, and it is difficult to determine from such studies whether changes in circulating levels of glucagon are due to the direct effect of an experimental manipulation or to an indirect effect.

Glucagon secreted *in vivo* from the pancreas is extracted by the liver prior to delivery of the hormone into the systemic circulation (Brockman *et al.*, 1976; Jaspan *et al.*, 1977; Röjdmark *et al.*, 1978a). In some instances, changes in glucagon secretion which would be evident from portal venous sampling may not be evident from arterial or peripheral venous sampling (Blackard *et al.*, 1974; Felig *et al.*, 1974; Dencker *et al.*, 1975). Moreover, hepatic extraction of glucagon may be altered under certain experimental (Röjdmark *et al.*, 1978b) or pathological (Marco *et al.*, 1973b) conditions. Finally, interpretation of *in vivo* studies is confounded by immunoheterogeneity and extrapancreatic sources of glucagon. Antibodies used in radioimmunoassays are polyclonal and thus recognize with varying affinity different antigenic sites in the glucagon molecule; such antibodies bind polypeptides other than the 3500-molecular-weight molecule (Conlon, 1980). There are four immunoreactive species present in plasma with apparent molecular weights of 40,000, 9000, 3500, and 2000 (Jaspan and Rubenstein, 1977) (Fig. 1). There is considerable individual and species variation in the proportion of each component found in plasma, although changes in plasma glucagon immunoreactivity during stimulation or suppression of A-cell secretion are primarily due to changes in the 3500-molecular-weight molecule (Jaspan and Rubenstein, 1977). In certain condi-

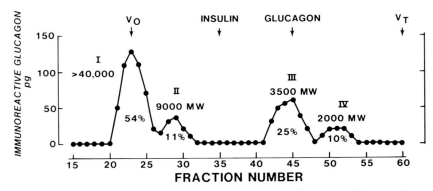

Fig. 1. Gel chromatography of glucagon immunoreactivity in normal human plasma. Plasma (5 ml) from a normal overnight-fasted subject was placed on a 0.9 × 110 cm BioGel P-10 column and eluted in 5-ml fractions with 50 mM ammonium bicarbonate buffer (pH 8.8). The column was equilibrated with dextran blue, I^{125}-labeled insulin, and I^{125}-labeled glucagon.

tions, such as renal failure (Kuku *et al.,* 1976) and liver disease (Müller, *et al.,* 1979b), an increased proportion of one of the high-molecular-weight species occurs. Thus comparisons based on absolute levels of total glucagon immunoreactivity may be misleading.

In dogs and in man and probably in other species, the pancreas is not the sole source of circulating immunoreactive glucagon; A cells, similar to those in pancreatic islets, have been found in the stomach and in the small intestine (Sasaki *et al.,* 1975; Munoz-Barragan *et al.,* 1977). These cells contain a peptide which has immunological, physiochemical, and biological characteristics similar or identical to those of pancreatic A-cell glucagon (Sasaki *et al.,* 1975; Srikant *et al.,* 1977; Doi *et al.,* 1979). The relative contribution of pancreatic and extrapancreatic A cells to plasma glucagon remains to be established. Furthermore, control of extrapancreatic glucagon secretion appears to differ from that of pancreatic glucagon (Müller *et al.,* 1974; Mashiter *et al.,* 1975; Miyata *et al.,* 1976; Munoz-Barragan *et al.,* 1976; Lefebvre and Luyckx, 1978; Wener and Palmer, 1978; Marre *et al.,* 1979; Muller *et al.,* 1979a).

Because of the above considerations, numerous *in vitro* systems have been devised to study glucagon secretion and pancreatic A-cell function. These include incubation of freshly isolated islets, cultured islets, or monolayers of fetal or newborn pancreas (Marliss *et al.,* 1973), perifusion of isolated islets, and finally perfusion of pancreases *in situ* or *in vitro.* Although insulin release has been studied *in vitro* using incubated (Ono *et al.,* 1977) or perifused (Idahl *et al.,* 1976a) isolated islet cells, this technique has not been as yet applied to the study of glucagon release. Since the endocrine portion of the mammalian pancreas consists of individual islets scattered throughout the acinar parenchyma and, since the volume of islets comprises only a small percentage of the entire pancreas, direct studies on the metabolism of islets require isolation of islets from the exocrine pancreas. Islets can be isolated by microdissection (Hellerström, 1964) or by enzymatic digestion with collagenase, the most frequently used method (Lacy and Kostianovsky, 1967). Variations in the enzyme composition of commercially available collagenase preparations frequently lead to overdigestion of islets and damage to peripherally located A cells. In some species, it is difficult to obtain sufficient quantities of viable islets for study (Scharp *et al.,* 1980). Modifications of the original method of Lacy and Kostianovsky have thus been described in efforts to increase the yield of islets from individual pancreases (Lindall *et al.,* 1967; Scharp *et al.,* 1973, 1975; Shibata *et al.,* 1976).

Incubation of isolated islets has been used to study islet A-cell metabolism, but it is difficult to extrapolate from overall islet metabolism to metabolism occurring specifically in islet A cells. Islets comparatively rich in A cells derived from animals given alloxan or streptozotocin have been employed in studying glucagon secretion and islet A-cell metabolism (Edwards and Taylor, 1970; Petersson *et al.*, 1970; Laube *et al.*, 1971; Edwards *et al.*, 1972; Buchanan and Mawhinney, 1973a,b; Pagliara *et al.*, 1975b; Matschinsky *et al.*, 1976). However, the secretion of glucagon and the metabolism of these cells may not necessarily be characteristic of normal A cells; agents used to destroy islet B cells may impair glucagon release and glucose oxidation by A cells (Pagliara *et al.*, 1977; Goto *et al.*, 1978; Östenson, 1980; Tomita, 1980). Moreover, a lack of B cells and increases in islet D cells (Orci *et al.*, 1976; Patel and Weir, 1976; Hara *et al.*, 1979) may also result in the secretion of glucagon which differs from that of intact islets.

Another problem associated with using incubated islets to study hormone secretion is the high background generally observed. Thus, in contrast to the perfused pancreas preparation in which arginine may stimulate glucagon secretion severalfold above baseline and in which glucose can inhibit glucagon secretion virtually to zero values, with isolated islets stimulation of glucagon secretion by arginine is at most 1.5- to 2-fold above baseline and suppression of glucagon secretion is usually difficult to demonstrate and rarely exceeds 50–70% (Itoh *et al.*, 1980a). In some instances, agents demonstrated to influence glucagon release from the perfused pancreas and *in vivo* have not uniformly altered glucagon release from isolated islets (Vance *et al.*, 1971; Buchanan and Mawhinney, 1973a,b; Norfleet *et al.*, 1975). These discrepancies may be due to damage of A cells by collagenase digestion. Maintaining islets in tissue culture prior to study has been employed to circumvent this problem (Fujimoto *et al.*, 1974; Turcot-Lemay *et al.*, 1975). Another possible explanation is that the glucagon content and number of A cells per islet varies in different parts of the pancreas (Gingerich *et al.*, 1978; Orci, 1980). The latter drawback also applies to perifusion of isolated islets used to examine dynamic changes in glucagon secretion *in vitro* (Ashby and Speake, 1975; Oliver *et al.*, 1976; Eisenstein and Strack, 1978a; Sorenson *et al.*, 1979; Tomita, 1980). Results with this system also tend to be more variable than those obtained employing the perfused pancreas. Although perifused islets have been used to examine concomitant changes in insulin release and calcium efflux, there have been no comparable studies with glucagon secretion. It is difficult of course to extrapolate changes in overall islet calcium efflux to changes in A-cell calcium efflux, since A cells form only a small portion of the islet cell mass.

Perfused pancreases of several species including the rat, dog, mouse, Chinese hamster, and cat (Fig. 2) have been used to study the dynamics of glucagon secretion *in vitro*. This technique (Grodsky and Fanska, 1975)

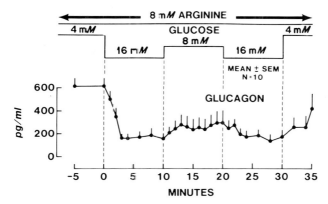

Fig. 2. Glucagon release from the perfused cat pancreas. Effect of alterations in perfusate glucose concentration.

avoids the potential problems associated with collagenase digestion and the differing cellular composition of islets located in different parts of the pancreas. Moreover, results with this preparation are generally less variable than those obtained with other preparations, and greater increments or decrements from the baseline are observed. Isolation of the pancreas and perfusion of it *in situ* with a defined medium (Penhos *et al.*, 1969) allow direct study of pancreatic glucagon secretion during neural stimulation, studies not possible with pancreases perfused *in vitro*. The shortcomings and limitations discussed above must be borne in mind in evaluating the body of experimental data to be subsequently reviewed.

II. DETERMINANTS OF GLUCAGON SECRETION

Glucagon secretion is under complex regulation, several aspects of which have been discussed in previous reviews (Fajans and Floyd, 1972; Gerich *et al.*, 1976a; Smith and Porte, 1976; Unger and Orci, 1976; Gerich and Lorenzi, 1978). As a major hormone involved in homeostatic regulation of metabolic fuels, the secretion of glucagon is influenced by changes in the extracellular concentrations of various substrates; moreover, glucagon secretion can be modulated by ionic, hormonal, neuronal, and local factors (insulin, somatostatin, monoamines, prostaglandins). In discussing potential influences on A-cell function, an effort will be made to distinguish between data derived from *in vivo* studies and those derived from *in vitro* studies.

A. Substrates

1. Glucose

Glucose inhibits glucagon secretion, an effect first demonstrated *in vivo* (Ohneda *et al.,* 1969) and extensively studied with rat pancreases as perfused *in vitro* (Gerich *et al.,* 1974a; Pagliara *et al.,* 1974) and *in situ* (Weir *et al.,* 1974). *In vitro,* the values for threshold, half-maximum, and maximum suppression of glucagon secretion by glucose are approximately 2.5, 5.0, and 10.0 m*M* glucose, respectively, whereas the corresponding values for stimulation of insulin release are 4.5, 8.0, and 25.0 m*M* (Fig. 3). Thus it appears that the A cell is more sensitive to glucose than the B cell. These observations contrast with the relative insensitivity of A cells to glucose seen in studies employing isolated rat islets (Chesney and Scofield, 1969; Edwards and Taylor, 1970; Buchanan and Mawhinney, 1973a).

In vitro a rapid decrease in glucose concentration from 5.5 to 1 m*M* stimulates glucagon release (Weir *et al.,* 1974; Pagliara *et al.,* 1974) from perfused rat pancreas; in some instances, a biphasic response has been observed (Weir *et al.,* 1974). Although it is well established that hypoglycemia (plasma glucose less than 3 m*M*) stimulates glucagon secretion *in vivo* (Ohneda *et al.,* 1969; Gerich *et al.,* 1974b; Garber *et al.,* 1976), controversy exists as to whether absolute hypoglycemia is necessary (DeFronzo *et al.,* 1977; Lilavivathana *et al.,* 1979); decrements below euglycemia and decrements from hyperglycemia have been reported to increase plasma glucagon in man (Gerich *et al.,* 1974b; Santiago *et al.,* 1980). Moreover, a

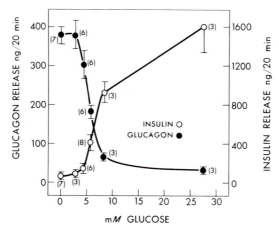

Fig. 3. Dose–response curves for glucose-induced suppression of glucagon release and stimulation of insulin release from the perfused rat pancreas. (From Gerich *et al.,* 1974a reproduced with permission.)

decrease in perfusate glucose concentration from 16 to 8 mM increases glucagon release from the cat pancreas *in vitro* (Fig. 2).

Since suppression of glucagon release by glucose occurs at glucose concentrations too low to stimulate insulin release (Gerich *et al.,* 1974a; Pagliara *et al.,* 1974), it is likely that glucose can suppress glucagon release independently of its stimulation of insulin release. Glucose suppresses glucagon release *in vitro* when B cells have been destroyed by streptozotocin or alloxan so that insulin release is not possible (Palgiara *et al.,* 1975b; Matschinsky *et al.,* 1976). However, suppression of glucagon release under these conditions is not normal, suggesting a permissive role for insulin. Metabolism of glucose may be required for the suppression of glucagon release, since increases in glucagon secretion have been observed *in vivo* (Müller *et al.,* 1979a) and *in vitro* (Edwards, 1973; Weir *et al.,* 1974; Pagliara *et al.,* 1975a) when glucose metabolism is inhibited. Moreover, glyceraldehyde, a metabolite of glucose, inhibits glucagon release *in vitro* (Hahn *et al.,* 1974). However, glucose may also act through a glucoreceptor mechanism independently of or in additon to the consequences of its metabolism; the α anomer of D-glucose is more effective than the β anomer in suppressing glucagon release (Rossini *et al.,* 1974: Grodsky *et al.,* 1975; Matchinsky *et al.,* 1975), despite the apparent lack of stereospecificity of glucose uptake and phosphorylation in islets (Idahl *et al.,* 1976b). Correlation of the suppression of glucagon release from A-cell preparations with glucose metabolism and studies on the effects of nonmetabolizable hexoses would be of interest.

2. Amino Acids

Amino acids stimulate biphasic glucagon secretion *in vivo* (Assan *et al.,* 1967; Ohneda *et al.,* 1968; Pek *et al.,* 1968; Müller *et al.,* 1971b; Rocha *et al.,* 1972; Wise *et al.,* 1973a; Müller *et al.,* 1975) and *in vitro* (Assan *et al.,* 1972; Gerich *et al.,* 1974a; Pagliara *et al.,* 1974; Assan *et al.,* 1977). The relative potency of amino acids as glucagon secretagogues varies among species: In the dog, asparagine, glycine, and phenylalanine are the most potent secretagogues (Rocha *et al.,* 1972). In man arginine is more potent than alanine and glycine, while leucine, valine, and isoleucine are inactive (Wise *et al.,* 1973a; Müller *et al.,* 1975; Gerich *et al.,* 1977). *In vitro,* arginine and structurally related amino acids such as ornithine and homoarginine are the most potent stimulators of glucagon release from the perfused rat pancreas (Assan *et al.,* 1977).

Arginine stimulates biphasic glucagon secretion at concentrations less than 1 mM; the dose–response curve is sigmoidal (Fig. 4), with half-maximal release and maximal release occurring at approximately 3–4 and 12–13 mM, respectively (Gerich *et al.,* 1974a). In contrast, half-maximal

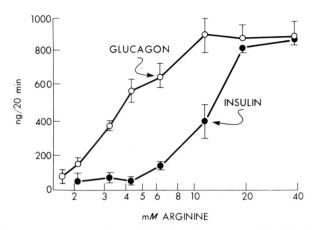

Fig. 4. Dose–response curves for arginine-induced glucagon and insulin release from the perfused rat pancreas. (From Gerich *et al.,* 1974a reproduced with permission.)

release and maximal release of insulin occur at 12–13 and 19–20 mM, respectively, indicating that the A cell is more sensitive to arginine than the B cell; since glucose decreases glucagon responses to arginine noncompetitively, glucose and arginine probably affect pancreatic A-cell function via different mechanisms (Gerich *et al.,* 1974a). Prior addition and subsequent removal of glucose from the perfusing medium results in the suppression of subsequent glucagon responses to arginine, indicating that glucose exerts a "memory" effect on the A cell similar to that described for the B cell (Grill *et al.,* 1979). Although α-ketoisocaproate, a metabolite of leucine, stimulates glucagon release (Leclerq-Meyer *et al.,* 1979b), the fact that nonmetabolizable analogues of leucine (Fajans *et al.,* 1971) and arginine (Assan *et al.,* 1977) also stimulate glucagon release suggests that amino acids may interact with receptors to trigger the release of glucagon independent of their metabolism. It thus seems to be of interest to examine the binding and metabolism of amino acids in A-cell preparations.

3. Free Fatty Acids and Ketone Bodies

Increases in plasma free fatty acids (FFAs) decrease plasma glucagon in the dog (Seyffert and Madison, 1967; Madison *et al.,* 1968; Luyckx and Lefebvre, 1970), duck (Gross and Miahle, 1974), and human (Gerich *et al.,* 1974c; Andrews *et al.,* 1975); decreases in plasma FFAs increase plasma glucagon in dogs (Luyckx and Lefebvre, 1970) and man (Gerich *et al.,* 1974c). These changes in circulating glucagon concentration appear to be mediated by direct effects of FFAs on islets, since octanoate (5 mM)

diminishes glucagon release from guinea pig islets incubated *in vitro* and physiological concentrations of oleate (1500 μM) diminish arginine-induced glucagon release from the perfused rat pancreas (Campillo *et al.,* 1979). Metabolism of FFAs may be essential for these effects, since inhibition of octanoate oxidation prevents suppression of glucagon release by this FFA (Edwards and Taylor, 1970). Ketone bodies also inhibit glucagon release *in vitro,* an effect dependent on their metabolism (Edwards and Taylor, 1970). The observation that hyperketonemia does not suppress hypoglycemia-induced glucagon release in the dog (Müller *et al.,* 1976) does not necessarily conflict with the above *in vitro* results, since hypoglycemia is an extremely potent stimulus for glucagon release *in vivo.* Both FFAs and ketone bodies augment insulin release (Gerich *et al.,* 1976a); thus these substrates, like glucose, cause reciprocal changes in A- and B-cell function.

4. *Meals and Dietary Influences*

The A-cell response to a meal is dependent on the relative carbohydrate and protein content of the meal (see Chapter 18). Plasma glucagon concentration increases in humans after ingestion of a high-protein meal and decreases after ingestion of a high-carbohydrate meal (Müller *et al.,* 1970; Wahren *et al.,* 1976; Day *et al.,* 1973, Raskin *et al.,* 1978). Following ingestion of a mixed meal in a normal man (Fig. 5), glucagon concentrations in peripheral venous plasma increase gradually by 40–60 pg/ml, reaching a maximum after 2 hr and returning to basal levels by 4–5 hr (Gerich *et al.,* 1975a). Portal plasma glucagon increases within 5 min following a mixed meal in man (Dencker *et al.,* 1975); since this increase precedes increases in plasma amino acids following meal ingestion (Unger *et al.,* 1969), humoral or neural factors may be involved.

Antecedent diet also influences A-cell function. A period of carbohydrate restriction increases both fasting and postmeal plasma glucagon in man (Müller *et al.,* 1971c). In rats fed a high-protein, carbohydrate-free diet, plasma glucagon is increased (Eisenstein and Strack, 1976). Glucagon release from islets obtained from such rats is apparently nonsuppressible by glucose (Eisenstein and Strack, 1976), and the stimulatory effect of arginine is enhanced; refeeding a normal diet to the rats returns arginine-stimulated glucagon secretion to normal within 5 days (Eisenstein and Strack, 1978a,b). A low-protein diet does not alter plasma glucagon in rats (Kabadi *et al.,* 1976).

Fasting increases plasma glucagon in man (Marliss *et al.,* 1970) and in rats (Van Lan *et al.,* 1974). It has been suggested that this may be due to a reduction in the clearance of glucagon (Fisher *et al.,* 1976), but enhanced secretion of glucagon from islets obtained in fasting rats has been observed *in vitro* (Oliver *et al.,* 1977; Prieto *et al.,* 1978).

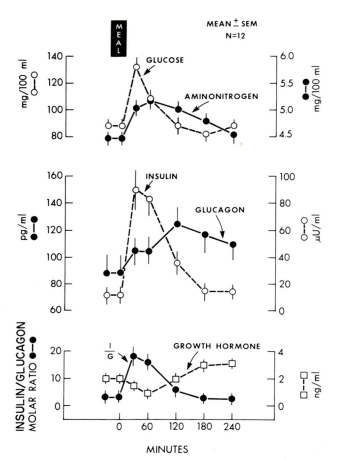

Fig. 5. Plasma glucagon, insulin and growth hormone responses to ingestion of a mixed meal in normal man. (From Gerich *et al.,* 1975a reproduced with permission from the American Medical Association.)

B. Ionic Milieu

Extracellular calcium is essential for insulin release (Grodsky and Bennett, 1966; Milner and Hales, 1967; Malaisse, 1973), but the effects of this cation on glucagon secretion are controversial. In some studies, increased secretion of glucagon from rat islets (Edwards, 1973; Leclercq-Meyer *et al.,* 1973, 1975, 1976) and cell monolayers (Wollheim *et al.,* 1975) incubated in the absence of added calcium has been observed; in other studies, no effect on glucagon release from incubated Syrian hamster islets (Nonaka *et al.,* 1971) or an inhibition of glucagon release from perfused canine (Iversen and Hermansen, 1977) and rat (Gerich et al., 1974d; Lundquist et al., 1976) pancreases has been found (Fig. 6).

These discrepancies may be due to the fact that it is difficult to remove extracellular calcium totally under static incubation conditions. In immunocytochemical studies using the freeze-fracture technique, the paradoxical release of glucagon provoked by calcium deprivation was not associated with exocytosis in spite of a significant depletion of A-cell granules; in contrast, arginine-stimulated glucagon release was associated with exocytosis; these observations suggest that the paradoxical increase in basal glucagon release during calcium deprivation may be artifactual (Carpentier et al., 1977). Interpretation of the effect of calcium deprivation is complicated by the fact that, in addition to altering intracellular coupling processes, removal of calcium may alter the physical and chemical properties of surface membranes (Loewenstein, 1966; Orci et al., 1974). However, verapamil, which inhibits the transport of calcium into many tissues (Fleck-

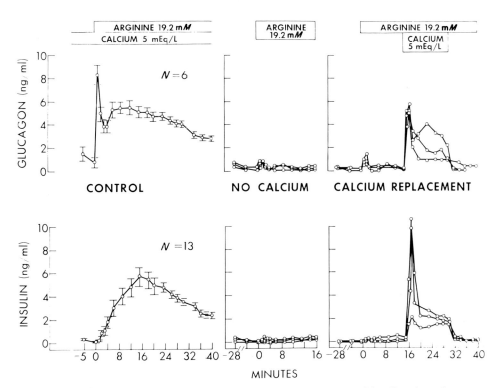

Fig. 6. Effects of calcium depletion and repletion on glucagon and insulin release from the perfused rat pancreas. (From Gerich et al., 1974d reproduced with permission.)

enstein, 1971) decreases arginine-stimulated glucagon release from perfused rat (Leclercq-Meyer *et al.,* 1978, 1979a) and canine (Hermansen and Iverson, 1977) pancreases.

The induction of hypercalcemia has had a variable effect on plasma glucagon (Boettger *et al.,* 1972; Kuzuya *et al.,* 1974). However, *in vitro* increases in extracellular calcium consistently augment glucagon release from perfused rat (Lundquist *et al.,* 1976) and dog (Iversen and Hermansen, 1977) pancreases, and from islet cell monolayer cultures (Fujimoto and Ensinck, 1976). The divalent cation ionophores A23187 and X537a, both of which increase the permeability of cell membranes to calcium, also increase glucagon release *in vitro* (Ashby and Speak, 1975; Wollheim *et al.,* 1974, 1976).

In general, most experimental data are consistent with the concept that calcium uptake by the A cell is an essential requirement for glucagon release (Gerich *et al;.,* 1976a; Leclercq-Meyer *et al.,* 1977; Grodsky *et al.,* 1977; Berggren *et al.,* 1979) and that calcium availability may play a similar role in islet A and B cells. Islet A-cell calcium fluxes have not been extensively studied independently of whole-islet calcium flux. However, in one series of experiments using islets from streptozotocin-treated guinea pigs, increases in extracellular glucose concentration reduced incorporation of $^{45}Ca^{2+}$ into the residual islet cell population, suggesting that glucose-induced suppression of glucagon release may involve an alteration in A-cell calcium uptake (Berggren *et al.,* 1979). Further work is needed in this area; for example, it would be of interest to know whether arginine enhances calcium uptake by islet A cells.

The effect of magnesium on A-cell function has not been extensively examined; in one study, a low concentration of magnesium increased and high concentrations decreased glucagon release from pieces of rat pancreas (Leclercq-Meyer *et al.,* 1973). Calcium and magnesium are thought to play antagonistic roles in secretory processes (Milner and Hales, 1967; Lambert *et al.,* 1969; Hales and Milner 1968; Bennett *et al.,* 1969; Rubin, 1970); thus the inhibitory effect of magnesium on insulin and glucagon release may be mediated by competition of magnesium with calcium for a common carrier; magnesium inhibits glucose-induced $^{45}Ca^{2+}$ net uptake by isolated islets (Malaisse-Lagae and Malaisse, 1971).

The effects of physiological alterations in extracellular potassium concentration on glucagon release have not been systemically investigated. Intravenous infusion of potassium increased plasma insulin and glucagon in the dog (Santeusanio *et al.,* 1972a; Kuzuya *et al.,* 1974). The supraphysiological potassium concentrations studied *in vitro* may affect A-cell function by causing depolarization or secondary changes in calcium fluxes (Dean and Matthews, 1970). Potassium (> 11 mM) has been reported to augment (Epstein *et al.,* 1978) or to inhibit (Bhathena *et al.,* 1976) arginine-stimulated glucagon release from perfused rat pancreases. Valinomycin, which is thought to increase tissue potassium permeability and to hyperpolarize cells (Hoffman and Lavis, 1974), inhibits both arginine- and potassium-induced insulin and glucagon release *in vitro* (Epstein *et al.,* 1978), suggesting that depolarization and hyperpolarization may affect islet A- and B-cell function similarly. To date, there have been no studies examining potassium fluxes in A cells, although such fluxes have been studied in whole islets and have been inferred to be linked with B-cell secretory events (Sehlin and Täljedal, 1975; Henquin, 1979; Boschero and Malaisse, 1979).

C. Neural Regulation

Pancreatic islets are richly innervated by both sympathetic and parasympathetic nerve fibers. Evidence for neural regulation of glucagon release has been derived from *in vivo* experiments involving stimulation or section of autonomic nerves, stimulation or lesion of various regions of the hypothalamus, and infusion of neurotransmitter substances, and from studies *in vitro* in which putative neurotransmitter substances have been added to pancreatic islets or perfused pancreas preparations. Infusions of epinephrine increase plasma glucagon concentrations in humans (Gerich *et al.,* 1973), baboons (Chideckel *et al.,* 1977), and dogs (Gray *et al.,* 1980). This can be attributed to a direct effect on A cells, since epinephrine (or norepinephrine) stimulates glucagon release *in vitro* from perfused rat and dog pancreases and from incubated and perifused rat islets (Iversen, 1973a; Weir *et al.,* 1974; Sorenson *et al.,* 1979). Electrical stimulation of the pancreatic sympathetic inflow (splanchnic nerves) increases plasma glucagon in the dog and calf (Bloom *et al.,* 1973; Kaneto *et al.,* 1975a; Bloom and Edwards, 1978; Miller and Horton, 1979). Release of norepinephrine induced by scorpion toxin, which blocks sodium channel deactivation in excitable membranes (Catteral, 1980), also increases glucagon release from perfused rat pancreas (Johnson and Ensinck, 1976). Section of the splanchnic nerves decreases glucagon secretion in the dog (Miller and Horton, 1979).

There are conflicting observations concerning the adrenergic receptor mechanisms affecting glucagon secretion. The prevention of epinephrine stimulation of glucagon secretion by propranolol *in vitro* and *in vivo* (Iversen, 1973a; Gerich *et al.,* 1976b; Samols and Weir, 1979) and the mimicking of the effect of epinephrine by isoproterenol (Gerich *et al.,* 1975b; Iversen, 1973a; Kaneto *et al.,* 1975b) provide evidence for beta-adrenergic stimulation of glucagon release. An inhibitory alpha-adrenergic effect on glucagon release has been observed in man (Gerich *et al.,* 1974e) and in dogs (Miller and Horton, 1979), but other studies have not found such an effect in the dog *in vivo* or when dog or rat pancreases were perfused *in vitro* (Samols and Weir, 1979; Iversen, 1973a; Kaneto *et al.,* 1975b). It has been reported that neither alpha- nor beta-adrenergic blockage prevents the enhancement of glucagon secretion following splanchnic nerve stimulation in the dog (Kaneto *et al., 1975a,b)* and in the calf (Bloom and Edwards, 1978), suggesting that norepinephrine may not be the sole neurotransmitter affecting islet A-cell function under these conditions.

The role of the sympathetic nervous system in the regulation of plasma glucagon has been investigated under various physiological and pathological conditions. Plasma glucagon concentrations are increased in numerous stress situations (hemorrhage, myocardial infarction, hypoglycemia) (Gerich *et al.,* 1977). Stimulation of glucagon release by hypoglycemia does not appear to be mediated through the adrenergic system, since the response occurs in adrenalectomized (Ensinck *et al.,* 1976) and sympathectomized individuals (Palmer *et al.,* 1976) as well as during pharmacological blockage of adrenergic receptors (Rizza *et al.,* 1979). Both alpha- and beta-adrenergic mechanisms have been suggested as being involved in exercise-induced hyperglucagonemia in the rat (Luyckx and Lefebvre, 1973; Harvey *et al.,* 1974), although propranolol failed to modify this response in humans (Galbo *et al.,* 1976). Hypoxia-induced hyperglucagonemia in the puppy is attenuated by phenoxybenzamine, but not propranolol, suggesting involvement of the sympathetic nervous system through an alpha-adrenoreceptor mechanism (Baum *et al.,* 1979). In contrast, hyperglucagonemia following exsanguination in the dog appears to be a beta-adrenergic event (Lindsey *et al.,* 1975).

Acetylcholine stimulates glucagon release from the canine pancreas *in vitro* (Iversen, 1973b) and *in situ* (Kaneto and Kosaka, 1974). Since this response is blocked by atropine, a muscarinic receptor mechanism appears to be involved. Electrical stimulation of the vagus increases plasma glucagon in dogs (Kaneto *et al.,* 1974); atropine decreases plasma glucagon in man (Bloom *et al.,* 1974).

The role of the parasympathetic nervous system in modulating glucagon responses to hypoglycemia is unclear. There is evidence in the calf (Bloom *et al.,* 1973) for such involvement, but a report that patients with truncal vagotomy have markedly impaired plasma glucagon responses to insulin-induced hypoglycemia compared with patients with selective vagotomy (Russel *et al.,* 1974) has not been confirmed (Palmer *et al.,* 1979). Moreover, atropine does not modify insulin-induced hyperglucagonemia in humans (Palmer *et al.,* 1979). Postprandial hyperglucagonemia may be under parasympathetic influence; atropine but not a splanchnic nerve section blunts this response in the calf (Bloom *et al.,* 1978).

Electrical or chemical stimulation of the hypothalamus (Frohman and Bernardis, 1971; Frohman *et al.,* 1974; DeJong *et al.,* 1977; Helman *et al,*

1980) and hypothalamic lesions (Chikamori et al., 1980) alter plasma glucagon in the rat, but the precise nature of the link between the hypothalamus and the A cell remains to be determined, since studies employing ganglionic blockers, receptor antagonists, and adrenalectomized and sympathectomized animals have failed to identify a neural or humoral mechanism. Although it is clear that the autonomic nervous system can influence glucagon secretion, the relative importance of sympathetic versus parasympathetic nerves remains to be determined. It is possible that some of the responses reported to be resistant to conventional receptor-blocking drugs may be shown eventually to be mediated through noncholinergic, nonadrenergic nerves. For example, islets have a rich network of vasoactive intestinal peptide-containing nerves (Bishop et al., 1980), and this peptide has been found to stimulate glucagon secretion in vitro (Schebalin et al., 1977; Adrian et al., 1978).

D. Hormonal Influences

Altered glucagon secretion occurs following administration of various hormones and in a number of clinical states associated with endogenous hormone excess or deficiency. In most instances whether such changes represent direct effects of the hormones in question on the A cell is unclear. The following discussion will emphasize studies reported since this topic was last reviewed (Gerich et al., 1976a) and pay particular attention to those examining direct effects of hormones on glucagon secretion in vitro (Table I).

With regard to hypothalamic hormones, a peptidelike substance has been isolated from rat ventromedial hypothalamus (Moltz et al., 1979) which stimulates glucagon release when added to rat islets in vitro. This peptide appears to be different from substance P and neurotensin which also directly stimulate glucagon secretion (Brown and Vale, 1976; Ukai et al., 1977; Dolais-Kitabgi et al., 1979).

In acromegaly, basal and arginine-stimulated glucagon release is increased (Goldfine et al., 1972; Seino et al., 1978a; Trimble et al., 1980). Recently, an immediate stimulatory effect of physiological concentrations of growth hormone on glucagon release from perfused rat pancreases (Tai and Pek, 1976) and on portal venous glucagon concentrations in dogs (Sirek et al., 1979) has been reported. However, the transitory responses observed make it unlikely that these direct actions of growth hormone can explain the hyperglucagonemia found in acromegaly. The increased plasma glucagon levels found in growth hormone-deficient man (Blackard et al., 1973; Seino et al., 1978b) and in hypophysectomized rats (Van Lan et al., 1974) may be due in part to concomitant hypoglycemia and insulinopenia.

TABLE I

Direct Effect of Various Hormones on Glucagon Secretion

Hormone	Effect	Reference
Hypothalamic hormones		
N-terminal-extended somatostatin peptides	−	Mandarino *et al.* (1981)
Somatostatin	−	Weir *et al.*, (1976); Gerich *et al.*, (1975)
Ventromedial hypothalamus extract	+	Moltz *et al.*, (1979)
Substance P	+	Kaneto *et al.*, (1978); Brown and Vale (1976)
Neurotensin	+	Dolais-Kitabgi *et al.*, (1979); Kaneto *et al.*, (1978); Ukai *et al.*, (1977)
Pituitary hormones		
Growth hormone	+	Tai and Pek, (1976); Sirek *et al.*, (1979)
Gastrointestinal hormones		
Gastric inhibitory polypeptide	+	Pederson and Brown, (1978)
Vasoactive intestinal peptide	+	Lindkaer-Jensen *et al.*, (1978); Schebalin *et al.*, (1977); Kaneto *et al.*, (1977); Ipp *et al.*, (1978a); Szecowka *et al.*, (1980); Adrian *et al.*, (1978)
Secretin	0	Iverson, (1971)
Gastrin	+	Iverson, (1971)
Pancreozymin	+	Iverson, (1971)
Adrenal steroid		
Corticosterone	+	Barseghian and Levine, (1980)

+ Stimulates; −, inhibits; 0, has no effect.

Although alterations in plasma glucagon have been found in hyper- and hypothyroid individuals, there are no studies examining the direct effect of thyroid hormones on glucagon secretion *in vitro*.

Hyperglucagonemia has been found in Cushing's syndrome and following glucocorticoid administration in man (Marco *et al.*, 1973a; Wise *et al.*, 1973b; Seino *et al.*, 1977). Islets obtained from prednisolone-treated mice showed increased basal and arginine-stimulated glucagon release, although addition of prednisolone to incubation medium was without immediate effect (Marco *et al.*, 1976). Corticosterone has recently been shown to have a direct and immediate stimulatory effect on glucagon release from rat pancreases perfused *in vitro* (Barseghian and Levine, 1980). Hyperglucagonemia has been found in adrenalectomized rats (Van Lan, 1974).

Moreover, there is excessive glucagon release from perfused pancreases of adrenalectomized rats; the latter was reversible after glucocorticoid treatment *in vivo* (Lentzen, 1976). Conceivably, chronic hypoglycemia and hypoinsulinemia may explain this phenomenon.

Numerous gastrointestinal hormones have been reported to affect glucagon secretion *in vivo* and *in vitro* (Gerich *et al.*, 1976a). However, in few studies have the effects of physiological concentrations of these hormones been examined. Whereas gastrin increases plasma glucagon at pharmacological but not at physiological concentrations (Rehfield *et al.*, 1978), physiological concentrations of gastric inhibitory polypeptide augment glucagon release from the perfused rat pancreas in the presence of low perfusate glucose concentrations (Pederson and Brown, 1978). However, in man, no effect of gastric inhibitory polypeptide has been found under hyperglycemic and euglycemic conditions (Elahdi *et al.*, 1979). Secretin suppresses plasma glucagon in dogs (Santeusanio, 1972b), but no effect was found in man when physiological increments in plasma secretin were induced by infusion of this hormone (Shima *et al.*, 1978); moreover, no effect was found in perfused canine pancreas (Iversen, 1971). Pharmacological concentrations of vasoactive intestinal peptide (VIP) consistently stimulate glucagon release *in vitro* (Kaneto *et al.*, 1977; Schebalin *et al.*, 1977; Adrian *et al.*, 1978; Lindkaer-Jensen *et al.*, 1978; Ipp *et al.*, 1978a; Szecowka *et al.*, 1980). Since VIP-containing neurons supply the pancreas, this peptide might affect islet A-cell function as a neurotransmitter.

E. Local Regulatory Factors

1. Insulin

There is considerable indirect evidence mainly derived from *in vivo* experiments suggesting that insulin exerts a suppressive effect on glucagon release. Acute insulin deficiency produced by the administration of antiinsulin serum in dogs (Müller *et al.*, 1971a) or withdrawal of insulin from diabetic humans (Gerich *et al.*, 1975a; Alberti *et al.*, 1975; Barnes *et al.*, 1977) results in hyperglucagonemia and excessive increases in plasma glucagon following arginine infusion (Gerich *et al.*, 1975a) (Fig. 7). These abnormalities can be readily normalized by the infusion of physiological quantities of insulin (Müller *et al.*, 1971c; Braaten *et al.*, 1974; Gerich *et al.*, 1975a; Raskin *et al.*, 1976; Kawamori *et al.*, 1980). Moreover, excessive increases in plasma glucagon following a protein meal in insulin-dependent human diabetics are corrected by physiological amounts of insulin (Raskin *et al.*, 1978). Other aspects of pancreatic A-cell function in diabetes are discussed in detail in Chapter 18.

242 M. Itoh *et al.*

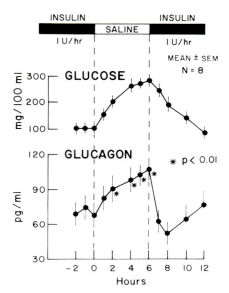

Fig. 7. Effect of acute withdrawal and reinfusion of insulin on plasma glucagon in insulin-dependent diabetic subjects. (From Gerich *et al.*, 1975a reproduced with permission.)

A suppressive effect of insulin on basal glucagon release from perfused pancreases of normal rats has been reported (Weir *et al.*, 1976), but in the same study arginine-stimulated glucagon release was unaffected, and inconsistent effects on basal and arginine-stimulated glucagon release from pancreases of streptozotocin-treated animals were observed. Moreover, in these experiments, insulin was used at concentrations of 2000 and 20,000 μU/ml which are probably greater than that to which A cells are exposed *in vivo* (Sorensen *et al.*, 1980). In another study, amino acid-stimulated glucagon release from perfused pancreases of alloxan diabetic rats was decreased by insulin (23,000 μU/ml), and suppression of glucagon release by glucose was enhanced (Pagliara *et al.*, 1975b). In other studies, insulin (1000 μU/ml) had no effect on basal glucagon release from perfused pancreases of streptozotocin diabetic rats (Laube *et al.*, 1971) but restored suppression of glucagon release by glucose from islets of streptozotozin diabetic rats while having no effect on islets from normal animals (Buchanan and Mawhinney, 1973a,b). Thus, to date, a direct effect of physiological quantities of insulin on glucagon release *in vitro* has not been consistently demonstrated; such an effect seems likely, since islets from streptozotocin-treated rats possess insulin receptors (Verspohl and Ammon, 1980). To some extent, in normal tissue this apparent lack of effect of insulin could be due to the fact that insulin is already exerting a maximal effect; if so, enhancement of glucagon release by insulin antiserum may be demonstrable. With respect to islets from animals treated with alloxan or streptozotocin, the results of such studies are difficult to interpret, since these drugs may damage A cells so as to render them less sensitive to insulin (Pagliara *et al.*, 1977; Goto *et al.*, 1978; Östenson, 1980).

2. Somatostatin

The interaction of this peptide with islet A and B cells is discussed in Chapters 11 and 18. Suffice it to say that there is considerable evidence that somatostatin probably acts as a local regulator of A- and B-cell function, since insulin and glucagon release from islets incubated with somatostatin antiserum is increased (Barden *et al.*, 1977; Taniguchi *et al.*, 1977; Itoh *et al.*, 1980a) (Fig. 8). It remains to be determined under what physiological conditions locally released somatostatin alters islet A- and B-cell function. Glucagon can stimulate somatostatin release (Patton *et al.*, 1977; Weir *et al.*, 1979); thus inhibition of glucagon by somatostatin release may be part of a feedback mechanism. Recently, two N-terminally extended somatostatin peptides, one a 28-amino-acid peptide and the other a 25-amino-acid peptide, have been isolated from hypothalamus and gut; these peptides suppress insulin and glucagon release more potently than somatostatin itself (Mandarino *et al.*, 1981); at a low concentration ($10^{-12}M$), both preferentially inhibit insulin release, whereas somatostatin preferentially inhibits glucagon release. If either of these two peptides is

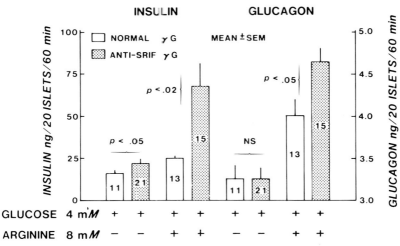

Fig. 8. Effect of antisomatostatin gamma globulin on arginine-stimulated glucagon and insulin release from rat islets incubated *in vitro*. (From Itoh *et al.*, 1980 reproduced with permission from the American Diabetes Association.)

present in islet D cells, its preferential release could provide a mechanism for selective inhibition of insulin and glucagon release.

3. Monoamines

Serotonin and dopamine are found in islets of several species (Woods and Porte, 1974), suggesting that these amines may influence islet function (see also Chapter 8). Variable effects of serotonin on insulin and glucagon release have been reported: Serotonin and its precursor 5-hydroxytryptophan inhibited glucagon release from pieces of rat pancreas (Pontirolli *et al.*, 1978), whereas 5-hydroxytryptophan increased plasma glucagon in rats (Jacoby and Bryce, 1979). Dopamine and its precursor L-dopa have been reported to diminish insulin release *in vitro* (Rossini and Buse, 1973; Itoh *et al.*, 1980b), to increase plasma glucagon in monkeys (George and Rayfield, 1974), rats (George and Bailey, 1978), and in man (Leblanc *et al.*, 1977; Lorenzi *et al.*, 1977, 1979), and to augment glucagon release from rat islets *in vitro* (Itoh *et al.*, 1980b). Although the effects of L-dopa and dopamine were not affected by either alpha- or beta-adrenergic blockage *in vivo* in monkeys or man (George and Rayfield, 1974: Lorenzi *et al.*, 1979), plasma glucagon responses to L-dopa in the rat were prevented by alpha-adrenergic blockage and blunted by beta-adrenergic blockage (George and Bailey, 1978). Furthermore, the stimulatory effect of dopamine *in vitro* was prevented by beta-adrenergic blockage (Itoh *et al.*, 1980b; Samols and Stagner, 1979). Finally, apomorphine, a dopaminergic agonist, did not affect plasma glucagon concentrations in man (Lorenzi *et al.*, 1977). Therefore most evidence seems to indicate that stimulation of glucagon release by dopamine or L-dopa is mediated by adrenergic receptors; this could occur as a result of their conversion to norepinephrine or of their causing the release of norepinephrine. Thus the physiological significance of islet serotonin and dopamine stores remains unknown.

4. Prostaglandins

Prostaglandins, which have been identified in the extracts of human pancreas (Karim *et al.*, 1967), theoretically might alter islet hormone release directly or could affect islet function indirectly by influencing the release and action of norepinephrine. The effects of prostaglandins on insulin secretion are discussed in Chapter 8. Glucagon release from perfused rat pancreas is stimulated by PGE_1, E_2, $F_{2\alpha}$, D_2, and H_2 (Pek *et al.*, 1978). Infusion of PGE_1 increases plasma glucagon in rats (Sacca and Perez, 1976; Akpan *et al.*, 1979) and in man (Giugliano *et al.*, 1979), while the infusion of PGA_1 has no effect in the rat (Sacca and Perez, 1976). The relationship between PGE_1-induced hyperglucagonemia and the sympathetic nervous system is unclear: Increases in plasma glucagon during PGE_1 infusion were observed in rats pretreated with a beta-adrenergic antagonist and in sympathectomized rats (an adrenal medullectomy plus reserpine treatment) (Sacca and Perez, 1976) but were prevented by pretreatment with propranolol in man (Giugliano et al., 1979).

Acetylsalicylic acid, which inhibits prostaglandin synthesis, increases basal plasma glucagon and diminishes the suppression of plasma glucagon following oral glucose in man (Micossi et al., 1978). However, indomethacin and isopropyl-2-nicotinoyl-3-indole (L8027), other inhibitors of prostaglandin synthesis, decrease glucagon responses to arginine and norepinephrine in vitro (Luyckx and Lefebvre, 1978) but do not affect glucagon responses to arginine in man (Vierhapper et al., 1980). These conflicting reports make it difficult to assess the precise effect of prostaglandins on glucagon release; perhaps the application of inhibitors of specific pathways of prostaglandin synthesis and the determination of changes in islet prostaglandin concentrations under different experimental conditions will yield a more consistent view.

5. Opiates

Immunohistochemical studies indicate that rat islets contain endorphin-like substances (Grube et al., 1978); morphine and β-endorphin enhance glucagon release from the isolated perfused dog pancreas and islet monolayer cultures (Ipp et al., 1978b; Kante et al., 1980), an effect completely abolished by naloxone, a specific opioid antagonist (Ipp et al., 1978b). Although various enkephalins inhibit glucagon release in vitro (Kante et al., 1980), no effect of infusion of a long-acting enkephalin on plasma glucagon was observed in man (Stubbs et al., 1978). Thus a physiological role of opiates in glucagon release remains to be elucidated; endogenous opiates could affect islet A-cell function by acting as neurotransmitters or by modulating the release or effect of other neurotransmitters..

F. Cyclic Nucleotides

Cyclic nucleotide concentrations, guanylate and adenylate cyclase activity, and cyclic AMP (cAMP)-dependent protein kinase activity have been determined in whole islets of the mouse, guinea pig, and rat (Cooper et al., 1973; Howell and Montague, 1974; Howell et al., 1974; Charles et al., 1975) but not in pure preparations of islet A, B, or D cells. Thus data regarding the role of the cAMP system in glucagon release have involved studies using agents presumed to act through increases in cellular cAMP concentrations. Exogenous cAMP (Jarrousse and Rosselin, 1975; Wollheim et al., 1976), adenylate cyclase activators such as isoproterenol (Leclercq-Meyer et al., 1971; Iversen, 1973; Marliss et al., 1973; Howell et al., 1974; Weir et

al., 1974), cholera toxin (Wollheim *et al.,* 1976), and phosphodiesterase inhibitors (Howell *et al.,* 1974b; Wollheim *et al.,* 1976) all increase glucagon
release *in vitro.* In B-cell-deficient islets epinephrine, theophylline, and
dibutyryl cAMP activate cAMP-dependent protein kinase and enhance glucagon release (Howell *et al.,* 1974).

Thus it seems likely that alterations in A-cell cAMP can affect glucagon
release; how cyclic nucleotides modulate glucagon secretion is unknown.
cAMP is probably not a universal second messenger for all A-cell secretagogues, since arginine, a potent stimulator of glucagon release does not
alter cAMP concentrations (Charles *et al.,* 1975). Conceivably, cyclic
nucleotides and cAMP in particular may affect glucagon release by altering
A-cell calcium fluxes and the A-cell microtubular system. Vinblastine and
colchine, which specifically bind tubulin (Lacy and Malaisse, 1973), increase glucagon secretion from isolated guinea pig islets, without affecting
islet glucose metabolism (Edwards and Howell, 1973), and from the perfused rat pancreas in a dose-dependent manner (Assan *et al.,* 1978).
Moreover, islets contain calmodulin, a calcium-dependent phosphodiesterase modulator (Valverde *et al.,* 1979), and a calmodulin-sensitive adenylate
cyclase (Scharp *et al.,* 1980).

III. FUTURE RESEARCH DIRECTIONS

Studies on pancreatic A-cell function *in vivo* have been limited by the immunoheterogeneity of glucagon, the presence of extrapancreatic glucagon,
potential variations in the hepatic extraction of glucagon, and considerable
differences in responses among species. These factors may explain certain
discrepancies between the results of *in vitro* and *in vivo* experiments, especially in the area of adrenergic influences on A-cell function. Although
there is substantial evidence that the nervous system may modulate glucagon secretion, there is a need to establish the physiological circumstances
under which the autonomic nervous system affects A-cell function; in addition, the role of peptidergic neurons needs to be considered. Pancreatic
A-cell function in diabetes, as described in Chapter 18, will continue to be
an area of interest, especially with respect to the question of the relative
contributions of insulin deficiency and a glucoreceptor defect as causes of
hyperglucagonemia.

Although perfused pancreases have provided an excellent preparation for
examining the dynamics of glucagon secretion *in vitro,* studies on the
cellular mechanisms leading to glucagon secretion have been hampered by
an inability to determine fluxes of cyclic nucleotides and ions such as calcium and potassium and to assess substrate metabolism in A cells under

conditions which simulate the physiological islet microenvironment. The use of pure A-cell preparations in the presence of somatostatin and insulin might be a worthwhile approach. The mechanism of glucose action on A cells and those of other substrates deserve further examination, as well as the question of whether calcium has the same role in the A cell as in the B cell; for example, glucose-induced suppression of glucagon release may involve inhibition of A-cell calcium uptake; it would thus be of interest to determine whether FFA- or ketone body-induced suppression and amino acid-induced stimulation of glucagon release are also associated with alterations in A-cell calcium fluxes. Studies examining the effects of nonmetabolizable hexoses on glucagon release and other A-cell parameters also seem of interest.

To date there have been no studies on potassium fluxes and on the electrical activity of A cells, areas which would be available for examination if suitable A-cell preparations could be developed. Little definitive information is available on the role of local factors in the regulation of glucagon release, especially those of insulin, somatostatin, prostaglandins, and monoamines; a search for receptors for these agents and the use of antisera against them appear to be endeavors which may yield important insights in this area. Finally, despite considerable interest in the mathematical modeling of insulin release, comparable characterization of islet A-cell function has yet to be undertaken. To be sure, there are many unanswered questions regarding glucagon secretion; improvement in the methods for the study of A-cell function will be required for these questions to be answered.

ACKNOWLEDGMENTS

Brian Furman was in receipt of a Wellcome Travel Grant.

REFERENCES

Adrian, T., Bloom, S., Hermansen, K., and Iversen, J. (1978). *Diabetologia* **14**, 413–417.
Akpan, J., Hurley, M., Pek, S., and Lands, W. (1979). *Can. J. Biochem.* **57**, 540–547.
Alberti, K., Christensen, N., Iversen, J., and Orskov, H. (1975). *Lancet* **1**, 1307–1311.
Andrews, S., Lopez, S., and Blackard, W. (1975). *Metabolism* **24**, 35–44.
Ashby, J., and Speake, R. (1975). *Biochem. J.* **150**, 89–96.
Assan, R., Rosselin G., and Dolais, J. (1967). *In* "Journ. Ann. Diabetol," pp. 25–41. Hotel Dieu, Flammarion Ed, Paris.
Assan, R., Boillot, J., Attali, J., Soufflet, E., and Ballerio, G. (1972). *Nature New Biol.* **239**, 125–126.
Assan, R., Attali, J., Ballerio, G., Boillot, J., and Girard, J. (1977). *Diabetes* **26**, 300–307.

Assan, R., Soufflet, E., Ballerio, G., Attali, J., Boillot, J., and Girard, J. (1978). *Diabetologia* **14**, 121–127.

Barden, N., Lavoie, M., Dupont, A., Côté, J., and Côté, J. P. (1977). *Endocrinology* **101**, 635–638.

Barnes, A., Bloom, S., Alberti, K., Smythe, P., Alford, F., and Chisholm, D. (1977). *N. Engl. J. Med.* **296**, 1250–1256.

Barseghian, G., and Levine, R. (1980). *Endocrinology* **106**, 547–552.

Baum, D., Porte, D., Jr., and Ensinck, J. (1979). *Am. J. Physiol.* **237** E404–417.

Bennett, L., Curry, L., and Grodsky, G. (1969). *Endocrinology* **85**, 594–596.

Berggren, P.-O., Östenson, C.-G., Petersson, B., and Hellman, B. (1979). *Endocrinology* **105**, 1463–1468.

Bhathena, S., Perino, P., Voyles, N., Smith, S., Wilkins, S., Coy, D., Schally, A., and Recant, L. (1976). *Diabetes* **25**, 1031–1040.

Bishop, A., Polak, J., Green, I., Bryant, M., and Bloom, S. (1980). *Diabetologia* **18**, 73–78.

Blackard, W., Andrews, S., and Lazarus, E. (1973). *Proc. Soc. Exp. Biol. Med.* **163**, 1042–1044.

Blackard, W., Nelson, N., and Andrews, S. (1974). *Diabetes* **23**, 199–202.

Bloom, S., and Edwards A. (1978). *J. Physiol (London)* **280**, 25–35.

Bloom, S., Edwards, A., and Vaughan, N. (1973). *J. Physiol. (London)* **233**, 457–466.

Bloom, S., Vaughan, N., and Russell, R. (1974). *Lancet* **2**, 546–549.

Bloom, S., Edwards A., and Hardy, R. (1978). *J. Physiol.* **280**, 37–53.

Boettger, I., Faloona, G., and Unger, R. (1972). *J. Clin. Invest.* **51**, 831–836.

Boschero, A., and Malaisse, W. (1979). *Am. J. Physiol.* **236**, E139–146.

Braaten, J., Faloona, G., and Unger, R. (1974). *J. Clin. Invest.* **53**, 1017–1021.

Brockman, R., Manns, J., and Bergman, E. (1976). *Can. J. Physiol. Pharmacol.* **54**, 666–670.

Brown, M., and Vale, W. (1976). *Endocrinology* **98**, 819–822.

Buchanan, K., and Mawhinney, A. (1973a). *Diabetes* **22**, 797–800.

Buchanan, K., and Mawhinney, A. (1973b). *Diabetes* **22**, 801–803.

Campillo, J.-E., Luyckx, A., and Lefebvre, P. (1979). *Acta Diabetol. Lat.* **16**, 287–293.

Carpentier, J.-L., Malaisse-Lagae, F., Müller, W., and Orci. L. (1977). *J. Clin. Invest.* **60**, 1174–1182.

Catterall, W. (1980). *Annu. Rev. Pharmacol. Toxicol.* **20**, 15–43.

Charles, M., Lawecki, J., Pictet, R., and Grodsky, G. (1975). *J. Biol. Chem.* **250**, 6134–6140.

Chesney, T., and Schofield, J. (1969). *Diabetes* **18**, 627–632.

Chideckel, W., Goodner, C., Koerker, D., Johnson, D., and Ensinck, J. (1977). *Am. J. Physiol.* **232**, E464–470.

Chikamori, K., Nishimura, N., Suehiro, F., Sato, K., Mori, H., and Saito, S. (1980). *Horm. Metab. Res.* **12**, 56–69.

Conlon, J. (1980). *Diabetologia* **18**, 85–88.

Cooper, R., Ashcroft, S., and Randle, P. (1973). *Biochem. J.* **134**, 599–605.

Day, J., Johansen, K., Ganda, O., Soeldner, J., Gleason, R., and Midgley, W. (1978). *Clin. Endocrinol.* **9**, 443–454.

Dean, P., and Matthews, E. (1970). *J. Physiol.* **210**, 255–264.

DeFronzo, R., Andres, R., Bledsoe, T., Boden, G., Faloona, G., and Tobin, J. (1977). *Diabetes* **26**, 445–452.

DeJong, A., Strubbe, J., and Steffens, A. (1977). *Am. J. Physiol.* **233**, E380–388.

Dencker, H., Hedner, P., Holst, J., and Tranberg, K. (1975). *Scand. J. Gastroenterol.* **10**, 471–474.

Doi, K., Prentki, M., Yip, C., Muller, W., Jeanrenaud, B., and Vranic, M. (1979). *J. Clin. Invest.* **63**, 525-513.
Dolais-Kitabgi, J., Kitabgi, P., Brazeau, P., and Freychet, P. (1979). *Endocrinology* **105**, 256-260.
Edwards, J. (1973). *Postgrad. Med. J* **49**, 611-615.
Edwards, J., and Howell, S. (1973). *FEBS Lett.* **30**, 89-92.
Edwards, J., and Taylor, K. (1970). *Biochim. Biophys. Acta* **215**, 310-315.
Edwards, J., Hellerstrom, C., Peterson, B., and Taylor, K. (1972). *Diabetologia* **8**, 93-98.
Eisenstein, A., and Strack, I. (1976). *Diabetes* **25**, 51-55.
Eisenstein, A., and Strack, I. (1978a). *Diabetes* **27**, 370-376.
Eisenstein, A., and Strack, I. (1978b). *Proc. Soc. Exp. Biol. Med.* **158**, 578-581.
Elahdi, D., Andersen, D., Brown, J., Debas, H., Hershcopf J., Raizes, G., Tobin, J., and Andres, R. (1979). *Am. J. Physiol.* **237**, E185-191.
Ensinck, J., Walter, R., Palmer, J. Brodows, R., and Campbell, R. (1976). *Metabolism* **25**, 227-232.
Epstein, G., Fanska, R., and Grodsky, G. (1978). *Endocrinology* **103**, 2207-2215.
Fajans, S., and Floyd, J., Jr. (1972). *In* "The Handbook of Physiology and Endocrinology" (R. Greep and E. Ashwood, eds.), Vol. 7, pp. 473-494. Am. Physiol. Soc., Washington, D.C.
Fajans, S., Quibrera, R., Pek, S., Floyd, J., Jr., Christensen, H., and Conn, J. (1971). *J. Clin. Endocrinol.* **33**, 35-41.
Felig, P., Gusberg, R., Hendler, R., Gump, F., and Kinney, J. (1974). *Proc. Soc. Exp. Biol. Med.* **147**, 88-90.
Fisher, M., Sherwin, R., Hendler, R., and Felig, P. (1976). *Proc. Natl. Acad. Sci. U.S.A.* **73**, 1735-1739.
Fleckenstein, A. (1971). *In* "Calcium and the Heart" (P. Harris and L. Opic, eds.), pp. 135-188. Academic Press, New York.
Frohman, L., and Bernardis L. (1971). *Am. J. Physiol.* **221** E1596-1603.
Frohman, L., Bernardis, L., and Stachura, M. (1974). *Metabolism* **23**, 1047-1056.
Fujimoto, W., and Ensinck, J. (1976). *Endocrinology* **98**, 259-262.
Fujimoto, W., Ensinck, J., and Williams, R. (1974). *Life Sci.* **15**, 1999-2004.
Galbo, H., Holst, J., Christensen, N., and Hilsted, J. (1976). *J. Appl. Physiol.* **40**, 855-863.
Garber, A., Cryer, P., Santiago, J., Haymond, M., Pagliara, A., and Kipnis, D. (1976). *J. Clin. Invest.* **58**, 7-15.
George, D., and Bailey, P. (1978). *Proc. Soc. Exp. Biol. Med.* **157**, 1-4.
George, D., and Rayfield, E. (1974). *J. Clin. Endocrinol. Metab.* **39**, 618-621.
Gerich, J., and Lorenzi, M. (1978). *In* "Frontiers in Neuroendocrinology" (W. Ganong and L. Martin, eds.), Vol. 5, pp. 265-288. Raven, New York.
Gerich, J., Karam, J., and Forsham, P. (1973). *J. Clin. Endocrinol. Metab.* **37**, 479-481.
Gerich, J., Charles, M., and Grodsky, G. (1974a). *J. Clin. Invest.* **54**, 833-841.
Gerich, J., Schneider, V., Dippe, S., Langlois, M., Noacco, C., Karam, J., and Forsham, P. (1974b) *J. Clin. Endocrinol. Metab.* **38**, 77-82.
Gerich, J., Langlois, M., Schneider, V., Karam, J., and Noacco, C. (1974c). *J. Clin. Invest.* **53**, 1284-1289.
Gerich, J., Frankel, B., Fanska, R., West, L., Forsham, P., and Grodsky G. (1974d). *Endocrinology* **94**, 1381-1385.
Gerich, J., Langlois, L., Noacco, V., Schneider, P., and Forsham, P. (1974e). *J. Clin. Invest.* **53**, 1441-1446.
Gerich, J., Lorenzi, M., Karam, J., Schneider, V., and Karam, P. (1975a). *J. Am. Med. Assoc.* **234**, 159-165.
Gerich, J., Lovinger, R., and Grodsky, G. (1975b). *Endocrinology* **96**, 749-756.

Gerich, J., Charles, M., and Grodsky, G. (1976a) *Ann. Rev. Physiol.* **38**, 353–388.

Gerich, J., Lorenzi, M., Tsalikian, E., and Karam, J. (1976b). *Diabetes* **25**, 65–71.

Gerich, J., Tsalikian, E., and Lorenzi, M. (1977). *Clin. Res.* **25** 125A.

Gingerich, R., Lacy, P., Chance, R., and Johnson, M. (1978). *Diabetes* **27**, 96–101.

Giugliano, D., Torella, R., Sgambato, S., and D'Onofrio, F. (1979). *J. Clin. Endocrinol. Metab.* **48**, 302–308.

Goldfine, I., Kirstein, L.,and Lawrence A. (1972). *Horm. Metab. Res.* **4**, 97–100.

Goto, F., Seino, F., and Imura, H. (1978). *Endocrinology* **102**, 1496–1500.

Gray, D., Lickley, H., and Vranic, M. (1980). *Diabetes* **29**, 600–608.

Grill, V., Adamson, U., Rundfeldt, M., Anderson, S., and Cerasi, E. (1979). *J. Clin. Invest.* **64**, 700–707.

Grodsky, G., and Bennett, L. (1966). *Diabetes* **15**, 910–913.

Grodsky, G., and Fanska, R. (1975). *Methods in Enzymol.* **39**, 364–372.

Grodsky, G., Fanska, R., and Lundquist, I. (1975). *Endocrinology* **97** 573–580.

Grodsky, G., Lundquist, I., Fanska, R., and Pictet, R. (1977). *In* "Glucagon: Its Role in Physiology and Clinical Medicine" (P. Foà, J. Bajaj, and N. Foà, eds.), p. 215. Springer-Verlag, Berlin and New York.

Gross, R., and Mialhe, P. (1974). *Diabetologia* **10**, 277–283.

Grube, D., Voight, K., and Weber, E. (1978). *Histochemistry* **59**, 75–79.

Hahn, H.-J., Ziegler, M., and Mohr, E. (1974)). *FEBS Lett.* **49**, 100–102.

Hales, C., and Milner, R. (1968). *J. Physiol.* **194**, 725–743.

Harvey, W., Faloona, G., and Unger, R. (1974). *Endocrinology* **94**, 1254–1258.

Hara, M., Patton, G., and Gerich, J. (1979). *Life Sci.* **24**, 625–628.

Hellerström, C. (1964). *Acta Endocrinol.* **45**, 122–131.

Helman, A., Amira, R., Nicolaidis, S., and Assan R. (1980). *Endocrinology* **106**, 1612–1619.

Henquin, J. (1979). *Nature (London)* **280**, 66–68.

Hermansen, K., and Iversen, J. (1977). *Scand. J. Clin. Lab. Invest* **37**, 139–142.

Hoffman, J., and Lavis, P. (1974). *J. Physiol.* **239**, 519–522.

Howell, S., and Montague, W. (1974). *Biochem. J.* **142**, 379–384.

Howell, S., Edwards, J., and Montague, W. (1974). *Horm. Metab. Res.* **6**, 49–52.

Idahl, L.-A., Lernmark, Å., Sehlin, J., and Täljedal, I.-B. (1976a). *Pfluegers Arch.* **366**, 185–188.

Idahl, L., Rahemtulla, F., Sehlin, J., and Täljedal, I. (1976b). *Diabetes* **25**, 450–458.

Ipp, E., Dobbs, R., and Unger, R. (1978a). *FEBS Lett.* **92**, 33–35.

Ipp, E., Dobbs, R., and Unger, R. (1978b). *Nature (London)* **276**, 190–191.

Itoh, M., Mandarino, L., and Gerich, J. (1980a). *Diabetes* **29**, 693–696.

Itoh, M., Mandarino, L., and Gerich, J. (1980b). *Clin. Res.* **28**, 520A.

Iversen, J. (1971). *J. Clin. Invest.* **50**, 2123–2136.

Iversen, J. (1973a). *J. Clin. Invest.* **52**, 2102–2116.

Iversen, J. (1973b) *Diabetes* **22**, 381–387.

Iversen, J., and Hermansen, K. (1977). *Diabetologia* **13**, 297–303.

Jacoby, J., and Bryce, G. (1979). *Horm. Metab. Res.* **11**, 90–94.

Jarrousse, C., and Rosselin, G. (1975). *Endocrinology* **96**, 168–177.

Jaspan, J., and Rubenstein, A. (1977). *Diabetes* **26**, 887–902.

Jaspan, J., Huen, A., Morley, C., Moossa, A., and Rubenstein, A. (1977). *J. Clin. Invest.* **60**, 421–428.

Johnson, D., and Ensinck, J. (1976). *Diabetes* **25**, 645–649.

Kabadi, U., Eisenstein, A., and Strack, I. (1976). *J. Nutr.* **106**, 1247–1253.

Kaneto, A., and Kosaka, K. (1974). *Endocrinology* **95**, 676–681.

Kaneto, A., Miki, E., and Kosaka, K. (1974). *Endocrinology* **95**, 1005–1010.

Kaneto, A., Kajinuma, H., and Kosaka, K. (1975a) *Endocrinology* **96**, 143–150.

Kaneto, A., Miki, E., and Kosaka, K. (1975b) *Endocrinology* **97**, 1166–1173.

Kaneto, A., Kaneko T., Kajinuma, H and Kosaka, K. (1977). *Metabolism* **26**, 781–786.

Kaneto, A., Kaneko, T., Kajinuma, H., and Kosaka, K. (1978). *Endocrinology* **103**, 393–401.

Kante, R., Ensinck, J., and Fujimoto, W. (1980). *Diabetes* **29**, 84–86.

Karim, S., Sandler, M.,and Williams, E. (1967). *Br. J. Pharmacol. Chemother.* **31**, 340–344.

Kawamori, R., Shichiri, M., Kikuchi, M., Yamasaki, Y., and Abe, H. (1980). *Diabetes* **29**, 762–765.

Kuku, S., Jaspan, J., Emmanouel, D Zeidler, A., Katz, A., and Rubenstein, A. (1976). *J. Clin. Invest.* **58**, 742–750.

Kuzuya, T., Kajinuma, H., and Ide, T. (1974). *Diabetes* **23**, 55–60.

Lacy, P., and Kostianovsky, M. (1967). *Diabetes* **16**, 35–39.

Lacy, P., and Malaisse, W. (1973). *Res. Progr. Horm. Res.* **29**, 199–226, 1973.

Lambert, A., Jeanrenaud, B., Junod, A., and Renold, A. (1969). *Biochim. Biophys. Acta* **184**, 540–553.

Laube, H., Fussgänger, R., Goberna, R., Schröder, K., Straub, K., Sussman, K., and Pfeiffer, E. (1971). *Horm. Metab. Res.* **3**, 238–242.

Leblanc, H., Lachelin, G., Abu-Fadil, S., and Yen, S. (1977). *J. Clin. Endocrinol. Metab.* **44**, 196–198.

Leclercq-Meyer, V., Bisson, G., and Malaisse, W. (1971). *Nature (London)* **231**, 248–249.

Leclercq-Meyer, V., Marchand, V., and Malaisse, W. (1973). *Endocrinology* **93**, 1360–1370.

Leclercq-Meyer, V., Rebolledo, O., Marchand, J., and Malaisse, W. (1975). *Science* **189**, 897–899.

Leclercq-Meyer, V., Marchand, J., Malaisse, W. (1976). *Diabetologia* **12**, 531–538.

Leclercq-Meyer, V., Marchand, J., and Malaisse, W. (1977). *In* "Glucagon: Its Role in Physiology and Clinical Medicine" (P. Foà, J. Bajaj, and N. Foà, eds.), p. 185. Springer-Verlag, Berlin and New York.

Leclercq-Meyer, V., Marchand, J., and Malaisse, W. (1978) *Diabetes* **27**, 996–1004.

Leclercq-Meyer, V., Marchand, J., and Malaisse, W. (1979a). *Am. J. Physiol.* **236**, E98–104.

Leclercq-Meyer, V., Marchand, J., Leclercq, R., and Malaisse, W. (1979b). *Diabetologia* **17**, 121–126.

Lefebvre, P., and Luyckx, A. (1978). *Endocrinology* **103**, 1579–1582.

Lenzen, S. (1976). *Endokrinologie* **68**, 189–197.

Lilavivathana, U., Brodows, R., Woolf, P., and Campbell, R. (1979). *Diabetes* **28**, 873–877.

Lindall, A., Steffes, M., and Sorensen, R. (1967). *Endocrinology* **85**, 218–223.

Lindkaer-Jensen, S., Fahrenkrug, J, Holst, J., Vagn Nielsen, O., and Schaffalitzkyde-Muckadell, O. (1978). *Am. J. Physiol.* **235**, E387–391.

Lindsey, C., Faloona, G., and Unger, R. (1975). *Diabetes* **24**, 313–316.

Loewenstein, W. (1966). *Ann. N.Y. Acad. Sci.* **137**, 441–472.

Lorenzi, M., Tsalikian, E., Bohannon, N., Gerich, J., Karam, J., and Forsham, P. (1977). *J. Clin. Endocrinol. Metab.* **45**, 1154–1158.

Lorenzi, M., Karam, J., Tsalikian, N., Bohannon, N., Gerich, J., and Forsham, P. (1979). *J. Clin. Invest.* **63**, 310–317.

Lundquist, I., Fanska, R., and Grodsky, G. (1976). *Endocrinology* **99**, 1304–14312.

Luyckx, A., and Lefebvre, P. (1970) *Proc. Soc. Exp. Biol. Med.* **133**, 524–528.

Luyckx, A., and Lefebvre, P. (1973) *Postgrad. Med. J.* **49**, 620–623.

Luyckx, A., and Lefebvre, P. (1978). *Diabetologia* **15**, 411–416.

Madison, L., Seyffert, W, Unger, R., and Barker, B. (1968). *Metabolism* **17**, 301–304.

Malaisse, W. (1973). *Diabetologia* **9**, 167–173.

Malaisse-Lagae, F., and Malaisse, W. (1971). *Endocrinology* **88**, 72–80.

Mandarino, L., Blanchard, W., Stemner, D., and Gerich, J. (1981). *Clin. Res.* **29**, 57A.

Marco, J., Calle, C., Roman, D., Diaz-Fierros, M., Villanueva, M., and Valverde, I. (1973a) *N. Engl. J. Med.* **288**, 128-131.

Marco, J., Diego, J., Villanueva, M., Diaz-Fierros, M., Valverde, I., and Segovia, J. (1973b). N Engl. J. Med. **289**, 1107-1111.

Marco, J., Calle, C., Hedo, J., and Villaneuva, M. (1976). *Diabetologia* **12**, 307-311.

Marliss, E., Aoki, T., Unger, R., Soeldner, J., and Cahill, G. (1970). *J. Clin. Invest.* **49**, 2256-2270.

Marliss, E., Wollheim, C., Blondel, B., Orci, L., Lambert, A., Stauffacher, W., Like, A., and Renold, A. (1973). *Eur. J. Clin. Invest.* **3**, 16-26.

Marre, M., Bobbioni, E., Suarez, M., Reach, G., Dubois, M., and Assan R. (1979). *Diabetes* **28**, 213-220.

Mashiter, K., Harding, P., Cou, M., Mashiter, G., Strit, J., Diamond, D., and Field, J. (1975). *Endocrinology* **95**, 678-693.

Matschinsky, F., Pagliara, A., Hover, B., Haymond, M., and Stillings, S. (1975). *Diabetes* **24**, 369-372.

Matschinsky, F., Pagliara, A., Hover, B., Pace, C., Ferrendelli, J., and Williams. A. (1976). *J. Biol. Chem.* **251**, 6053-6061.

Micossi, P., Pontiroli, A., Baron, S., Tamayo, R., Lengel, F., Bevilacqua, M., Raggi, U., Norbiato, G., and Foà, P. (1978). *Diabetes* **27**, 1196-1204.

Milner, R., and Hales, C. (1967). *Diabetologia* **3**, 47-49.

Miller, R., and Horton, E. (1979). *Diabetes* **28**, 762-768.

Miyata, M., Yamamoto, T., Yamaguchi, M., Nakao, K., and Yoshida, T. (1976). *Proc. Soc. Exp. Biol. Med.* **152**, 540-543.

Moltz, J., Dobbs, R., McCann, S., and Fawcett, C. (1979). *Endocrinology* **105**, 1262-1268.

Müller, W., Faloona, G., Aguilar-Parad, E., and Unger, R. (1970). *J. Clin. Invest.* **283**, 109-115.

Müller, W., Faloona, G., and Unger, R. (1971a). *J. Clin. Invest.* **50**, 1992-1999.

Müller, W., Faloona, G., and Unger, R. (1971b). *J. Clin. Invest.* **50**, 2215-22 8.

Müller, W., Faloona, G.,and Unger, R. (1971c). *N. Engl. J. Med.* **285**, 1450-454.

Müller, W., Brennan, M., Tan, M., and Aoki, T. (1974). *Diabetes* **23**, 512-515.

Müller, W., Aoki, T., and Cahill, G. (1975). *J. Clin. Endocrinol. Metab.* **40**, 418-425.

Müller, W., Aoki, T., Flatt, J., Blackburn, G., Edgahl, R., and Cahill, G. (1976) *Metabolism* **25**, 1077-1086.

Müller, W., Berger, M., Suter, P., Cüppers, H., Reiter, J., Wyss, T., Berchtold, P., Schmidt, F., Assal, P.-P., and Renold, A. (1979a). *J. Clin. Invest.* **63**, 820-827.

Müller, W., Berger, M., Cüppers, H., Berchtold, P., Strohmeyer, G., Renold, A., Hofstetter, J., and Convers, J.-J. (1979b). *Gut* **20**, 200-204.

Munoz-Barragan, L., Blazquez, E., Patton, G., Dobbs, R., and Unger, R. (1976). *Am. J. Physiol.* **231**, E1057-1068.

Munoz-Barragan, L., Rufener, C., Srikant, C., Dobbs, R., Shannon, W. Jr., Baetens, D., and Unger, R. (1977). *Horm. Metab. Res.* **9**, 37-39.

Nonaka, K., Sugase, T., and Foà, P. (1971). *In* "Proc 7th Congr Int. Diabetes Fed." (R. Rodriguez and J. Vallance-Owen, eds.), vol. 231, pp. 625-635. Excerpta Medica, Amsterdam.

Norfleet, W., Pagliara, A., Haymond, M., and Matschinsky, F. (1975). *Diabetes* **24**, 961-970.

Ohneda, A., Parada, E., Eisentrant, A., and Unger, R. (1978). *J. Clin. Invest.* **47**, 2305-2322.

Ohneda, A., Aguilar-Parade, E., Eisentrant, A., and Unger, R. (1969). *Diabetes* **18**, 1-10.

Oliver, J., Williams, V., and Wright, P. (1976). *Diabetologia* **12**, 301-306.

Oliver, J., Williams, V., and Wright, P. (1977). *Proc. Soc. Exp. Biol. Med.* **154**, 210-214.

Ono, J., Takaki, R., and Fukuma, M. (1977). *Endocrinol. Jpn.* **24**, 265-270.

Orci, L. (1980). In "Current Views on Hypoglycemia and Glucagon" (D. Andreani, P. Le-febvre, and V. Marks, eds.) pp. 1-11 Academic Press, New York.
Orci, L., Blondel, B., Malaisse-Lagae, F., Ravazzola, M., Wollheim, C., Malaisse, W., and Renold, A. (1974). Diabetologia 10, 282 (Abstr.).
Orci, L., Baetens, D., Rufener, C., Amherdt, M., Ravazzola, M., Studer, P., Malaisse-Lagae, F., and Unger, R. (1976). Proc. Natl. Acad. Sci. U.S.A. 73, 1338-1342.
Östenson, C.-G. (1980). Biochem. J. 188, 201-206.
Pagliara, A., Stillings, S., Hover, B., Martin, D., and Matschinsky, F. (1974). J. Clin. Invest. 54, 819-832.
Pagliara, A., Hover, B., Ellerman, J.,and Matschinsky, F. (1975a). Endocrinology 97, 698-708.
Pagliara, A., Stillings, S., Haymond, M., Hover, B., and Matschinsky, F. (1975b). J. Clin. Invest. 55, 244-255.
Pagliara, A., Stillings, S., and Matschinsky, F. (1977). Diabetes 26, 973-979.
Palmer, J., Henry, D., Benson, J., Johnson, D., and Ensinck, J. (1976). J. Clin. Invest. 57, 522-525.
Palmer, J., Werner, P., Hollander, P , and Ensinck, J. (1979). Metabolism 28, 549-552.
Patel, Y., and Weir, G. (1976). Clin. Endocrinol. 5, 191-194.
Patton, G., Ipp, E., Dobbs, R., Orci, L., Vale, W., and Unger, R. (1977). Proc. Natl. Acad. Sci. U.S.A. 74, 2140-2143.
Pederson, R., and Brown, J. (1978). Endocrinology 103, 610-615.
Pek, S., Fajans, S., Floyd, J., Knopl, F., and Conn, J. (1968). J. Lab. Clin. Med. 72, 1003.
Pek, S., Tai, T.-Y., and Elster, A. (1978). Diabetes 27, 801-809.
Penhos, J., Wu, C., Basabe, J., Lopez, N., and Wolff, F. (1969). Diabetes 18, 733-738.
Petersson, B., Hellerström, C., and Gurnarsson, R. (1970). Horm. Metab. Res. 2, 313-317.
Pontirolli, A., Micossi, P., and Foà, P. (1978). Horm. Metab. Res. 10, 200-203.
Prieto, J., Ortiz, S., Sobrino, F., Henera, M., Bedoya, F., and Goberna, R. (1978). Rev. Esp. Fisiol. 34, 291-294.
Raskin, P., Aydin, I., and Unger, R. (1976). Diabetes 25, 227-229.
Raskin, P., Aydin, I., Yamamoto, T , and Unger, R. (1978). Am. J. Med. 64, 988-997.
Rehfeld, J., Holst, J., and Kühl, C. (1978). Eur. J. Clin. Invest. 8, 5-9.
Rizza, R., Cryer, P., and Gerich, J. (1979). J. Clin. Invest. 64, 62-71.
Rocha, D., Faloona, G., and Unger, R. (1972). J. Clin. Invest. 51, 2346-2351.
Röjdmark, S., Bloom, G., Chou, M., and Field, J. (1978a). Endocrinology 102, 806-813.
Röjdmark, S., Bloom, G., Chou, M., Jaspan, J., and Field, J. (1978b). Am. J. Physiol. 235, E88-96.
Rossini, A., and Buse, M. (1973). Horm. Metab. Res. 5, 26-28.
Rossini, A., Soeldner, J., Hiebert, J., Weir, G., and Gleason, R. (1974) Diabetologia 10, 795-799.
Rubin, R. (1970). Pharmacol. Rev. 22, 389-428.
Russell, R., Thomson, J., and Bloom, S. (1974). Br. J. Surg. 61, 821-824.
Sacca, L., and Perez, G. (1976). Metabolism 25, 127-130.
Samols, E., and Stagner, J. (1979). Excerpta Medica 481, 202, (Abstr.).
Samols, E., and Weir, G. (1979). J. Clin Invest. 63, 230-238.
Santeusanio, F., Faloona, G., Knochel, J., and Unger, R. (1972a). J. Clin. Invest. 51, 85a (Abstr.).
Santeusanio, F., Faloona, G., and Unger, R. (1972b). J. Clin. Invest. 51, 1743-1749.
Santiago, J., Clarke, W., Shah, S., and Cryer, P. (1980). Clin. Res. 28, 522a (Abstr.).
Sasaki, H., Rubalcava, B., Baetens, D., Blazquez, E., Srikant, C., Orci, L., and Unger, R. (1975). J. Clin. Invest. 56, 135-145.

Scharp, D., Kemp, C., Knight, M., Ballinger, W., and Lacy, P. (1973). *Transplantation* **16**, 686–689.

Scharp, D., Murphy, J., Newton, W., Ballinger, W.,and Lacy, P. (1975). *Surgery* **77**, 100–105.

Scharp, D., Downing, R., Merrell, R., and Greider, M. (1980). *Diabetes* **29**, Suppl. 1, 19–30.

Schebalin, M., Said, S., and Makhlouf, G. (1977). *Am. J. Physiol.* **232**, E197–200.

Sehlin, I., and Täljedal, I.-B. (1975). *Nature (London)* **253**, 635–636.

Seino, Y., Goto, Y., Kurahachi, H., Sakurai, H., Ikeda, M., Kadowaki, S., Inoue, Y., Mori, K., Taminato, T., and Imura, H. (1977). *Horm. Metab. Res.* **9**, 28–32.

Seino, Y., Taminato, T., Goto, Y., Inoue, Y., Kadowaki, S., Mori, K., and Imura, H. (1978a). *Clin. Endocrinol.* **9**, 577–581.

Seino, Y., Taminato, T., Goto, Y., Inoue, Y., Kadowaki, S., Hattori, M., Mori, K., Kato, Y., Matsukura, S.,and Imura, H. (1978b). *Clin. Endocrinol* **9**, 563–570.

Seyffert, W., and Madison, L. (1967). *Diabetes* **16**, 765–776.

Sharp, G., Wiedenkeller, D., Kaelin, D., Siegel, E., and Wollheim, C. (1980). *Diabetes* **29**, 74–77.

Shibata, A., Ludvigsen, C., Naber, S., McDaniel, M., and Lacy, P. (1976). *Diabetes* **25**, 667–672.

Shima, K., Kurokawa, M., Sawazaki, N., Tamaka, R., and Kumahara, Y. (1978). *Endocrinol. Jpn.* **25**, 461–465.

Sirek, A., Vranic, M., Sirek, O., Vigas, M., and Policova, Z. (1979). *Am. J. Physiol* **237**, E107–112.

Smith, P., and Porte, D., Jr. (1976). *Annu. Rev. Pharmacol. Toxicol.* **16** 269–285.

Sorenson, R., Elde, R., and Seybold, V. (1979). *Diabetes* **28**, 899–906.

Sorenson, R., Lindell, D., and Elde, R. (1980). *Diabetes* **29**, 747–751.

Srikant, C., McCorkle, K., and Unger, R. (1977). *J. Biol. Chem.* **252**, 1847–1851.

Stubbs, W., Jones, A., Edwards, C., Delitale, G., Jeffcoate, W., and Ratter, S. (1978). *Lancet* **2**, 1225–1227.

Szecowka, J., Sandberg, E., and Efendic, S. (1980). *Diabetologia* **19**, 137–143.

Tai, T., and Pek, S. (1976). *Endocrinology* **99**, 669–677.

Taniguchi, H., Utsumi, M., Hasegawa, M., Kobayashi, T., Watanabe, Y., Murakami, M., Seki, M., Tsutou, A., Makimura, M., Sakoda, M., and Baba, S. (1977). *Diabetes* **26**, 700–702.

Tomita, T. (1980). *Diabetologia* **19**, 154–157.

Trimble, E., Atkinson, A., Buchanan, K., and Hadden, D. (1980). *J. Clin. Endocrinol. Metab.* **51**, 626–631.

Turcot-Lemay, L., Lemay, A., and Lacy, P. (1975). *Biochem. Biophys. Res. Commun.* **63**, 1130–1138.

Ukai, M., Inoue, I., and Itatsu, T. (1977). *Endocrinology* **100**, 1284–1286.

Unger, R., Ohneda, A., Aguilar-Parad, E., and Eisentrant, A. (1969). *J. Clin. Invest.* **48**, 810–822.

Unger, R., and Orci, L. (1976). *Physiol. Rev.* **56**, 778–826.

Valverde, I., Vandermeers, A., Anjaneyulir, R., and Malaisse, W. (1979). *Science* **206**, 225–227.

Vance, J., Buchanan, K., and Williams, R. (1971). *Diabetes* **20**, 78–82.

Van Lan, V., Yamaguchi, N., Garcia, M., Ramey, E., and Penhos, J. (1974). *Endocrinology* **94**, 671–675.

Verspohl, E., and Ammon, H. (1980). *J. Clin. Invest.* **65**, 1230–1237.

Vierhapper, H., Bratusch-Marrain, and Waldhäusl, W. (1980). *J. Clin. Endocrinol. Metb.* **50**, 1131–1134.

Wahren, J., Felig, P., and Hagenfeldt, L. (1976). *J. Clin. Invest.* **57**, 987–999.

Weir, G., Knowlton, S., and Martin, D. (1974). *J. Clin. Invest.* **54**, 1403–1412.
Weir, G., Knowlton, S., Atkins, R., McKennan, K., and Martin, D. (1976). *Diabetes* **25**, 275–282.
Weir, G., Samols, E., Loo, S., Patel, Y., and Gabbay, K. (1979). *Diabetes* **28**, 35–40.
Werner, P., and Palmer, J. (1978). *Diabetes* **27**, 1005–1012.
Wise, J., Hendler, R., and Felig, P. (1973a). *N. Engl. J. Med.* **288**, 487–490.
Wise, J., Hendler, R., and Felig, P. (1973b). *J. Clin. Invest.* **52**, 2774–2782.
Wollheim, C., Blondel, B., and Sharp, G. (1974). *Diabetologia* **10**, 391 (Abstr.).
Wollheim, C., Blondel, B., Müller, W., and Sharp, G. (1975). *Eur. J. Clin. Invest.* **5**, 58.
Wollheim, C., Blondel, B., Renold, A., and Sharp, G. (1976). *Diabetologia* **12**, 269–277.
Woods, S., and Porte, D., Jr. (1974). *Physiol. Rev.* **54**, 596–619.

11

Somatostatin and Its Role in Insulin and Glucagon Secretion

S. EFENDIĆ and R. LUFT

I. INTRODUCTION

Somatostatin was originally extracted from the hypothalamus and was found to be a tetradecapeptide with the property of inhibiting the release of pituitary growth hormone (GH). It does so in the usual fashion after being transported by the hypothalamic-hypophyseal portal vessels to the pituitary

The Islets of Langerhans
Copyright © 1981 by Academic Press, Inc.
All rights of reproduction in any form reserved.
ISBN 0–12–187820–1

gland. The intense somatostatin research during the last few years has established that somatostatin is also produced in a number of endocrine cells in the periphery (Efendić et al., 1978a; Luft et al., 1978). Furthermore, one of the most interesting observations has been the discovery of somatostatin in the central and peripheral nervous systems as well as in the autonomic nervous system. This pattern of localization suggests that, in addition to its hormone action, somatostatin also modulates nervous functions.

The first endocrine tissue where the presence of somatostatin was established was the *pancreatic islets* (Luft et al., 1974; Dubois, 1975; Goldsmith et al., 1975; Hökfelt et al., 1975; Orci et al., 1975; Polak et al., 1975; Rufener et al., 1975; Erlandsen et al., 1976; Parsons et al., 1976). Islet cells containing somatostatin-like immunoreactivity (SLI) were identified as A_1 or D cells by electron microscopic immunohistochemistry (Goldsmith et al., 1975; Rufener et al., 1975), by correlative immunofluorescence and silver staining (Hökfelt et al., 1975; Polak et al., 1975), and by consecutive staining with antisera to somatostatin, glucagon, and insulin (Orci et al., 1975).

Most immunoreactive structures in the islets could be identified as cells with strong cytoplasmic fluorescence and a nonfluorescent nucleus, but fluorescent extensions of the cytoplasm were also observed, often in direct connection with cell bodies. In the rat, the positive elements were always localized to the periphery of the islets and occasionally formed a complete ring around them. In man and guinea pigs, they were spread all over the islets.

These reports of cells showing somatostatin in the pancreatic islets appeared particularly noteworthy in view of the demonstration that somatostatin exerted a direct inhibition of insulin and glucagon secretion (see below). Against this background, it was tempting to suggest that the close morphological association between, on the one hand, somatostatin-containing D cells and, on the other hand, A cells and B cells, reflected a mechanism for local intraislet regulation of insulin and glucagon release (Efendić et al., 1978a; Luft et al., 1978). Indeed, a mechanism of this kind had been previously suggested by Hellman and Lernmark (1969a,b). These authors had reported a marked *in vitro* inhibition of insulin release from isolated islets incubated in the presence of an extract obtained either from islets of obese hyperglycemic mice or from D-cell-rich islets from ducks.

II. ACTIONS OF SOMATOSTATIN ON THE RELEASE OF PANCREATIC HORMONES

The isolation and synthesis of somatostatin was soon followed by the finding that the peptide—in addition to inhibition of GH release—also suppressed the release of insulin (Alberti *et al.,* 1973; Efendić *et al.,* 1974; Koerker *et al.,* 1974; Mortimer *et al.,* 1974). In man somatostatin inhibited insulin release induced by glucose (Alberti *et al.,* 1973; Mortimer *et al.,* 1974: Efendić and Luft, 1975; Efendić *et al.,* 1976b), as well as by arginine, tolbutamide, and glucagon (Gerich *et al.,* 1974a; Leblanc *et al.,* 1975; Efendić *et al.,* 1976a,b). A vast literature already exists demonstrating similar effects in different species both under *in vitro* and *in vivo* conditions.

Recent studies show that there are considerable species differences in the sensitivity of B cells to the peptide. In man as little as 7 ng/kg/min inhibited glucose-induced initiation of insulin release, whereas in rats a dose of 700 ng/kg/min was required (Efendić *et al.,* 1978b, 1979c; Lins *et al.,* 1980c). On the other hand, somatostatin did not influence the potentiation or inhibition of insulin release mediated by prior administration of glucose (Efendić *et al.,* 1979c).

Prolongation of the infusion period in man for up to 24 hr was accompanied by continuous insulin suppression (Lins *et al.,* 1980a). In contrast, in rats infused for 24 hr, the peptide did not exert inhibition of glucose-stimulated insulin release (Lins *et al.,* 1980c). In addition, when the rats were infused for 4 days, there was no noticeable effect on basal insulin, glucagon, and GH, or on body weight gain, food consumption, and water intake. These findings suggest that rats, at least, develop mechanisms counteracting the peptide, e.g. tachyphylaxis. The latter idea is supported by the appearance of tachyphylaxis to the inhibitory effect of somatostatin on the electrically induced release of acetylcholine from the myenteric plexus of the guinea pig ileum (Guillemin, 1976).

Similarly, somatostatin inhibited basal and stimulated glucagon release *in vivo* in normal man (Gerich *et al.,* 1974b; Mortimer *et al.,* 1974; Leblanc *et al.,* 1975; Efendić *et al.,* 1976a) and in experimental animals (Koerker *et al.,* 1974, Chideckel *et al.,* 1975), as well as in perfused rat and dog pancreases (Gerich *et al.,* 1975: Iversen, 1974; Norfleet *et al.,* 1975; Efendić *et al.,* 1976a). The stimuli used were hypoglycemia, arginine, isoproterenol, and theophyllamine. Basal glucagon release was also suppressed by somatostatin (Christensen *et al.,* 1974; Efendić *et al.,* 1976a).

In our laboratory, somatostatin seemed to be a more potent inhibitor of insulin than of glucagon release. Thus, in the perfused rat pancreas, a dose of somatostatin as low as 100 pg/ml suppressed insulin and, if anything, enhanced glucagon release (unpublished).

The mode of action of somatostatin so far has not been clarified. Available data indicate that at least two effects may be involved: one is the level of cyclic adenosine 3′,5′-monophosphate (cyclic AMP) in the target cells, and the other is calcium uptake by these cells. Somatostatin suppressed basal as well as prostaglandin-, theophylline-, and thyrotropin-releasing hormone-stimulated levels of cyclic AMP in the pituitary gland and its cells (Kaneko *et al.,* 1973; Borgeat *et al.,* 1974a,b). Our studies on isolated pancreatic islets from the rat also demonstrated a decrease in the level of cyclic AMP (Claro *et al.,* 1977). In dose–response studies, the inhibition by somatostatin of the effect of glucose on ^{3}H-labeled cyclic AMP and insulin release could be overcome by a high concentration of glucose (44.9 mmol/liter), suggesting competitive inhibition. Somatostatin did not affect phosphodiesterase activity. These data indicate that somatostatin-induced inhibition of insulin release is, at least partially, mediated by cyclic AMP, probably through inactivation of islet adenylate cyclase.

As for the effect of calcium ions, the inhibitory effect of somatostatin on glucose-induced insulin release from the perfused rat pancreas (Curry and Bennet, 1974) as well as in man (Wajchenberg *et al.,* 1978) could be overcome by increasing the calcium concentration. However, controversy still exists regarding the influence of somatostatin on calcium uptake by the islets.

It has been suggested that the inhibitory effect of somatostatin on insulin release may, at least partially, be mediated by α-adrenergic receptors (Smith *et al.,* 1976, 1977). Our finding that the α-adrenergic blocking agent phentolamine did not counteract this inhibition either in humans *in vivo* (Efendić and Luft, 1975) or in the isolated rat islet (unpublished data) does not support the above concept. Recent data reported by Kaneto *et al.* (1978), Schmitt *ėt al.* (1979), and Järhult *et al.* (1979) also argue against the involvement of α-adrenergic receptors in the action of somatostatin.

In an attempt to dissociate the effect of somatostatin on glucagon and insulin release, we have investigated the effects of *analogues of somatostatin* on arginine-stimulated insulin and glucagon release from the perfused rat pancreas (Efendić *et al.,* 1975, 1977). In our studies, neither the amino terminal nor a free carboxyl terminal seemed to be essential for the activity of the cyclic peptide. The addition of amino acids to the amino terminal did not decrease the activity. On the other hand, minor changes in the structure of linear somatostatin, which led to loss of the ability to form a cyclic peptide, greatly impaired the activity. Deletion of the Asn^5 was accompanied by a marked inhibition of insulin release, whereas glucagon release was not suppressed but rather stimulated. Des-Asn^5-somatostatin also had a more marked effect on insulin release than on glucagon release when tested on rats *in vivo* (Sarantakis *et al.,* 1976). On the other hand, the analogues D-Cys^{14}-somatostatin (Brown *et al.,* 1976; Meyers *et al.,* 1977), Ala^2-D-Cys^{14}-somatostatin, D-Trp^8-D-Cys^{14}-somatostatin, and Ala^2-D-Trp^8-D-Cys^{14}-somatostatin (Meyers *et al.,* 1977) exerted more specific inhibition of arginine-induced glucagon than insulin release on rats *in vivo*. Moreover, the latter analogue (Ala^2-D-Trp^8-D-Cys^{14}-somatostatin), while inhibiting arginine-induced glucagon release in rats *in vivo* at a dose of 10 ng/kg/min, stimulated glucose-induced insulin release at a dose range of 10–100 ng (Lins *et al.,* 1980b).

A tentative explanation for the divergent effects of Des-Asn^5-somatostatin and Ala^2-D-Trp^8-D-Cys^{14}-somatostatin on insulin and glucagon release is that, while both analogues bind to A and B cells, the former exerts intrinsic activity only on B cells and the latter only on A cells. Accordingly, Des-Asn^5-somatostatin would counteract the effect of endogenous somatostatin on A cells, and Ala^2-D-Trp^8-D-Cys^{14}-somatostatin on B cells, the net effect being stimulation of glucagon and insulin release, respectively.

In addition to its inhibition of insulin and glucagon release, somatostatin also inhibited the release of pancreatic polypeptide (Marco *et al.,* 1977; Wilson *et al.,* 1978) (see Chapter 12).

III. RADIOIMMUNOASSAY FOR SOMATOSTATIN

The development of a sensitive radioimmunoassay (RIA) for somatostatin made it possible to investigate mechanisms controlling the release of this compound. Since somatostatin does not contain a tyrosine residue, N-Tyr-, 1-Tyr-, or 11-Tyr-somatostatin has been used for iodination (McIntosh and Arnold, 1978). Both the chloramine-T and lactoperoxidase methods have been used. In order to produce antibodies to somatostatin, the peptide was conjugated with various carrier proteins, such as α- and β-globulins, thyroglobulin, and hemocyanin, which were coupled to somatostatin using glutaraldehyde, carbodiimide, or bisdiazotized benzidine. Evaluation of the recognition sites of the antibodies revealed that the antisera raised against glutaraldehyde- or carbodiimide-coupled cyclic somatostatin were specific for the amino acid sequence 4–14 (Arimura *et al.,* 1977). They could not recognize changes at the N-terminus. In contrast, antibodies raised against bisdiazotized benzidine-coupled Tyr^{11}-somatostatin were N-terminal-directed (Vale *et al.,* 1976; Arimura *et al.,* 1978).

Although RIA of somatostatin in tissue extracts, culture media, and organ perfusates is relatively easy to perform, and the results obtained are reliable and reproducible, measurement of somatostatin in plasma is difficult because of interference by nonsomatostatin substances, including plasma proteins. Somatostatin is fairly strongly bound to some proteins. For this reason, it should be extracted from plasma before determination (Arimura *et al.,* 1978). Recently, Penman *et al.* (1979) have developed and validated a RIA for somatostatin in plasma using prior extraction of the peptide onto leached silica glass. They found a parallelism between standard synthetic cyclic somatostatin and extracted plasma samples. The fasting level of somatostatin in normal subjects was 17–81 pg/ml.

The sensitivity of our own RIA for somatostatin is about 5 pg/ml, with a coefficient of variation of 15%. Dilution of acid–ethanol extracts of pancreas and hypothalamus demonstrated binding parallel to that of somatostatin standards. This was also the case with dilutions of the perfusion solutions used for the isolated rat pancreas. The mean recovery of exogenous somatostatin from plasma was 90%. Cross-reactivity of the antibodies was less than 0.01% with insulin, glucagon, substance P, luteinizing hormone-releasing hormone, vasopressin, and oxytocin.

IV. RELEASE OF PANCREATIC SOMATOSTATIN

With the use of a sensitive RIA for somatostatin, the influence of certain factors on the *in vivo* and *in vitro* release of somatostatin has been studied: glucose and amino acids, hormones, the autonomic nervous system, ions, and drugs. The *in vitro* studies were performed on isolated rat islets and monolayer cultures of neonatal rat pancreas (Patel *et al.*, 1979), as well as on isolated perfused rat and dog pancreases.

A. Effect of Glucose

Most studies on the release of somatostatin, for obvious reasons, deal with the impact of nutrients. Under *in vitro* conditons, at least, high concentrations of glucose undoubtedly stimulated somatostatin release from isolated rat islets (Schauder *et al.*, 1976, 1977a,b) and from isolated dog (Ipp *et al.*, 1977a; Weir *et al.*, 1978) and rat pancreases (Efendić *et al.*, 1978c, 1979b). Moreover, even moderate doses of glucose seemed to enhance the release from dog pancreas (Ipp *et al.*, 1977a; Weir *et al.*, 1978).

In the *in vivo* studies, somatostatin was measured in portal and peripheral blood after orally or intravenously administered glucose. In rats, intragastric and intravenous administrations of glucose were accompanied by marked elevations of portal SLI, the patterns of SLI following closely those of portal glucose and insulin (Berelowitz *et al.*, 1978). In contrast, no changes were observed in somatostatin in peripheral blood using unextracted plasma. These data have been confirmed with extracted plasma after intravenous glucose loading (Efendić *et al.*, 1980).

In dogs, SLI was increased in blood collected from the pancreaticoduodenal vein and in peripheral blood after intragastric and intraduodenal glucose, whereas it fell in peripheral blood after intravenous loading (Schusdziarra *et al.*, 1978a,c). In man oral glucose loading was accompanied by increased somatostatin in peripheral plasma (Penman et al., 1979). In pigs, intravenous glucose administration was accompanied by a fall in somatostatin in the superior pancreaticoduodenal vein (Gustavsson and Lundqvist, 1978).

In all, the *in vitro* data strongly support the idea that glucose stimulates the release of pancreatic somatostatin. The inconsistency of the *in vivo* data may be accounted for by species differences and the procedures used. Moreover, it should be remembered that somatostatin in peripheral blood represents somatostatin produced anywhere in the body, and somatostatin in portal blood that from the whole splanchnic area. Furthermore, because of collaterals between veins draining the pancreas and the gastrointestinal tract, somatostatin in the pancreatic veins may not necessarily represent somatostatin from only the pancreas.

B. Effect of Amino Acids

Arginine markedly stimulated the release of somatostatin from the isolated pancreas of dogs (Patton et al., 1976b, Weir et al., 1979) and rats (Efendić et al., 1978c, 1979a; Gerich et al., 1979; Gotto et al., 1979; Hara et al., 1979; Kadowaki et al., 1979). In the former species, the release was also stimulated by leucine and a mixture of 10 amino acids (Ipp et al., 1977a). In addition, leucine stimulated somatostatin release from isolated rat islets (Schauder et al., 1977a). Intravenous arginine in rats increased somatostatin in portal and peripheral blood (Arimura et al., 1978; Efendić et al., 1980). Intragastric administration of a casein hydrolysate and a liver meal elicited a prompt increase in SLI in the pancreatic and peripheral veins (Schusdziarra et al., 1978a,c, 1979b). The liver meal had a more pronounced effect on SLI release at an antral pH of 2 than at a pH of 7. These findings were interpreted as indicating that, in the stomach, there are factor(s) which are stimulated by low pH and which are involved in the gastro-insular axis.

In the perfused rat pancreas arginine and glucose seemed to have an additive effect on the release of somatostatin (Efendić et al., 1980).

C. Effect of Hormones

Glucagon consistently stimulated somatostatin release from isolated pancreases of dogs (Patton et al., 1976a, 1977; Weir et al., 1978, 1979) and rats (Kadowaki et al., 1979). The insulin response to glucagon was markedly enhanced by increased perfusate glucose, unlike the somatostatin response which was little affected (Weir et al., 1979). Gastrointestinal hormones also stimulated release of the peptide somatostatin pancreozymin–cholecystokinin in the dog pancreas (Ipp et al., 1977a,b), gastrin and secretin in the dog pancreas (Ipp *et al.*, 1977b), gastric inhibitory polypeptide in dog (Ipp *et al.*, 1977b) and rat pancreases (unpublished), and vasoactive intestinal polypeptide in dog (Ipp *et al.*, 1978a) and rat pancreases (Szecówka *et al.*, 1980).

Studies on isolated rat islets revealed that neurotensin at low glucose concentrations stimulated insulin, glucagon, and somatostatin release. In contrast, it inhibited the effects of arginine and high glucose concentrations on the release of these hormones (Dolais-Kitabgi *et al.*, 1979). Perfusion of the dog pancreas with a somatostatin analogue (D-Trp^8-D-Cys^{14}-somatostatin) which did not cross-react with somatostatin antibodies, was accompanied by suppression of the somatostatin response to cholecystokinin and arginine (Ipp *et al.*, 1979). These results raise the possibility of a self-inhibiting action of the native hormone.

Perfusion of the isolated dog pancreas with large doses of insulin was without influence on somatostatin release (Patton *et al.*, 1977; Weir *et al.*, 1979). Furthermore, insulin did not alter basal somatostatin release and somatostatin responses to theophylline and glucose from monolayer cultures of neonatal rat pancreas (Patel *et al.*, 1979). On the other hand, insulin induced a rapid increase in somatostatin secretion in isolated perfused chicken pancreas–duodenum preparations (Honey and Weir, 1979).

D. Effect of the Autonomic Nervous System

Electrical stimulation of the vagal nerve in anesthetized cats induced a decrease in somatostatin in portal blood but an increase in somatostatin release into the antral lumen (Uvnäs-Wallensten *et al.*, 1980). Since somatostatin is released from several parts of the splanchnic area, the decrease in this compound in portal blood does not necessarily reflect the secretion of pancreatic somatostatin. It may be considered justified to attribute such a decrease in portal somatostatin to the activation of cholinergic fibers. Thus cholinergic ganglion cells are present within the islets (Woods and Porte, 1978), and acetylcholine inhibits somatostatin release from the perfused pancreas of normal dogs (Samols *et al.*, 1978).

Recently, the vagal nerve has been shown to contain several types of peptidergic fibers including gastrin, somatostatin, vasoactive intestinal peptide, substance P, and enkephalins (Uvnäs-Wallensten *et al.*, 1977, 1978; Lundberg *et al.*, 1978). Furthermore, β-endorphin has been shown to inhibit pancreatic somatostatin release (Ipp *et al.*, 1978b). Therefore a vagally induced decrease in portal somatostatin may be mediated via peptidergic fibers. It has also been suggested that the stomach influences pancreatic D-cell activity through atropine-sensitive pathways (Schusdziarra *et al.*, 1979b).

D cells also seem to be influenced by the adrenergic system. Thus D-cell secretion, like that of B cells, was inhibited by α-adrenergic agonism and stimulated by β-adrenergic agonism. However, β-adrenergic-induced changes in D-cell secretion were smaller in magnitude than those of B-cell secretion (Samols and Weir, 1979).

E. Effect of Drugs

So far, attention has concentrated on the effect of sulfonylureas on somatostatin release. Tolbutamide (Ipp et al., 1977a; Samols et al., 1978) and glibenclamide (Efendić et al., 1979b) markedly smulated somatostatin as well as insulin release from perfused dog and rat pancreases, respectively. Furthermore, in the presence of low glucose concentration, these drugs inhibited glucagon release (Samols et al., 1978; Efendić et al., 1979b).

As to the interaction between nutrients and sulfonylureas on somatostatin release, glucose, especially in low concentrations, inhibited glibenclamide-stimulated somatostatin release from the rat pancreas (Efendić et al., 1979b). In contrast, arginine and glibenclamide exerted a synergistic action on this release (Efendić et al., 1979a).

Diazoxide, in contrast to sulfonylureas, inhibited the release of both insulin and somatostatin (Samols et al., 1978).

F. Effect of Fasting

Perifused islets from 48-hr-fasted rats released more somatostatin in the presence of 3.3 mmol glucose than islets from fed controls. Simultaneously, the somatostatin content of the former islets was decreased (Schauder et al., 1979). On the other hand, neither fasting for 24 hr (unpublished data) or for 48 hr (Schauder et al., 1979) impaired the response of somatostatin to glucose, while the insulin response was markedly decreased. In rats in vivo, 72 hr of fasting was accompanied by a substantial decrease in SLI in portal blood, while the somatostatin content of the pancreas and gastrointestinal tract was elevated (Shapiro et al., 1979). In the same study, 15 hr of fasting was followed by only a minor decrease in portal blood SLI but a marked decrease in tissue somatostatin.

The above studies show that the amount of somatostatin released in fasted rats does not necessarily reflect tissue levels of the peptide.

G. Stimulus–Secretion Coupling in the Pancreatic D Cells

Since all studies on this aspect were performed on the islets or the perfused pancreas, the results obtained—besides direct interaction between experimental maneuvers and D cells—may also reflect processes in the A and B cells. In analogy to the situation in the B cells, it seems that both cyclic AMP and calcium ions play an important role in the mediation of somatostatin secretion. Glucagon (Patton *et al.,* 1976a,b, 1977; Weir *et al.,* 1978, 1979; Kadowaki *et al.,* 1979) and isoproterenol (Hermansen *et al.,* 1979), established stimulators of adenylate cyclase activity, as well as the phosphodiesterase inhibitor theophylline (Schauder *et al.,* 1977b; Barden *et al.,* 1978; Goto *et al.,* 1979), enhanced somatostatin release. In addition, the inhibitory effect of epinephrine on somatostatin secretion (Schauder *et al.,* 1976; Samols and Weir, 1979) may be, at least partially, mediated by a decrease in cyclic AMP in the D cells. The stimulatory effect of glucose on the release of somatostatin—like that on insulin secretion—was inhibited by mannoheptulose (Schauder *et al.,* 1976), suggesting that glucose metabolism in the D cells was a prerequisite for the effect of the hexose in this respect. In this connection, it is of interest that D-glyceraldehyde stimulated insulin release but diminished the secretion of somatostatin (Schauder *et al.,* 1977a). Calcium was shown to stimulate somatostatin release from the isolated canine pancreas in a typical biphasic response pattern (Hermansen *et al.,* 1979). Calcium ions were active also in the absence of glucose, but their effect was enhanced by increasing the glucose concentration in the perfusate. This finding implies that somatostatin secretion may be triggered by the accumulation of calcium ions at some critical site in the D cell.

V. PHYSIOLOGICAL ROLE OF SOMATOSTATIN IN THE PANCREAS

Three pieces of evidence support the physiological role of somatostatin in the endocrine pancreas: (1) its presence in D cells in the islets, (2) its marked inhibitory effect on the release of other pancreatic hormones, and (3) its release from the pancreas, which is modulated by factors known to control the secretion of insulin and glucagon.

Two aspects of the physiological function of islet somatostatin may be envisaged: a classical hormone action on the islets and on remote target cells and tissues via the blood circulation, and a local paracrine regulation of islet functions (see Chapter 18).

The question of a *classical hormone action* was approached, e.g., by means of somatostatin antibodies. This antiserum increased GH and glucagon-like immunoreactivity but not insulin and glucagon release in rats and dogs (Tannenbaum *et al.,* 1978; Schusdziarra *et al.,* 1978b). These findings suggest that any influence of somatostatin on insulin and glucagon release has to take place via a pathway inaccessible to intravenously administered antisomatostatin serum, i.e., within the islets themselves.

The finding in rats that, on the one hand, large doses of somatostatin were required to inhibit glucose- and arginine-stimulated insulin release and arginine-induced glucagon release (Efendić *et al.*, 1979c; Lins *et al.*, 1980c), whereas, on the other hand, the same glucose and arginine loads were accompanied by only minor increases in somatostatin in plasma, also supports this idea (Efendić *et al.*, 1980).

However, it should be emphasized that exogenous somatostatin was a considerably more potent inhibitor of insulin and glucagon release in man than in rats (Lins *et al.*, 1980c). Therefore it cannot be excluded that, at least in some species, islet somatostatin may modulate A and B cells also by acting as a classical hormone via the circulation (Efendić *et al.*, 1980).

A hormonal action of pancreatic somatostatin on remote tissues has been indirectly approached by several groups. Somatostatin injected into the portal vein of dogs at a rate of 50 ng/min reduced the rise in plasma triglycerides after a fat–protein meal, whereas neither fasting nor postprandial insulin or glucagon levels were reduced (Schusdziarra *et al.*, 1979a). Furthermore, minute amounts of somatostatin (1–3 μg/hr) administered intravenously to humans decreased intestinal motility and prolonged the absorption of oral glucose (Johansson *et al.*, to be published). These results are compatible with a physiological role for splanchnic somatostatin in the homeostasis of nutrients.

A *paracrine* interaction of pancreatic hormones was suggested by Samols *et al.* (1965), who also reported that glucagon stimulated insulin secretion and that insulin inhibited glucagon secretion (Samols *et al.*, 1976). The idea of intraislet interplay gained further recognition when somatostatin entered the picture and when cytochemical evidence for this interplay was presented. Thus studies on the topographic interrelationships of A, B, and D cells in humans and rats have defined a heterocellular region in the islets in which these cell types are in direct contact with one another (Orci *et al.*, 1975, 1976). Furthermore, intercellular communications were demonstrated in monolayer cultures of neonatal rat pancreas microinjected with fluorescein and scanned topographically by microfluorimetry (Kohen *et al.*, 1979). Fluorescein spread from an injected islet cell directly into neighboring islet cells and, in the presence of 16.7 mmol glucose, significantly more islet cells communicated with the injected cell than in glucose-free medium.

When discussing a paracrine action of somatostatin, it is important to consider whether the somatostatin concentration in the extracellular fluid reaches concentrations sufficient for the modulation of insulin and glucagon release. As little as 50–100 pg of somatostatin per milliliter of perfusate suppressed insulin and glucagon release in the isolated dog pancreas (Hermansen *et al.*, 1979) and insulin release in the rat pancreas (to be published). These levels are easily achieved in the efflux from isolated pancreases in response to physiological stimuli, and therefore the above pre-requisite for a paracrine action seems to be fulfilled. A paracrine action of somatostatin in pancreatic islets is supported by the finding that the addition of somatostatin antibodies to isolated rat islets enhances glucose- and leucine-induced insulin release (Taniguchi et al., 1977, 1979) and arginine-induced glucagon release (Barden et al., 1978).

In addition, there are other findings suggesting a paracrine interaction between D and B cells. Thus, after a fasting period of 48 hr, glucose-induced insulin release from perifused rat islets was diminished, while somatostatin release was increased (Schauder et al., 1979). It is conceivable that the high secretory activity of the D cell might be one of the reasons why insulin release is diminshed in the fasting state. Furthermore, the addition of glucagon caused a dose-related increase in somatostatin release from the perfused rat pancreas (Kadowaki et al., 1979). In contrast, insulin release, especially its first phase, was suppressed when the concentrations of glucagon were increased.

In this connection, we have studied the effect of glibenclamide on glucose-induced release of insulin and somatostatin (Efendić et al., 1979b). The lowest glucose load applied, 6.7 mM, clearly stimulated insulin release. This was even more pronounced with 16.0 mM glucose, whereas infusion of 33.3 mM glucose was accompanied by only a minor further increase. Somatostatin release was not affected by 6.7 mM glucose, whereas 16.7 and 33.3 mM were stimulatory. The infusion of 1 μg of glibenclamide per milliliter with 6.7 mM glucose produced an additive effect on insulin release. The drug had no effect on insulin release stimulated by 16.7 and 33.3 mM glucose. The increase in somatostatin release produced by gliben-clamide was markedly inhibited by 6.7 mM glucose. This inhibiton was less pronounced at 16.7 mM glucose and almost absent at 33.3 mM. This finding that a moderate glucose load enhances the effect of glibenclamide on insulin release while inhibiting its effect on somatostatin release supports a paracrine interaction between D and B cells.

Recent observations on the perfused rat pancreas suggest a paracrine interaction between D and A cells also. Thus under four experimental conditions enhancement of somatostatin release was accompanied by suppression of glucagon release: (1) Glucose suppressed arginine-induced glucagon release. On the other hand, glucose and arginine exerted an additive action on somatostatin release (Efendić et al., 1980). Their effect on insulin release was a synergistic one. (2) Priming with glucose modulated the effect of a consecutive arginine load; the release of insulin and somatostatin was enhanced, whereas glucagon release was suppressed (Grill et al., in press). (3) Sulfonylurea (glibenclamide) enhanced arginine-stimulated soma-tostatin release and suppressed the effect of arginine on glucagon release

(Efendić *et al.*, 1979a). (4) In pancreases perfused with medium without glucose or with only a low concentration of glucose, glibenclamide markedly enhanced somatostatin and inhibited glucagon release (Efendić *et al.*, 1979b).

The suggestion that, in rat islets, somatostatin exerts its physiological action by paracrine interaction with B and A cells is further supported by our recent finding that prolonged intravenous administration of somatostatin leads to the development of tachyphylaxis for the peptide: After 24 hr of continuous infusion of 700 ng/kg/min of somatostatin, the peptide could no longer inhibit glucose-induced insulin release (Lins *et al.*, 1980c).

In a patient with a somatostatinoma, the response of pancreatic B cells but not of A cells to nutrient stimuli was inhibited, while GH release was suppressed, which also suggests somatostatin resistance, at least in some target tissues (Krejs *et al.*, 1979).

VI. CONCLUSIONS

Somatostatin is widely distributed in the body, in a number of endocrine cells as well as in the nervous system. In the pancreas, it is produced in the D cells. Most likely, the peptide plays a role in control of the secretion of the other islet hormones: insulin, glucagon, and pancreatic polypeptide. An important question in this context involves how somatostatin exerts its effects on the other islet cells. So far, a number of findings indicate that somatostatin acts in a paracrine fashion, i.e., through intercellular or direct cell-to-cell contacts. However, the possibility remains that islet somatostatin also exerts its effects as a classical hormone, via the circulation. The latter action would include effects on the islets as well as on remote tissues. In this context, special interest has been focused on the possibility that somatostatin plays an important role in the control of fluxes of nutrients by influencing the motility of the gastrointestinal tract.

REFERENCES

Alberti, K. G. M., Christensen, S. E., Iversen, J., Seyer-Hansen, K., Christensen, N. J., Prange-Hansen, A., Lundbaek, K., and Ørskov, H. (1973). *Lancet* **2**, 1299–1301.

Arimura, A., Lundqvist, G., Rothman, J., Chang, R., Fernandez-Durango, R., Elde, R., Coy, D. H., Meyers, C., and Schally, A. V. (1978). *Metabolism* **27**, Suppl. 1, 1139–1144.

Barden, N., Cote, J. P., Lavoie, M., and Dupont, A. (1978). *Metabolism* **27**, Suppl. 1, 1215–1218.

Berelowitz, M., Kronheim, S., Pimstone, B., and Shapiro, B. (1978). *J. Clin. Invest.* **61,** 1410–1414.

Borgeat, P., Drouin, J., Bélanger, A., and Labrie, F. (1974a). *Fed. Am. Soc. Exp. Biol.* **33,** 263A.

Borgeat, P., Labrie, F., Drouin, J., Bélanger, A., Immer, H., Sestanj, K., Nelson, V., Gotz, M., Schally, A. V., Coy, D. H., and Coy, E. J. (1974b). *Biochem. Biophys. Res. Commun.* **56,** 1052–1059.

Brown, M., Rivier, J., and Vale, W. (1976). *Metabolism* **25,** Suppl. 1, 501–503.

Chideckel, E. W., Palmer, J., Koerker, D. J., Ensinck, J., Davidson, M. B., and Goodner, C. J. (1975). *J. Clin. Invest* **55,** 754–762.

Christensen, S. E., Prange-Hansen, A. A., Iversen, J., Lundbaek, K., Örskov, H., and Seyer-Hansen, K. (1974). *Scand. J. Clin. Lab. Invest.* **34,** 321–325.

Claro, A., Grill, V., Efendić, S., and Luft, R. (1977). *Acta Endocrinol.* **85,** 379–388.

Curry, D. L., and Bennett, L. L. (1974). *Biochem. Biophys. Res. Commun.* **60,** 1015–1019.

Dolais-Kitabgi, J., Kitabgi, P., Brazeau, P., and Freychet, P. (1979). *Endocrinology* **105,** 256–260.

Dubois, M. P. (1975). *Proc. Natl. Acad. Sci. U.S.A.* **72,** 1340–1343.

Efendić, S., Claro, A., and Luft, R. (1976a). *Acta Endocrinol.* **81,** 753–761.

Efendić, S., Enzmann, F., Nylén, A., Uvnäs-Wallensten, K., and Luft, R. (1979a). *Acta Physiol. Scand.* **108,** 231–233.

Efendić, S., Enzmann, F., Nylén, A., Uvnäs-Wallensten, K., and Luft, R. (1979b). *Proc. Natl. Acad. Sci. U.S.A.* **76,** 5901–5904.

Efendić, S., Hökfelt, T., and Luft, R. (1978a). *In* "Advances in Metabolic Disorders" (R. Levine and R. Luft, eds.), Vol. 9, pp. 367–424. Academic Press, New York.

Efendić, S., Lins, P. E., and Cerasi, E. (1979c). *Acta Endocrinol.* **90,** 259–271.

Efendić, S., Lins, P. E., and Luft, R. (1978b). *Metabolism* **27,** Suppl. 1, 1275–1281.

Efendić, S., Lins, P. E., Luft, R., Sievertsson, H., and Westin-Sjödahl, G. (1977). *Acta Endocrinol.* **85,** 579–586.

Efendić, S., Lins, P. E., Luft, R., Uvnäs-Wallensten, K., and Szecówka, J. (1980). *In* "Frontiers of Hormone Research" (Tj. B. van Wimersma Greidanus, ed.), Vol. 7, pp. 41–51. Karger, Basel.

Efendić, S., and Luft, R. (1975). *Acta Endocrinol.* **78,** 516–523.

Efendić, S., Luft, R., and Claro, A. (1976b). *Acta Endocrinol.* **81,** 743–752.

Efendić, S., Luft, R., and Grill, V. (1974). *FEBS Lett.* **42,** 169–172.

Efendić, S., Luft, R., and Sievertsson, H. (1975). *FEBS Lett.* **58,** 302–305.

Efendić, S., Nylén, A., Roovete, A., and Uvnäs-Wallensten, K. (1978c). *FEBS Lett.* **92,** 33–35.

Erlandsen, S. L., Hegre, O. D., Parsons, J. A., McEvoy, R. C., and Elde, R. P. (1976). *J. Histochem. Cytochem.* **24,** 883–897.

Gerich, J. E., Lorenzi, M., Schneider, V., and Forsham, P. H. (1974a). *J. Clin. Endocrinol. Metab.* **39,** 1057–1060.

Gerich, J. E., Lorenzi, M., Schneider, V., Kwan, C. W., Karam, J. H., Guillemin, R., and Forsham, P. H. (1974b). *Diabetes* **23,** 876–880.

Gerich, J. E., Lovinger, R., and Grodsky, G. M. (1975). *Endocrinology* **96,** 749–754.

Gerich, J., Greene, K., Hara, M., Rizza, R., and Patton, G. (1979). *J. Lab. Clin. Med.* **93,** 1009–1017.

Goldsmith, P. C., Rose, J. C., Arimura, A., and Ganong, W. F. (1975). *Endocrinology* **97,** 1061–1064.

Goto, Y., Seino, Y., Taminato, T., Kadowaki, S., Chiba, T., Note, S., and Imura, H. (1979). *Diabetes* **28,** 457–459.

Grill, V., Rundfeldt, M., and Efendić, S. (1981). *Diabetologia* (in press).

Guillemin, R. (1976). *Endocrinology* 99, 1653–1654.
Gustavsson, S., and Lundqvist, G. (1978). *Biochem. Biophys. Res. Commun.* 82, 1229–1235.
Hara, M., Patton, G., and Gerich, J. (1979). *Life Sci.* 24, 625–628.
Hellman, B., and Lernmark, Å. (1969a) *Diabetologia* 5, 22–24.
Hellman, B., and Lernmark, Å. (1969b). *Endocrinology* 84, 1484–1488.
Hermansen, K., Christensen, S. E., and Ørskov, H. (1979). *Diabetologia* 16, 261–266.
Hökfelt, T., Efendić, S., Hellerström, C., Johansson, O., Luft, R., and Arimura, A. (1975). *Acta Endocrinol.* 80, Suppl. 200.
Honey, R. N., and Weir, G. C. (1979). *Life Sci.* 24, 1747–1750.
Ipp, E., Dobbs, R. E., Arimura, A, Vale, W., Harris, V., and Unger, R. H. (1977a). *J. Clin. Invest.* 60, 760–765.
Ipp, E., Dobbs, R. E., Haris, V., Arimura, A., Vale, W., and Unger, R. H. (1977b). *J. Clin. Invest.* 60, 1216–1219.
Ipp, E., Dobbs, R. E., and Unger, R. H. (1978a). *FEBS Lett.* 90, 76–78.
Ipp, E., Dobbs, R., and Unger, R. H. (1978b). *Nature (London)* 276, 190–191.
Ipp, E., Rivier, J., Dobbs, R. E., Brown, M., Vale, W., and Unger, R. H. (1979). *Endocrinology* 104, 1270–1273.
Iversen, J. (1974) *Scand. J. Clin. Lab. Invest.* 33, 125–129.
Järhult, J., Ahrén, B., and Lundquist, I. (1979). *Acta Endocrinol.* 92, 166–173.
Kadowaki, S., Taminato, T., Chiba, T., Mori, K., Abe, H., Goto, Y., Seino, Y., Matsukura, S., Nozawa, M., and Fujita. T. (1979). *Diabetes* 28, 600–602.
Kaneko, T., Oka, H., Saito, S., Munemura, M., Musa, K., Oda, T., Yanaihara, N., and Yanaihara, C. (1973). *Endocrinol. Jpn.* 20, 535–538.
Kaneto, A., Kajinuma, H., Kaneko, T., and Kosaka, K. (1978). *Metabolism* 27, 901–910.
Koerker, D. J., Ruch, W., Chideckel, E., Plamer, J., Goodner, C. J., Ensinck, J., and Gale, C. C. (1974). *Science* 184, 482–484.
Kohen, E., Kohen, C., Thorell, B., Mintz, D. H., and Rabinovitch, A. (1979). *Science* 204, 862–865.
Krejs, G. J., Orci, L., Conlon, J. M., Ravazzola, M., Davis, G. R., Raskin, P., Collins, S. M., McCarthy, D. M., Baetens, D., Rubenstein, A., Aldor, T. A. M., and Unger, R. H. (1979). *N. Engl. J. Med.* 301, 285–292.
Leblanc, H., Anderson, J. R., Sigel, M. B., and Yen, S. S. C. (1975). *J. Clin. Endocrinol. Metab.* 40, 568–572.
Lins, P. E., Efendić, S., and Hall, K. (1980a). *Acta Med. Scand.* 206, 441–445.
Lins, P. E., Efendić, S., Meyers, C. A., Coy, D. H., Schally, A., and Luft, R. (1980b). *Metabolism.* 29, 728–731.
Lins, P. E., Petersson, B., and Efendić, S. (1980c). *Acta Physiol. Scand.* 110, 267–275.
Luft, R., Efendić, S., Hökfelt, T., Johansson, O., and Arimura, A. (1974). *Med. Biol.* 52, 428–430.
Luft, R., Efendić, S., and Hökfelt, T. (1978). *Diabetologia* 14, 1–13.
Lundberg, J. M., Hökfelt, T., and Nilsson, G. (1978). *Acta Physiol. Scand.* 104, 499–501.
McIntosh, C., and Arnold, R. (1979). *Z. Gastroenterol.* 16, 330–340.
Marco, J., Hedo, J. A., and Villanueva, M. L. (1977). *Life Sci.* 21, 789–792.
Meyers, C., Arimura, A., Gorcin, A., Fernandez-Durango, R., Coy, D. H., Schally, A. V., Drouin, J., Ferland, L., Beaulieu, M.,and Labrie, F. (1977). *Biochem. Biophys. Res. Commun.* 74, 630–636.
Mortimer, C. H., Carr, D., Lind, T., Bloom, S. R., Mallinson, C. N., Schally, A. V., Tunbridge, W. M. G., Yeomans, L., Coy, D. H., Kastin, A., Besser, G. M., and Hall, R. (1974). *Lancet* 1, 697–701.

Norfleet, W. T., Pagliara, A. S., Haymond, M. W., and Matschinsky, F. (1975). *Diabetes* **24**, 961–970.

Orci, L., and Unger, R. H. (1975). *Lancet* **2**, 1243–1244.

Orci, L., Baetens, D., Dubois, M. P., and Rufener, C. (1975). *Horm. Metab. Res.* **7**, 400–402.

Orci, L., Baetens, D., Rufener, C., Amherdt, M., Ravazzola, M., Studer, P., Malaisse-Lagae, F., and Unger, R. H. (1976). *Proc. Natl. Acad. Sci.* **73**, 1338–1342.

Parsons, J., Erlandsen, S., Hegre, O., McEvoy, R., and Elde, R. P. (1976). *J. Histochem. Cytochem.* **24**, 872–882.

Patel, Y. C., Amherdt, M., and Orci, L. (1979). *Endocrinology* **104**, 676–679.

Patton, G. S., Dobbs, R., Orci, L., Vale, W., and Unger, R. H. (1976a). *Metabolism* **25**, Suppl. 1, 1499.

Patton, G. S., Ipp, E., Dobbs, R. E., Orci, L., Vale, W., and Unger, R. H. (1976b). *Life Sci.* **19**, 1957–1960.

Patton, G. S., Ipp, E., Dobbs, R. E., Orci, L., Vale, W., and Unger, R. H. (1977). *Proc. Natl. Acad. Sci. U.S.A.* **74**, 2140–2143.

Penman, E., Wass, J. A. H., Lund, A., Lowry, P. J., Stewart, J., Dawson, A. M., Besser, G. M., and Rees, L. H. (1979). *Ann. Clin. Biochem.* **16**, 15–25.

Polak, J. M., Grimelius, L., Pearse, A. G. E., Bloom, S. R., and Arimura, A. (1975). *Lancet* **1**, 1220–1222.

Rufener, C., Amherdt, M., Dubois, M. P., and Orci, L. (1975). *J. Histochem. Cytochem.* **23**, 866–869.

Samols, E., and Harrison, J. (1976). *Metabolism* **25**, Suppl. 1, 1443–1447.

Samols, E., and Weir, G. C. (1979). *J. Clin. Invest.* **63**, 230–238.

Samols, E., Marri, G., and Marks, V. (1965). *Lancet* **2**, 415–416.

Samols, E., Weir, G. C., Ramseur, R., Day, J. A., and Patel, Y. C. (1978). *Metabolism* **27**, Suppl. 1, 1219–1221.

Sarantakis, D., McKinley, W. A., Jaunakais, J., Clark, D., and Grant, N.H. (1976). *Clinical Endocrinol.* **5**, 275–278.

Schauder, P., McIntosh, C., Arends, J., Arnold, R., Frerichs, H., and Creutzfeldt, W. (1976). *FEBS Lett.* **68**, 225–227.

Schauder, P., McIntosh, C., Arends, J., Arnold, R., Frerichs, H., and Creutzfeldt, W. (1977a). *Biochem. Biophys. Res. Commun.* **75**, 630–635.

Schauder, P., McIntosh, C., Panten, U., Arends, J., Arnold, R., Frerichs, H., and Creutzfeldt, W. (1977b). *FEBS Lett.* **81**, 355–358.

Schauder, P., McIntosh, C., Arends, J., and Frerichs, H. (1979). *Diabetes* **28**, 204–207.

Schmitt, J. K., Lorenzi, M., Gerich, J. E., Bohannon, N. V., Karam, J. H., and Forsham, P. H. (1979). *J. Clin. Endocrinol. Metab.* **48**, 880–882.

Schusdziarra, V., Harris, V., Conlon, J. M., and Arimura, A. (1978a). *J. Clin. Invest.* **62**, 509–518.

Schusdziarra, V., Rouiller, D., Arimura, A., and Unger, R. H. (1978b). *Endocrinology* **103**, 1956–1959.

Schusdziarra, V., Rouiller, D., Harris, V., Conlon, J. M., and Unger, R. H. (1978c). *Endocrinology* **103**, 2264–2273.

Schusdziarra, V., Harris, V., Arimura, A., and Unger, R. H. (1979a). *Endocrinology* **104**, 1705–1708.

Schusdziarra, V., Rouiller, D., Harris, V., and Unger, R. H. (1979b). *Diabetes* **28**, 658–663.

Shapiro, B., Berelowitz, M., Pimstone, B. L., Kronheim, S., and Sheppard, M. (1979). *Diabetes* **28**, 182–184.

Smith, P. H., Woods, S. C., and Porte, D., Jr., (1976). *Endocrinology* **98**, 1073–1076.

Smith, P. H., Woods, S. C., Ensinck, J. W., and Porte, D., Jr., (1977). *Metabolism* **26**, 841–845.

Szecówka, J., Sandberg, E., and Efend ć, S. (1980). *Diabetologia,* **19,** 137–142.

Taniguchi, H., Utsumi, M., Hasegawa M., Kobayashi, T., Watanabe, Y., Murakami, S., Seki, M., Tsutou, A., Makimura, M., Sakoda, M., and Baba, S. (1977). *Diabetes* **26,** 700–702.

Taniguchi, H., Hasegawa, M., Kobayashi, T., Watanabe, Y., Murakami, K., Seki, M., Tsutou, A., Utsumi, M., Makimura, H., Sakoda, M., and Baba, S. (1979). *Horm. Metab. Res.* **11,** 23–26.

Tannenbaum, G. S., Epelbaum, J., Colle, E., Brazeau, P., and Martin, J. B. (1978). *Metabolism* **27,** Suppl. 1, 1263–1267.

Uvnäs-Wallensten, K., Rehfeldt, J. F Larsson, L. J., and Uvnäs, B. (1977). *Proc. Natl. Acad. Sci. U.S.A.* **74,** 5707–5710.

Uvnäs-Wallensten, K., Efendić, S., and Luft, R. (1978). *Acta Physiol. Scand.* **402,** 248–250.

Uvnäs-Wallensten, K., Roovete, A., Johansson, C., and Efendić, S. (1980). *Acta Physiol. Scand.* **109,** 393–398.

Vale, W., Ling, N., Rivier, J., Villarreal, J., Rivier, C., Douglas, C., and Brown, M. (1976). *Metabolism* **25,** 1491–1494.

Wajchenberg, B. L., Cesar, F. P., Leme, C. E.., Silva, H. B., Lerario, A. C., Coy, D. H., and Schally, A. V. (1978). *Clin Endocrinol.* **9,** 515–521.

Weir, G. C., Samols, E., Day, Jr., J. A., and Patel, Y. C. (1978). *Metabolism* **27,** Suppl. 1, 1223–1226.

Weir, G. C., Samols, E., Loo, S., Patel, Y. C., and Gabbay, K. H. (1979). *Diabetes* **28,** 35–40.

Wilson, R. M., Boden, G., and Ower, O. E. (1978). *Endocrinology* **102,** 859–863.

Woods, S. C., and Porte, D. (1978). *In* "Advances in Metabolic Disorders" (R. Levine and R. Luft, eds.), Vol. 9, pp. 283–312. Academic Press, New York.

12

Synthesis, Storage, Secretion, and Significance of Pancreatic Polypeptide in Vertebrates

R. L. HAZELWOOD

The Islets of Langerhans
Copyright © 1981 by Academic Press, Inc.
All rights of reproduction in any form reserved.
ISBN 0-12-187820-1

I. INTRODUCTION

The suggestion that a "third hormone of the pancreas" exists has been offered by workers many times since the turn of the century. Early studies indicated clearly that several cell types possessing endocrine characteristics, other than A and B islet cells, existed in significant numbers in the vertebrate pancreas. In 1968 a chance observation by Kimmel and colleagues opened the door to investigations which, over the last 12 yr, have led to approximately 170 reports relative to the origin, chemistry, release, and function of the third pancreatic hormone. (The secretion of the D cell was later identified as somatostatin.) Thus Kimmel *et al.* (1968) reported the existence of a basic polypeptide found as a contaminant of preparations of chicken insulin from fresh pancreases. As it was first isolated with and subsequently separated from chicken insulin, it was tentatively named avian pancreatic polypeptide (APP). Within 3 yr, a better appreciation of the physiochemical characteristics of APP was gained, as were some of the physiological effects of this peptide when injected into recipient vertebrates. In 1972, Chance's laboratory reported the existence of homologous pancreatic polypeptides (PPs) in extracts obtained from sheep (OPP), beef (BPP), and human (HPP) pancreata (Lin and Chance, 1972; Lin *et al.* 1973). The search for the cellular origin, release mechanism(s), and function of the various PPs had commenced.

II. CELLULAR ORIGIN

It had been established early that in certain vertebrates (e.g., chickens) the origin of PP secretion was restricted to the pancreas, there being no detectable immunoassayable interaction with extracts of other digestive or paradigestive organs (Langslow *et al.*, 1973). As more and more tissues of various animal species were surveyed for immunologically positive reactions with antibodies to PP, it became clear that the initial observations were not absolute; thus the identification of extrapancreatic PP-secreting cells was recognized in a number of vertebrates (e.g., dog, opposum, and monkey). Today, the anatomical localization of PP-secreting cells is well established in most vertebrate species. Also established and appreciated is the topographical distribution of PP cells within each species of pancreas.

A. Primates

Histochemical and ultrastructural identification of PP-secreting cells in human pancreases obtained at surgery has been made, and for the most part the observations agree with those of workers who employed peroxidase–antiperoxidase and/or immunofluorescent antibody techniques. Thus HPP cells are found at both exocrine and endocrine pancreatic loci, the latter being more prominent in the normal human pancreas. Like the A-and D-cell populations of islet tissue, HPP-secreting cells are located primarily at the periphery of the islets in smaller numbers than either of their neighbors (Bergstrom et al., 1977; Gersell et al., 1976, 1979; Larsson et al., 1975a; Pelletier and Leclere, 1977). The B cells of course occupy the majority of the central islet area. The PP cells appear to possess all the characteristics of endocrine-type cells and to have cytoplasmic granules with diameters approaching 130–180 nm in fairly elongated cells (Bergstrom et al., 1977; Baetens et al., 1977; Larsson et al., 1975b; also see Chapter 1). Human PP cells have the capability to take up and decarboxylate amine precursors (Larsson et al., 1975b) and, after correlative staining, PP-containing cells yield a faint argyrophilic reaction to the Grimelius silver method and a negative reaction to the aldehyde–fuchsin–trichrome tinctorial stain (Gersell et al., 1976). Thus HPP cells appear to be a population distinct from neighboring A, B, and D cells of the islets (Gersell et al., 1976; Larsson et al., 1975a), most closely resembling the so-called F cell described by Munger or the type V cell described by Deconinck (see Chapter 1).

A reasonable number of HPP cells are found in exocrine areas of the pancreas, as well as within epithelium of small to middle-sized ducts (Gersell et al., 1979; Larsson et al., 1975a). Usually these cells are single entities or small clusters of cells and are likely to increase in number in a wide variety of chronic pancreatic diseases (Gersell et al., 1976; also see Section VI,B and C). Often HPP cells are more populous in the duodenal (uncinate, right lobe or head) regions of the human pancreas (Gersell et al., 1979), but this feature is not as consistent as that observed in the canine organ (Larsson et al., 1975b). Human fetuses (18–22 weeks) contain pancreatic HPP-staining cells in localized aggregates which differ greatly from the more generalized distribution pattern seen in adulthood (Larsson et al.,

1975a; Malaisse-Lagae *et al.,* 1979). Cellular quantitation of PP cells cor-relates significantly with regional tissue concentrations of PP and once again identifies the previously described F cell as the cell species responsible for secreting HPP (Gersell *et al.,* 1979).

A single case report recently indicated the presence of an hepatic PP-apudoma in a 62-year-old man; it was suggested that this tumor (detected by immunofluorescent staining) was of intrahepatic bile duct origin (Warner *et al.,* 1980).

B. Other Mammals

The location of PP-secreting cells has been described for a wide variety of nonprimate mammals, including the dog, cat, rat, mouse, guinea pig, chinchilla, and opossum. In all these species, the candidate cells are local-ized in the islet periphery and, to a lesser extent, in the exocrine and ductile elements. Usually the duodenal (right lobe, or in the dog the uncinate pro-cess) contains four to five times more PP than other regions (Baetens *et al.,* 1976; Gersell *et al.,* 1976; Larsson *et al.,* 1976a; Orci *et al.,* 1976; Gingerich *et al.,* 1978a; Lundquist *et al.,* 1979). [Insulin and glucagon (B and A) cells predominate in the body and tail of the canine pancreas.] Most workers have employed antibodies to BPP to establish the location of these cell aggregates by immunofluorescent methods and, in doing so, have ob-served that lower mammals frequently have extrapancreatic PP cells dis-tributed in various regions of the gastrointestinal tract. Thus in dogs a CPP cell population of reasonable size has been described in the antral, pyloric, and certain ileal regions in addition to the pancreatic islet and exocrine areas (Baetens *et al.,* 1976).

Studies in the opposum indicate that, like the dog, this mammal has a reasonable representation of PP cells in the gastric mucosa and that these cells respond with a dopamine-like formaldehyde-induced fluorescence. Such fluorescence is not detectable in PP cells of the rat, mouse, or guinea pig, species in which the PP cells exhibit uptake and decarboxylation of amine activity (Larsson *et al.,* 1976).

The origin of PP-secreting cells has been studied in the neonatal rat by Sundler's group (1977a), and their results indicate that, while at birth the preponderance of PP-containing cells appear to have exocrine locations, 5–7 days later the islet content (as a peripheral halo) of these PP cells is in-creased markedly, while that of nonendocrine tissue decreases (Sundler *et al.,* 1977a). Ten days after parturition, the adult-type distribution of rat PP cells is attained. The fact that PP-containing cells are not identified in the rat pancreas prior to parturition implies that this peptide is the last of the four hormones to appear during embryogenesis. A restricted few PP cells can be identified in the rat antrum the first few days after birth though, unlike somatostatin and glucagon cells, they are not observed elsewhere in the gut. Like man, PP cells of the rat, guinea pig, and chinchilla contain relatively small, fairly electron-dense cytoplasm-located granules (Larsson et al., 1976a). The PP cells of the dog and cat contain fairly large electron-lucent granules. (See Chapter 1 for electron microscopic details of PP cells.)

Because of the above studies, caution should be exercised in comparing PP-containing cell populations of one animal with those of another, whether such a comparison is made within species, between species, or even within the same organism. The suggestion has been made by several workers, and most recently emphasized by Orci (Baetens et al., 1979; Orci et al., 1976; Malaisse-Lagae et al., 1979), that most mammals have an unequal distribution of PP-containing cells within the endocrine pancreas and that the aging process further tends to modify this topographical distribution and content (Fig. 1). Thus comparisons of one tissue with another, especially if one source is of a pathophysiological nature, may not be valid unless extreme care is taken to evaluate the same anatomical regions of the two pancreases under examination, or one attempts the monumental task of *total* pancreatic comparison. This caution is even more applicable to cross-species comparisons. Generally speaking, there is an inverse relationship between PP-containing and glucagon- (and probably somatostatin)-containing cells, regardless of location within the mammalian pancreas (Orci et al., 1976; Baetens et al., 1979; Fig. 1).

C. Submammalian Forms

Probably the best studied submammalian forms as far as pancreatic localization of PP-secreting cells is concerned are members of the class Aves. Embryological differentiation of endocrine cell types in the developing chick pancreas occurs such that, as in the rat pancreas at birth, APP elements are not prevalent until the last 2 days of incubation, at which time the immunoassayable polypeptide content increases about 1500% in just a 24-hr period (3.2 versus 44.8 pmol per pancreas). Unlike PP, both insulin and somatostatin increase markedly several days earlier, though the final-day (day 21) concentrations of these two hormones also either double (insulin) or increase 1000-fold (somatostatin). Glucagon concentrations of the embryonic chick pancreas fluctuate in a bimodal fashion with the immunoreactive glucagon (IRG) peak observed at day 18 and again at day 21 (Goldman et al., 1978).

The APP cells in adult birds have been reported to be spindle-shaped or polygonal, with numerous elongated processes extending a reasonable dis-

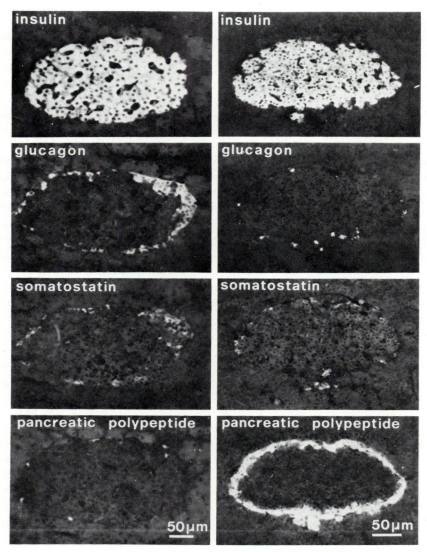

Fig. 1. (Left) Series of four consecutive sections of a rat pancreatic islet stained, respectively, with antiinsulin, antiglucagon, antisomatostatin, and anti-PP antisera. The pattern is characteristic of islets situated in the body and tail of the pancreas (the so-called splenic region). Compare with the section on the right. (Right) Series of four consecutive sections of a rat pancreatic islet stained, respectively, with antiinsulin, antiglucagon, antisomatostatin, and anti-PP antisera. The pattern is characteristic of islets situated in the lower part of the head of the pancreas. Compare with the sections on the left panel. (Courtesy of L. Orci.)

tance. This is especially true for the PP cells in exocrine regions, a feature which to some extent distinguishes birds from most mammals (Larsson *et al.*, 1974a). Thus a large proportion of APP cells reside in exocrine areas, and in some birds the majority of these cells are either exocrine or ductule-affiliated. The numerous cytoplasmic granules, the ability of the PP cells to decarboxylate L-dopa, and the tendency for APP cells to be more numerous at hatching time collectively confirm similar observations made in the rodent pancreas (Larsson *et al.*, 1974a). Immunoassay of tissue extracts of pancreatic-enteric structures in young birds has established that, unlike the situation in many mammals, the pancreas is the sole source of APP in Aves (Langslow *et al.*, 1973).

Association of PP with both the central (CNS) and peripheral nervous systems (PNS) has been reported in species as diverse as the blow fly (brain), various higher mammals (CNS and PNS), and chicken (CNS and PNS). Positive immunocytochemical identification of nerve fibers containing PP was made in the cerebral cortex and stria terminalis, as well as in nuclei in the para- and periventricular hypothalamic nuclei, and in the medial preoptic area (Loren *et al.*, 1979). Additionally, immunoreactive perikarya were demonstrated in the gut, particularly associated with the submucosal and myenteric plexus. Neuronal PP reactivity appeared to be dissociable from that of pancreatic PP-like peptides by use of different antisera raised against various (species) different PPs (Loren *et al.*, 1979).

Data on the origin and distribution of PP-active tissue in lower vertebrates are scarce. Falkmer has made a careful examination of the evolutionary distribution and topographical organization of endocrine cell types in the alimentary tract and discrete pancreases of cephalochordates (amphioxus), cyclostomes (river lamprey), holocephalons (rat- and rabbitfish), elasmobranchian cartilaginous and teleostian bony fish, and anuran amphibians. By use of the indirect immunofluorescence technique (using antisera to mammalian insulin, glucagon, somatostatin, and PP) Falkmer concluded that, during evolution, all four islet hormone cells migrated from intestinal mucosa sites via the pancreatic ducts to form discrete islets of Langerhans. The phylogenetic sequence of appearance in pancreatic islets of these cell types probably was insulin first, followed by somatostatin, then by glucagon, and last by polypeptide cells (Stefan and Falkmer, 1978). Fluorescent PP cells are absent from amphioxus and lamprey primitive guts, but the mucosa of the straight digestive tube of the primitive rat- and rabbitfish react positively (Falkmer and Stefan, 1978). While immunoreactive PP cells were not found in the compact pancreas of these fish (Falkmer and Stefan, 1978), such a cell type has been identified by the special tinctorial method of A. Epple (personal communication). In more highly developed animal groups (cartilaginous and bony fish, amphibians) cells immunoreactive with antisera to BPP were found both in the mucosa of the alimentary tract and in pancreatic endocrine cell clusters. In sharks and rays all four islet hormone cell types were found either in pancreatic ductal elements or in duct-associated islet parenchyma. Also, such cell types were found as isolated cell aggregates within the exocrine pancreas (Falkmer and Stefan, 1978; Stefan and Falkmer, 1978). The topographical distribution of PP cells characteristic of most adult mammals is not evident until the teleost level is reached. Thus PP appears early in evolution but is the last of the four endocrine peptides to appear in the discrete pancreas. The PP cells appear to be located where there is exocrine pancreatic tissue contiguous with the gastrointestinal tube (Stefan and Falkmer, 1978).

III. SYNTHESIS AND CHEMISTRY

The initial report on the isolation of PP was the result of a fortuitous, then unappreciated, observation that this polypeptide was a contaminant of all chicken insulin preparations (Kimmel et al., 1968). The only other information offered by Kimmel and his colleagues at that time was the amino acid composition and a postulated molecular weight of 4200. Since this report in 1968, only a handful of papers have appeared dealing with the physiochemical characteristics of the PP molecule (Chance et al., 1975; Kimmel et al., 1971, 1975; Langslow et al., 1973: Noelken et al., 1977). Appropriately, these reports have emanated from only two laboratories, wherein the basic chemistry of the avian (Kimmel) and mammalian (Chance) homologues was first elucidated.

A. Pro-Form and General Chemistry:
Isolation and Characterization

Employing modifications of classical acid–alcohol extraction methods for insulin isolation from fresh pancreases, the PP component of the supernatant can then be separated (after clarification and lipid removal) by gel filtration with Sephadex G-50 followed by chromatography (Kimmel et al., 1968, 1975). Final purification commonly is then performed by countercurrent distribution or rechromatography on DEAE in urea-containing buffers. Homogeneity has been established by paper chromatography, polyacrylamide electrophoresis, and amino acid composition studies (Kimmel et al. 1968, 1975).

The results of the above methodology yield a polypeptide which, in the case of Aves, contains 36 amino acid residues and has a molecular weight of 4240 and an isoelectric point of pH 6–7 (Kimmel et al., 1971, 1975). The molecule appears to be composed of three distinctive peptide segments (Fig. 2). (Mammalian PPs also have 36 residues and similar chemical characteristics—see Section III,B for comparative data.) As can be seen, the molecule contains four proline residues fairly equally spaced from the N-terminus, four side-chain carboxyl groups, and essentially no residues with hydrophobic side chains. Thus segment 1 (residues 1–16 from the N-terminus) differs from the middle segment (residues 17–31), wherein alternating hydrophobic pairs or singlets appear and constitute favorable conformational conditions for the existence of a stable helical or β structure (Kimmel et al., 1975). The final segment (residues 32–36) is polar, basic, and too short for a helical arrangment; the high proline content of the N-terminus also obviates a helical structure. Subsequent work by Noelken et al. (1977) employing optical rotatory dispersion and circular dichroism methods confirms that approximately 50% of the 36 residues of APP, BPP, and CPP are in an α-helical conformation.

The possibility of the existence of higher molecular weight PPs in plasma has been suggested by immunoreactivity studies on eluates (gel filtration) of human plasma. Also, a precursor of PP has been identified in extracts of chicken pancreases. Thus a prohormone has been isolated from avian pancreases which is more basic than intact APP_{1-36}. This addition to the intact molecule contains one lysine, three arginine, and two half-cystine residues which, along with 19 others, are connected to the N-terminus of APP (Kimmel and Rafferty, 1980). Sequence data are yet to be reported.

B. Comparative Molecular Structures

While the avian pancreas yields approximately 4 mg APP/100 g fresh pancreas (Kimmel et al., 1975), beef, pork, and human pancreases apparently contain much less (Chance et al., 1975). Also, while in most avian species assayed the PP content or concentration is equal to or greater than the insulin levels in the same pancreas (Langslow et al., 1973; Kimmel et

```
        1        3        5        7        9        11
    [GLY•PRO•SER•GLN•PRO•THR•TYR•PRO•GLY•ASP•ASP•ALA•

       13       15       17       19       21       23
     PRO•VAL•GLU•ASP•LEU•ILE•ARG•PHE•TYR•ASP•ASN•LEU•

       25       27       29       31       33       35
     GLN•GLN•TYR•LEU•ASN•VAL•VAL•THR•ARG•HIS•ARG•TYR–NH₂]
```

Fig. 2. Structure of APP as reported by Kimmel et al. (44). The brackets indicate the three contiguous fragments that appear to have distinctive physicochemical characteristics (see text).

al., 1975), the reverse appears to be true in all mammalian species so far investigated.

Pork pancreatic peptide (PPP), BPP, OPP, and HPP have been isolated by Chance and colleagues (Lin *et al.,* 1973, 1974; Chance *et al.,* 1975), though the quaternary structure of each is yet to be reported or compared with that of avian polypeptide. What few studies have been done with canine pancreatic polypeptide (CPP) indicate that it is molecularly and structurally very similar to BPP (Noelken *et al.,* 1977; J. R. Kimmel, personal communication). All mammalian PPs contain 36 amino acid residues, and each has a molecular weight approximating 4200 (Chance *et al.,* 1975; Lin *et al.,* 1973, 1974). The bovine and canine peptides have single, uninterrupted α helices in the middle portion (residues 14–30 or 31) of the molecule (Noelken *et al.,* 1977); both exhibit pH-dependent dimerization, and the predicted α helices (of both) exhibit a hydrophobic face (Chang *et al.,* 1980; Noelken *et al.,* 1980). The bovine peptide may need to aggregate to bury and protect (helical) hydrophobic side chains. Residues 1–10 appear to be involved in a collagen-like helix which, through the aid of a bend at residues 10–13 of the polypeptide, may align alongside the α helix.

The structures of several PPs are compared to HPP in Fig. 3 where it can be seen that excellent homology exists among the structures of all mammalian polypeptides. At best only three positions within the molecule(s) appear to show substituted residues in the mammalian forms: these replacements at positions 2, 6, and 23 are conservative, indeed. The APP structure, however, has 15 identities with that of BPP and HPP, indicating remarkable homology despite phylogenetic origin. In comparing APP with mammalian PPs one sees that conservative substitutions prevail, such as polar side chain for polar side chain (at 16), hydrophobic group for hydrophobic group (at 17, 18, 21, 30, and 31), and even replacements involving basic and neutral amino acids (25 and 26). Such amino acid replacements within various vertebrate species would not be expected to have a profound effect on the three-dimensional structure of the PP molecule. If one accepts the average value of 0.72 mutation per amino acid pair, the calculated value for random pairing of amino acids from two separate pools having the composition of APP and BPP, respectively, is 1.49 mutations per pair. The number of mutations required for the conversion of APP to BPP is less than that expected by chance (Kimmel *et al.,* 1975).

Along similar lines of reasoning, a structural comparison of APP with chicken glucagon indicates possible homology when the latter structure is aligned with that of APP as shown in Fig. 3. The Tyr-NH$_2$ C-terminus may be essential for some of the mammalian PP action as a gastrointestinal secretogogue, but the hexapeptide at this end is not incorporated within

Residue No:	1		3		5		7		9		11	
Man:	ALA·PRO·LEU·GLU·PRO·VAL·TYR·PRO·GLY·ASP·ASN·ALA·
Beef:	ALA·PRO·LEU·GLU·PRO·GLU·TYR·PRO·GLY·ASP·ASN·ALA·
Sheep:	ALA·SER·LEU·GLU·PRO·GLU·TYR·PRO·GLY·ASP·ASN·ALA·
Pig:	ALA·PRO·LEU·GLU·PRO·VAL·TYR·PRO·GLY·ASP·ASP·ALA·
Chicken:	GLY·PRO·SER·GLN·PRO·THR·TYR·PRO·GLY·ASP·ASP·ALA·
Glucagon(chick):	HIS·SER·GLN·GLY·THR·PHE·THR·SER·ASP·TYR·SER·

Residue No:	13	15	17	19	21	23
Man:	THR·PRO·GLU·GLN·MET·ALA·GLN·TYR·ALA·ALA·ASP·LEU·
Beef:	THR·PRO·GLU·GLN·MET·ALA·GLN·TYR·ALA·ALA·GLU·LEU·
Sheep:	THR·PRO·GLU·GLN·MET·ALA·GLN·TYR·ALA·ALA·GLU·LEU·
Pig:	THR·PRO·GLU·GLN·MET·ALA·GLN·TYR·ALA·ALA·GLU·LEU·
Chicken:	PRO·VAL·GLU·ASP·LEU·ILE·ARG·PHE·TYR·ASP·ASN·LEU·
Glucagon(chick):	LYS·TYR·LEU·ASP·SER·ARG·ARG·ALA·GLN·ASP·PHE·VAL·

Residue No:	25	27	29	31	33	35
Man:	ARG·ARG·TYR·ILE·ASN·MET·LEU·THR·ARG·PRO·ARG·TYR−NH$_2$
Beef:	ARG·ARG·TYR·ILE·ASN·MET·LEU·THR·ARG·PRO·ARG·TYR−NH$_2$
Sheep:	ARG·ARG·TYR·ILE·ASN·MET·LEU·THR·ARG·PRO·ARG·TYR−NH$_2$
Pig:	ARG·ARG·TYR·ILE·ASN·MET·LEU·THR·ARG·PRO·ARG·TYR−NH$_2$
Chicken:	GLN·GLN·TYR·LEU·ASN·VAL·VAL·THR·ARG·HIS·ARG·TYR−NH$_2$
Glucagon(chick):	GLN·TRP·LEU·MET·SER·THR

Fig. 3. Comparative structures of human, bovine, ovine, porcine, and avian PPs. Underscoring of residues in the chicken structure indicates identity with the human structure, while the dashed underscoring in the chicken glucagon structure indicates homologies with chicken PP. Note the similarity of all mammalian structures except at positions 2, 6, and 23.

that of the glucagon structure (Chance *et al.*, 1975; Kimmel *et al.*, 1975; Lin and Chance, 1972; Lin *et al.*, 1974).

In summary, the primary structural features of APP largely have been retained in the mammalian homologues, that is, the number and location of the four proline residues in the first segment, the α-helical arrangement with alternating polar-hydrophobic side chains in the middle segment, and the polar, highly basic C-terminus. There is no obvious structural similarity between any of the PPs and any gastrointestinal or pancreatic hormone other than that described between avian glucagon and APP.

C. Immunoreactivity

The original report dealing with the distribution of PP among various avian species and other lower vertebrates included the first description of a radioimmunoassay technique which could be applied successfully both to tissue extracts and to plasma (Langslow *et al.,* 1973). Tissue extracts were prepared by homogenization and double extraction with acid–alcohol, clarified and the pH adjusted to 7.9–8.0, filtered, and stored at $-20°C$ prior to assay (Pettinga, 1958). Plasma was freshly prepared, or previously frozen plasma which had been thawed only once was used.

The similarity in PP structure among mammals has allowed the use of a non-isologous antibody in assaying mammalian tissue and plasma for PP concentrations. The most frequently used antibody is that to BPP because of the latter's ready availability and excellent cross-reactivity features. All PPs have been found to be antigenic in rabbits, and high-titer antibody development is readily achieved. The assay described by Langslow (1973) for avian preparations has been employed by most other workers for mammalian tissues and plasma with little or no modification. The technique is based mainly on method C of Hales and Randle (1963) which employs a double-antibody approach [guinea pig anti-PP serum and rabbit (or goat) anti-guinea pig serum]. The sensitivity thus achieved with the double-antibody method ranges within 17–25 pg/tube (170–250 pg/ml). Separation of free hormone from bound hormone can be achieved on dextran-coated charcoal with experimental sensitivities ranging down to 5 pg/tube (Weir *et al.,* 1979). Trasylol does not interfere, but excessive amounts of heparin do interfere with the assay.

With these methods basal (nonfasted) dog and human plasma PP levels have been established as 150–200 pg/ml and 60–110 pg/ml, respectively. The extreme values within the foregoing ranges usually represent variations due to species of antibody and source of PP standard employed in the assay. Adult monkeys (*Macaca mulatta*) have been reported to have basal plasma PP levels of 200–225 pg/ml (Hansen *et al.,* 1978). While mammalian antibodies appear to cross-react well with most—if not all—mammalian PPs, avian antibody (anti-APP) cross-reacts poorly (less than 14%) with mammalian plasma containing PP. Chicken pancreas contains 3–5 mg/100 g fresh tissue, 4 hr postprandial plasma levels range from 6 to 10 ng/ml, and fasted plasma levels range from 2 to 4 ng/ml in young birds (Hazelwood and Langslow, 1978; Kimmel *et al.,* 1971, 1975; Langslow *et al.,* 1973).

Rat pancreatic polypeptide is yet to be isolated in quantity and in pure enough form to permit immunological characterization.

Computer analysis of the primary structure of the various PPs and other gastrointestinal hormones does not support the suggestion that homology exists therein. Consistent with such a statement is the fact that there is no detectable cross-reactivity of antibody to any PP and serum containing (over a wide concentration range) somatostatin, proinsulin, C peptide, insulin, proglucagon, glucagon, cholecystokinin (CCK), gastroinhibitory peptide, secretin, gastrin, or vasoactive intestinal peptide (VIP) (Floyd *et al.*, 1977; Kimmel *et al.*, 1975; Langslow *et al.*, 1973). The immunological characteristics of various PPs and salient points regarding structure versus immunoreactivity have been reviewed by Chance *et al.* (1979).

IV. SECRETION: PRANDIAL, NEURAL, AND HORMONAL CORRELATES

The release of PP has been studied in man and other mammalian species, as well as in chickens, and for the most part the results have proven to yield wide areas of general agreement. Such studies also have yielded valuable associative data on perturbations of the plasma levels with prandial state, age, sex, and metabolism of PP.

Plasma levels of HPP vacillate between 50 and 80 pg/ml plasma in young, healthy, adult human subjects (Floyd *et al.*, 1977). These levels increase modestly with an overnight fast (Villaneuava *et al.*, 1978), rise rapidly to levels considerably above basal levels with food ingestion (Floyd *et al.*, 1977), and are subject to graduated gerontological effects as each decade of life is reached (Eaetens *et al.*, 1976; Berger *et al.*, 1978a; Bergstrom *et al.*, 1977; Floyd *et al.*, 1977). Thus the basal plasma level of HPP approximates 50 pg/ml in 30-yr-old human subjects, rises by age 55 to approximately 110 pg/ml, and subsequently reaches levels exceeding 200 pg/ml in septagenarians (Floyd *et al.*, 1977). Caution is required therefore in comparing group data obtained from human subjects who differ widely in age.

Levels of PP in well-fed, normal adult dogs usually range with those of 50- to 60-yr-old humans, that is, approximately 125–175 pg/ml and, like man will increase approximately 50% with a 12- to 18-hr fast.

Avian (mainly chicken) plasma levels of PP are the highest reported for vertebrates, being about 8–11 ng/ml in nonfasted young adults, and *decrease* with a 24-hr fast to approximately 2–4 ng/ml. Total pancreatectomy in chickens reduces these levels to 1–2 ng/ml, observations which percentagewise are similar to those in the pancreatectomized dog and possibly man (Adrian *et al.*, 1977; Floyd *et al.*, 1977). Older birds appear to have higher levels than males. However, no definitive study relating sex differences to possible plasma PP concentration differences has been reported to our knowledge, and those cited above for the bird are random observations at best.

A. Circadian Effects on Release

In vertebrates PP circulates probably with rapid oscillations occurring on a minute-to-minute basis. This is true also of other pancreatic hormones and C-peptide. Thus Hansen *et al.* (1978) reported rapid oscillations with an average frequency of 9.5 min for PP in monkeys. The amplitude of oscillation was ± 30% of basal PP levels in 75% of the monkeys studied. These oscillations are out of phase with those of insulin and glucagon. However, the relatively constant phase relationships between and among glucagon, insulin, somatostatin, and PP probably indicate close coordination of the secretory machinery of the various islet cells. Even in the face of constant glucose perfusion, the isolated canine pancreas demonstrates an intrinsic rhythm of hormone secretion, one which may suggest a high degree of coordination of communication between islets by a paracrine system (Stagner *et al.,* 1979). Alternatively, a hormone-to-hormone feedback system may exist, which is coordinated by a pancreatic neuronal pacemaker. Thus the suggestion has been made that "intrinsic pancreatic hormone oscillations during the post-absorptive state may serve to stimulate both the release and synthesis of pancreatic hormones" (Stagner *et al.,* 1979). Oscillations in HPP levels in humans appear to be synchronous with oscillations in spontaneous gastric acid secretion (Schwartz *et al.,* 1979a) and, as such, may be an indicator of tonic vagal nerve activity (see below).

Circadian variations in circulating HPP in man have been reported, both in the fed and in the fasted state (Floyd *et al.,* 1976; Villanueva *et al.,* 1978). The lowest levels of HPP appear shortly after arising (by 0900) and progressively rise to levels double or triple earlier values by late afternoon or evening (1800–2100) even during fasting (Floyd *et al.,* 1977; Villanueva *et al.,* 1978), only to decrease rapidly during sleep. The possibility that oscillations in vagal tone and/or circulating glucose underlie the observed perturbations in HPP has been suggested but not explored in any systematic manner (Section IV,A and B).

Adiposity is correlated positively with insulin levels in adult humans, but not with HPP or glucagon when age is taken into account (Berger *et al.,* 1978a). Obese subjects also respond in the normal manner to the presence of a known stimulus (such as a protein meal) to HPP (Wahl *et al.,* 1979; also see Section VI,A).

The liver appears to be the major site of PP metabolism in mammals. Pharmacokinetic studies on BPP injected into man indicated that the steady-state metabolic clearance was 4.5 ± 0.2 ml/kg/min, the apparent distribution space 47 ± 4 ml/kg, which approximates to the estimated plasma volume (Adrian *et al.,* 1978a; Bloom *et al.,* 1977). The *in vivo* half-life value of 7.4 ± 0.4 min in man is approximated by that found for APP in chickens, namely, 6.1 ± 0.3 min. In dogs, the $t\frac{1}{2}$ for infused PPP was reported as 5.5 ± 1 min, with a metabolic clearance rate of 25.6 ± 1 ml/kg/min and a volume distribution of 209 ± 42 ml/kg (Taylor *et al.,* 1979b).

B. Physical-Neural Triggers of Release

Though a few disparate reports exist, the vast majority of pertinent literature supports the postulate that vagal activity is important in effecting release of PP in vertebrates, particularly in response to a meal. This is true in dogs, humans, and probably pigs and birds.

Cephalic induction of PP release has been demonstrated in sham feeding experiments in man (Schwartz *et al.,* 1979b) and has been inferred from other similar experiments in chickens (Johnson and Hazelwood, 1979). Thus an initial very rapid increase in HPP is observed in human subjects requested to "chew and spit," but the amount of peptide released over the first few minutes represents only a small percentage of the total PP released in response to a test meal. This initial response in plasma HPP is markedly reduced by premedication with atropine or by truncal vagotomy (Schwartz *et al.,* 1979b; Taylor *et al.,* 1978a). If the chewed food is swallowed but diverted prior to reaching the upper gastrointestinal tract, the initial HPP release is again seen, but full expression of the HPP response to the presence of digesta again is blunted, even though gastric acid production is increased. Schwartz and Rehfeld (1977) and Schwartz *et al.* (1979b) feel that the PP response is totally independent of the acid production coincident with chewing and swallowing (sham feeding). Thus it appears that tasting, chewing, and swallowing food provoke a rapid rise (2–4 min) in HPP levels, four to sixfold, an effect which is blocked by antimuscarinic agents or surgical intervention of vagal activity (Schwartz *et al.,* 1979b; Taylor *et al.,* 1978a). However, full expression of the HPP elevation in response to a meal usually lasts 3–4 hr and thus relies on continued stimulation by similar or other mechanisms.

Gastric distention in humans and in chickens definitely encourages PP release, a response which is more prolonged than that seen in the sham feeding experiments. Thus intubation of the stomach with distilled water, saline, or glucose to the point that obvious distention occurs causes an abrupt increase in HPP release which is greater and lasts 20–30 min longer than that observed as a result of chewing food (Taylor *et al.,* 1978a; Schwartz *et al.,* 1979b). The effects of gastric distension are severely obtunded by truncal vagotomy or atropine. Duodenal distention by rapid injection of water or saline in human subjects has been reported to cause a rapid release of HPP, which reaches a peak within 2 min, only to return to basal levels shortly thereafter (Fink et al., 1979). Since such distension circumvents the problem of simultaneous gastrin secretion, the results again may be viewed as indicative of a physical inducement of HPP release involving cholinergic (vagal) afferent paths. Regardless of the amount of nonnutritive test substance, or the gut locus at which distension occurs, the observed PP response is less in magnitude and in duration than when digesta of the same volume appears at the same loci.

Stimulation of the vagus (0.5–8.0 Hz) in anesthetized pigs, acetylcholine injection or infusion (half-maximal dose 0.19 μM) in dogs, insulin-induced hypoglycemia in man, infusion of either bethanechol or metoclopramide into dogs and humans, and of course the presence of food, stimulate release of the respective PP in vertebrates (Adrian et al., 1977; Feldman et al., 1979; Floyd et al., 1977; Glaser et al., 1979; Schwartz et al., 1978, 1979b; Spitz et al., 1979; Taylor et al., 1978a,b). All these experimentally induced results are greatly reduced by pretreatment with atropine and usually abolished by bilateral vagotomy. Atropinization does not appear to alter basal PP levels in normal subjects, however, but is effective in reducing the abnormally high (two- to fourfold) HPP levels in duodenal ulcer patients (Schwartz et al., 1978). After a standard meal, duodenal ulcer victims show the same biphasic release of HPP as normal subjects (Adrian et al., 1979; Schwartz et al., 1976); however, after truncal vagotomy, the initial spike in PP release is abolished and the associated protracted secondary rise in HPP markedly attenuated (Adrian et al., 1979; Schwartz et al., 1978). Evidence has been presented indicating that extravagal cholinergic afferents may participate also in the release of HPP in humans. Thus atropine effects are not always duplicated by bilateral vagotomy, suggesting alternate cholinergic pathways (Glaser et al., 1979; Taylor et al., 1978a,b). The availability of Ca^{2+} in the extracellular fluid may be important to the vagal release of PP, though the PP cells do not appear to be as dependent on the presence of this cation as insulin and glucagon are (Hermansen and Schwartz, 1979b).

Attempts to implicate sympathetic adrenergic regulation of PP release in mammals have been few in number, yet consistent in negative results. Neither α-nor β-receptor blockage influences the secretion of PPP in vagally stimulated pigs (Schwartz et al., 1978), nor does the infusion of either catecholamine significantly modify basal HPP levels in man (Hedo et al., 1978). While insulin secretion and clearance decrease in man during strenuous bicycle exercise, marked increases in circulating levels of PP, somatostatin, secretin, and vasoactive intestinal polypeptide are found (Hilsted et al., 1980). β-adrenergic blockage prevents the elevation usually observed in HPP levels in exercise-stressed human subjects (Berger et al., 1978b). Maturity-onset diabetic patients who concomitantly exhibit autonomic neuropathy have basal HPP levels similar to those of other age-matched diabetics, but they are reported to exhibit delayed HPP responses to meal ingestion (Levitt *et al.,* 1979).

In summary, it appears that an intact vagal system must exist for observation of the normal PP response to upper tract distention and/or the presence of digesta within the alimentary canal. Thus, the cephalic-vagal and enteric-vagal neural reflexes appear as preliminary effectors of PP release, which are largely responsible for the initial PP peak observed after a meal, and to which is added the impact of secretogogues released from the intestinal mucosa, absorbed nutrients per se, or non-vagal cholinergic input to PP cells.

C. Nutritive Triggers of PP Release

The biphasic response in PP secretion immediately following food intake has been reported for all vertebrates studied. The response observed in various animal species differs only quantitatively, depending on the amount and (chemical) nature of the ingredients. Typical of earlier studies, the temporal relationships reported among HPP, insulin, glucagon, and glucose following a test meal of 500 g cooked ground beef are those shown in Fig. 4. It is apparent from this figure that, while glucose levels are virtually stable for 4 hr postprandially, both insulin and glucagon levels double after 60 min. However, the increase in HPP in response to the same meal is striking, beginning 1–4 min after intake and remaining elevated for at least 4 hr at levels averaging six to eight times basal, pre-food intake levels. The question whether it is the proteinaceous nature of the test meal or merely a generalized response to food has been examined in man (Floyd *et al.,* 1977), dogs (Wilson *et al.,* 1978), and chickens (Colca and Hazelwood, unpublished).

Infusion of an individual amino acid such as arginine or leucine for 30 min into healthy subjects produces a very mild, if any, increase in HPP immediately and a very slow rise in this level about 60 min after the infusion is stopped (Floyd *et al.,* 1977). Actually, the onset of this delayed rise in HPP is temporally related to the nadir in plasma glucose, a rather consistent finding (see below). When 10 essential amino acids are infused as a mixture into humans, an immediate transient peak in HPP occurs, which returns to normal basal levels after 15 min only to rise significantly after the infusion is stopped. Once again, although the accumulative amount of HPP released far exceeds that observed in saline-infused subjects, in no way does it compare with that seen after a meal as presented in Fig. 4. Individual amino acids infused intraduodenally into dogs more than double the basal CPP levels of 195 pg/ml almost immediately, but the plasma peak levels of the absorbed amino acid follow the CPP response (Wilson *et al.,* 1978).

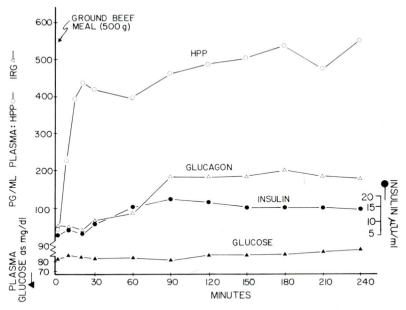

Fig. 4. Effects of ingestion of 500 g cooked beef on plasma glucose, insulin, glucagon, and HPP. Note the relative stability of plasma glucose. (Modified with permission from Floyd *et al.,* 1977.)

These results, in conjunction with those for full meal stimulation of PP release versus the relative ineffectiveness of intravenously infused amino acids (Floyd *et al.,* 1976, 1977), strongly suggest that the gastrointestinal tract is important as an intermediate structure in the release of PP from the pancreas. Furthermore, assessment of whether or not amino acids act directly on the pancreas has been made in *in vitro* studies in which pieces of pancreas were incubated with a variety of media containing different nutrient substrates. At 15 m*M*, individual amino acids are without effect in releasing CPP from the dog pancreas into the medium (Gingerich, 1977). However, a mixture of 16 amino acids (in relative proportions to dog plasma) caused a 30% increase over the basal release of CPP. [Invariably, when regional pancreatic secretion was compared within the same dog pancreas, pieces taken from the uncinate (duodenal, head) process released over 10-fold more CPP than pieces obtained from the tail (spleen) area (Gingerich, 1977; Gingerich *et al.,* 1976, 1978a).]

A modest stimulation of the release of HPP in healthy subjects was observed by Floyd *et al.* (1977) who fed them a commercial lipid-laden dietary supplement. The increment in HPP which developed was of a much lesser magnitude (triple the basal levels) after 20–30 min than when a mixed diet or a high-protein diet was fed (Floyd *et al.*, 1977). Thus fat appears to have a modest stimulatory effect in releasing human PP, an effect not observed when equivalent amounts are infused intravenously over a 90-min period. In contrast to the ingestion of lipid-rich materials, the intravenous infusion of emulsions, with or without heparin added, causes a marked, progressive decline in HPP in healthy subjects. Thus a fasting HPP level of 65 ± 10 pg/ml is driven by acute high plasma free fatty acid levels (over 5000 μEq/liter) down to 25 ± 7 pg/ml (Hedo *et al.*, 1979). This depression of HPP by elevated free fatty acid levels is of such quality and metabolic force that it is capable of producing marked attenuation of the usual rise observed in HPP after a protein-rich meal (Hedo *et al.*, 1979). Evidence is still somewhat unclear as to whether or not acute decreases in plasma free fatty acids increase HPP levels. Dogs prepared with gastric and duodenal fistulas and subsequently infused with an oleate preparation through a duodenal cannula respond with an increase in CPP 2.5 times the basal levels in the first 15 min, a sustained rise which lasts over 65 min and is paralleled to some extent by an increment in plasma CCK levels (Deviff *et al.*, 1979; Wilson *et al.*, 1978).

The role of glucose as an effector of PP release has been studied by many workers (Floyd *et al.*, 1977; Hedo *et al.*, 1978; Marco *et al.*, 1978; Waldhausl *et al.*, 1979; J. Colca, unpublished). Glucose ingested by healthy subjects causes a modest transient rise in HPP release into the plasma (Floyd *et al.*, 1976, 1977). The initial HPP peak (130 pg/ml) occurs within 15 min after glucose is administered *per os* and is followed much later, approximately 180 min, by a very large secondary HPP release (400 pg/ml). Growth hormone fluctuations are similar on the same time coordinate in response to glucose (Floyd *et al.*, 1977). Intravenous infusion of glucose (30 g) causes a modest depression in HPP which quickly rebounds upward as soon as the infusion is stopped (Floyd *et al.*, 1977; Marco *et al.*, 1978). The induction of acute hypoglycemia by tolbutamide or insulin invariably causes a rapid increase in HPP release in humans, the rising PP levels being coincident with the glycemic nadir. Invariably, the onset and peak of HPP release are most closely related to establishment of the glycemic nadir (Marco *et al.*, 1978). Tissue glucopenia (as may be produced by intravenous 2-deoxy-D-glucose) similarly evokes a rapid, marked HPP release in healthy subjects (Hedo *et al.*, 1978), a response which is greatly reduced by prior injection of atropine. While the inverse relationship of plasma glucose and PP appears established, caution should be offered at this time regarding the postulate that the polypeptide is important, or even necessary, to mammalian glucose homeostasis.

Attempts to estimate the production rate of HPP in the basal and in the glucose-loaded state have been made (Waldhausl *et al.*, 1979). Splanchnic production of HPP in the preglucose ingestion state has been reported at 14.76 ng/min and increases within 2 hr to 24.15 ng/min.

In general, investigators have found that, regardless of the manner in which the glycemia is altered, PP responses are very similar to the responses documented for growth hormone and glucagon. This certainly appears to be the case during fasting, exercise, induced hypoglycemia, etc. (Floyd *et al.,* 1976, 1977). Typical data are presented in Fig. 5. The increment(s) in PP following a mixed meal therefore appears to require an intermediary involvement of the gastrointestinal tract. Protein is the major component stimulus of PP release; lipid and glucose are much less efficacious in this respect. Comparative responses to these three nutrients are shown in Fig. 6. The presence of food, but not the presence of gastric or duodenal acid, is a requisite for the release of HPP or CPP (Floyd *et al.,* 1976, 1977; Wilson *et al.,* 1978). Double vagotomy abolishes the immediate PP response to the presence of food in the alimentary tract and obtunds the (otherwise expected) secondary, protracted release of polypeptide (Schwartz *et al.,* 1976; Taylor *et al.,* 1978b, 1979b). The fact that atropine, in addition to vagotomy, obliterates the secondary PP release, suggests that

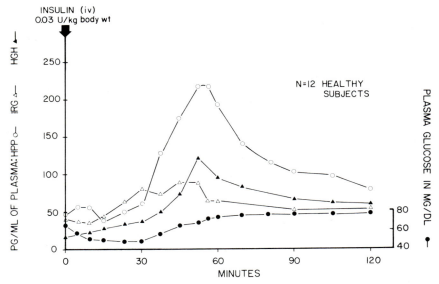

Fig. 5. Effects of intravenous injection (time 0) of 0.03 U insulin/kg body weight in 12 healthy subjects on plasma HPP, glucagon, human growth hormone (HGH), and glucose. All plasma hormones are in picograms per milliliter plasma (left ordinate) and glucose in in milligrams per deciliter (right ordinate). Plasma glucose nadir of 50 mg/dl occurred at 30 min postinjection. (Modified with permission from Floyd *et al.,* 1977.)

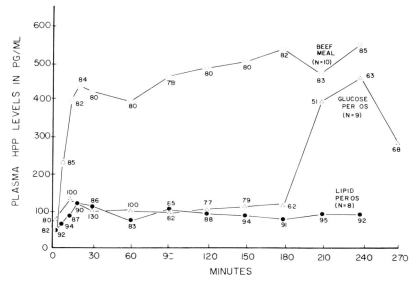

Fig. 6. Effects of ingestion of 500 g of a beef meal, 100 ml of a commercial dietary supplement containing 70 g fat (lipid), and 1.75 g glucose/kg ideal body weight on HPP levels in healthy adult subjects (N = 8–10 at each point). Numbers next to each point indicate (in milligrams per deciliter) the plasma glucose levels obtained for the same blood sample. Thus compensatory hypoglycemia following glucose ingestion occurred at approximately 180–210 min, concomitant with the surge in release of HPP. (Modified with permission from Floyd *et al.*, 1977.)

cholinergic pathways other than vagal pathways also may be involved (Taylor *et al.*, 1978a). Of course, the failure of proteinaceous substrates to effect the release of PP from isolated islets *in vitro* emphasizes the role the intestinal tract plays in mediating the PP response to a meal, a role which may involve the release of endogenous gut hormones and/or peptides.

D. Hormonal Triggers of Release

The probability that the gut mucosa was responsible for responding to resident digesta by releasing a factor, or factors, into the bloodstream to excite pancreatic release of PP was apparent from the discordant data obtained from studies employing alimentation as opposed to those wherein potential nutrients were either intravenously infused or incubated *in vitro* with pancreatic pieces. To this possibility is to be added absorbed nutrient stimulation of pancreatic insulin, glucagon, or somatostatin. The improbable role of insulin as a regulator of PP release is documented by the fact that, when insulin is infused into humans along with glucose to prevent experimental hypoglycemia, HPP levels remain undistrubed (Floyd *et al.*, 1977). These observations have been confirmed in the isolated canine pancreas (with duodenal exclusion) even at high insulin perfusion levels (Weir *et al.*, 1979). Moreover, PP has no effect on mammalian insulin release (Ipp *et al.*, 1978).

In his survey of potential secretogogues for CPP release, Gingerich (1977) has bioassayed many enteric-pancreatic peptides in an *in vitro* system employing dog pancreatic pieces in a bicarbonate-buffered medium. Gastrin (2 μg/ml) and secretin (5 U/ml) both elevate CPP release significantly, by 33 and 79%, respectively. Pentagastrin, injected at 0.5 μg/kg body wt into human subjects, produces a very sharp increase in HPP release, reaching a peak 300% above basal levels within 2–3 min only to subside quickly to preinjection levels 15 min later (Floyd *et al.*, 1977). Not all studies with gastrin agree with the foregoing, there being reports that intravenous gastrin-17 in humans is without effect on HPP release (Taylor *et al.*, 1978a). Bombesin, a known gastrin releaser, has been reported to increase CPP release when infused into dogs prepared with gastric fistulas; atropine greatly reduces this effect (Taylor *et al.*, 1979a).

Boot's secretin has been reported to be potent in releasing HPP (Adrian *et al.*, 1977; Glaser *et al.*, 1979), but caution should be exercised in data evaluation because of the suspect purity of the preparation. Pure (GIH) secretin also markedly increases PP release in humans, a response which is blocked by atropine but not by vagotomy (Glaser *et al.*, 1979). Thus the possibility of an extravagal cholinergic pathway to release HPP is again indicated.

Cholecystokinin induces a rapid and almost three- to fivefold increase in HPP in human subjects (Adrian *et al.*, 1977; Lonovics *et al.*, 1979) but, regardless of dose variation, the magnitude of response did not equal that of an ingested hospital meal (Lonovics *et al.*, 1979). Caerulein, an analogue of CCK which possesses both gastrin and CCK-like biological activities, is a peptide extracted from the skin of certain Australian frogs. This peptide markedly increases PP in human subjects as well as CPP from isolated perfused dog pancreases (Adrian *et al.*, 1977; Baetens *et al.*, 1977; Linare and Linari, 1976) and incubated pieces of dog pancreas (Gingerich, 1977). Since oleate infusion through a duodenal cannula in dogs leads to CCK release concomitant with that of CPP (Devitt *et al.*, 1979), the suggestion may be made that CCK, which also causes CPP release when given in physiological doses, is a significant afferent signal in the PP response to meal ingestion.

In vitro studies evaluating the efficacy of pancreatic insulin and glucagon in releasing PP from pancreatic pieces have been consistent in the negative results accumulated (Gingerich, 1977; Weir *et al.*, 1979). Somatostatin, a known inhibitor of both insulin and glucagon release from the pancreas in mammals, rapidly suppresses basal fasting HPP levels and abolishes the otherwise expected postprandial rise in HPP (Marco et al., 1977). These results have been confirmed in dogs (Wilson et al., 1978). However, in comparing the efficacy of somatostatin as a suppressor of all three pancreatic hormones, the PP cell appears to be least sensitive as judged by studies on the isolated dog pancreas (Hermansen and Schwartz, 1979b). Diazoxide, a known inhibitor of insulin release, also inhibits the release of PP from the isolated canine pancreas. A 10-min perfusion with diazoxide inhibits pancreatic glucagon and somatostatin release as well (Samols et al., 1977).

Glucocorticoids (short-term, in high doses) appear to suppress basal HPP levels as well as insulin-induced increases in HPP levels (Lantigua et al., 1979). Volunteers in an exercise–conditioning program responded with HPP levels five times greater than basal levels after 90 min of treadmill work. However, 2 months later, when subjected to the same work load, plasma HPP levels increased only twofold (Gingerich et al., 1979a). Thus the increases in HPP observed as a result of treadmill exercise bouts are more likely to be autonomically regulated than ACTH stress-related (Berger et al., 1978b). Isoproterenol, epinephrine, norepinephrine, and prostaglandin (PGE$_2$) are without effect in vitro in releasing PP from canine pancreatic pieces (Gingerich, 1977). Gastric inhibitory peptide (GIP) and VIP stimulate CPP release from the isolated dog pancreas (Adrian et al., 1978b).

In overall summary, therefore, significant in vivo data from the isolated perfused organ and in vitro data have accumulated indicating that the release of PP under normal conditions is regulated by both neural and hormonal pathways. Prehension, chewing, swallowing of food, and distention of certain gut regions produce an immediate, transient release of PP, which is vagus-mediated. A larger, more sustained release of PP follows as a result of contact of the digesta with the gastrointestinal mucosa, probably through the release of CCK, gastrin, and possibly secretin, GIP, and VIP. These hormonal agents then may act as a battery of regulators at the PP cell (F cell), reinforcing previous vagal release mechanisms. The possibility of other cholinergic, nonvagal contributions to meal-induced PP release is yet to be ruled out. It is evident that an enteric-pancreatic axis exists as an essential component for full expression of meal-induced PP release.

E. Comparative Studies

Even though the existence of PP as a potential third (at that time) pancreatic hormone was first established in birds (Hazelwood et al., 1973; Kimmel et al., 1968, 1971; Langslow et al., 1973), very few studies have been reported relative to PP release and/or physiology in species other than humans and dogs. The notable exception is the chicken, concerning which species the earliest suggestions were made relative to the possible role of neural elements and the quality of digesta as probable physiological triggers of importance in APP release (discussion after Floyd *et al.,* 1977; Kimmel and Pollock, 1975; Langslow *et al.,* 1973). To the author's knowledge, no other physiological reports of studies on PP in classes other than Mammalia and Aves have appeared to date.

Kimmel and his colleagues quickly identified the fluctuation in APP with the prandial state of young chickens (Langslow *et al.,* 1973; Kimmel and Pollock, 1975). Of curious interest, however, is that the catabolic state of fasting *decreases* plasma APP levels markedly from basal levels of 8–10 ng/ml plasma to 3–4 ng/ml within 24 hr. This reponse may appear to "make sense" (Section V,A) when certain physiological actions of the polypeptide are considered but is in stark contrast to the elevated levels observed both in man and dogs (Section IV,A). In mammals, the peptide appears to increase with both induced anabolic *and* catabolic conditions (fasting, meal eating, stress, exercise, etc.). Casein hydrolysate administered *per os* is the most effective nutrient stimulus of APP release in 6-week-old chickens, glucose and oil being less effective (Kimmel and Pollock, 1975). Actual intake of food is required, rather than merely the sight of food, to initiate the pronounced biphasic APP response (discussion to Floyd *et al.,* 1977). Not only are basal levels of APP 40–50 times greater than those of CPP and HPP, but the initial rise observed postprandially is usually of much greater magnitude, sometimes eightfold, within the first 20 min after food ingestion. Intravenous injection of glucose evokes a transient decrease in APP, the nature of which differs depending on whether the nutrient is given as a bolus or during an infusion. Thus, as in mammals, an enteric role appears evident in the regulation of APP release.

The contribution of the vagus to meal-induced APP release has been studied, and the data obtained are in accord with those reported for mammals. Thus both sodium pentobarbital and atropine reduce or abolish the postprandial release of APP in chickens (discussion to Floyd *et al.,* 1977). If taut ligatures are placed around the gut of fasted chickens at different locations and the birds allowed to feed *ad libitum* for 60 min, APP is released to varying extents and magnitudes depending on where the blockage is established. Of significance is the observation that merely filling the crop, a nonabsorptive structure in birds, releases APP quickly, accounting for ~30% of the APP release observed in normal, nonligated control animals (Johnson and Hazelwood, 1979). Thus the early partial, transient APP release in reponse to food prehension and swallowing appears to be vagally mediated in chickens, as has been established in man and dogs (Hazelwood, 1973; Johnson and Hazelwood, 1979). Approximately 60% of the full APP response to a 60-min refeeding regimen is observed in chickens in which the gut blockage is midjejunum, an area which is virtually unstretched by the digesta volume, suggesting that absorbed factors rather than distensible forces are more important in an area early in the small intestine.

Evaluation of the efficacy of various individual amino acids in releasing APP from isolated microfragments of chicken pancreas has been made. The most powerful stimulus appears to be a combination (10 mM as percent of chicken feed composition) of amino acids when added to a perifusate of microfragments of chicken pancreas. Glucose, glucagon, insulin, and long-chain fatty acids apparently are without effect as potential APP secretogogues in the perifusion system. In fact, the injection of a glucagon bolus *in vivo* decreases APP release by 25% (Hazelwood and Langslow, 1978). Overall therefore and with the exception of the effects of fasting on plasma APP levels, the bird, as represented by *Gallus domesticus,* appears to be quite similar to man in that protein is probably a major stimulus of release of APP, particularly if taken by mouth. The intermediary role of a "gut factor," as in man, also is highly likely, but this does not mean that high levels of individual amino acids given intravenously will fail to cause APP release. They will, but like glucose as a potential modulator of PP release, normal food intake and absorption in birds is not accompanied by such exaggerated plasma fluctuations in these nutrients as to affect the PP cell release mechanism(s).

Bombesin, when injected into intact chickens, is known to increase "gastric acid" secretion. This effect is abolished by surgical removal of the gizzard–duodenum junction but not by previous pancreatectomy. Thus APP apparently is not an intermediary in bombesin-induced gastric secretion, although it may act as such in caerulein-induced acid secretion (Linare and Linari, 1976).

V. FUNCTION OF PANCREATIC POLYPEPTIDE

In contrast to the apparent plethora of reports in the literature devoted to regulators of PP release in vertebrates, there exists at this time a virtual dearth of literature devoted to the basic function of PP. Those studies available mainly emanate from less than five or six laboratories and are thus reviewed in the following paragraphs irrespective of the experimental approach or the animal species employed in each investigation.

A. *In Vivo* Studies

1. *Secretogogue Studies*

Probably the best documented physiological effect of PP is its secreto-gogical effect in mammals and birds. Thus in relatively low concentrations APP provokes almost instant increased secretion of fluid volume, free hydronium ion, pepsinogen, and total protein from the chicken proventri-culus (Fig. 7; Hazelwood, 1973; Hazelwood and Langslow, 1978; Hazel-wood *et al.*, 1973). This effect on the "secretory stomach" of birds appears to be direct, not requiring the release of histamine (Turner and Hazelwood 1973). Also, this biological action, unlike the relationship of pentagastrin to gastrin-17, appears to require more of the native molecule than the C-terminal pentapeptide. Synthetic avian C-pentapeptide acts as an in-hibitor of an otherwise APP stimulus in birds, indicating recognition by the proventriculus receptor but loss of biological activity (Kanellis *et al.*, 1979). Chance and his colleagues have reported the essentiality of the Tyr-NH$_2$ at the terminal position 36 in the BPP molecule for biological effects in dogs (Chance *et al.*, 1975; Lin and Chance, 1972; Lin *et al.*, 1974, 1977).

Secretogogical action of BPP apparently depends on the basal gastric se-cretion rate, as well as the rate and dose at which BPP is infused into surgi-

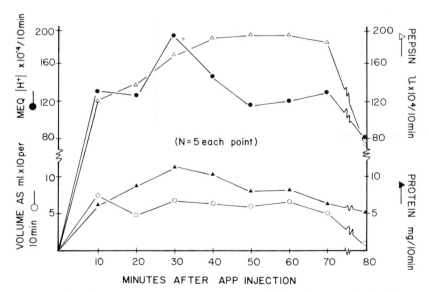

Fig. 7. Effect of APP (25 μg/kg body wt) on proventricular volume secretion and the pro-duction of free acid, pepsin, and total protein in chickens. Birds were 6 to 8 weeks old, fasted, SCWL. All data expressed as above control levels. (Modified from Hazelwood *et al.*, 1973.)

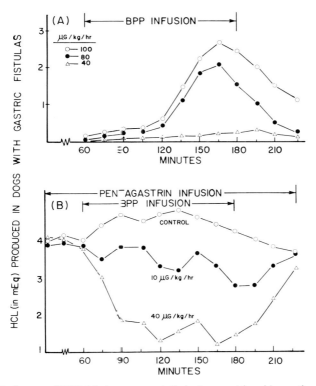

Fig. 8. Influence of BPP (via intravenous infusion) on gastric acid secretion in adult dogs with gastric fistulas. (A) Effects of graded doses of BPP on basal (nonprimed) acid secretion. (B) Effects of BPP on acid secretion in dogs previously and simultaneously stimulated with an infusion of pentagastrin (0.5 μg/kg/hr). (Modified with permission from Lin *et al.,* 1977.)

cally prepared dogs (Fig. 8). Thus, with a low basal secretion of gastric acid in dogs, the infusion or bolus injection of BPP stimulates acid secretion (Lin *et al.,* 1973, 1977). However, at high basal secretory rates, or in canine preparations wherein steady-state pentagastrin stimulation of gastric acid is induced, BPP infusions have a profound inhibitory action (Chance *et al.,* 1975; Lin and Chance, 1972; Lin *et al.,* 1973, 1974, 1977). Neither stimulation nor inhibition of gastric acid occurs in human volunteers when BPP is infused at dose ranges bracketing those normally found after a mixed meal (Bloom *et al.,* 1977). A very consistent inhibitory effect of BPP on exocrine pancreatic function is observed when it is infused into dogs. Thus, after an initial transient increase in water and bicarbonate secretion, there follows a profound, protracted decrease in these parameters together with a marked depression in enzyme release (Fig. 9; Chance *et al.,* 1975; Lin *et al.,* 1973,

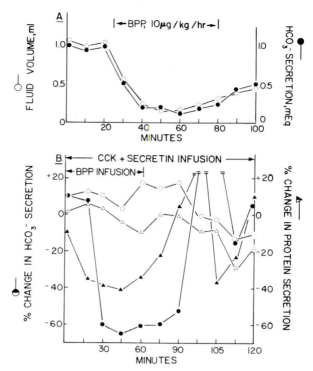

Fig. 9. Effect of BPP on pancreatic exocrine function in dogs. (A) Effect of BPP infused at 10 μg/kg/hr on basal water and HCO_3^- secretion in dogs with chronic pancreatic fistulas. (B) Effect of superimposing a BPP infusion (2 μg/kg/hr) on the stimulated exocrine pancreas of dogs with chronic pancreatic fistulas. CCK (0.5 U) and secretin (0.2 U) were infused continuously on a body weight basis, while BPP was infused only for the first 60 min. Open symbols represent control dogs (CCK and secretin only); solid symbols represent dogs receiving BPP (2 μg/kg/hr) in addition to CCK and secretin. (Modified with permission from Lin *et al.,* 1977.)

1977; Taylor *et al.,* 1979b). In man, intravenous infusion of BPP causes a reduction in pancreatic secretion (assayed from duodenal juice) of approximately 25% if concentrations of the peptide are employed equaling those seen in plasma after a meal (Adrian *et al.,* 1978c). The stimulation of exocrine pancreatic secretion with low doses of BPP, and inhibition with high doses, are actions which parallel closely those of CCK or CCK analogues on pancreatic enzymes and fluid volume flow (Otsuki *et al.,* 1979). Trypsin secretion is also reduced in man when BPP (60–300 pmol/kg/hr) is infused (Greenberg *et al.,* 1978, 1979). Exocrine pancreatic inhibition by BPP definitely requires an intact BPP molecule, as removal of Tyr-NH$_2$ at the C-terminus and infusion of the resulting BPP$_{1-35}$ augments water, bicarbonate, and trypsin secretion in dogs (Lin *et al.,* 1974). Of curious interest is the finding of endogenous HPP, like that of insulin and glucagon, in significant amounts in pancreatic ductal fluid (Carr-Locke and Track, 1979; Lawrence *et al.,* 1979). The significance of this finding, other than that it is a potential local inhibitor of exocrine pancreatic secretion, is yet to be established. Thus, while HPP and BPP tentatively may be considered so-called pancreogastrones, agreement has not been reached as to the role they play when present at physiological levels in man and dog (Bloom *et al.,* 1977; Parks *et al.,* 1979; Taylor *et al.,* 1979b). In dogs, gastric acid secretion may be totally unrelated to prevailing plasma CPP levels, though the regulation of pancreatic secretion may be correlated positively to such levels (Parks *et al.,* 1979).

In addition to the powerful inhibitory effect of PP on mammalian (not demonstrated in avian) pancreatic fluid and enzyme secretion is the effect the peptide has on the mechanics of bilirubin secretion into the duodenal fluid. Thus, unlike CCK, BPP when infused into dogs prepared with appropriate fistulas relaxes gallbladder smooth muscle and increases choledochal tone but has little if any effect on bile flow (Chance *et al.,* 1975; Lin and Chance, 1972, 1974; Lin *et al.,* 1973). In man, BPP infusion causes an abrupt reduction (60–80%) in the bilirubin content of duodenal juice, evidence suggesting decreased bile flow. These effects have been reported by several groups of workers (Adrian *et al.,* 1978c; Bloom *et al.,* 1977; Greenberg *et al.,* 1978, 1979).

Intestinal muscle tone also is altered by the presence of exogenous BPP. Implantation of miniature induction coils in the gut wall of conscious dogs, which are subsequently infused with BPP, allows gut motility to be monitored at several loci simultaneously. Pyloric, duodenal, and colonic muscle motility is increased (Lin and Chance, 1972). Retching, vomiting, and defecation are common side effects observed at higher (50–100 μg/kg body wt) doses of BPP infused intravenously. The rate of BPP infusion and the concentration of the peptide dictate whether general increases or decreases in gut motility are observed (Chance *et al.,* 1975). In contrast to these observations in dogs, other workers have reported a consistent decrease in gut motility, which is dose-related when APP is infused into young turkeys (Duke *et al.,* 1979). However, postprandial APP levels rarely reach the plasma levels required to demonstrate this reduction in contractile activity, requiring some caution in assessing the physiological significance of these findings.

Intraarterial infusion of BPP into the opossum induces increased contractility of the lower esophageal sphincter, an effect which is virtually linear and dose-related (Rattan and Goyal, 1979). This increase in sphincter pressure in response to BPP is partially blocked by tetrodotoxin and atropine but not by adrenergic, serotoninergic, or histaminergic antagonists (Rattan and Goyal, 1979). Thus BPP stimulation of sphincter closure in the opossum may be due partially to direct action of the peptide on the muscle or may occur via cholinergic nerve elements.

In partial summary, therefore, action of PP on enteric-pancreohepatic structures is normally stimulated by meal eating. The activity of PP appears unique among gastrointestinal hormones in that the action of this putative hormone contrasts with that of gastrin, CCK, and secretin in that it does not stimulate bile and pancreatic exocrine secretion, does not increase gallbladder tone, and does not reduce resistance to flow within the common bile duct. In its effects on pancreatic electrolyte secretion BPP differs from insulin and glucose also. Equally significant differences (from glucagon) are apparent in BPP lacking diuretic, hyperkalemic, hyperglycemic, and inhibition of motility effects (Lin and Chance, 1972: Lin et al., 1974). Thus, when these differences in the action of BPP are considered in light of the fact that PP molecular structures are totally different from all known gastrointestinal polypeptides as well as that of insulin and somatostatin, the peptide remains somewhat of an enigma. At circulating levels commensurate with those observed immediately after meal eating, PP may play a role (check-and-balance?) in controlling pancreatic fluid, bicarbonate, and enzyme release concomitant with regulating bile storage within the gallbladder.

2. Metabolic Studies

The examination of metabolic parameters which may be important in obtaining further understanding of PP molecular action has failed to present a well-defined picture. The very first reports on the spectrum of biological effects of PP came from an evaluation of APP activity in young chickens (Hazelwood, 1973; Hazelwood et al., 1973; Kimmel et al., 1971). Over a wide range of doses, APP is without effect on blood glucose levels (Hazelwood et al., 1973; Kimmel et al., 1971), an effect which has been confirmed in birds (Hayden 1976) and with BPP in dogs (Lin et al., 1977). Despite this lack of a glycemic effect, liver glycogen of fed chickens is decreased rapidly (Hayden, 1976; Hazelwood et al., 1973), suggesting that the mobilized glucose is siphoned quickly into either a glycolytic or a lipogenic pathway. No information is available on the former possibility, but exogenous APP has been reported to have a hypoglycerolemic effect (Hayden, 1976; Hazelwood et al., 1973) occurring concomitantly with a marked lowering of α-amino acids, especially alanine (Hayden, 1976). The liver lipid content of birds decreases in the presence of APP, while plasma triglycerides increase (Hayden, 1976). Thus PP may act as a "fed hormone" in birds, encouraging lipogenesis in liver and its transport (with lipoprotein) to adipose rests. The large influx of carbohydrate with (continual) meal eating in chickens offers an adequate substrate for the above-suggested sequence of events. More work is needed to clarify the precise metabolic influence APP may exert, though at this time it appears to fall into the category of an anabolic hormone. The marked decrease in plasma APP with overnight fasting and the rapid increase to plasma levels about 6–10 times greater than basal levels within 10 min of refeeding (Johnson and Hazelwood, 1979; Kimmel and Pollock, 1975) may emphasize the role this polypeptide plays in Aves.

In the fasting chicken, APP administration exerts less clear effects, though once again those which appear most profound involve lipid metabolism. Plasma glycerol and free fatty acids are reduced, but phospholipid and triglyceride levels are unperturbed (Hayden, 1976). When injected as a bolus into adult chickens APP appears to be antilipolytic, as plasma free fatty acid levels decrease by at least 20% within minutes after injection (Hazelwood and Langslow, 1978; Langslow and Hazelwood, 1975). This observation has been confirmed *in vitro* (McCumbee and Hazelwood 1977, 1978; see Section B,2). However, APP is without effect on insulin, glucose, and uric acid levels, therein differing markedly from other pancreatic hormones (Hazelwood and Langslow, 1978).

Generally, PP has been reported to be without effect on insulin release (Ipp *et al.,* 1978; Hazelwood and Langslow, 1978) and glucose production or uptake (e.g., Hazelwood and Langslow, 1978; Lin *et al.,* 1977; McCumbee and Hazelwood, 1977), but recent evidence has been presented indicating that it may inhibit glucose-induced insulin release in mice, an effect similar to that observed with somatostatin and low doses of substance P (Lundquist *et al.,* 1979). Thus the nature of the stimulus presented to the B cell may in some way determine the magnitude of the peptide effect.

That gastrin and its synthetic analogue pentagastrin exert trophic effects on the maturation and maintenance of gastrointestinal structures in mammals is well known and accepted. A possible similar role for PP has been suggested by studies on APP in developing chick embryos. Not only does pancreatectomy lead to a quick "thinning" of the secretory stomach organ, the proventriculus, within 4 days after the operation, but also single injections of APP on days 12–14 of incubation lead to increased growth and development of the proventriculus of the embryonic gut (Laurentz and Hazelwood, 1979). Increases in nucleic acid content and incorporation of [^{14}C]leucine also have been observed in gastric, but not intestinal or hepatic, structures when APP is administered to developing chick embryos. Interestingly, the sensitivity of embryonic structures appears to be greatest on the days (days 12–14) when endogenous PP is the lowest (the release greatest?) and endogenous gastric secretion commences (Goldman *et al.,*

1978; Laurentz and Hazelwood, 1979). Thus, in addition to its gastrin-like secretogogical action in birds, APP may exert anabolic regulation of the developing avian gut. Comparable studies in mammals are lacking.

Recently, attempts have been made to evaluate a possible role for mammalian PPs in regulating food intake, thereby leading to faulty lipid metabolism in some cases. Thus intraperitoneal injections (three times a day) of either APP or BPP into New Zealand genetically obese mice have been reported to repair the diabetes-type glucose tolerance curve normally observed for these rodents. Also, when such injections are carried out for 30 days, there is a return to normal of the preexisting hyperglycemia, hyperinsulinemia, and abnormal weight gain characteristic of this obese mouse strain (Gates and Lazarus, 1977). Since amelioration of this diabetes-type condition can be achieved by transplantation of a pancreas either from normal or from alloxan-diabetic white mice, the suggestion was made that the New Zealand obese mouse is normally deficient in PP (Gates and Lazarus, 1977). Unfortunately, this report did not present food intake or plasma PP data.

Addressing this suggestion or problem more directly, Orci's laboratory observed that genetically obese mice (*ob/ob*, C57BL/6J) have reduced numbers of PP cells in their pancreatic islets (Malaisse-Lagae *et al.*, 1978). The question may be asked, Are they obese because of lack of a satiation factor which may stimulate the appropriate hypothalamic hunger–satiety center? Injection of BPP into these obese hyperphagic mice reduced food intake and suppressed body weight gain (Malaisse-Lagae *et al.*, 1978). The regulation of food intake therefore may fall within the sphere of PP physiological action. Unanswered is the question, however, whether the genetically obese hyperphagic hyperglycemic mouse suffers from a paucity of circulating PP or, alternatively, from an excess of this peptide. Thus the observation that hyperglycemic obese (*ob/ob*) mice have elevated (300%) numbers of PP cells per islet, as well as an increased (60–70%) concentration of the peptide in the pancreas, when compared with homozygous (+ / +) control mice, suggests either a deficiency in the PP release mechanism or elevated plasma PP levels in the diabetic murine pancreas (Gingerich *et al.*, 1978b). More work is needed on this intriguing subject before the exact position PP plays in the metabolism of vertebrates can be established.

B. *In Vitro* Studies: Metabolic, Adipocytic, and Hepatocytic

Glucagon-stimulated lipolysis is inhibited by APP in isolated chicken adipocytes *in vitro* by as much as 45%. Such an antilipolytic effect is probably due to the suppression of glucagon-induced cyclic adenosine 3′,5′-monophosphate (cyclic AMP) accumulation (McCumbee and Hazelwood, 1977). In the avian adipocyte, BPP also acts as an antilipolytic agent, though it is not as effective as equal amounts of APP (McCumbee and Hazelwood, 1978). Neither APP nor BPP inhibits glucagon-stimulated lipolysis in rat adipocytes. Two orders of receptor sites have been described for APP in the isolated adipocyte (McCumbee and Hazelwood, 1977). Thus the decrease in plasma free fatty acid levels observed *in vivo* (Hayden, 1976) conceivably could be a result of the dual action of APP in favoring the lipogenic machinery concomitant with an antilipolytic effect at the adipocyte level by interfering with the adenylate cyclase system. Plasma APP fluctuations have not been associated with the increased activity of various hepatic lipogenic enzymes during the first few hours after a meal, although ATP-citrate lyase, malic enzyme, and fatty acid synthetase levels are elevated 3 hr later (M. Adamo and R. Hazelwood, unpublished).

C. Tentative Conclusions as to Action

Briefly, therefore, any summarization of the probable *in vivo* metabolic effects of PP should include the statement that the hormone is a conservative one; that is, it is anabolic-like in most actions. Its fluctuations with the prandial state of the organism are associated with the ultimate degradation of food and distribution of the absorbed nutrients, the latter most probably by playing some role (yet to be defined at the molecular level) in lipid metabolism. The possibility that PP plays a regulatory role in the prehension of food by acting on hypothalamic centers is yet to be established with certainty, but it is a suggestion which is consonant with the earlier finding of specific receptors in the hypothalamus for a myriad of gastrointestinal hormones such as CCK, VIP, and gastrin.

VI. PATHOPHYSIOLOGICAL CORRELATES

A. Deficiency versus Excess States

A major hindrance in furthering our understanding of the true significance of PP is the blatant fact that a genuine deficiency state is yet to be described in humans. Also, no tumor secreting *only* PP has been described. Supplies of PP are not luxurious enough to allow investigators to "load" an animal, seeking to determine the physiological impact of the consequences of PP excess, and chronic preparations employing continuous administration of anti-PP serum in addressing the question of the impact or consequences of a deficiency in PP are not practical at this time. Relative deficiencies in PP can be achieved only by surgical extirpation of the pancreas, but even with such a procedure circulating PP levels, although mark-edly reduced, are not abolished.

Obese humans (> 20% over ideal weight) not only have normal basal levels of plasma HPP (36 ± 4 pmol/liter) but also respond quickly and equally to the challenge of food intake by a three- to fourfold increase after 30 min. Though the reported response is not significantly different from the response to the same meal stimulus observed in normal subjects of ideal weight, the 30-min HPP levels of the obese are almost twice those of the control group (Wahl et al., 1979). A more intense study may be necessary to isolate various nuances suggested by such data. Similar studies have been carried out in the obese Pima Indians of the southwestern United States. This population is characterized by a strong tendency to become obese and/or diabetic by the age of 40, although one condition may exist in the absence of the other. Obese Pimas with basal (fasting) HPP levels (151 ± 25 pg/ml) in excess of those seen either in Caucasians or in diabetic, nonobese Pima Indians, respond to a meal with 15-min postpran-dial HPP levels significantly greater (1440 ± 257 pg/ml) than those ob-served in the other two groups (Gingerich et al., 1979b). While more study of these interrelationships is necessary to elucidate cause versus effect, the need to normalize and/or differentiate nutritional, age, ethnic, and body weight factors in future studies on PP function appears essential (Gingerich et al., 1979b). Thus these reports on human subjects add to the conjecture raised as to the relationship of obesity to circulating levels of PP, and the latter to pancreatic islet PP distribution and content discussed in Section V,A,2 (Gingerich et al., 1978b; Malaisse-Lagae et al., 1978). They also raise a question about the role played, if any, by the diseased pancreas as seen in diabetes mellitus in the function of PP.

Metabolism of HPP may be a function of normal kidney (but not liver) physiology. Thus, while PP levels are elevated both in patients with cir-rhosis and with chronic renal failure (CRF), only in the latter is there demonstrable significant reduction in PP extraction (Boden et al., 1980). It is suggested by the author that PP contributes to the uremic syndrome associated with CRF. The conclusions relative to the role of the kidney dif-fer considerably from those presented by Adrian et al. (1978a) and Taylor et al. (1979b).

B. Diabetes Mellitus

Probably the most complete assessment of plasma HPP levels in a dis-ease state is that carried out by Floyd and colleagues in 282 patients with di-abetes mellitus (Floyd et al., 1977; Floyd, 1979). Most diabetic patients screened had markedly elevated plasma HPP levels, ranging from 400 to over 10,000 pg/ml, which is to be compared with the normal range of 60–90 pg/ml in healthy control subjects. Also, most of these diabetic patients possessed the ability to bind HPP, a finding which indicated normal antibody response to components of exogenous commercial insulin (Floyd et al., 1977). Such insulin preparations are not subjected to an isolation–purification step which specifically removes PP. Patients treated with insulin for many years inevitably develop anti-BPP, anti-OPP, and anti-PPP antibodies. It has been estimated that, after 10 yr of insulin at least 87% of the diabetic population will have serum with the capacity to bind HPP because of the excellent cross-reactivity between HPP and antisera to other mammalian PPs (Fitz-Patrick, 1979). The same is true to a greater extent for antiinsulin antibodies, and to a lesser extent for antiglucagon and antisomatostatin antibodies in the same insulin-treated diabetic population (Fitz-Patrick, 1979).

When age and previous clinical history of diabetic populations are taken into consideration (normalized), the absolute values of plasma HPP in nontreated diabetic patients are still considerably elevated over those of healthy controls by approximately 40–50% (85 versus 120 pg/ml). This difference is statistically significant, as is the 100% difference in plasma glucose levels in the two groups (82 versus 158 mg/dl). Generally speaking, when comparisons are made between and among various diabetic subjects grouped as to uncontrolled, diet-controlled receiving oral therapy, and insulin-treated juvenile- and maturity-onset-type diabetes, the elevated HPP levels parallel closely the elevations observed also in circulating glucagon and growth hormone in each case (Floyd et al., 1977). Diet-controlled diabetic subjects usually have the lowest—yet elevated—HPP levels of all diabetic groups; sulfonylurea-treated diabetics have somewhat higher HPP levels, and by comparison insulin-treated juvenile-onset-type diabetics appear to have the highest plasma HPP levels. Thus, as the clinical severity of diabetes increases, plasma HPP, glucagon, and growth hormone levels apparently increase also (Floyd and Fajans, 1976; Floyd et al., 1977).

The observation has been made in experimentally induced diabetes that, concomitant with a decrease in islet cell mass (volume) and an increase in glucagon-producing cell volume, there occurs a significant increase in PP cell number and volume. Thus alloxan-induced diabetes in rats reduces B-cell mass by 50%, simultaneous with an approximate doubling of PP cell volume (Sundler et al., 1977b). Hyperplasia of PP-type cells in diabetic humans has been reported, the major source of new cells emanating from small and medium ductal elements (Gepts et al., 1977). Such increases in PP cell types are claimed to appear as "ribbons" of cells (first described in juvenile diabetes by Cecil in 1911) in an atypical islet regeneration (Gepts and DeMay, 1978; Gepts *et al.,* 1977). Attractive as such postulates are, and with the apparent existent corollary of elevated plasma HPP levels in diabetic subjects, caution should be exercised in accepting that diabetes in man "produces atypical islet mass enlargement and volume increase." Recently, as a result of reports from several laboratories, a better appreciation of the nonuniform distribution of islet or acinar cell populations in normal pancreases has been gained. Thus, in addition to reports of nonrandom localization of PP cells in dog and human pancreases (Gersell *et al.,* 1976, 1979; Gingerich *et al.,* 1978a) there appears to be recent evidence that at least two islet populations exist within the same rat pancreas (Orci *et al.,* 1976). A three-dimensional reconstruction of the rat pancreas by the use of serial sections (3 μm) and specific immunofluorescent techniques has been accomplished (Baetens *et al.,* 1979). Results of such cytological studies indicate unequivocally that two types of islets exist which are situated at different anatomical locations of the pancreas and located in exocrine areas drained by different excretory ducts. As indicated in Section II, islets in the area of the duodenum–head region are sparse in glucagon A cells but very rich in PP cells which form a "halo effect" at the islet periphery. The reverse is true in islets from the body or tail (splenic) region of the mammalian pancreas (Orci *et al.,* 1976; Baetens *et al.,* 1979). Morphometrical analysis of pancreases from juvenile diabetics indicate that, quantitatively, HPP cells do not differ from those examined in nondiabetic subjects *if* care is taken to evaluate identical topographical regions of each pancreas (L. Orci, personal communication). Thus earlier reports of increased cell numbers in diabetes mellitus (but not necessarily the transitional form of ductal epithelial cells) must be viewed with caution because of a likely sampling bias. Equal caution must therefore be exercised when interpreting functional or morphological observations using different pancreatic tissue fractions (Orci *et al.,* 1976; Baetens *et al.,* 1979).

C. Other Pancreatic Dysfunctions

The existence of diabetes mellitus is not a requisite for increased circulating PP levels and, as Floyd *et al.* (1977) have pointed out, an increase in HPP cell number is not specific for genetic diabetes. Evidence is accumulating indicating that increased plasma PP levels attend virtually any stress on the vertebrate pancreas. Thus pancreatitis, benign islet tumors, multiple endocrine adenomatosis, microatherosclerosis involving the pancreas, etc., most frequently are associated with elevated plasma HPP levels. Subcutaneous lipoma cases have been reported to have elevated basal HPP levels and to respond to meal eating with a grossly exaggerated PP response (Floyd *et al.,* 1977), while cystic fibrotic patients have normal basal HPP levels but fail to respond to the known stimulus of food ingestion (J. R. Kimmel, personal communication).

The presence of insulin-secreting tumors in the human pancreas frequently is associated with elevated plasma HPP levels. However, removal of these growths, while lowering plasma insulin, actually increases HPP levels. Assay of the tumor tissue (after removal) indicates lower or equal concentrations of HPP on a unit tissue weight basis, as is found in tissue obtained from normal, healthy subjects (Floyd *et al.*, 1977). Thus the source of the elevated plasma HPP must not be the tumor per se. The evaluation of other forms of islet pathology also provides evidence that the sources of the elevated plasma levels observed in such cases are most probably nontumorous sites or possibly nonpancreatic sites (Floyd *et al.*, 1975, 1977).

Patients with chronic pancreatitis (exhibiting steatorrhea) exhibit normal basal HPP levels but fail to respond to the meal-eating stimulus (Adrian *et al.*, 1979). In contrast, patients with active coeliac disease or with acute tropical sprue (with steatorrhea) respond to the meal-eating stimulus with a normal, rapid, protracted elevation in plasma HPP levels.

Elevated plasma HPP levels are not a specific marker for the existence of a pancreatic tumor (Floyd and Fajans, 1976). This statement includes the tumor associated with the Zollinger–Ellison syndrome (Taylor *et al.*, 1977b). Yet, in a survey of a variety of endocrine neoplasms of the pancreas (including gastrinomas, insulinomas, glucagonomas, and vipomas), over half the afflicted patients exhibited elevated basal plasma HPP levels (Polak *et al.*, 1976). In addition, extracts of tumor tissue, as well as hepatic and lymph node metastases, were found to contain HPP-secreting cells (Larsson *et al.*, 1976b; Polak *et al.*, 1976). (Notable exceptions in this regard were insulin-secreting tumors.) Of particular note, however, has been the finding of both HPP- and VIP-producing cells in tumors removed from patients suffering from the watery diarrhea (Verner–Morrisson) syndrome. While plasma VIP levels may be normal or elevated, most frequently plasma HPP levels are excessively high (Larsson, 1976; Larsson *et al.*, 1976b). Such an aberration is neither absolute nor a requisite. (Extra-tumor (pancreatic) hyperplasia of HPP-secreting cells has been reported also.) Thus the finding of elevated circulating HPP levels concomitant with VIP-producing tumors and/or nontumorous HPP hyperplasia of the pancreas may indeed implicate the latter polypeptide as an accessory (or a major factor) in expression of the debilatating watery diarrhea syndrome (Larsson, 1976). Unfortunately, a tumor, regardless of location, producing only HPP is yet to be described. Yet the observation exists that extirpation of "mixed" pancreatic tumors does not usually restore plasma HPP levels to normal (Floyd *et al.*, 1977). The role established so far for HPP in gastroenteric-pancreatic exocrine function in vertebrates, with or without concomitant VIP release, may be a factor contributing to the diarrhea syndrome more so than any other disease so far investigated within this area (Larsson, 1976).

VII. SUMMARY OF CURRENT INFORMATION

Development of a relatively specific radioimmunoassay for PP, as well as the use of radioimmunofluorescent antibody techniques, leads us to certain useful conclusions, some of which can be stated more pontifically than others.

A. Certainties versus Putative Functions

Pancreatic polypeptide is a 36-amino-acid structure with an approximate molecular weight of 4200 which is synthesized as a larger promolecule and secreted from apparent endocrine-type cells in the pancreas of all vetebrates so far studied. Cells secreting PP are always located in the vertebrate pancreas, usually at the periphery of the endocrine islets, and, depending on the species, to varying degrees throughout the sea of exocrine tissue. Topographical identification of PP cells indicates that the largest population exists in the head or uncinate process, and the smallest in the tail or splenic area, in contrast to the distribution of glucagon-secreting cells in the same pancreas. A few nonprimate mammals have PP-secreting cells in the gastric mucosa.

Circulating levels of PP are readily detected by a double-antibody immunoassay technique, the use of which has established that in the basal state HPP ranges from 60 to 100 pg/ml plasma. Fasting elevates mammalian PP levels but lowers avian levels. Elevated PP levels also are found as a result of hypoglycemia, exercise, and stress, and particularly after meal eating. The proteinaceous content of food appears most important as a secretogogue elevating PP levels, although vagal cholinergic afferent release mechanisms have been described in fair detail. Thus the presence of food at a nonabsorptive mucosal site initiates a spike release of PP within minutes, which is followed subsequently by a prolonged PP release (several hours), probably as a result of the interaction of nutrients with hormone-releasing cells of the gut, or with actual absorption of these nutrients.

Once released, PP has been shown to have a variety of apparently unrelated effects resulting in hepatic glycogenolysis without hyperglycemia, hypoglycerolemia, hypoaminoacidemia and, depending on the prandial state, various perturbations in plasma triglyceride and free fatty acid levels.

Depending on the dosage (low doses stimulate, high physiological doses inhibit) PP has a profound effect on gastric acid (in mammals and birds) and pepsin secretion (in birds), as well as a dual action, the inhibitory portion being more prominent on exocrine pancreatic secretion of enzymes, water, and HCO_3^- (in dogs).

Isolated cell preparations have not been employed by many workers studying the function of PP, but what has been reported indicates that PP may have insulin-like antilipolytic activity at the adipocyte. This action would be a result of PP interference with the adenylate cyclase system. There are many pieces of evidence implicating PP somehow, some way, in lipid metabolism in mammals and birds. Thus a possible action of PP on hypothalamic hunger–satiety centers has been postulated based on the observation that chronic injections of PP into genetic obese mice restore to normal plasma glucose and insulin levels as well as the otherwise abnormal laying down of body adipose tissue. Finally, the powerful secretogogic effect of PP on the gastropancreatic-intestinal tract may implicate this polypeptide in the etiology of the debilitating watery diarrhea syndrome. Since a total deficiency state of PP has never been reported and, because a specific tumor elaborating only PP has never been identified, the putative hormone appears at this time to be a PP in search of a disease.

B. Further Research

The plethora of investigations directed at the spectrum of factors and/or conditions which provoke release of PP from the vertebrate pancreas contrast sharply with the dearth of reports devoted to elucidating the molecular action—and thus the basic physiological effects—of PP. Although there appears to be a metabolic response to exogenous PP, the evidence currently at hand does not allow establishment of a meaningful common thread tying such observations together and explaining the cellular expression of this PP. Obviously, more work should be directed toward the basic physiology of PP, in particular toward determining the fate of mobilized liver glycogen and the role it may (or may not) play in lipid synthesis, mobilization of lipid, and/or the fate of lipid. An intensification of effort also should be directed toward establishing PP receptors in CNS structures known to be involved in hunger–satiety phenomena. Are certain types of obesity causes, or are they effects of excessive or insufficient amounts of endogenous PP? Finally, in conjunction with the above, there appears a need to evaluate what impact, if any, elevated plasma PP levels exert in diseases such as diabetes and the Verner–Morrison syndrome. Are these elevated levels coincidental with a metabolically stressed pancreas, or are they truly indicative of participating PP cell types which in some way play a heretofore unrecognized significant role in the etiology of pancreatic pathophysiology?

Until considerable more fundamental work is completed and reported relative to the effects and molecular action of PP this polypeptide will remain a putative hormone awaiting the proper credentials essential for it to join the fraternity of recognized hormones.

ACKNOWLEDGMENT

The author acknowledges with appreciation critical review of Section III of this chapter by Dr. J. R. Kimmel.

SIGNIFICANT REVIEWS

1. General Chemistry: "Isolation and Characterization of a New Pancreatic Polypeptide" by J. R. Kimmel, L. J. Hayden, and H. G. Pollock. *J. Biol. Chem.* **250,** 9369–9376, 1975.
2. Radioimmunoassay and Distribution of PP in Vertebrates: "Studies of the Distribution of A New Avian Pancreatic Polypeptide and Insulin Among Birds, Reptiles, Amphibians and Mammals" by D. R. Langslow, J. R. Kimmel, and H. G. Pollock. *Endocrinology* 93, 558–565, 1973.
3. Gastric and Pancreatic Function: "Bovine Pancreatic Polypeptide: Action on Gastric and Pancreatic Secretion in Dogs" by T. Lin, D. C. Evans, R. E. Chance, and G. F. Spray. *Am. J. Physiol.* **232,** E311–E315, 1977.
4. Pancreatic Polypeptide in Health and Disease: "A Newly Recognized Pancreatic Polypeptide: Plasma Levels in Health and Disease" by J. C. Floyd, Jr., S. S. Fajans, S. Pek, and R. E. Chance. *Rec. Prog. Hormone Res.* **33,** 519–570, 1977.
5. Comparative Studies on Pancreatic Polypeptide: No single review article appears available. The interested reader may glean most information from a collation of *Gen. Comp. Endocrinol.* **21,** 485–497, 1973; *J. Endocrinol.* **76,** 449–460, 1978; *Gen. Comp. Endocrinol.* **33,** 518–525, 1977; and *Gen. Comp. Endocrinol.* **34,** 421–427, 1978.

REFERENCES

Adrian, T. E., Besterman, H. S., Cooke, T. J. C., Bloom, S. R., Barnes, A. J. Russell, R. C. G., and Faber, R. G. (1977). *Lancet* **1,** 161–163.

Adrian, T. E., Greenberg, G. R., Besterman, H. S., and Bloom, S. R. (1978a). *Gut* **19,** 907–908.

Adrian, T. E., Bloom, S. R., Hermanson, K., and Iversen, J. (1978b). *Diabetologia* **14,** 413–417.

Adrian, T. E., Besterman, H. S., Mallinson, C. N., Greenberg, G. R., and Bloom, S. R. (1978c). *Gut* **20,** 37–40.

Adrian, T. E., Besterman, H. S., Mallinson, C. N., Garalotis, C., and Bloom, S. R. (1979). *Gut* **20**, 98–101.

Baetens, D., Rufner, C., and Orci, L. (1976). *Experientia* **32**, 785 (Abstr.).

Baetens, D., De Mey, J., and Geots, W. (1977). *Cell Tissue Res.* **185**, 239–246.

Baetens, D., Malaisse-Lagae, F., Perrelet, A., and Orci, L. (1979). *Science* **206**, 1323–1325.

Berger, D., Crowther, R., Floyd, J., Jr., Pek, S., and Fajans, S. (1978a). *J. Clin. Endocrinol. Metab.* **47**, 1183–1188.

Berger, D., Floyd, J. C., Jr., Pek, S., Lampman, R., and Fajans, S. (1978b). *Diabetes* **27** (2), 468 (Abstr.).

Bergstrom, B. H., Loo, S., Hirsch, H. J., Schutzengel, D., and Gabbay, K. H. (1977). *J. Clin. Endocrinol. Metab.* **44**, 795–799.

Bloom, S., Greenberg, G. R., Adrian, T. E., Besterman, H. S., Mallinson, C. N., McCloy, R. F., Chadwick, V. S., and Baron, J. H. (1977). *Irish J. Med. Sci.* **146**(1), 15 (Abstr.).

Boden, G., Master, R. W. Owen, D. E., and Rudnick, M. R. (1980) *J. Clin. Endocrinol. Metab.* **51**, 573–579.

Carr-Locke, D. L., and Track, N. S. (1979). *Lancet* **1**, 151–152.

Chance, R. E., Lin, T. M., Johnson, M. G., Moon, N. E., Evans, D. C., Jones, W. E., and Koffenberger, J. E. (1975). *Endocrinology* **96**, Suppl., 183 (Abstr.).

Chance, R. E., Moon, N. E., and Johnson, M. G. (1979). *In* "Methods of Hormone Radioimmunoassay," 2nd ed., Chapter 33. Academic Press, New York.

Chang, P. J., Noelken, M. E., and Kimmel, J. R. (1980). *Biochem.* **19**, 1832–1837.

Devitt, P., Ayalon, S., Lonovics J., Hejtmancik, K., Rayford, P. L., and Thompson, J. C. (1979). *Physiologist* **22**, 29 (Abstr.).

Duke, G. E., Kimmel, J. R., Redig, P. T., and Pollock, H. G. (1979). *Poult. Sci.* **58**, 239–246.

Falkmer, S., and Stefan, Y. (1978). *Scand. J. Gastroenterol.* **13**, Suppl. 59 (Abstr.).

Feldman, M., Richardson, C. T. Taylor, I. L., and Walsh, J. H. (1979). *J. Clin. Invest.* **63**, 294–298.

Fink, A. S., Floyd, J. C., Jr., and Fiddian-Green, R. G. (1979) *Metabolism* **28**, 339–342.

Fitz-Patrick, D. (1979). *Diabetes* **28**, 349 (Abstr.).

Floyd, J. C., Jr. (1979). *In* "Clinic in Endocrinology and Metabolism" (K. D. Buchanan, (ed.), Vol. 8, pp. 379–399. Saunders, Philadelphia, Pennsylvania.

Floyd, J. C., Jr., and Fajans, S. S. (1976). *Diabetes* **25**, Suppl., 330 (Abstr.).

Floyd, J. C., Jr., Chance, R. E. Hayashi, M., Moon, N. E., and Fajans, S. S. (1975). *Clin. Res.* **23**, 535A (Abstr.).

Floyd, J. C., Jr., Fajans, S. S., and Pek, S. (1976). *Trans. Assoc. Am. Phys.* **89**, 146–158.

Floyd, J. C., Jr., Fajans, S., Pek, S., and Chance, R. E. (1977). *Recent Prog. Horm. Res.* **33**, 519–570.

Gates, R. J., and Lazarus N. R. (1977). *Hormone Res.* **8**, 189–202.

Gepts, W., and De May, J. (1978). *Diabetes* **27**, Suppl., 251–261.

Gepts, W., De May, J., and Marichal-Pipeleers, M. (1977). *Diabetologia* **13**, 27–34.

Gersell, D. J., Greider, M. H., and Gingerich, R. L. (1976). *Diabetes* **25**, Suppl, 364 (Abstr.).

Gersell, D. J., Gingerich, R. L. and Greider, M. H. (1979). *Diabetes* **28**, 11–15.

Gingerich, R. L. (1977). *Diabetes* **26**, 375 (Abstr.).

Gingerich, R., Greider, M., Chance, R., and Johnson, M. (1976) *Diabetes* **25**, Suppl., 329 (Abstr.).

Gingerich, R., Lacy, P. E., Chance, R. E., and Johnson, M. G. (1978a) *Diabetes* **27**, 96–101.

Gingerich, R. L., Gersell, D. J., Greider, M. H., Finke, E. H., and Lacy, P. E. (1978b). *Metabolism* **27**, 1526–1532.

Gingerich, R. L., Hickson, C., Hagberg, J. M., and Winder, W. W. (1979a). *Metabolism* **28**, 1179–1182.

Gingerich, R. L., Nagulesparan, M., and Dye, E. (1979b). *Diabetes* **28**, 404 (Abstr.).

Glaser, B., Vinik, A. I., Sive, A. A., Floyd, J. C., Jr., Fajans, S. S., and Pek, S. (1979). *Diabetes* **28**, 434 (Abstr.).

Goldman, J., Pugh, W., Yuen, A., and Kimmel, J. R. (1978). *Diabetes* **24**, 478 (Abstr.).

Greenberg, G. R., McCloy, R. F., Adrian, T. E., Chadwick, V. S., Baron, J. H., and Bloom, S. R. (1978) *Gut* **19**, A961–962.

Greenberg, G. R., McCloy, R. F., Chadwick, V. S., Adrian, T. E., Baron, J. H., and Bloom, S. R. (1979). *Digest. Dis. Sci.* **24**, 11–14.

Hales, C. N., and Randle, P. J. (1963). *Biochem J.* **88**, 137–146.

Hansen, B. W., Pek, S., and Floyd, J. C., Jr., (1978). *Endocrinology* **102**, Suppl., 196 (Abstr.).

Hayden, L. J. (1976). Ph.D. Dissertation. Univ. Kansas Medical School.

Hazelwood, R. L. (1973). *Am. Zool.* **13**, 699–709.

Hazelwood, R. L., and Langslow, D. R. (1978). *J. Endocrinol.* **76**, 449–459.

Hazelwood, R. L., Turner, S. D., Kimmel, J. R., and Pollock, H. G. (1973). *Gen. Comp. Endocrinol.* **21**, 485–497.

Hedo, J. A., Villanueva, M. L., and Marco, J. (1978). *Endocrinology* **102**, Suppl. 155 (Abstr.).

Hedo, J. A., Villanueva, M. L., and Marco, J. (1979). *J. Clin. Endocrinol. Metab.* **49**, 73–78.

Hermansen, K., and Schwartz, T. W. (1979a). *Endocrinology* **105**, 1469–1474.

Hermansen, K., and Schwartz, T. W. (1979b). *Metabolism* **28**, 1229–1233.

Hilsted, J., Galbo, H., Sonne, B., *et al.* (1980). *Am. J. Physiol.* **239**, G136–140.

Ipp, E., Dobbs, R. E., McCorkle, K., Harris, V., and Unger, R. H. (1978). *Clin. Res.* **26**, 33A (Abstr.).

Johnson, E. M., and Hazelwood, R. L. (1979). *Physiologist* **22**, 63 (Abstr.).

Kanellis, P., Dyckes, D. F., and Hazelwood, R. L. (1979). *Int. J. Pept. Protein Res.* **13**, 201–206.

Kimmel, J. R., and Pollock, H. G. (1975). *Fed. Proc. Fed. Am. Soc. Exp. Biol.* **34**, 454 (Abstr.).

Kimmel, J. R., and Rafferty, M. R. (1980). *Endocrinology* **106**, Suppl., 217 (Abstr.).

Kimmel, J. R., Pollock, H. G., and Hazelwood, R. L. (1968). *Endocrinology* **83**, 1323–1380.

Kimmel, J. R., Pollock, H. G., and Hazelwood, R. L. (1971). *Fed. Proc. Fed. Am. Soc. Exp. Biol.* **30**, 1318 (Abstr.).

Kimmel, J. R., Hayden, L. J., and Pollock, H. G. (1975). *J. Biol. Chem.* **250**, 9369–9376.

Langslow, D. R., and Hazelwood, R. L. (1975). *Diabetologia* **11**, 357 (Abstr.).

Langslow, D. R., Kimmel, J. R., and Pollock, H. G. (1973). *Endocrinology* **93**, 558–565.

Lantigua, R. A., Streck, W. F., Lockwood, D. H., and Jacobs, L. S. (1979). *Endocrinology* **104**, Suppl., 142 (Abstr.).

Larsson, L-I (1976). *Lancet* **2**, 149.

Larsson, L.-I., Sundler, F., Hakanson, R., Pollock, H., and Kimmel, J. (1974a). *Histochemistry* **42**, 377–382.

Larsson, L.-I., Sundler, F., and Hakanson, R. (1975a). *Cell Tissue Res.* **156**, 167–171.

Larsson, L.-I., Sundler, F., and Hakanson, R. (1975b). *Diabetologia* **11**, 357 (Abstr.).

Larsson, L.-I., Sundler, F., and Hakanson, R. (1976a). *Diabetologia* **12**, 211–226.

Larsson, L.-I., Schwartz, T., Lundquist, G., Chance, R., Sundler, F., Rehfeld, J., Grimelius, L., Fahrenkrug, J., Schaffalitzky de Muckadell, O., and Moon, N. (1976b). *Am. J. Pathol.* **85**, 675–684.

Laurentz, D. A., and Hazelwood, R. L. (1979). *Proc. Soc. Exp. Biol. Med.* **160**, 144–149.

Lawrence, A. M., Prinz, R. A., Paloyan, E., and Kokal, W. A. (1979). *Lancet* **1**, 1354.

Levitt, N. S., Sive, A. A., and VanTonder, S. (1979). *Diabetes* **28**, 414 (Abstr.).

Lin, T. M., and Chance, R. E. (1972). *Gastroenterology* **62**, 852 (Abstr.).

Lin, T. M., and Chance, R. E. (1974). *Gastroenterology* **67**, 730–738.

Lin, T. M., Chance, R. E., and Evans, D. (1973). *Gastroenterology* **64**, 865 (Abstr.).

Lin, T. M., Evans, D., and Chance, R. E. (1974. *Gastroenterology* **66**, 852 (Abstr.).

Lin, T. M., Evans, D., Chance, R. E., and Spray, G. F. (1977). *Am J. Physiol.* **232**, E311–E315.

Linare, G., and Linari, M. B. (1976). *Arch. Int. Pharmacol.* **224**, 283–290.

Lonovics, J., Guzman, S., Devitt, P., Hejtmancik, Suddith, R. S., Rayford, P. L., and Thompson, J. C. (1979). *Physiologist* **22**, 79 (Abstr.).

Loren, I., Almets, J., Hakanson, R. and Sundler, F. (1979) *Cell Tissue Res.* **200**, 179–186.

Lundquist, I., Sundler, F., Ahren, B., Alumets, J., and Hakanson, R. (1979). *Endocrinology* **104**, 823–838.

McCumbee, W., and Hazelwood, R. L. (1977). *Gen. Comp. Endocrinol.* **33**, 518–525.

McCumbee, W., and Hazelwood, R. L. (1978). *Gen. Comp. Endocrinol.* **34**, 421–427.

Malaisse-Lagae, F., Carpentier, J. L. Patel, Y. C., Malaisse, W. I., and Orci, L. (1978). *Experientia* **33**, 915–917.

Malaisse-Lagae, F., Stefan, Y., Cox, J., Perrelet, A., and L. Orci (1979). *Diabetologia* **17**, 361–365.

Marco, J., Hedo, J., and Villanueva, M. (1977). *Life Sci.* **21**, 789–792.

Marco, J., Hedo, J., and Villanueva, M. (1978). *J. Clin. Endocrinol. Metab.* **46**, 140–145.

Noelken, M. E., Dyckes, D. F., and Kimmel, J. R. (1977). *Fed. Proc. Fed. Am. Soc. Exp. Biol.* **36**, 838 (Abstr.)

Noelkin, M. E., Chang, P. J., and Kimmel, J. R. (1980). *Biochem. J.* **19**, 1838–1843.

Orci, L., Baetens, D., Ravazolla, M., Stefan, Y., and Malaisse-Lagae, F. (1976). *Life Sci.* **19**, 1811–1816.

Otsuki, M., Sakamoto, C., Maeda, M., Yuu, H., Morita, S., and Baba, S. (1979). *Endocrinology* **105**, 1396–1399.

Parks, D. L., Gingerich, R. L., Jaffe B. M., and Akande, B. (1979). *Am. J. Physiol.* **236**, E488–494.

Pettinga, C. W. (1958). *Biochem. Prep.* **6**, 28–31.

Pelletier, G., and Leclere, R. (1977). *Gastroenterology* **72**, 569–571.

Rattan, R., and Goyal, R. K. (1979). *Gastroenterology* **77**, 672–676.

Polak, J., Adrian, T., Bryant, M., Bloom, S., Heitz, P., and Pearse, A. (1976). *Lancet* **1**, 328–330.

Samols, E., Weir, G. C., Patel, Y. C. Fernandez-Durango, R., Arimura, A., and Loo, S. W. (1977). *Diabetes* **26**, 375 (Abstr.).

Schwartz, T. W., and Rehfeld, J. F. (1977). *Lancet* **1**, 697–698.

Schwartz, T., Stadil, F., Chance, R., Rehfeld, J., Larsson, L-I, and Moon, N. (1976). *Lancet* **1**, 1102–1105.

Schwartz, T. W., Holst, J. J., Fahrenkrug, J., Jensen, S., Nielsen, O. V., Rehfeld, J. F., De Muckadell, O. B., and Stadil, F. (1978). *J. Clin. Invest.* **61**, 781–789.

Schwartz, T., Stenquist, B., Olbe, L., and Stadil, F. (1979a). *Gastroenterology* **76**, 14–19.

Schwartz, T., Stenquist, B., and Olbe, L. (1979b). *Scand. J. Gastroenterol.* **14**, 313–320.

Stagner, J., Samols, E., and Weir, G. (1979) *Endocrinology* **104**, Suppl., 75 (Abstr.).

Stefan, Y., and Falkmer, S. (1978). *Diabetologia* **15**, 272.

Spitz, I. M., Zylber, E., Jersky, J., and Leroith, D. (1979). *Metabolism* **28**, 527–530.

Sundler, F., Hakanson, R., and Larsson, L-I. (1977a). *Cell Tissue Res.* **178**, 303–306.

Sundler, F., Hakanson, R., Lundquist, I., and Larsson, L-I. (1977b). *Cell Tissue Res.* **178**, 307–312.

Taylor, I. L., Walsh, J. H., Rotter, J., and Passaro, E. P. (1977). *Gastroenterology* **72,** 1139–1142.

Taylor, I. L., Feldman, M., Richardson, C. T., and Walsh, J. H. (1978a). *Gastroenterology* **75,** 432–437.

Taylor, I. L., Impicciatore, M., Carter, D. C., and Walsh, J. H. (1978b). *Am. J. Physiol.* **235,** E443–447.

Taylor, I. L., Walsh, J. H., Carter, D., Wood, J., and Grossman, M. I. (1979a). *Gastroenterology* **77,** 714–718.

Taylor, I. L., Solomon, T. E., Walsh, J. H., and Grossman, M. I. (1979b). *Gastroenterology* **76,** 524–528.

Turner, S. D., and Hazelwood, R. L. (1973). *Proc. Soc. Exp. Biol. Med.* **144,** 852–856.

Villanueva, M. L., Hedo, J. A., and Marco, J. (1978). *Proc. Soc. Exp. Biol. Med.* **159,** 245–248.

Wahl, T. O., Schimke, R. N., Kyner, J. L., and Kimmel, J. R. (1979). *Diabetes* **28,** 436 (Abstr.).

Waldhausl, A., Bratusch-Marrain, P., Gasic, S., Korn, A., and Nowotny, P. (1979). *Diabetes* **28,** 352 (Abstr.).

Warner, T. F. C. S., Seo, I. S., Madura, J. A., Polak, J. M., and Pearse, A. G. E. (1980). *Cancer* **46,** 1146–1151.

Weir, G., Samols, E., Loo, S., Patel, Y., and Gabbay, K. H. (1979). *Diabetes* **28,** 35–40.

Wilson, R., Boden, G., and Owen, O. E. (1978). *Endocrinology* **102,** 859–863.

III

PATHOLOGY OF THE ISLETS OF LANGERHANS

13

Islet Changes in Human Diabetes

W. GEPTS

I. HISTORICAL BACKGROUND

Although the diabetic syndrome was recognized early in the history of mankind, it was not until the nineteenth century that its relationship to the

321

The Islets of Langerhans
Copyright © 1981 by Academic Press, Inc.
All rights of reproduction in any form reserved.
ISBN 0–12–187820–1

pancreas was firmly established. In 1845, Bouchardat expressed the opinion, based on autopsy findings, that diabetes was a disease of the pancreas. In 1880, Lancereaux reported the existence in man of a form of diabetes (*diabète maigre ou pancréatique*) which was accompanied by lesions of this organ. Frerichs (1884) similarly stated that there were gross changes in the pancreas in a high percentage of diabetic patients. However, it remained for Von Mering and Minkowski (1889) to demonstrate beyond any doubt the cardinal importance of the pancreas in carbohydrate metabolism by showing that total pancreatectomy in dogs caused severe diabetes.

The endocrine nature of this pancreatic function was proved by Hedon (1892), who showed that the blood sugar remained normal in totally pancreatectomized dogs when part of the pancreas was transplanted subcutaneously or into the spleen, whereas severe diabetes developed as soon as the transplant was removed. Laguesse (1893) located this endocrine function in the peculiar cell groups (*Zellhaufen*) described by Langerhans in 1869, for which he therefore proposed the designation "islands of Langerhans."

Starting from these findings, the early students of the diabetic pancreas (Ssobolew, 1900, 1902; Opie, 1901; Weichselbaum, 1910; for a complete review of these early studies see Kraus, 1929) concentrated their attention on the endocrine pancreatic islets. They reported that in diabetes these islets were frequently abnormal, whereas they appeared unaltered in pancreatic diseases not associated with hyperglycemia. In 1911, Heiberg proclaimed that islet lesions were present in all diabetics and that these lesions afforded an adequate explanation of the disease. The discovery of insulin by Banting and Best in 1922, and the observation that treatment with this hormone apparently was able to correct the metabolic disturbance characteristic of diabetes, seemed to provide decisive confirmation of the pancreatic origin of the disease.

However, the insular theory of diabetes never achieved unanimous acceptance. Several authors denied that islet changes were constantly present in the pancreas of diabetics. It was even emphasized that 30% of diabetics showed no demonstrable pathology in the islets of Langerhans. Moreover, it was also pointed out that the insular changes described in diabetics also occurred in nondiabetics, albeit more rarely.

In the ensuing years, the concept that insulin is not the only regulator of carbohydrate metabolism, but that other hormones, such as growth hormone and glucocorticoids, also play an important role in this respect gradually obtained recognition. Therefore the attention of investigators was diverted from the pancreas to extrapancreatic factors capable of eliciting insulin insufficiency through β-cell exhaustion. Not only hormonal but many other factors were investigated, such as insulin antibodies, excessive destruction of insulin, and anomalies of a supposed protein vehicle of circulating insulin. For none of these factors, however, could a role in the origin of the common types of diabetes be decisively demonstrated.

An important turning point in the history of diabetes research occurred in 1960. That year, Yalow and Berson (1960) described a method for measuring the minute amounts of circulating insulin. With the help of this method it was confirmed that insulin secretion was strongly reduced or completely abolished in juvenile diabetics, but that the insulin levels in many elderly diabetics, far from being lower than those found in nondiabetics, were often higher. However, in these elderly diabetics it was also shown that β cells responded more slowly than those of nondiabetics to the same glucose stimulation. The same radioimmunological technique was applied later to evaluation of the receptors for insulin on the surface of the target cells (Kahn, 1976; De Meyts et al., 1976). These studies revealed that the number of receptors was not fixed but varied under physiological and pathological circumstances, suggesting that defects in the peripheral action of insulin may play a role of variable importance in the pathogenesis of diabetes. In recent years, the application of electron microscopy and immunocytochemistry, the refinement of biochemical techniques and of methods of tissue culture, the phenomenal burgeoning of immunology, further developments in genetics and epidemiology, and many other investigations in the field of clinical and experimental diabetes, have produced a vast amount of new information on the morphology, physiology, and physiopathology of the endocrine pancreas. At the same time, new concepts were proposed. The demonstration of structural specializations of cell membranes (gap and tight junctions) between neighboring islet cells of the same as well as of different types (Orci et al., 1973) inspired the concept of an integrated islet function and of a possible derangement of this function in diabetes (Unger and Orci, 1977). The paracrine system of Feyrter (1952) and the APUD cell system of Pearse (1968, 1978), although still controversial in some of their aspects, have profoundly influenced our thinking in the field of endocrine pathology.

Although little has been added to the remarkable descriptions of the diabetic pancreas published early in this century, a reevaluation of the significance of islet changes in the light of our present understanding of islet physiology and physiopathology appears justified. For many of the classical morphological descriptions we shall rely heavily on several excellent reviews of these subjects (Kraus, 1929; Warren et al. 1966; Volk and Wellmann, 1977).

Although the author, as a pathologist, cannot entirely endorse the view that insulin-dependent diabetes appearing late in life is the same disease as classical juvenile diabetes, the recommendation of the National Diabetes Data Group that the terms "juvenile diabetes" and "maturity-onset diabetes'' be abandoned and replaced, respectively, by ''type I diabetes'' and ''type II diabetes,'' has been largely followed in this chapter.

II. QUANTITATIVE ISLET CHANGES

A. Methodological Problems

A quantitative study of islet tissue is made difficult by its dispersion in a large exocrine gland of which it represents only 1 or 2% in volume. The number and size of the islets, as well as their cytological composition, are not the same in different parts of the pancreas. This heterogeneity is accentuated in diabetes. At least in large mammalian species, precise determinations of the number of islets, of the total volume of islet tissue, and of its principal components are therefore impossible.

B. Reduction in the Number of Islets

Despite the fact that only crude methods could be applied, converging results were obtained by all the pathologists who counted the islets in the pancreases of diabetics. The number of islets is reduced in diabetics, and this reduction is much more pronounced in type I than in type II diabetics (MacLean and Ogilvie, 1955, 1959; Gepts, 1957; Kraus, 1929; Volk and Wellmann, 1977). There have even been reports of alleged aplasia of the islets in young diabetics (Conroy, 1922; Moore, 1936; Dodge and Laurence, 1977).

Although, in view of the converging conclusions, the general trend toward a numerical reduction in the islets in diabetics appears dificult to deny, valid criticism of these studies has been expressed. Indeed, all of them were performed with methods of low specificity and sensitivity. There is little doubt that with these methods many islets escaped detection. This is especially the case in long-standing type I diabetes, in which the islets are almost invariably composed of small cells that were difficult to stain even with the granule-staining techniques of Gomori commonly used before more sensitive immunocytochemical methods became available. Moreover, as for the other quantitative parameters, there was a large degree of overlap in the number of islets in the diabetic and nondiabetic groups.

C. Changes in Islet Size

Considerable variation in the size of the islets exists in the pancreas of normal individuals. The largest diameter of 70% of the islets in mature normal individuals varies between 100 and 225 μm (Heiberg, 1906). Hellmann (1959a) plotted the number of islets in relation to their size; he noted a highly asymmetric curve, the number of islets decreasing progressively with an increase in diameter. According to Burkhardt (1936), islets with a diameter exceeding 500 μm should be considered giant in size, but other authors put the limit at 300 μm (Weichselbaum, 1908) or 400 μm (Warren and LeCompte, 1952).

In diabetics both atrophy and hypertrophy of the islets occur. An increased proportion of small islets is characteristic of the pancreas of type I diabetics, especially those with a disease of long duration (Weichselbaum, 1910; Kraus, 1929; MacLean and Ogilvie, 1959; Gepts, 1965). However, hypertrophic islets have been described in recent-onset as well as in long-standing cases (MacLean and Ogilvie, 1959; Gepts, 1965). According to MacLean and Ogilvie these large islets might result from an insular stimulation of extrapancreatic origin; however, a compensatory hypertrophy of some of the islets as a result of the atrophy of the others is an alternative and more likely explanation.

In a study on the islands of Langerhans in 19 cases of pronounced obesity, Ogilvie (1933) noticed an increase of 65% in the average size of the islets and of 56% in the proportion of islet tissue in the pancreas. These findings are of interest because hyperinsulinism has been demonstrated in many obese individuals.

D. Changes in the Proportion of Islet Tissue in the Pancreas

In view of the crudeness of the applied methods of measurement, remarkably close figures have been obtained by the numerous investigators who have calculated the percentage of endocrine tissue in the pancreatic parenchyma. The proportion of pancreatic tissue occupied by islets in the adult varies between 0.5 and 4% with an average value of 2% (Susman, 1942; MacLean and Ogilvie, 1955; Gepts, 1957; for earlier studies, see Kraus, 1929). In diabetics, this proportion is reduced, and this reduction is more pronounced in type I than in type II diabetics (MacLean and Ogilvie, 1955, 1959; Gepts, 1957, 1965).

E. Changes in the Cytological Composition of the Islets

After preliminary observations by several early students of the islands of Langerhans (Lazarus and Volk, 1962). Lane (1907) and Bensley (1911–1912) were the first to show that the islet cells constituted a heterogeneous population. Using an alcoholic and nonalcoholic fixative, Lane (1907) demonstrated respectively, α and β cells. Subsequently, Bensley (1911–1912) described a method for staining both cell types in a single preparation. In 1931, an additional cell type was described in human islets by Bloom and termed the D cell. The introduction of electron microscopy and especially of immunocytochemistry into the study of islet histology has led to the discovery of other types of cells. Presently, not less than eight different types of cells have been recognized in the pancreatic islets (Solcia *et al.*, 1978; see also Chapter 1). However, in this review of islet pathology in diabetes only the four main types will be taken into consideration: insulin-secreting β cells, glucagon-secreting α cells, somatostatin-secreting D cells, and PP cells, which secrete the pancreatic polypeptide of Kimmel *et al.* (1968, 1971) and Chance (1972).

Additional difficulties have been added to the quantitative studies on the changes in islet cytology in diabetes by the recent demonstration of heterogeneous distribution of the different islet cell types (Larsson *et al.*, 1975a,b; Orci *et al.*, 1976b, 1978; Paulin and Dubois, 1978; Gersell *et al.*, 1979; Baetens *et al.*, 1979; Malaisse-Lagae *et al.*, 1979; Rahier *et al.*, 1979) and of changes in this distribution with aging (Orci *et al.*, 1979). It is generally agreed that PP cells represent the prevailing cell type in the lobules composing the posterior part of the juxtaduodenal segment of the pancreas, whereas these cells are rare in the rest of the pancreas, at least under normal conditions. On the other hand, somatostatin cells are nearly eight times more numerous in infants than in adults in all regions of the pancreas (Orci *et al.*, 1979; Rahier *et al.*, 1980). The physiological significance of the heterogeneous distribution of islet cell types in the pancreas and the instability of the islet cell population throughout life are still poorly understood. However, their importance should not be underestimated in view of the functional and morphological interrelationships shown to exist between islet cells.

All the earlier studies on the changes in cytological composition of the islets in diabetes were performed with staining techniques of limited specificity and without an awareness of the sampling problems. Despite these methodological reservations, a number of conclusions drawn from these studies are still valid:

1. The proportion of β cells is lower in the islets of diabetics than in those of nondiabetics of the same age (Gepts, 1957, 1958; Warren *et al.*, 1966; Volk and Wellmann, 1977).

2. This difference is more marked in type I than in type II diabetics (MacLean and Ogilvie, 1955, 1959; Gepts, 1957, 1965).

3. In type I diabetics, the majority of the islets are composed of non-β cells. β cells can still be found in a few islets in young diabetics who died shortly after the clinical onset of the disease; the number of β cells containing islets decreases rapidly with longer survival.

One remarkable exception to these general rules has been reported by Evans (1972) who described the autopsy findings in a 22-yr-old female insulin-dependent diabetic who died of renal failure after a disease of 9 yr duration. Quantitative studies gave an islet area of 10% and sections stained with Gomori's aldehyde–fuchsin revealed that the majority of the cells in the islets were β cells. The author suggested dyshormonogenesis as a possible explanation for this unusual finding. This is one indication among others that the syndrome of juvenile diabetes may be heterogeneous.

In type II diabetes, numerous studies on the cytological composition of the islets, after staining of the sections with silver impregnation or with one of the Gomori techniques, have been reported (Gepts, 1957, 1958; Seifert, 1959; Lazarus and Volk, 1962; Warren et al., 1966; Volk and Wellmann, 1977). Investigators agree that the percentage of β cells is usually decreased in diabetics. However, they all point out that the cytological composition of the islets is extremely variable in adult diabetics as well as in adult nondiabetics. Although the difference between the two groups is statistically significant, there is a large degree of overlap. In our own study (Gepts, 1957), performed with the chromium hematoxylin technique of Gomori on 95 nondiabetics and 47 diabetics, the proportion of β cells varied between 45 and 90% (average, 60%) in the former, and between 28 and 78% (average, 53%) in the latter group. The variability within each of the groups was probably due to the fact that they were composed of patients who suffered from various diseases in addition to or in the absence of diabetes. Anyhow, it is clear that a decreased proportion of β cells and an increased proportion of non-β cells do not represent specific changes linked to diabetes. Moreover, in all these studies the non-β cells were designated α cells, whereas it has now become clear that they represent a heterogeneous population composed of glucagon-secreting as well as somatostatin- and pancreatic polypeptide-secreting cells. The contribution of these respective cell populations to the increased proportion of non-β cells could not be studied at that time. Only Fujita (1968), using a silver impregnation technique, believed to be specific for α_1 or D cells, has reported an increased proportion of these cells in the islets of type II diabetics.

Only recently have more specific, sensitive staining methods been applied to study of the diabetic pancreas. In the pancreas of two chronic type I diabetics, Orci et al. (1976a) showed that two-thirds of the islet cells were glucagon cells and the remaining one-third somatostatin cells. They were unable to find any insulin cells. In a more recent study (Gepts and De Mey, 1978) on pancreatic specimens from 58 diabetics with onset of the disease before age 40, the following conclusions were reached:

1. β cells are present in small numbers in the pancreas of almost every recent-onset type I diabetic. They can still be found, but in even smaller numbers, in 50% of young diabetics with a survival time between $\frac{1}{2}$ and 10 yr,

and in 18% of diabetics with a disease of longer duration. The few pre-served β cells are as a rule no longer contained within the islets; many of them occur as single cells amid the exocrine cells.

2. The majority of the islets in the pancreas of type I diabetics are com-posed of small cells containing either glucagon or somatostatin. These cells are present in large numbers throughout the course of the disease. As for the insulin cells, their distribution becomes increasingly irregular with time. The glucagon cells in particular occur in large numbers outside the islets.

3. In cases of type I diabetes of long duration, a large proportion of the islets are composed exclusively of PP cells (Gepts *et al.*, 1978). These PP islets often occur in a lobular distribution.

Since this last observation was made on pancreatic samples collected without regard to the heterogeneous distribution of PP cells in the normal pancreas, it remains for further studies performed with a more adequate sampling technique to decide whether hyperplasia of the PP cells is char-acteristic of the pancreas in long-term type I diabetes.

A quantitative study on the cellular composition of the islets, using im-munocytochemical techniques and taking into account the heterogeneous distribution of the different islet cell types, has yet to be performed in type II diabetes. However, it is evident from simple observation that well-granulated β cells remain present in large numbers in the islets of almost every type II diabetic.

F. Changes in the Total Mass of α and β Cells

In view of the many difficulties involved in the quantitative evaluation of the pancreatic endocrine tissue, it is hardly surprising that no precise data are available on the total mass of the respective types of endocrine cells. The inconvenience of this lack of information is attenuated by the fact that only marked changes in total cell mass are likely to be of functional signifi-cance.

In recent-onset type I diabetics the total number of β cells has been estimated to be less than 10% of normal (Gepts 1965). This profound nu-merical reduction is consistent with the severe insulin deficiency character-istic of this type of diabetes. Until recently it was generally assumed that in most cases of type I diabetes the β cells disappeared completely shortly after the onset of the disease. However, recent studies have demonstrated that a significant proportion of insulin-dependent diabetics are able to pre-serve some β cells (Gepts and De Mey, 1978) and some insulin secretion (Block *et al.*, 1972; Heding and Rasmussen, 1976; Ludvigsson and Heding, 1976; Beischer *et al.*, 1976) for many years after clinical onset of the disease.

Crude estimations of the total mass of β and non-β cells have been performed in type II diabetics. A reduction of 50–60% of the normal total mass of β cells was reported in two studies (Maclean and Ogilvie, 1955; Gepts, 1957). The total mass of non-β cells was found to be slightly reduced in one study (Maclean and Ogilvie, 1955) and unchanged in the other (Gepts, 1957). These findings showed that the increased proportion of non-β cells demonstrated in the islets of many maturity-onset diabetics was not due to a true hyperplasia of these cells but to a reduction in the number of β cells. In any event, there exists a considerable overlap of the values in the diabetic and the nondiabetic series.

III. QUALITATIVE ISLET CHANGES

A. Cytological Changes in Islet Cells

1. Hydropic Changes in β Cells

In young diabetics, mainly those who die in a coma after disease of short duration, many β cells are swollen and show complete degranulation and an empty-appearing cytoplasm (Fig. 1). In elderly diabetics this lesion is rarer and affects only a few β cells.

Weichselbaum and Stangl (1901) were the first to describe this change. They attached considerable importance to it, regarding it as degenerative in nature and as a forerunner of islet cell atrophy. They noted that, in its early stages, it was frequently associated with peri- and intrainsular lymphocytic infiltration, and in later stages with fibrosis.

Divergent opinions have been expressed about the nature of this lesion. Earlier pathologists interpreted it as a liquefaction of the cell cytoplasm, but this interpretation became unlikely when Toreson (1951) demonstrated that, at least in many cases, the empty appearance of the cytoplasm was due to glycogen deposits. Lazarus and Volk (1962) have pointed out that vacuolar changes in the β cells either can be the result of a harmless glycogen deposition in the cytoplasm or represent a truly degenerative lesion (ballooning degeneration). In the latter it is associated with nuclear pycnosis. In the pancreas of human diabetics, true hydropic degeneration is not easily distinguished from vacuolization due to glycogen deposits, but it appears to be a rare change.

2. Hypertrophy of the β Cells

In juvenile diabetics with disease of short duration, the few preserved β cells are hypertrophic and largely degranulated (Fig. 2). Their cytoplasm contains irregular particles with vague outlines; these particles were first

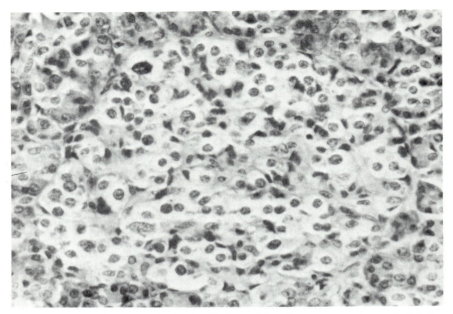

Fig. 1. Hydropic change in the β cells in an islet of a recent-onset type I diabetic. Hemalum–erythrosin–saffron. × 400.

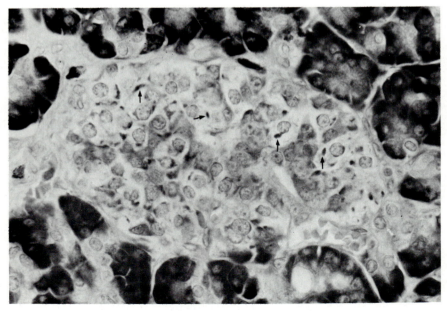

Fig. 2. Hypertrophy of the β cells in an islet of a recent-onset type I diabetic. Arrow indicates *Körnchen*. Toluidine blue–erythrosin. × 600.

described by Weichselbaum (1910) who called them *Körnchen* (granules), but it later became clear that they were not secretion granules. With histochemical techniques, they can be shown to be largely composed of ribonucleic acid (Gepts, 1965). They represent the light microscopic equivalent of a well-developed endoplasmic reticulum, indicative of enhanced protein synthesis.

3. Degranulation of β Cells

In type I diabetics the preserved β cells are markedly degranulated; in older diabetics, β-cell degranulation is much less marked and is often completely absent, especially in patients over 60 yr of age (Bell, 1953). It is striking that, in many type II diabetics, the β cells maintain a normal amount of insulin granules despite the fact that they have been subjected to hyperglycemia for a long time (Fig. 3).

4. Atrophy of Islet Cells

A reduction in the size of islet cells is a constant characteristic of the prevailing type of islets in the pancreas of type I diabetics. These islets (Fig. 4) are of variable size and often irregular in outline; they are composed of thin cords of small cells with dark nuclei and scanty cytoplasm. It was formerly

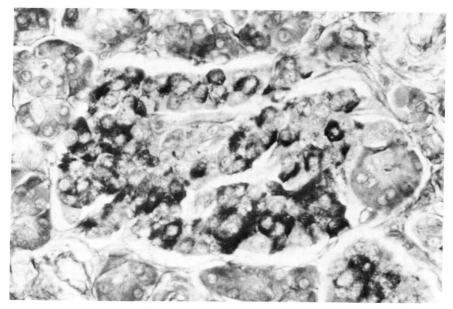

Fig. 3. Islet of a type II diabetic. The β cells are numerous and well granulated. Aldehyde–thionine–trichrome. × 400.

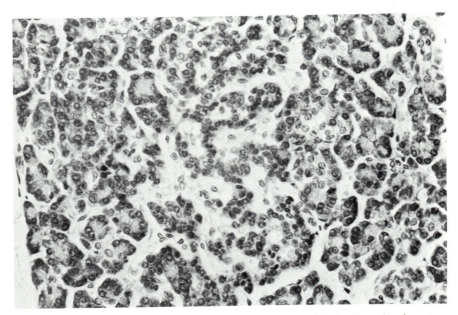

Fig. 4. Atrophy of the islet cells in the pancreas of a type I diabetic. Chromium hematox-ylin–phloxin. × 300.

believed that these atrophic islet cells were undifferentiated or functionally inactive, but the application of immunocytochemical techniques has revealed that they contain either glucagon or somatostatin (Orci *et al.,* 1976a; Gepts and De Mey, 1978).

5. Nuclear Changes

Nuclear hypertrophy is one indication of functional hyperactivity in the small number of surviving pancreatic β cells in recent-onset type I diabetics. In some cases, this simple hypertrophy is replaced by more profound nuclear abnormalities such as irregularity, hyperchromatism, and pycnosis (Gepts, 1965). In cases of longer duration all but a few islets are composed of non-β cells; their nuclei are small and round and contain dense chromatin.

In type II diabetics, β cells show little or no sign of functional hyperactivity, despite the persistent hyperglycemia to which they have been subjected for a long period of time. On the contrary, the nuclei are often small and have dense chromatin. Westermark and Grimelius (1973) performed karyometric studies on islet cells and found a significant decrease in nuclear size in the α and β cells in type II diabetics.

6. Lipid Deposits

The presence of tiny lipid deposits in the cytoplasm of β cells is a normal finding (Ssobolew 1902, Weichselbaum and Stangl, 1901; Like, 1967; Deconinck et al., 1971), especially in older individuals. Weichselbaum and Stangl (1901) claimed that a greater amount of fat was more often present in the β cells of diabetics than in those of nondiabetics of corresponding age, and this finding was confirmed by other authors (Wilder, 1926; Hartroft, 1960). However, an increased amount of fat in the cytoplasm is not a specific change, since this is also found in the β cells of patients dying from conditions unrelated to diabetes (Symmers, 1909; Warren et al., 1966; Gepts, 1972).

7. Perinuclear Inclusions

With the electron microscope, Greider et al. (1977) observed unusual perinuclear inclusions in pancreatic duct cells in 23 diabetic pancreases, in 9 pancreases with islet hyperplasia, and in 10 of 27 pancreases without islet pathology. The origin and significance of these inclusions could not be determined, but the authors suggested that they may be of viral origin or represent a cellular response to an unknown stimulus.

B. Changes in the Islet Stroma

1. Fibrosis of the Islets

Fibrosis is the most frequent lesion in the islets of diabetics. It is present in 60% of diabetics in early-onset as well as maturity-onset cases (Gepts, 1957; Warren et al., 1966). In chronic type I diabetes and in type II diabetes, insular fibrosis is always associated with diffuse pancreatic fibrosis. In late-onset diabetes and partly in chronic juvenile diabetes, islet fibrosis is related to interacinar fibrosis. When interacinar fibrosis involves the endocrine islets, it divides them into lobules of irregular size (Fig. 5). With silver staining techniques it can be seen that an increased number of connective tissue fibrils also develop alongside the islet capillaries (Gepts, 1972).

The cause of interacinar and islet fibrosis does not appear to be singular. Infiltration of the connective tissue with lymphocytes and plasma cells occasionally suggests an inflammatory etiology, but chronic pancreatitis can account for only a small number of cases. Vascular etiology seems to play a predominant role; conspicuous arterio- and arteriolosclerosis is always present in the pancreas of diabetes of long duration. Lazarus and Volk (1962) attributed an important role to islet fibrosis of vascular origin in the pathogenesis of type II diabetes. According to them, the increased amounts

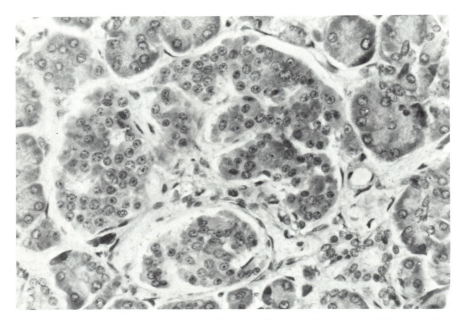

Fig. 5.   Fibrosis in an islet of a type II diabetic. Chromium hematoxylin–phloxin. × 400.

of connective tissue in the islets could represent an obstacle to normal exchanges between β cells and the blood and explain the sluggishness of insulin secretion in elderly diabetics. However, similar degrees of vascular and islet fibrosis also exist in 40% of nondiabetics of the same age. Therefore type II diabetes appears difficult to explain on this basis.

In recent-onset type I diabetes, islet fibrosis is associated with neither vascular changes nor fibrosis of the exocrine tissue. Instead, it affects mainly the seemingly atrophic islets in which a few hydropic β cells are still present but where there is evidence of a collapse of the reticular framework of the islets after the disappearance of a number of β cells (Fig. 6). In many cases lymphocytic infiltration is present in these islets as well. Experimental observations (Toreson *et al.*, 1968; LeCompte *et al.*, 1966) support the role of an immunological process in the development of this type of islet fibrosis. Also, Heydinger and Lacy (1974) produced fibrosis with rare lymphocytic infiltration in the islets of rats by repeated injections of islets isolated from the same species.

2. Hyalinization (Amyloidosis) of the Islets

Hyalinization of the islets consists of deposition of a hyalin substance between the capillaries and the islet cells. As this accumulation increases in

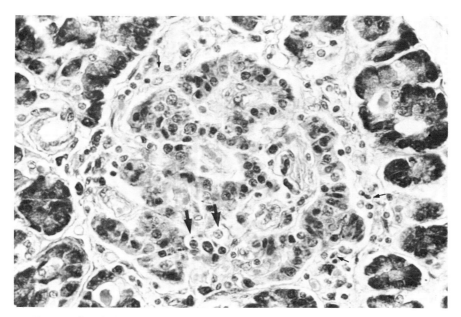

Fig. 6. Fibrosis in an islet of a type I diabetic. Large arrow indicates hydropic β cells; small arrow indicates lymphocytic infiltration. Chromium hematoxylin-phloxin. × 400.

size, it compresses the islet cells, which in an advanced stage may almost completely disappear (Fig. 7).

Hyalinization of the islets in the pancreas of diabetics was first described simultaneously but independently by Opie and by Weichselbaum and Stangle in 1901. It is rare in type I diabetes. In type II diabetes it is much more common, but the figures reported in the literature for its exact frequency vary widely. Weichselbaum (1911) observed it in 28%, Seyfarth (1920) in 20%, and Kraus (1929) in 10% of diabetic pancreases. Ehrlich and Ratner (1961) noticed it in 50% of diabetic patients over 50 yr of age. Bell (1959) observed a progressive increase in the frequency and intensity of islet hyalinization with advancing age. He found no hyalinized islets in diabetics under the age of 20, but noticed them in 10% of subjects between the ages of 20 and 40, in 25% of those between the ages of 40 and 60, and in 46% of those over 60 yr. He also observed that the development of hyalinization of the islets was unrelated to the duration or the severity of the disease. Recently, Westermark and Wilander (1978) reported the surprising fact that they were able to detect islet amyloidosis in the pancreas of every type II diabetic they examined.

The earlier pathologists considered hyalin islets as strongly suggestive, if

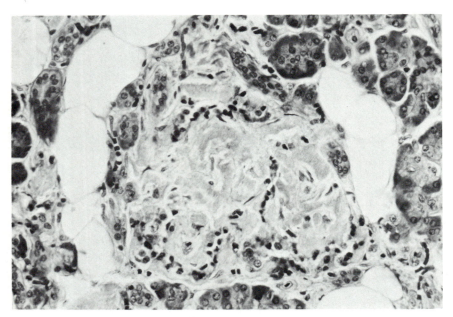

Fig. 7. Extensive hyalinization of an islet in a type II diabetic. Chromium hematoxylin-phloxin. × 260.

not diagnostic, of diabetes, but it was soon recognized that they also occurred (although much more rarely) in the pancreas of elderly nondiabetics (Arey, 1943; Ahronheim, 1943; Bell, 1959). However, since in most of these cases blood sugar levels were not determined and glucose tolerance tests were not carried out, the possibility that these patients may have been unrecognized diabetics cannot be excluded. In any event, the frequency of hyalinized islets is so much greater in diabetics than in nondiabetics that the relationship of this change to the diabetic state cannot be doubted.

Several investigators have stressed the similarity between islet hyalin and amyloid (Warren *et al.,* 1966; Volk and Wellmann, 1977). They have many staining reactions and ultrastructural characteristics in common. Both are metachromatic with methyl violet, stain with Congo red, and exhibit birefringence after this staining. Ultrastructurally hyalin, as well as classical amyloid, is composed of wavy bundles of nonbranching 100-Å-thick fibrils (Lacy, 1964; Kawanashi *et al.,* 1966; Westermark, 1973). On the other hand, differences have been pointed out: acid mucopolysaccharides (Rinehart *et al.,* 1954) and lipids (Hartroft, 1956) are present in islet hyalin but not in systemic amyloid, whereas tryptophan, a typical constituent of amyloid, cannot be demonstrated in islet hyalin (Pearse *et al.,* 1972). Under the electron microscope, the fibrils of islet hyalin are thinner and more wavy than those of ordinary amyloid (Westermark, 1977).

The earlier concept of Opie (1901) that islet hyalin was a product of degeneration of β cells has long been abandoned in view of the fact that it is rarely found in the islets of type I diabetics. The ultrastructural characteristics of islet hyalin argue against the interpretation that it might result from a hyalin transformation of the pericapillary fibrosis or from an intrainsular extension of arteriolar hyalinosis, which are common findings in the pancreas of elderly diabetics (Lacy, 1964). Because deposits identical to islet hyalin also occur in insulin-secreting and in other polypeptide-secreting tumors (Westermark et al., 1977), it has been suggested that it represents a polypeptidic secretion product. Electron microscopic observations are consistent with this view; the fibrils are so oriented as to be perpendicular to the surface of the β cells (Lacy, 1964), and their presence has also been detected in membrane-limited pockets inside these cells (Westermark, 1974). Material that reacts with antibodies to insulin has been extracted from islet hyalin but represents only a small proportion of such material. By submitting crystallized insulin to dilute acid, Westermark (1974) obtained a gel which showed the tinctorial characteristics of amyloid. Recent studies have suggested that amyloid shares antigenic properties with cytoskeletal intermediate (10-nm) filaments (Starger and Goldmann, 1977; Linder et al., 1979). The physiological role of cytoskeletal filaments and the mechanism of their occasional extracellular deposition are still poorly understood. Further investigation of these subjects might prove of interest in view of the secretory deficiency of the β cells in type II diabetes.

3. Calcium Deposits

Selective calcification of the islets of Langerhans is extremely rare. Only a few examples have been reported (Mallory, 1914; Fischer, 1915; Von Meyenburg, 1940; Cotelingam and Hellstrom, 1978). In most of the cases the calcium deposits were located in a hyalinized islet stroma. In the case reported by Fischer (1915) the islets were numerous, many were enlarged, and fibrosis as well as hyalinization was present. Increased islet size and hyalinization were not observed in the case reported by Cotelingam and Hellstrom (1958), but this case was associated with myeloma and hypercalcemia. These authors rightly pointed out that pancreatic islets were not among the tissues affected by metastatic calcification in hypercalcemia. Indeed, all these authors agree that calcification of the islets is of the dystrophic type, but the events leading to islet injury and necrosis are not clear. Although all the reported cases of islet calcification have occurred in diabetics, this lesion clearly represents a secondary phenomenon and is of such rarity that its importance in the explanation of diabetes appears to be negligible.

4. Inflammatory Infiltration of the Islets (Insulitis)

Inflammatory infiltration of the islets (Fig. 8), for which von Meyenburg (1940) coined the name "insulitis," was described early in this century by the first pathologists to perform studies on the pancreas (Kraus, 1929). These investigators regarded it as a rare change and therefore did not attach much importance to it. However, they did notice that inflammatory changes were more common in the islets of young diabetics than in those of elderly patients. Warren and co-workers (Warren and Root, 1925; Stanfield and Warren, 1928) were the first to point out that insulitis occurred almost exclusively in the pancreas of juvenile diabetics. However, this fact was ignored until 1958, when LeCompte again drew attention to it and suggested that insulitis in juvenile diabetics may not be as rare as had been previously reported. This suggestion was confirmed when we detected insulitis in the pancreas of 15 of 22 type I diabetics who died within 6 months of the first symptoms of the disease (Gepts, 1965). Many isolated reports have confirmed the occurrence of lymphocytic infiltration in the pancreatic islets of young diabetics with disease of short duration (Gepts and Pipeleers, 1976). However, the exact frequency of insulitis is still uncertain.

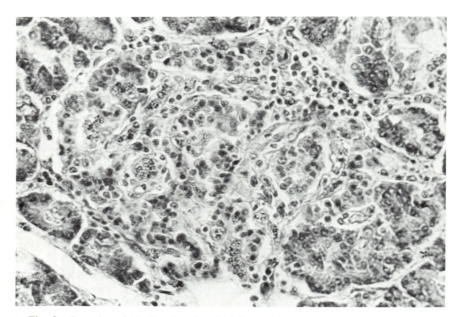

Fig. 8. Lymphocytic infiltration (insulitis) in an islet of a type I diabetic. Chromium hematoxylin–phloxin. × 360.

Ogilvie (1964) reported it as rare. Doniach and Morgan (1973) did not find it at all in a group of 13 recent-onset juvenile diabetics. On the other hand, Junker et al. (1977) noticed it in 6 of 11 young diabetics who died within 2 months after the onset of diabetes.

No straightforward explanation can be offered for these discrepant reports. The inflammatory infiltration of the islets is often discrete and can be missed if not sought specifically. A pancreas with insulitis is never uniformly affected: The lesion may be entirely absent in large areas, while present in a florid phase in a few lobules. Sampling may therefore represent one obstacle to a correct evaluation of the frequency of insulitis. Differences in age distribution of the cases might be another partial explanation, as suggested by Junker et al. (1977). In their and in our material, the majority of diabetics with insulitis were younger than 10 yr of age, whereas Doniach and Morgan (1973) had only one case below this age. However, insulitis also occurs, albeit less frequently, in older insulin-dependent diabetics (Gepts, 1965; LeCompte and Legg, 1972). It is rarely seen in type I diabetics who have survived the first symptoms of the disease for more than a year.

Insulitis has also been described in an infant with a cytomegalic virus infection (Hultquist et al , 1973). Another case report records the presence of insulitis accompanied by structures suggestive of viral particles (Goldman et al., 1976). Lymphocytic infiltration of the islets has also been observed in spontaneously diabetic animals namely, in cows (Christensen and Schambye, 1950; Barboni and Manocchio, 1962), in a cat (Gepts and Toussaint, 1967), and in rats (Nakhooda et al., 1977; Rossini et al., 1979; Like et al., 1979).

In the majority of cases, the inflammatory infiltrate is composed of lymphocytes, occasionally with a few larger cells, perhaps macrophages and mast cells. A few cases have been reported in which the cellular infiltrate consisted predominantly of polymorphonuclear leukocytes. It should be emphasized that, in many cases, the inflammatory cells do not invade the islets but remain localized at their periphery (Fig. 9). Sometimes the affected islets are large and predominantly composed of hypertrophic β cells, but more often they begin to show the pattern of cords of small cells, with few or no β cells, incipient collapse of the insular framework and fibrosis (Fig. 6).

C. Regeneration

1. Mitotic Divisions of Islet Cells

Despite the intense stimulation as evidenced by the cytological appearance of the surviving β cells in the pancreas of recent-onset juvenile

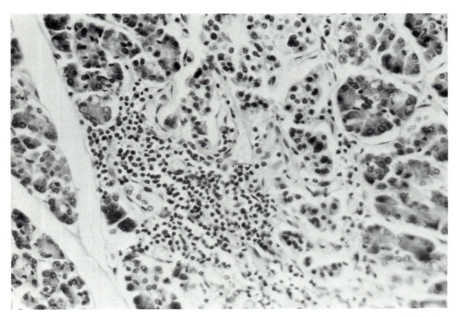

Fig. 9. Lymphocytic infiltration localized at the periphery of an islet in a type I diabetic. Hemalum–erythrosin–saffron. × 360.

diabetics, mitoses are extremely rare. On the other hand, in nondiabetics and in elderly diabetics, mitoses may appear in relatively large numbers under certain pathological conditions (Lecompte and Merriam, 1962; Potvliege *et al.*, 1963).

2. Islet Neoformation

Islet regeneration or neoformation is not a specific characteristic of the diabetic pancreas, and it is more prominent in the pancreas of recent-onset juvenile diabetes (Gepts, 1965). It is represented by a proliferation and endocrine differentiation of ductal and ductular cells (Fig. 10). The newly formed islets are at first predominantly composed of β cells; α and D cells increase in number later on (Gepts and De Mey, 1978). These foci of islet regeneration are irregularly distributed in the pancreas: they may appear in large numbers in a few lobules and may be completely absent in the rest of the pancreas. In one such example, many of the newly formed islets were heavily infiltrated with lymphocytes (Fig. 11), whereas such infiltrates were much more discrete in islets devoid of β cells. With prolonged duration of disease, images of focal islet neoformation become increasingly rare.

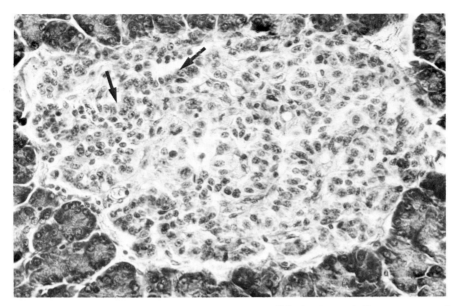

Fig. 10. Newly formed islet in a recent-onset type I diabetic. Arrows indicate remnants of ductal epithelium. Alum hematoxylin–phloxin. × 400.

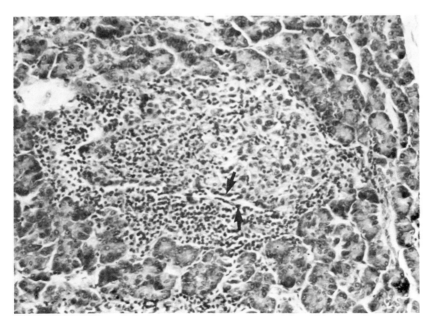

Fig. 11. Severe insulitis affecting an islet in an area of islet neoformation. Arrows indicate remnants of ductal epithelium. Chromium hematoxylin–phloxin. × 320.

IV. CHANGES IN THE EXOCRINE PANCREAS

There are no characteristic macroscopic changes in the pancreas in idiopathic diabetes. In type I diabetics with disease of long duration, the pancreas is often reduced in weight. This reduction cannot be attributed to congenital hypoplasia, because in patients who died shortly after the onset of diabetes the pancreatic weight was normal (Gepts, 1965). In type II diabetics, the weight of the pancreas is quite variable; fatty infiltration and fibrosis are common, but no more so than in nondiabetics. Lipomatosis appears to be more closely related to obesity than to diabetes.

In acute cases of juvenile diabetes, focal lesions of necrotizing pancreatitis are common (Gepts, 1965). They are usually centered around distended ducts. They probably represent terminal complications resulting from dehydration in comatose patients.

Intralobular and perilobular sclerosis, whether or not accompanied by focal inflammatory infiltrates, is a regular finding in chronic type I as well as in type II diabetes. In type I diabetes of long duration the acinar cells are usually small and have relatively few zymogen granules. In a study on the exocrine pancreatic function in type I diabetics, Frier *et al.* (1976) reported a reduction in the secretory capacity in 80% of the patients; the severity of the reduction was related to the duration of the diabetes.

In both chronic type I and type II diabetes, lesions of arterio- and arteriolosclerosis are common. Although these vascular changes are on the average more severe in elderly diabetics than in nondiabetics of the same age, the difference is not clear-cut enough for one to conclude that they play a role in the development of diabetes.

Olsen (1978) found a significantly higher incidence of chronic inflammation in the pancreas of elderly diabetics than in nondiabetics. The lesions were always mild and had not produced clinical symptoms. However, a slight deterioration of the exocrine pancreatic function in maturity-onset diabetes has been reported (Barron and Nabarro, 1972).

V. MORPHOLOGICAL ASPECTS OF THE PATHOGENESIS OF HUMAN DIABETES

In spite of the fact that great variation is observed in the appearance of the endocrine pancreas in diabetes, two distinct pathological entities emerge roughly corresponding to the classical subdivision of idiopathic diabetes into a juvenile-onset and a maturity-onset type. Impressive evidence has been accumulating in recent years that these two types of diabetes differ in etiology, genetic background, and pathogenesis.

The subdivision of idiopathic diabetes on the basis of age at onset has been criticized. It is true that insulin-dependent diabetes sometimes develops late in life; conversely, in young individuals a milder type of disease may occur. However, in most cases of maturity-onset diabetes, including many genuine insulin-requiring cases, the appearance of the endocrine pancreas is distinctly different from that in early-onset cases, both quantitatively and qualitatively.

A. Early-Onset Insulin-Dependent Diabetes (Type I Diabetes, Juvenile Diabetes)

Classical type I diabetes is characterized by a severe insulin deficiency resulting from a profound numerical reduction in β cells. At the time of clinical onset, the number of β cells is reduced to less than 10% of normal, and this number decreases further with time. In most patients the β cells disappear completely, but in a significant number of cases a few β cells survive for many years (Gepts and De Mey, 1958). These morphological findings are consistent with clinical studies performed with C-peptide radioimmunoassay, which have followed the secretory capacity of the β cells in a number of juvenile diabetics and have demonstrated the preservation of some β-cell function for several years after clinical manifestation of disease (Block et al., 1973; Heding and Rasmussen, 1975; Beischer et al., 1976; Ludvigsson et al., 1977).

The cause of the progressive disappearance of β cells from the pancreas of young diabetics has not yet been entirely elucidated. Whether this cause is the same in all cases of juvenile diabetes appears questionable. Pathological observations suggest that in at least some cases β cells are destroyed by an inflammatory process which selectively affects the pancreatic islets (insulitis). The proportion of cases of juvenile diabetes in which insulitis is responsible for the destruction of β cells remains uncertain, because the frequency of this lesion is still controversial. In some studies (Gepts, 1965; Junker et al., 1977) it has been reported as a frequent finding, and in others it has been stated to be rare (Ogilvie, 1964) or could not be detected at all (Doniach and Morgan, 1973). Recently, cases of insulin-dependent diabetes have been described after accidental or suicidal ingestion of a rodenticide (Prosser and Karam, 1978; Pont et al., 1979); severe lesions of the β cells were found in autopsy cases, but no insulitis was apparent. In light of these reports and of experimental work with alloxan and streptozotocin, alternative mechanisms of β-cell destruction by still unidentified toxic agents must be considered a possibility (see chapter 15).

Insulitis has generated considerable interest in recent years because it might offer a clue to the etiology of juvenile diabetes. Unfortunately, lymphocytic infiltration is a change of low specificity, which occurs in a variety of pathological conditions of unrelated etiology. In the case of insulitis, three possible etiologies are commonly favored at the present time: (1) Insulitis results directly from a viral infection of the β cells; (2) it is the expression of an autoimmune reaction, and (3) it results from an autoimmune reaction triggered by a viral infection. The clinical, epidemiological, and experimental evidence supporting each of these hypotheses has been thoroughly reviewed in Chapters 16 and 17. Pathological evidence suggests that viral infections and autoimmune reactions may play a part of variable importance in the etiology of juvenile diabetes.

At one end of the spectrum there are cases in which viruses seem to be directly responsible for the destruction of β cells. The number of well-documented cases of this type is extremely small. These include the case of a 5-yr-old girl who developed severe myocarditis and insulin-dependent diabetes 19 days after operative suture of an atrial septum defect (Gladisch *et al.,* 1976), three cases of acute ketotic diabetes with myocarditis of suspected viral etiology described by Gibbs (1974), and one case of a 10-yr-old boy suffering from an influenza-like illness (Yoon *et al.,* 1979) (see Chapter 16). In all cases severe diabetes was present, with evidence of infection of islet cells with coxsackie virus. At the autopsy, insulitis and necrosis of the β cells were found. However, these cases do not prove that the lymphocytes composing the inflammatory infiltrate in the patient's islets were responsible for destruction of the β cells. In viral models of experimental diabetes (Craighead, 1977) and *in vitro* (Yoon *et al.,* 1978; Prince *et al.,* 1978), β-cell necrosis can occur in the absence of lymphocytes. Since antibodies to coxsackie B_4 are present in a large proportion of the population, it is clear that this virus cannot be a common cause of acute-onset diabetes and that other factors must play a role in its pathogenicity.

Apart from these rare cases of fulminant viral infection associated with acute diabetes, there is a much larger group in which the disease has a more insidious onset, characterized by progressive weight loss, polydipsia, and polyuria. In the past such cases often remained undiagnosed until, as a result of some trivial infection, the patient developed ketoacidosis and coma. When death occurs, which fortunately no longer happens that often nowadays, the pancreas shows clear evidence of a pathological process that has been smoldering subclinically for some time. Indeed, nearly all the islets have an abnormal appearance. Some of them still contain β cells but show collapse of their framework and incipient fibrosis. The majority of the islets are composed of thin cords of small cells which, with immunocytochemical techniques, appear to be α or D cells; β cells are no longer present. Insulitis, when present in such cases, predominantly affects the β-cell-containing islets; after the disappearance of the β cells, it is much more discrete or totally absent in the residual islets. These observations suggest that the lymphocytes of insulitis have been attracted by some antigen specifically present in β cells. The precise nature of this antigen is unknown. Cell-mediated (Nerup et al., 1971) and humoral (Bottazzo et al., 1974) autoimmunity have been well documented in insulin-dependent early-onset diabetes. The respective parts played by these immune reactions in development of the disease are not yet clear. A pathogenic role for islet cell antibodies is unlikely, since these antibodies react with all types of endocrine islet cells and only the β cells are destroyed. Raised levels of K (killer lymphocyte) cells have been found in recent-onset juvenile diabetes (Pozilli et al., 1979); these levels returned to normal in chldren who had had diabetes for more than a year. Lymphocytes from juvenile diabetes have been found to kill cultured human insulinoma cells (Huang and Maclaren, 1976). These and other findings are consistent with the hypothesis that immune mechanisms contribute to the destruction of β cells, although the precise mechanism of this effect remains to be clarified.

Experimental studies (Logothetopoulos and Bell, 1966; Marx et al., 1970; Logothetopoulos et al., 1970; Logothetopoulos, 1972; Hellerström et al., 1976) have shown that pancreatic tissue is capable of regenerating islets, particularly β cells. However, this capacity is not unlimited, and species differences have been demonstrated. In rats (Marx et al., 1970) subtotal pancreatectomy is followed by intense islet regeneration, but this decreases as time goes on, and after 1 or 2 months permanent diabetes develops. In steroid-treated rabbits, Lazarus and Volk (1959) have observed increased mitotic activity of β cells, ductular proliferation, and marked hyperplasia. In dogs and cats, the regenerative capacity appears to be much more limited, and in these species subtotal pancreatectomy rapidly leads to permanent diabetes (Homans, 1915; Allen, 1922). In humans, the capability of the islet tissue to regenerate is not known. Islet regeneration is a prominent feature of the pancreas of some juvenile diabetics in the early clinical stage of the disease and probably explains the temporary remission which often follows the clinical manifestation. As time goes by, images of islet regeneration become more difficult to find and eventually disappear. In animals, a strong genetic influence on the capacity for regeneration of β cells has been demonstrated (Boquist et al., 1974; Hellerström et al., 1976), and this may also be the case in man. The clinical manifestation of type I diabetes may well be determined by exhaustion of the regenerative capacity of the pancreas under the effects of continuous immune aggression of the β cells.

Paradoxical hyperglucagonemia is a characteristic feature of juvenile diabetes (Unger, 1976) (see Chapter 18). In view of the classical concept of total islet atrophy in the pancreas of chronic juvenile diabetics, the source of the high levels of circulating glucagon has for some time remained problematic. An extrapancreatic source was suggested by the observation that totally depancreatized dogs maintained high levels of serum glucagon believed to be produced by α cells located in the fundic part of the gastric mucosa (Baetens *et al.*, 1976). In man, however, very few if any pancreatic glucagon cells can be detected in the gastrointestinal mucosa (Larsson *et al.*, 1975c; Grimelius *et al.*, 1976). This apparent discrepancy has now been resolved by the demonstration, with new immunocytochemical techniques, that the seemingly atrophic islets in the pancreas of juvenile diabetics are actually composed of cells actively secreting glucagon or somatostatin and that these cells are preserved in large numbers throughout the course of the disease (Orci *et al.*, 1976a; Gepts and De Mey, 1978). The observation that glucagon cells are no longer always contained within the islets, but are dispersed between the exocrine cells, could perhaps account for the functional abnormality of these cells in type I diabetes (Unger, 1976).

B. Type II Diabetes (Insulin-Independent Diabetes, Maturity-Onset Diabetes)

There have been conflicting reports as to whether a deficiency in insulin secretion plays a primary role in the pathogenesis of type II diabetes. It has been repeatedly shown that circulating insulin levels are often higher in late-onset diabetics than in nondiabetics of corresponding age. In many elderly diabetics, amounts of extractable insulin similar to those present in nondiabetics can be found in the pancreas (Hartroft and Wrenshall, 1955), but is has also been shown that, in type II diabetics, insulin rises at a slower rate than in nondiabetics in response to the same glucose stimulation (Yalow and Berson, 1960; Pfeiffer, 1963; Cerasi and Luft, 1967) and that the insulin secretion is not always correctly adjusted to the high levels of glycemia (Seltzer *et al.*, 1967).

In spite of the great variety of changes found in the pancreas in type II diabetics, pathology can offer no explanation for this secretory deficiency. Although a numerical reduction in β cells can be demonstrated in many elderly diabetics, this reduction is much more moderate than in juvenile diabetics. On the average, it amounts to only 50% of normal. This reduction is in itself insufficient to account for the diabetes since, in experimental animals, 80–90% of the pancreas must be removed in order for the disease to develop. Indeed, the same amount of β-cell reduction has been found in many elderly individuals without clinical evidence of diabetes. However, it has been well demonstrated that there is a deterioration of glucose tolerance with age (Burgess, 1976; Reaven, 1977; Williams, 1978).

Therefore it is not always easy to decide whether a degree of glucose intolerance at a certain age represents true diabetes or an acceptable physiological aging process.

Perhaps the most striking abnormality of the islets in type II diabetics is that the β cells fail to develop the cytological evidence of hyperactivity which would be expected from them if they were attempting to compensate for their numerical inferiority and the high levels of glycemia to which they have been subjected over a long period of time. On the contrary, and in striking constrast to the β cells of recent-onset type I diabetics, the β cells of type II diabetics are often small and well-granulated. In a study on 995 diabetic pancreases, Bell (1953) found β-cell degranulation in all patients under the age of 20 but only in 34% of those over 60 yr of age. This pathological observation strongly supports the concept that type II diabetes at least partly results from failure of the β cells to recognize adequately the stimulus of hyperglycemia.

Pathologists have attempted to attribute this failure of β-cell response to a decreased availability of glucose to the islets as a result of either vascular sclerosis or islet fibrosis. But these changes are neither constant nor specific. Moreover, they follow rather than precede the diabetic state. Perhaps more importance should be attached in this respect to islet hyalinosis, since Westermark and Wilander (1978) have reported that they have detected this change in the pancreas of every elderly diabetic they examined. They emphasize that β cells close to hyalin deposits are usually heavily granulated; they believe that β cells involved in amyloid (hyalin) secretion are not capable of releasing insulin normally. The significance of Westermark and Wilander's observation is slightly diminished by the fact that they also found islet hyalin in 60% of aged nondiabetics. However, it has already been pointed out that there is no sharp border between the secretory dysfunction of the β cells in overt type II diabetes and the reduced glucose tolerance of aging individuals. Recent biochemical and morphological investigations have illustrated the role of fibrillary proteins in the cytoskeleton, in cellular motility, and in intracellular transport of secretory products. Linder et al. (1979) have recently demonstrated that cytoskeletal intermediate (10-nm) filaments have staining characteristics identical to those of amyloid. If this finding could be applied to islet amyloid, it would link the secretory dysfunction of the β cells in type II diabetes to some abnormality in the intracellular organization of these cells.

It has been pointed out that decreased sensitivity of β cells to glucose does not occur in man only. It has been demonstrated also in aging rats, *in vitro* as well as *in vivo* (Gommers, 1971; Andres and Tobin, 1975; Hauser *et al.*, 1975; Gold *et al.*, 1976; Kitahara and Adelman, 1979; Reaven *et al.*,

1979). It has likewise been impossible to establish a precise anatomical basis for this phenomenon in rats. Hellman (1959b) and Remacle *et al.* (1977) have shown that, in rats, increasing age results in an increase in islet tissue mass. Reaven *et al.* (1979) have confirmed this finding and demonstrated that this hyperplasia is due to an absolute increase in the number of β cells. Kitihara and Adelman (1979) found a diminished functional capacity in small islets and a compensatory increase in the proportion of larger islets in older rats. An ultrastructural stereological study on β cells (Remacle *et al.*, 1977, 1980; Delaere *et al.*, 1978) revealed decreased development of the endoplasmic reticulum and of the Golgi apparatus (the organelles involved in insulin synthesis) in senescent rats. The same findings were described in the β cells of human type II diabetics by Kawanishi *et al.* (1966), whereas Lacy (1964) found no differences between normal β cells and those of elderly diabetics.

A relative preponderance of α cells in the islets of type II diabetics has been demonstrated by many investigators. This preponderance results not from a true hyperplasia of these cells as contended by Ferner (1972) but from a reduction in the number of β cells (Maclean and Ogilvie, 1955; Gepts, 1957). However, in light of the possible physiological importance of an intercellular relationship within the islets (Orci and Unger, 1977), it could be argued than even a relative preponderance of α cells might be responsible for the secretory dysfunction of the islets in type II diabetes. But the same abnormality in the cytological composition of the pancreatic islets has been demonstrated in elderly nondiabetics as well. However, it should be pointed out that all earlier cytological studies on pancreatic islets were performed with nonspecific staining methods which were unable to distinguish the different types of non-β cells. The possible importance of disturbed intercellular relationships within the pancreatic islets in the etiology of type II diabetes must therefore await renewed investigations with more specific staining techniques and more refined stereological methods, and with an increased awareness of the heterogeneous distribution of the endocrine cells in the pancreas.

Recent research has clarified some of the many steps involved in the biosynthesis, storage, and release of insulin (Gepts and Pipeleers, 1976; Lacy, 1977). Several potential sites of defects in the cellular machinery could be responsible for the secretory dysfunction of the β cells in type II diabetes: deficient glucoreceptors in the β cell membrane, a defective adenylate cyclase system, impairment of calcium flux into the β cells, and last but not least derangement of the microtubule–microfilament system. It remains for future research to determine which of these factors is actually responsible for human insulin-independent diabetes.

C. Late-Onset Insulin-Dependent Diabetes

There are cases of genuine insulin-dependent diabetes, developing in elderly individuals, in which the pancreatic islets do not show the profound alterations characteristic of type I diabetes (W. Gepts, unpublished). In some of the cases, insulin dependency appears to have been triggered by some infection or vascular complication. However, there are other cases in which high insulin requirements had been present for years. In some of these cases, I found numerous islets containing many well-granulated β cells. Identical observations were described by Evans (1972) in a 22-yr-old female insulin-dependent diabetic who died of renal failure after a disease of 9 yr duration. Such observations suggest that a severe degree of functional deficiency of the β cells, rather than a destruction of these cells, may be responsible for some cases of insulin-dependent diabetes.

D. Secondary Diabetes

In this subclass, diabetes forms part of certain other conditions and syndromes that have many clinical features not generally associated with the diabetic state (National Diabetes Data Group, 1979). It represents a very large and heterogeneous group in which an etiological relationship between the disease or syndrome and the diabetes is evident in only a small minority of cases. In the majority of these varieties of diabetes, the information on the pancreatic changes associated with glucose intolerance is either incomplete, confusing, or lacking entirely. Only the diabetes occurring with pancreatitis and with hemochromatosis will be briefly considered here.

1. Pancreatitis and Diabetes

Severe pancreatitis is often associated with glucose intolerance. In acute pancreatitis this association is not surprising, because the pancreatic gland is nearly entirely destroyed by enzymatic digestion. Yet, hyperglycemia is not a constant feature of acute pancreatitis, and when diabetes does develop, it is often mild, nonketotic, and reversible. In patients who have survived the acute phase, permanent diabetes is present in only 2–10% of the cases (Barbier et al., 1967; Dérot et al., 1970)

Chronic pancreatitis only rarely starts with an acute phase. In the Western world, alcoholism is the most important etiological factor in chronic relapsing calcifying pancreatitis (Sarles, 1974). In tropical countries an association of malnutrition and food cyanogens (tapioca) seems to play a predominant role (Volk and Wellmann, 1977; McMillan and Geevarghese, 1979). The pathological changes seem to be identical in the two etiological varieties. Diffuse inter- and intralobular sclerosis, inspissated calcified plugs in the excretory ducts, more-or-less advanced acinar atrophy, and widespread inflammatory infiltrates are the most prominent features. Because of the extensive parenchymal sclerosis, resulting in pronounced architectural derangement, quantitative studies on the endocrine tissue are even more difficult to perform than in normal individuals or in cases of idiopathic diabetes. Many authors have described hypertrophy, hyperplasia, and neoformation of islets (Sarles and Sarles, 1964; Barbier *et al.*, 1967; Seifert, 1966; Potet *et al.*, 1970). Klöppel *et al.* (1978) performed a careful immunocytochemical quantification of the distribution of the four principal endocrine cell types in six cases of severe primary chronic pancreatitis, in six cases of chronic pancreatitis secondary to duct obstruction by a carcinoma, and in six nondiabetic control pancreases. They found a decrease in the number of β cells and an increase in the number of α cells in the cases of both primary and of secondary pancreatitis. The number of PP cells was significantly increased in primary chronic pancreatitis only. The authors consider the hyperplasia of α and PP cells a secondary phenomenon due to the loss of β cells. An impairment in PP secretion has been demonstrated in chronic pancreatitis (Häcki *et al.*, 1977; Sive *et al.*, 1978), suggesting a functional defect in the hyperplastic PP cells. According to Seifert and Klöppel (1974) the degree of pancreatic sclerosis determines the severity of the insulin deficiency and the resulting diabetic state. In cases showing only mild chronic pancreatitis but overt diabetes, an additional genetic predisposition to diabetes might be present.

2. Hemochromatosis and Diabetes

According to Sheldon (1935) diabetes is present in 80% of patients with hemochromatosis. In this metabolic disease, the pancreas is characterized by brown pigmentation and a firm consistency. Histologically, there is marked inter- and intralobular sclerosis with a variable degree of acinar atrophy. The iron pigment, mainly hemosiderin, is predominantly deposited in the ductal and acinar cells and in the connective tissue. The islets of Langerhans are variably affected, but generally less than the other components of the pancreatic tissue. Hartroft (1956) was the first to point out that the pigment was deposited almost exclusively in the β cells, whereas it spares the α cells. This finding was recently confirmed in our laboratory (F. Warson and W. Gepts, unpublished) with the aid of a combination of a histochemical reaction for hemosiderin (Perls) and an immunocytochemical demonstration of the four principal islet cell types. Iron pigment was found only in β cells, but not in α, D, or PP cells. On the other hand, we could not confirm the finding of Hartroft (1956) and MacGavran and Hartroft (1956) that the α cells were markedly reduced in number in the islets of patients with hemochromatosis. In our cases, the proportion of α cells was about 40%, a figure at the upper limits of the range of variation in diabetics and nondiabetics of same age. Neither could we find, contrary to McGavran and Hartroft (1956), an inverse relationship between the degree of pigmentation and β-cell granulation. Degranulation of β cells may occur without pigment deposition. Bell (1955) reported that hyalin deposits were rare in the islets of patients with hemochromatosis.

The etiology of diabetes in hemochromatosis has not been satisfactorily explained as yet. Bell (1955) firmly rejected the idea that it might result from destruction of the β cells by intracellular iron deposits. Indeed, there is no relationship between the degree of pigmentation and the severity of the diabetes. There are cases of hemochromatotic diabetes in which the islets show only minor changes. Clinical and biological observations (Saddi et al., 1978) suggest that in such cases an additional predisposition to diabetes might be present.

ACKNOWLEDGMENTS

The work by the author included in this chapter was supported by the Nationaal Fonds voor Geneeskundig Wetenschppelijk Onderzoek and by the Nationale Banke van België.

The author is indebted to Ms. Nicole Buelens, Ms. Marie-Jeanne de Cock, and Ms. Sonja Pieters for expert technical and secretarial assistance, and to Mr. Paul Alpert for his thorough proofreading of the manuscript.

REFERENCES

Ahronheim, J. H. (1943). Am. J. Pathol. 19, 873–882.
Allen, F. M. (1922). J. Metab. Res. 1, 5–41.
Andres, R., and Tobin, J. D. (1975). Adv. Exp. Biol. Med. 61, 239–249.
Arey, J. B. (1943). Arch. Pathol. 36, 32–38.
Baetens, D., Rufener, C., Unger, R. Renold, A., and Orci, L. (1976). C. R. Acad. Sci. 282, 195–197.
Baetens, D., Malaisse-Lagae, F., Perrelet, A., and Orci, L. (1979). Nature (London) 206, 1323–1325.
Barbier, P., Berge, S., and Jacobs, E. (1967). Acta Gastroenterol. Belgica 30, 329–342.
Barboni, E., and Manocchio, I. (1962). Arch. Vet. Ital. 13, 477–489.
Barron, J. H., and Nabarro, J. D. N. (1972). Br. Med. J. 4, 25–27.
Beischer, W., Rapis, S., Keller, L., Heinze, E., Schröder, D. E., and Pfeiffer, E. F. (1976). Diabetes 25, Suppl , 322 (Abstr.).
Bell, E. T. (1953). Diabetes 2, 125–129.
Bell, E. T. (1955). Diabetes 4, 435–446.

Bell, E. T. (1959). *Am. J. Pathol.* **35**, 801–805.

Bensley, R. R. (1911–1912). *Am. J. Anat.* **12**, 297–388.

Block, M. B., Mako, M. E., Steiner, D. F., and Rubenstein, H. (1972). *J. Clin. Endocr.* **35**, 402–406.

Bloom, W. (1931). *Anat. Rec.* **49**, 363–371.

Boquist, L., Hellmann, B., Lernmark, A., and Täljedal, I. B. (1974). *J. Cell. Biol.* **62**, 77–89.

Bottazzo, G. F., Florin-Christensen, A., and Doniach, D. (1974) *Lancet* **2**, 1279

Bouchardat, A. (1845). Quoted by Kraus, E. J. (1929).

Burgess, J. A. (1976). *In* "Hypothalamus, Pituitary, and Aging" (A. V. Everett and J. A. Burgess, eds.), p. 497. Thomas, Springfield, Illinois.

Burkhardt, L. W. (1936). *Virchows Arch.* **296**, 655.

Cerasi, E., and Luft, R. (1967). *Acta Endocrinol.* **55**, 278–304.

Chance, R. E. (1972). *Diabetes* **21**, Suppl. 2, 536.

Christensen, N. O., and Schambye, P. (1950). *Nord. Vet. Med.* **2**, 863–900.

Conroy, M. J. (1922). *J. Metab. Res.* **2**, 367–384.

Cotelingam, J. D., and Hellstrom, H. R. (1978). *Diabetes* **27**, 620–624.

Craighead, J. E. (1977). *In* "The Diabetic Pancreas" (B. W. Volk and K. F. Wellmann, eds.), p. 467. Plenum, New York.

Deconinck, J., Potvliege, P. R., and Gepts, W. (1971). *Diabetologia* **7**, 266–282.

Delaere, P., Remacle, C., and De Clercq, L. (1978). *Diabetologia* **15**, 226.

De Meyts, P., Bianco, A. R., and Roth, J. (1976). *J. Biol. Chem.* **251**, 1877–1888.

Dérot, M., Bour, H., Tutin, M., and Grand, G. (1970). *Diabète* **18**, 93–96.

Dodge, J. A., and Laurence, K. M. (1977). *Arch. Dis. Child.* **52**, 411–413.

Doniach, I., and Morgan, A. G. (1973). *Clin. Endocrinol.* **2**, 233–248.

Ehrlich, J. C., and Ratner, J. M. (1961). *Am. J. Pathol.* **38**, 49–59.

Evans, D. J. (1972). *Diabetes* **21**, 114–116.

Ferner, H. (1952). "Das Inselsystem des Pankreas." Thieme, Stuttgart.

Feyrter, F. (1952). *Frankf. Z. Pathol.* **63**, 259–266.

Fischer, B. (1915). *Frankf. Z. Pathol.* **17**, 218–275.

Frier, B. M., Saunders, J. H. B., Wormsley, K. G., and Boucher, I. A. D. (1976). *Gut* **17**, 685–691.

Frerichs, F. T. (1884). "Über den Diabetes." Hirschwald, Berlin. Quoted by B. W. Volk and K. F. Wellmann (1977).

Fujita, T. (1968). *Arch. Histol. Jpn.* **29**, 1–40.

Gepts, W. (1957). *Ann. Soc. Roy. Sci. Med. Nat.* **10**, 1–10.

Gepts, W. (1958). *Endokrinologie* **36**, 185–211.

Gepts, W. (1965). *Diabetes* **14**, 619–633.

Gepts, W. (1972). *In* "Handbook of Physiology—Endocrinology I. Endocrine Pancreas" (D. F. Steiner and N. Freinkel, eds.), p. 289–303. American Physiological Society, Washington, D.C.

Gepts, W., and Toussaint, D. (1967). *Diabetologia* **3**, 249–265.

Gepts, W., and Pipeleers, D. (1976). *Acta Med. Scand.* **601**.

Gepts, W., De Mey, J., and Marichal-Pipeleers (1977). *Diabetologia* **13**, 2.

Gepts, W., and De Mey, J. (1978). *Diabetes* **27**, Suppl. 1, 251–261.

Gersell, D., Gingerich, R. L., and Greider, M. H. (1979). *Diabetes* **28**, 11–15.

Gibbs, Ph. (1974). *Br. Med. J.* **3**, 781–783.

Gladisch, R., Hofmann, W., and Waldherr, R. (1976). *Z. Kardiol.* **65**, 838–849.

Gold, G., Karoly, K., Freeman, C., and Adelman, R. C. (1970). *Biochem. Biophys. Res. Commun.* **73**, 1003–1010.

Goldman, H., Bollande, R., Colle, E., and Marks, M. (1976). *Diabetes* **25**, suppl. 1, 365 (Abstr.).

Gommers, A. (1971). *Gerontologia* 17, 228-235.

Greider, M. H., Lacy, P. E., Kissane, J. M., Rieders, E., and Thomas, G. (1977). *Diabetes* 26, 793-797.

Grimelius, L., Capella, C., Buffa, R., Polak, J. M., Pearse, A. G. E., and Solcia, E. (1976). *Virchows Arch. B* 20, 217-228.

Häcki, W. H., Kayasseh, L., and Gyr, K. (1977). *Irish J. Med. Sci.* 146 (suppl.), 12-13.

Hartroft, W. S. (1956). *Diabetes* 5, 98-104.

Hartroft, W. B. (1960). *In* "Diabetes". (R. H. Williams, ed), p. 350. Hoeber Medical Division. Harper and Row, New York.

Hartroft, W. S., and Wrenshall, G. A. (1955). *Diabetes* 4, 1-7.

Hauser, N., Henquin, J. C., and Gommers, A. (1978). *Proc. 10th Intern. Congr. Gerontol. Jerusalem* 2, 18.

Heding, L. G., and Rasmussen, S. M. (1976). *Diabetologia* 11, 201-206.

Hedon, E. (1892). *C. R. Soc. Biol.* 44, 678-680.

Heiberg, K. A. (1906). *Anat. Anz.* 29, 49. Quoted by B. W. Volk and K. F. Wellmann (1977).

Heiberg, K. A. (1911). *Virchows Arch.* 204, 175-189.

Hellerström, G., Andersson, A., and Gunnarson, R. (1976). *Acta Endocrinol.* 205, Suppl. 145-158.

Hellman, B. (1959). *Acta Pathol. Microbiol. Scand.* 47, 21.

Heydinger, D. K., and Lacy, P. E. (1974). *Diabetes* 23, 579-582.

Homans, J. (1915). *J. Med. Res.* 33, 1-51.

Huang, S. W., and Maclaren, N. K. (1976). *Science* 192, 64-66.

Hultquist, G., Nordvall, S., and Lundström, C. (1973). *Upsala J. Med. Sci.* 78, 139-144.

Junker, K., Egeberg, J., Kromann, H., and Nerup, J. (1977). *Acta Pathol. Microbiol. Scand. Sect. A* 85, 699-706.

Kahn, C. R. (1976). *J. Cell Biol.* 70, 261-286.

Kawanishi, H., Akazawa, Y., and Machii, B. (1966). *Acta Pathol. Jpn.* 16, 177-197.

Kimmel, J. R., Pollock, H. G., and Hazelwood, R. L. (1968). *Endocrinology* 83, 1323-1330.

Kimmel, J. R., Pollock, H. G., and Hazelwood, R. L. (1971). *Fed. Proc. Fed. Am. Soc. Exp. Biol.* 30, 1318.

Kitihara, A., and Adelman, R. C. (1979). *Biochem. Biophys. Res. Commun.* 87, 1207-1213.

Klöppel, G., Bommer, G., Commandeur, G., and Heitz, Ph. (1978). *Virchows Arch. A* 377, 157-174.

Kraus, E. J. (1929). *In* "Handbuch der Speziellen Pathologische Anatomie und Histologie" (F. Henke and O. Lubarsch, eds.), Vol. 2, p. 622-747. Springer-Verlag, Berlin and New York.

Lacy, P. E. (1964). *In* "Ciba Foundation Colloquia on Endocrinology" (M. P. Cameron and M. J. O'Connor, eds.), Vol. 13, p. 82. Churchill, London.

Lacy, P. E. (1977). *In* "The Diabetic Pancreas" (B. W. Volk and K. F. Wellmann, eds.), p. 211. Plenum, New York.

Laguesse, E. I. (1893). *C. R. Soc. Biol.* 5, 819-820.

Lancereaux, E. (1880). *Union Méd Paris* 161-167.

Lane, M. A. (1907). *Am. J. Anat.* 7, 409-421.

Larsson, L. I., Sundler, F., and Håkanson, R. (1975a). *Cell Tissue Res.* 156, 167-171.

Larsson, L. I., Sundler, F., and Håkanson, R. (1975b). *Diabetologia* 12, 211-226.

Larsson, L. I., Holst, J., Håkanson, R., and Sundler, J. (1975c). *Histochemistry* 44, 281-290.

Lazarus, S. S., and Volk, B. W. (1959). *Arch. Pathol.* 67, 456-467.

Lazarus, S. S., and Volk, B. W. (1962). "The Pancreas in Human and Experiemental Diabetes." Grune & Stratton, New York.

LeCompte, P. M. (1958). *Arch. Pathol.* 66, 450-457.

LeCompte, P. M., and Merriam, J. C., Jr. (1962). *Diabetes* 11, 35-39.

LeCompte, P. M., Steinke, J., Soeldner, J. S., and Renold, A. E. (1966). *Diabetes* **15,** 586–596.

LeCompte, P. M., and Legg, M. A. (1972). *Diabetes* **21,** 762–769.

Like, A. A. (1967). *Lab. Invest.* **16,** 937–951.

Like, A. A., Rossini, A. A., Gubenski, D. L., and Appel, M. C. (1979). *Science* **206,** 1421–1423.

Linder, E., Lehto, V. P., and Virtanen, I. (1979). *Acta Pathol Microbiol. Scand. Sect. A* **87,** 299–306.

Logothetopoulos, J. (1972). *In* "Handbook of Physiology, Section 7. Endocrinology" (R. O. Grup and E. B. Astwood, eds.), Vol. 1, p. 67–76. Williams & Wilkins, Baltimore, Maryland.

Logothetopoulos, J., and Bell, E. G. (1966). *Diabetes* **15,** 205–211.

Logothetopoulos, J., Brosky, G., and Kern, H. (1970). *In* "The Structure and Metabolism of the Pancreatic Islets" (S. Falkmer, B. Hellman, and I. Täljedal, eds.), p. 15. Pergamon, Oxford.

Ludvigsson, J., and Heding, L. G. (1976). *Diabetologia* **12,** 627–630.

McGavran, M. H., and Hartroft, W. S. (1956). *Am. J. Pathol.* **32,** 631 (Abstr.).

Maclean, N., and Ogilvie, R. F. (1955). *Diabetes* **4,** 367–376.

Maclean, N., and Ogilvie, R. F. (1959). *Diabetes* **8,** 83–91.

McMillan, D. E., and Geevarghese, P. J. (1979). *Diabetes Care* **2,** 202–208.

Malaisse-Lagae, F., Orci, L., and Perrelet, A. (1979). *N. Engl. J. Med.* **300,** 436.

Marx, M., Schmidt, W., and Goberna, R. (1970). *Z. Zellforsch. Mikrosk. Anat.* **110,** 569–587.

Mallory, F. B. (1914). "The Principles of Pathologic Histology." Saunders, Philadelphia, Pennsylvania.

Moore, A. A. (1936). *Am. J. Dis. Child.* **52,** 627–632.

Nakhooda, A. F., Like, A. A., Chappel, C. I., Murray, F. T., and Marless, E. B. (1977). *Diabetes* **26,** 100–112.

National Diabetes Data Group (1979). *Diabetes* **28,** 1039–1057.

Nerup, J., Andersen, O. O., Bendixen, G., Egeberg, J., and Poulsen, J. E. (1971). *Diabetes* **20,** 424–427.

Ogilvie, R. F. (1933). *J. Pathol. Bacteriol.* **37,** 473–481.

Ogilvie, R. F. (1964). *In* "Aetiology of Diabetes Mellitus and Its Complications" (M. P. Cameron and M. J. O'Connor, eds.), Vol. 15, p. 49. Ciba Foundation Colloquia on Endocrinology. Churchill, London.

Olsen, T. S. (1978). *Acta Pathol. Microbiol. Scand. Sect. A* **86,** 361–365.

Opie, E. L. (1901). *J. Exp. Med.* **5,** 527–540.

Orci, L., and Unger, R. H. (1977). *Diabetes* **26,** 241–244.

Orci, L., Perrelet, A., Ravazzola, M., Malaisse-Lagae, F., and Renold, A. E. (1973). *Eur. J. Clin. Invest.* **3,** 433–445.

Orci, L., Baetens, D., Rufener, Cl., Amherdt, M., Ravazzola, M., Studer, P., Malaisse-Lagae, F., and Unger, R. H. (1976a). *Proc. Nat. Acad. Sci U.S.A.* **73,** 1338–1342.

Orci, L., Baetens, D., Ravazzola, M., Stefan, L., and Malaisse-Lagae, F. (1976b). *Life Sciences* **19,** 1811–1816.

Orci, L., Malaisse-Lagae, F., Baetens, D., and Perrelet, A. (1978). *Lancet* **2,** 1200–1201.

Orci, L., Stefan, Y., Malaisse-Lagae, F., and Perrelet, A. (1979). *Lancet* **1,** 615–616.

Paulin, C., and Dubois, P. M. (1978). *Cell Tissue Res.* **188,** 251–257.

Pearse, A. G. E. (1968). *Proc. Roy. Soc.* B **170,** 71–80.

Pearse, A. G. E. (1978). *In* "Peripheres, Dissemuniertes Endokrines Zellsystem (APUD System)" (G. Dhom, ed.), pp. 2–6. Fischer, Stuttgart.

Pearse, A. G. E., Ewen, S. W. B., and Polak, J. M. (1972). *Virchow Arch. B* **10**, 93–107.

Pfeiffer, E. F. (1963). *In* "Fortschritte der Diabetesforschung." Stuttgart.

Pont, A., Rubino, J. M., Bishop, D., and Peal, R. (1979). *Arch. Int. Med.* **139**, 185–187.

Potet, F., Barge, J., and Duclert, N. (1970). *Arch. Anat. Pathol.* **18**, 219–222.

Potvliege, P. R., Carpent, G., and Gepts, W. (1963). *Beitr. Pathol. Anat. Allg. Pathol.* **128**, 335–346.

Pozilli, P., Sensi, M., Gorsuch, A., Bottazzo, G. F., and Cudworth, A. G. (1979). *Lancet* **2**, 173–175.

Prince, G. A., Henson, A. B., and Billups, L. C. (1978). *Nature (London)* **271**, 158–161.

Prosser, P. R., and Karam, J. H. (1978). *J. Am. Med. Assoc.* **239**, 1148–1150.

Rahier, J., Wallon, J., Gepts, W., and Haot, J. (1979). *Cell Tissue Res.* **200**, 359–366.

Rahier, J., Wallon, J., Henquin, J. C (1980). *Diabetologia* (in press).

Remacle, C., Hauser, N., Jeanjean, M., and Gommers, A. (1977). *Exp. Gerontol.* **12**, 207–214.

Remacle, C., De Clercq, L., Delaere, P., Many, M. O., and Gommers, P. (1980). *Cell Tissue Res.* **207**, 429–448.

Reaven, G. M. (1977). *Geriatrics* **32**, 51–54.

Reaven, E. P., Gold, G., and Reaven, G. M. (1979). *J. Clin. Invest.* **64**, 592–599.

Rinehart, J. F., Toreson, W. E. and Abul-Haj, S. K. (1954). *Am. J. Med.* **17**, 124.

Rossini, A. A., Williams, R. M., Mordes, J. P., Appel, M. C., and Like, A. A. (1979). *Diabetes* **28**, 1031–1032.

Saddi, R., Hamon, B., Feingold, J., Eschwege, E., and Fagard, R. (1978). *In* "Journées Annuelles de Diabétologie" (M. Rathery, ed.). Flammarion, Paris.

Sarles, H. (1974). *Gastroenterology* **66**, 604–616.

Sarles, H., and Sarles, J. S. (1964). *Eur. Pancreas Symp. Erlangen, Schattauer, Stuttgart 1963* p. 191.

Seifert, G. (1959). *Verh. Dtsch. Ges. Pathol.* 50–84.

Seifert, G. (1966). *Langenbecks Arch. Chir.* **316**, 264–276.

Seifert, G., and Klöppel, C. (1974). *In* "Gastroenterologie und Stoffwechsel Aktionen und Interaktionen" (V. Becker, ed.) p. 119. Witzrock, Baden-Baden, Brussel.

Seyfart, C. (1920). Quoted by B. W. Volk and K. F. Wellmann (1977).

Seltzer, H. S., Allen, E. W., Heren, A. L., and Brennan, M. T. (1967). *J. Clin. Invest.* **46**, 323–335.

Sheldon, J. H. (1935) "Haemochromatosis." Oxford Univ. Press, London and New York.

Sive, A., Vinik, A. I., Van Tonder, S., and Lund, A. (1978). *J. Clin. Endocrinol. Metab.* **47**, 556–559.

Solcia, E., Polak, J. M., Pearse, A. G. E., Forssmann, W. G., Larsson, L. I., Sundler, F., Lechago, J., Grimelius, L., Fujita, T., Creutzfeldt, W., Gepts, W., Falkmer, S., Lefranc, G., Heitz, Ph., Hage, E., Buchan, A. M. J., Bloom, S. R., and Grossman, M. I. (1978). *In* "Gut Hormones" (S. R. Bloom, ed.), pp. 40–48. Livingstone, Edinburgh.

Ssobolew, L. W. (1900). *Cbl. Allg. Path. Path. Anat.* **11**, 202.

Ssobolew, L. W. (1902). *Virchows Arch.* **168**, 91–128.

Stansfield, O., and Warren, S. (1928). *N. Engl. J. Med.* **198**, 686–687.

Starger, J. M., and Goldmann, R. D. (1977). *Proc. Nat. Acad. Sci. U.S.A.* **74**, 2422–2426.

Susman, W. (1942). *J. Clin. Endocrinol.* **2**, 97–106.

Symmers, D. (1909). *Arch. Int. Med.* **3**, 379. Quoted by B. W. Volk and K. F. Wellman, 1977.

Toreson, W. E. (1951). *Am. J. Pathol.* **27**, 327–347.

Toreson, W. E., Lee, J. C., and Grodsky, G. M. (1968). *Am. J. Pathol.* **52**, 1099–1115.

Unger, R. H. (1976). *Diabetes* **25**, 136–151.

Unger, R. H., and Orci, L. (1977). *Diabetes* **26**, 241–244.

Volk, B. W., and Wellmann, K. F. (1977). "The Diabetic Pancreas." Plenum Press, New York and London.

Von Mering, J., and Minkowski, O. (1889). *Arch. Exp. Pathol. Pharmacol.* **26**, 371–387.

Von Meyenburg, H. V. (1940). *Schweiz. Med. Wochenschr.* **21**, 554–557.

Warren, S., and LeCompte, P. M. (1952). "The Pathology of Diabetes Mellitus." Lea & Febiger, Philadelphia, Pennsylvania.

Warren, S., and Root, H. F. (1925). *Am. J. Pathol.* **1**, 415–430.

Warren, Sh., LeCompte, P. M., and Legg, M. A. (1966). "The Pathology of Diabetes Mellitus." Lea & Febiger, Philadelphia, Pennsylvania.

Weichselbaum, A. (1908). *Sitzungsber, Akad. Wiss. Wien Math. Naturwiss. Kl. Abt.* **117**, 211.

Weichselbaum, A. (1910). *Sitzungsber. Dtsch. Akad. Wiss. Berlin Kl. Math. Allg. Naturwiss. Kl.* **119**, 73–281.

Weichselbaum, A. (1911). *Wien. Klin. Wochenschr.* **24**, 153.

Weichselbaum, A., and Stangl. E. (1901). *Wien. Klin. Wochenschr.* **14**, 968–972.

Wellmann, K. F., and Volk, B. W. (1977). *In* "The Diabetic Pancreas" (B. W. Volk and K. F. Wellmann, eds.), p. 291. Plenum, New York.

Westermark, P. (1973). *Virchows Arch. A* **359**, 1–18.

Westermark, P. (1974). *Histochemistry* **38**, 27–33.

Westermark, P. (1977). *Virchows Arch. A* **373**, 161–166.

Westermark, P., and Grimelius, L. (1973). *Acta Pathol. Microbiol. Scand. Sect. A* **81**, 291–300.

Westermark, P., and Wilander, E. (1978). *Diabetologia* **15**, 417–421.

Westermark, P., Grimelius, L., Polak, J. M., Larsson, L. I., Van Noorden, S., Wilander, E., and Pearse, A. G. E. (1977). *Lab. Invest.* **37**, 212–215.

Wilder, R. M. (1926). *S. Med. J.* **19**, 241. Quoted by B. W. Volk and K. F. Wellmann (1977).

Williams, T. F. (1978). *In* "Geriatric Endocrinology" (R. B. Greenblatt, ed.). Raven, New York.

Yalow, R. S., and Berson, S. A. (1960). *J. Clin. Invest.* **39**, 1157.

Yoon, J. W., Onodera, T., and Jenson, A. B. (1978). *Diabetes* **27**, 778–781.

Yoon, J. W., Austin, M., Onodera, T., and Notkins, A. L. (1979). *N. Eng. J. Med.* **300**, 1173–1179.

14

Animal Models of Spontaneous Diabetes

M. G. SORET and W. E. DULIN

The Islets of Langerhans
Copyright © 1981 by Academic Press, Inc.
All rights of reproduction in any form reserved.
ISBN 0-12-187820-1

I. INTRODUCTION

Spontaneous diabetes exists in a variety of animal species as well as in man. Studies on diabetic animals may be important, since they could provide important clues to the pathogenesis of diabetes in man.

The species described in this chapter where chosen because they clearly represent examples which demonstrate the wide physiological, morphological, and genetic heterogeneity of diabetes. This aspect of the discussion is considered important, since it is now recognized that human diabetes exhibits considerable heterogeneity and, if we expect to solve the inherent problems of this serious metabolic disease, we must be able to understand the basic characteristics of the various types. Since the phenotype of any genetic lesion represents the results of the interaction of genes and the environment, we must appreciate this interaction when we evaluate the available knowledge in our attempts to sort out the relative contributions of the genes and the environment.

It is highly probable that many different genetic lesions are involved in human diabetes, since the diseases we define as diabetes in man are extremely variable. The heterogeniety of diabetes represented in the animal models we will discuss, as in man, results from a variety of genetically controlled lesions. If we hope eventually to understand diabetes in man, we must begin with the more easily studied animal models in order to discover reasonable guidelines for the more complex problems of human studies. If we expect to unravel the mysteries of diabetes, we must discover the basic lesions under the control of the various genes. One important organ to begin with is the islet of Langerhans, which undoubtedly plays a central key role in the pathogenesis of this disease.

In this chapter we will describe the function and structure of the islets of Langerhans for several animal models of spontaneous diabetes and attempt to define the pathogenesis of this disease in each of the species discussed. Functional aspects of the islets will be based on data on the secretion of islet hormones, as determined by plasma levels and *in vitro* release and, when possible, hormone synthesis and pancreatic content. The structural changes characteristic of each of the experimental models will be described as they develop in the diabetic animal. The pathogenesis of diabetes in the various animal species will be discussed based on a correlation of the functional and structural changes observed. We will also highlight the observations we consider the most important in each of the species and correlate this information with the situation in man. In addition, we will describe the unresolved problems which need to be solved in the future in order to define more precisely the role of the islets of Langerhans in the pathogenesis of diabetes.

II. THE CHINESE HAMSTER *(CRICETULUS GRISEUS)*

A. Introduction

Diabetes was first described in the Chinese hamster by Meier and Yerganian in 1959 (96), and islet pathology was described by these authors in 1960 (97). Diabetes in this species was not related to obesity, and severity ranged from very mild to ketotic and insulin-requiring. When the disease was first described, the age of onset varied from preweaning to two or more years (45, 97), presumably as a result of genetic heterogeneity. With continued inbreeding, the age of onset became more predictable (45). Prior to 1975 most studies with diabetic Chinese hamsters involved animals from mixed lines usually inbred for less than 10–12 generations. Since 1975 the availability of animals from inbred lines has progressed to the state where data on specific lines can be obtained. At the present time the Upjohn colony consists of three inbred non-diabetes-producing lines designated M, AA, and AV, and seven primary diabetes-producing lines designated L, Z, X, XA, AC, AH, and AB. These lines have been inbred up to 37 generations, and some breed true for diabetes (43). Data obtained from these animals clearly indicate genetic heterogeneity, since phenotypic differences exist in animals from different nondiabetic lines as well as from different diabetic lines. The inheritance of diabetes in the Chinese hamster has been defined as multifactorial and may involve at least four recessive genes (14).

The prediabetic hamsters (phenotypically normal but genetically diabetic) discussed in this section were derived from two sources. One source was the offspring of two ketotic diabetic parents, since they produce 100% diabetic offspring (34, 49). Others were obtained from highly inbred diabetes-producing lines that breed true for diabetes. It should also be noted that, while diabetes was predictable, it was not possible to predict if prediabetics would develop mild or severe disease.

B. Islet Function

Prediabetics derived from two ketotic diabetics or from inbred lines (L and XA) have plasma insulin levels similar to those of nondiabetics (M line) until at least 25 days of age (22,24,44,46,47). Plasma insulin levels of animals from mixed lines show that recently diagnosed diabetics may have either normal or increased plasma insulin (36,45,88). Nonfasted plasma insulin levels of established diabetics from a mixture of inbred lines show considerable variability, ranging from decreased to increased (22,36,45, 48,128). Severe ketotic diabetics have relatively normal fasted plasma insulin levels but always extremely low nonfasting levels (45,48,88,128). The variability of plasma insulin levels reported in early studies may have resulted from genetic heterogeneity, since recent studies comparing animals from inbred lines of diabetics and nondiabetics showed that considerable variation also existed between lines (139). Data were obtained from nonfasting, nondiabetic hamsters from three inbred lines (M, AA, and AV) and from diabetics from seven inbred lines (L, Z, X, XA, AC, AH, and AB), which were 6–17 months old (19). Animals from one of the nondiabetic lines (M) had consistently lower plasma insulin levels than those of the other two nondiabetic lines (AV and AA). Diabetics from the AH line possessed plasma insulin levels equal to those of high-level nondiabetics (AA and AV). Diabetics from some lines (L, Z, XA, and AB) had plasma insulin levels equal to those of low-level nondiabetics (M), while others had extremely low plasma insulin levels (AC and X).

Pancreatic and plasma insulin levels of prediabetics from two ketotic diabetic parents were normal until at least 25 days of age. Prediabetics from the inbred XA line had normal pancreatic insulin levels at 14 days, but they were decreased by 23 days of age (24). Diabetics, however, always had decreased pancreatic insulin levels. Pancreatic insulin levels of ketotic diabetics were always considerably less than those of the milder diabetics (19,21,36,48,84,115,128). Isolated islets from diabetics from mixed lines contained less insulin than islets from nondiabetics (20,121).

Insulin synthesis by isolated islets of diabetics (20), and glucose-induced insulin release from islets, whole perfused pancreas, or pieces of pancreas of diabetics, were decreased (20,23,40,41,95,121).

Pancreatic or islet insulin levels of diabetics, as measured by insulin storage, release, or synthesis, showed less variation than plasma insulin levels, thus implying that whatever causes diabetes in the hamster has a uniformly detrimental effect on beta cells.

Plasma glucagon was elevated in prediabetic animals from the inbred diabetes-producing XA line as compared with nondiabetic M-line animals at 3 weeks of age. Plasma glucagon from 6 to 17-months-old animals of inbred diabetic lines (19) and from mixed diabetic lines (140) was increased compared to that of nondiabetic animals. Plasma glucagon was not increased in 3 to 4- or 10 to 12-months-old diabetics from line L as compared with nondiabetics from line M. Pancreatic glucagon on the other hand was found to be elevated in all the inbred diabetic lines of 6 to 17-months-old hamsters as compared with animals from nondiabetic lines (21,22,24,139).

The release of glucagon was not as effectively suppressed by glucose in the perfused whole pancreas from the diabetic animal as in the nondiabetic animal (54). Arginine caused greater glucagon release from whole perfused pancreases of diabetics as compared with those of nondiabetics (41,54). However, *in vivo* there was no greater release of glucagon in diabetics as measured by plasma glucagon levels following arginine treatment (143).

The somatostatin content of the pancreas was less in diabetic than in nondiabetic Chinese hamsters (115). Somatostatin did not decrease arginine-induced glucagon release in diabetics as measured by plasma glucagon levels (143), but it did inhibit insulin release equally well in diabetics and nondiabetics.

C. Morphology

The pancreatic islets of spontaneously diabetic Chinese hamsters show a number of alterations which (1) may appear early (17), (2) may vary in degree depending on severity and duration (17,130), and (3) may affect many cells in the islets (8,96,131).

At 1 day of age there was degranulation of beta cells in prediabetics as compared to nondiabetics, and this degranulation progressed to a more severe condition by 10 days of age. By 14 days of age and in weanlings, islets of prediabetics were hyperplastic, beta cells were degranulated, and some beta cells had glycogen deposits (17,97). Prediabetic Chinese hamsters derived from inbred lines under 14 days of age had larger and more numerous islets consisting almost entirely of beta cells derived from small ducts (97). It is not clear whether the hyperglycemic maternal environment contributed to these early changes in the offspring of diabetic mothers. Decreased beta-cell mass, islet volume, beta-cell degranulation, and glycogen infiltration of the islets of nondiabetic siblings of diabetics have been reported (18). The degranulation is evidenced by sparse staining with aldehyde–fuchsin (88,95,97), which is confirmed by an almost total absence of granulation in ultrastructural studies (8,9,89,91,130,137). The degranulated beta cell usually has an expanded rough endoplasmic reticulum (RER) (8,9,89,130). Frequently occurring hydropic changes, i.e., vacuolation of the cytoplasm in routine histological preparations, or red hyalin masses in periodic acid–Schiff (PAS)-stained material, represent cytoplasmic glycogen deposits which can be demonstrated by electron microscopy (8,11,17,18,31,88,89,91,96,97,130,137). The deposition of glycogen in beta cells has been correlated in some cases with the degree of hyperglycemia (89,137) associated with degranulation of the beta cells (137) and with the severity of the diabetes (8,17,130). However, it has also been reported that there is no clear association between decreased granulation and glycogen deposition (8,17). Glycogen deposition may occur concomitantly with, rather than as a consequence of, degranulation (137). However it should be emphasized that glycogen deposition probably results from hyperglycemia which is likely to result from insulin deficiency which would be expected to be manifested by beta-cell degranulation. If this is true, then it can be reasoned that degranulation probably precedes glycogen deposition.

Pancreatic islet hypertrophy and hyperplasia as reported in spontaneous diabetes in other species (122) have not been found in the Chinese hamster. Replication of preexisting beta cells in the diabetic Chinese hamster, as measured by [³H]thymidine uptake, has been reported (89). However, it has not been demonstrated that this labeling represents cell multiplication.

Since the diabetic syndrome is progressive in the Chinese hamster, the size of the pancreatic islet diminishes continuously through a steady loss of beta cells as the diabetic hamster ages (17,18,31,88,91,96,115,116). This loss of beta cells results in islets consisting mostly of alpha (α_2) cells, which causes the islet alpha-cell population to be increased relative to other cell types (88,89,91,96,130). Although some workers have reported no noteworthy changes in alpha cells (31,137), the number of autophagosomes is increased in alpha cells of diabetics (89,130) and there is a corresponding disposal of the excess of secretory granules through granulolysis (112,131).

Somatostatin-producing D (α_1) cells in diabetic Chinese hamsters have been reported to show no noteworthy changes (8,31), no difference from normal D cells (89), and no decrease in cell mass paralleling the decrease in islet volume (115). The PP cells recently described in the pancreatic islets of other species including humans (6,32,79,101,129) have not been described in the normal or diabetic Chinese hamster. Newer immunological techniques and morphometric analysis will have to be used to evaluate the cell populations of the islets of normal and diabetic hamsters quantitatively.

D. Pathogenesis

At 1 day of age the beta cells of prediabetics are degranulated, and this progresses to a more severe condition by 10 days of age. By 14 days, degranulation, hyperplasia, and glycogen deposits are seen. Since no abnormalities are observed in blood sugar, plasma, or pancreatic insulin levels, no correlation between morphological changes in prediabetes and physiological changes can be made at this early age. It is not clear whether the diabetic maternal environment contributes to these early morphological changes, although if this were the case, one would expect that the more severe changes would occur early and that the islets would recover after birth and with increasing age.

The picture is clearer after the onset of diabetes in the Chinese hamster. There are many morphological changes which correlate with the duration and severity of diabetes. Degranulation is almost total in the beta cells, and this correlates with the marked decrease in pancreatic insulin. The expanded RER and enlarged Golgi complex probably relate to the attempt of the beta cell to meet insulin demands, but the lack of stored insulin and, in most cases, a decrease in the plasma and pancreatic insulin surplus indicates that the beta cells cannot produce enough insulin. As the disease progresses, the size of the islets diminishes through a steady loss of beta cells, with a corresponding decrease in the ability to produce insulin. Although differences may occur among animals from inbred lines, all diabetic hamsters show depletion of pancreatic insulin, which correlates with a reduced number of beta cells, a marked reduction in secretory beta granules, and a decrease in measured stored pancreatic insulin. Since the degree of these changes correlates with the severity of the diabetes, there is little doubt that the loss of beta-cell function is an important factor in the pathogenesis of diabetes in the Chinese hamster.

The role of glucagon in diabetes in the Chinese hamster is not clear. There is no doubt that glucagon levels are increased in the plasma of diabetic Chinese hamsters. This increase probably results from the combined effects of increased pancreatic glucagon and abnormal control of glucagon secretion, as evidenced by the inability of glucose and somatostatin to suppress release and the *in vitro* increased release of glucagon by arginine stimulation. Further, abnormally elevated glucagon or the increase in the glucagon/insulin ratio in the diabetic is supported by the observed increased disposal of glucagon by granulolysis in α_2 cells. However, this role of granulolysis has not been proven by adequate experimental studies.

The role of somatostatin or of any other pancreatic islet hormones is not clear. These hormones have not been studied sufficiently, and perhaps future investigations will clarify their relative importance in the pathogenesis of diabetes in this species.

III. THE db MOUSE (C57BL/KsJdb)

A. Introduction

Diabetes, a mutation in the db mouse resulting from an autosomal recessive gene, was first reported by Hummel *et al.* (68) and was characterized by a metabolic disturbance resembling that in the maturity-onset diabetic human (68). All diabetic db mice were obese before the age of 1 month, after which they developed hyperglycemia. The hyperglycemia progressed rapidly to very high levels at about 8–12 weeks of age, after which time the animals became severely diabetic, lost weight, and generally died before they were 10 months old. During the weight loss stage, the animals may exhibit ketosis.

B. Islet Function

Plasma insulin levels of db mice were normal at 8 days of age but increased by 10–14 days (28,30). These levels then increased progressively until approximately 6–8 weeks of age and then decreased to near normal (5,25,27,28,30,36,55,86,114,132). During food restriction to normal intake, plasma insulin remained at a high level (36,141).

Basal pancreatic insulin release in perfused whole pancreases from diabetics 7–27 weeks of age was elevated over that of normals (7,80). Glucose-stimulated release of insulin in perfused pancreases was reported to be slower, equal to, or greater than normal at 7–12 weeks of age (7,80), perhaps because at this age animals were in variable stages of diabetes, with some progressing more rapidly than others. By 27 weeks of age, the perfused pancreas from db mice failed to respond to high glucose with increased insulin release (7). Studies have also been performed on insulin release by isolated islets from db mice 5, 10, and 20 weeks of age under high-glucose stimulation. Insulin release by islets of db mice at 5 weeks of age was high, at 10 weeks of age was normal, and at 20 weeks of age was lower than normal. Insulin release by islets from older diabetics (28–36 weeks) was also less than normal when incubated with 3, 20, or 40 mM glucose (10).

The pancreatic insulin content of db mice 1 month old was normal, but was decreased at all ages thereafter (28,33,114,132,141). Isolated islets from diabetics had less than normal amounts of insulin at all ages from 5 to 20 weeks of age (11,55).

Insulin and proinsulin synthesis as measured by [³H]leucine incorporation at a low glucose concentration was increased over that of controls at 5 weeks, but at 10 and 20 weeks incorporation rates of diabetics and controls were equal. With high glucose levels, insulin synthesis was similar in diabetic and control islets at 5 and 10 weeks, but at 20 weeks diabetic islets synthesized significantly less insulin than nondiabetic islets (55).

The plasma glucagon levels of 2-month-old db mice were normal when the mice were fasted but, when the mice were fed, increased to four times that of nondiabetic animals (140). The pancreatic glucagon levels of db mice 2–6 months old were two to four times those of nondiabetic mice (92,114,140). In the isolated perfused whole pancreas, the basal release of glucagon was higher from db pancreases, and glucose did not suppress glucagon in diabetics as well as in nondiabetics (80). Glucagon release during arginine infusion was slow in the pancreas of db mice but increased at about the same rate on a percentage basis as in nondiabetics (80).

Pancreatic somatostatin was increased by approximately twofold in 11-to 28-week-old db mice (92,114).

C. Morphology

The original report on diabetic db mice described decreased granulation of the pancreatic beta cells at 3–4 weeks of age, which continued to an almost total beta-cell degranulation at 3–5 months of age (25,27,67,68). Persistent hyperglycemia led to labeling of beta and duct cells with [^{3}H]thymidine (27,86). At this time RER expansion (87), beta-cell polyploidy (12,37), and increased contact of D and beta cells were observed in relation to alpha cell–D-cell contacts (83). Enlargement of the islet (86) and hypertrophic changes in individual beta cells (10) were also observed with continuous hyperglycemia, although Coleman and Hummel (27) reported no hypertrophy or hyperplasia in db mice. It was reported that in severely diabetic db mice the decrease in insulin-producing cells was accompanied by increased glucagon- and somatostatin-containing cells (5,111), as well as an increased number of pancreatic polypeptide-containing cells (5).

Polyploidy in pancreatic cells was confined to beta cells in normal and db mice (12,37). Alpha cells were always diploid (37). The percentage of tetraploid nuclei in diabetics was found to be elevated 220% over that in controls at 4 ½ weeks of age, and the percentage increased for a period of 12–14 weeks. This elevation was suggested to be "one of the earliest indications of impending disease" (118). In the very late stage of the diabetic syndrome, exhaustion of beta cells, including preexisting and neoformed cells, was observed (27). The exhaustion of beta cells was followed by degeneration (10,25,67) and necrosis (67,87), which resulted in a reduction in the beta-cell mass (67,87) and in the atrophic appearance of the islets (26,29, 67,111).

At 3–5 months of age the pancreatic ducts were dilated, and many ductular cells appeared to be transforming into beta cells, which suggested neo-

genesis (25,27,67,86). Duct proliferation within the islets (87) and neogenesis of islet cells from duct cells (68) has also been reported.

D. Pathogenesis

Diabetes in the db mouse is characterized by three stages. By 10–14 days
of age, db mice have elevated plasma insulin levels, and by 2–3 weeks of
age they are already becoming obese. During this early stage there is beta-
cell degranulation, but normal quantities of pancreatic insulin, suggesting
that the beta cells can meet the apparent increased demand for insulin.

By the second or third month, blood sugar has risen to a high level, the
animals are grossly obese, and plasma insulin is at its highest level. The
beta cells are degranulated, and the pancreatic and islet insulin levels are
decreased, which suggests that insulin production is incapable of meeting
the demand. Although the demand is greater, insulin synthesis is only at
normal levels in each islet. Evidence exists, however, that the animals attempt to increase insulin by increasing DNA synthesis, as evidenced by increased [³H]thymidine incorporation and the formation of new islet beta
cells as shown by the transition of ductular epithelium into islet cells.

A third stage of diabetes develops in the db mouse between 3 and 10
months, when the plasma and pancreatic insulin decreases. All beta cells
are degranulated and become exhausted, as evidenced by degeneration and
necrosis, with a resulting loss of beta cells. The decreased ability of islets to
synthesize normal amounts of insulin correlates with the morphological
changes. The cause of these events is not clear, but these mice develop
severe insulin resistance which places extreme demands on insulin production. The animals lose weight and die. The genetic characteristics of db
mice must determine the inability of these animals to produce new beta
cells to maintain this increased demand indefinitely.

The possible role of glucagon in diabetes in the db mouse is not clear.
The only evidence suggesting a role for glucagon is that, although the
fasting plasma glucagon level is normal, it is elevated in fed animals and
glucose does not seem to suppress glucagon release in the diabetic. Arginine
does not cause an abnormal increase in glucagon release by isolated islets
from diabetic db mice. Studies designed to decrease plasma glucagon levels
independently of changes in circulating insulin are required to learn the
possible role of glucagon in diabetes in this animal. However, since glucagon is not likely to counteract insulin activity in a variety of tissues, and
since the major problem in the db mouse seems to be insensitivity to insulin, a contribution of glucagon to diabetes in the db mouse is doubtful.

There is no evidence that any other pancreatic hormones have a role in
diabetes in this species.

IV. THE KK MOUSE

A. Introduction

The KK strain of mice was established in 1957 by Kondo *et al.* and was characterized by moderate obesity, polyphagia, and polyuria (76). These animals were recognized as diabetic on the basis of abnormal glucose tolerance, hyperglycemia, and persistent glycosuria (103). Fasting blood sugar levels were generally normal or only slightly elevated (142), but nonfasting blood sugar levels were usually increased at about 2 months of age and remained increased until 8–9 months when the animals lost weight and the glucose level normalized (35). The inheritance of diabetes in this strain is not clear but has been proposed to result from a dominant gene with recessive modifiers (14).

B. Islet Function

Plasma insulin was elevated by 1 month of age in KK mice, after which it continued to increase to a level 50–100 times normal by 5–6 months; then it decreased toward normal, reaching a value of about 2 times normal by 13 months (4,15,33,35,36,69,110,127,142,146). Three months of diet limited to normal intake reduced plasma insulin to essentially a normal level (36). Pancreatic insulin was increased by $3-3\frac{1}{2}$ months and remained elevated throughout various ages, reaching a highly elevated level of about 20 times normal when plasma insulin had returned to about 2 times normal (4,33,35,103,105).

The insulin content of isolated islets was also significantly (two times) increased over that of islets from C57/BL mice at 6 months of age (3). [1-^{14}C]- or [6-^{14}C] glucose oxidation by isolated islets was increased when islets were incubated in 100 mg% glucose. When incubated at 300 mg% glucose concentration, both nondiabetic and diabetic islets oxidized more glucose than at 100 mg%, but the increase in diabetic islets was considerably greater (142). Baseline insulin release by perfused isolated islets of KK mice was elevated over normal, and at 375 mg% glucose the release of insulin by diabetic islets was considerably more than that from islets of normal mice (4). Insulin synthesis as measured by [^{3}H]leucine incorporation by islets from KK mice was elevated over that by islets from C57/BL6J mice (4). There were no studies involving the measurement of glucagon in KK mice.

C. Morphology

In the early reports spontaneous diabetes in the KK strain of mice was morphologically characterized by beta-cell degranulation and hypertrophy of the pancreatic islets (103,104,105). Degranulation of beta cells and glycogen deposition were observed from 5 to 14 weeks of age and were followed by hypertrophy and central cavitation of the islets (69). After 16 weeks of age beta cells became well granulated and were free of glycogen deposition, although the islets were hypertrophied. During the period of hypertrophy mixed exoendocrine cells were observed, as well as aldehyde-fuchsin-positive cells in the pancreatic ducts, which indicated the transformation of extrainsular cells into beta cells (127).

In the spontaneously diabetic KK mouse islet hyperplasia and hypertrophy are prominent features of the disease (17).

D. Pathogenesis

The KK mouse develops only a mild form of diabetes at about 3 months of age as a result of hyperphagia, obesity, and insulin resistance. It produces large amounts of insulin, which is reflected in high levels of pancreatic and plasma insulin. Early in the disease the islets are hypertrophic but degranulated, even though total pancreatic insulin is high. The islets continue to hypertrophy and become well granulated as the animal compensates for increased insulin needs. An additional phenomenon aiding in meeting the increased insulin demand is an increase in the number of beta cells by neoformation from extrainsular cells. This animal reverts to a normal state of glucose metabolism at about 9–12 months, the plasma insulin normalizes, and the pancreas has 20 times the normal quantity of insulin. Apparently the KK mouse is genetically able to increase the number of beta cells at a rate sufficient to meet the total insulin requirement and prevent the overwork exhaustion seen in other species.

V. THE SPINY MOUSE (ACOMYS CAHIRINUS)

A. Introduction

The spiny mouse is a small rodent living in desert areas of eastern Mediterranean regions (52,53). In captivity, when fed *ad libitum,* most of these animals become obese and mildly hyperglycemic (52), and 15% of those that exhibit gross obesity become frankly diabetic, showing moderate hyperglycemia, glucosuria, and sometimes ketonuria, weight loss, and death (53). It should be noted, however, that under laboratory conditions spiny mice may be normoglycemic, intermittent diabetic, nonketotic diabetic, or ketotic diabetic (51,71). Characteristic of the spiny mouse is remarkable congenital hyperplasia and an abundance of pancreatic islets (50).

B. Islet Function

It has been reported that there are two populations of normoglycemic spiny mice based on plasma insulin levels. Some have normal or slightly decreased insulin levels, while others have high plasma insulin levels after intravenous glucose administration (132). Compared with other species, fed normoglycemic spiny mice have elevated insulin levels (71). However, it has been reported that plasma insulin is decreased in spiny mice with normal fasting blood sugar levels but with abnormal glucose tolerances at 2–3, 8, or 21 months of age (57).

Intermittent diabetics had either increased or normal plasma insulin (51,71). Nonketotic and ketotic diabetics had decreased plasma insulin (51,71).

In comparison with Swiss albino mice, the plasma insulin level after glucose (16,120), arginine, glucagon, isoprenaline, aminophylline, and dibutyryl cyclic adenosine 3′,5′-monophosphate (cyclic AMP) showed that spiny mice, 8–12 weeks old and with a normal fasting blood sugar level and decreased glucose tolerance, had a defect in insulin release (16). The abnormality in insulin release was more apparent with glucagon, isoprenaline, aminophylline, and dibutyryl cyclic AMP than with glucose (16). Severely diabetic spiny mice showed no increase in plasma insulin following a glucose load (57).

From islets perifused with 150, 300, or 1000 mg% glucose, compared with rat and albino mouse islets, *Acomys* did not release any insulin during the first 5 min, released less than rats and mice at 15 min, but released equal amounts at 30 min (119). Glucose-induced insulin release by isolated islets was the same as for rats at 2.8 and 5.6 mM glucose. At high glucose levels (8.4–56 mM) insulin release by *Acomys* islets was less over a 15-min period (56). At 2 hr of incubation, *Acomys* and rat islets had equal insulin releases with 2.8, 28, or 56 mM glucose, but at 5.6, 8.4, 11.2, and 16.7 the *Acomys* islets released less insulin (56).

Pancreatic insulin of glycosuric spiny mice was increased over that in other normal species (2,51,71,132), and those with intermittent glucosuria had normal pancreatic insulin levels (71). Ketotics had lower (one-fifth those of normal spiny mice) pancreatic insulin levels than normal glycemic spiny mice but were relatively normal compared to other normal species (51,71).

The individual islet insulin content was reported to be the same in islets of *Acomys* and of rats.

C. Morphology

The islets of Langerhans of diabetic spiny mice showed beta-cell degranulation (52,53) and, in the later stages of the syndrome, glycogen degeneration of beta cells (53).

Ultrastructurally, beta cells showed a highly developed Golgi apparatus, gross degranulation, and variable deposition of glycogen. Mixed endocrine-exocrine cells in the pancreatic islets of diabetic animals were also frequently seen. (117). Granulolysis in alpha cells was another ultrastructural finding (112). It was suggested that the purpose of granulolysis was to destroy unneeded secretory granules (113). Also observed was the presence in beta cells of secretory granules in various stages of degradation and of granule-digesting vacuoles. These vacuoles were considered to be lysosomes necessary for the disposal of undischarged secretory granules of insulin (2). The accumulation of beta secretory granules has been suggested to be related to defective insulin release (16) due to an apparent abnormality in the beta-cell microtubular system (94).

D. Pathogenesis

It is generally concluded that diabetes in the spiny mouse results from defective insulin release, since pancreatic insulin is abundant in these animals and there is no evidence of beta-cell destruction or loss since beta cells are abundant at all stages of diabetes. In addition, plasma insulin levels after the administration of glucose, arginine, glucagon, and other secretagogues were lower in spiny mice than in other mice even though pancreatic insulin levels were adequate. *In vitro,* insulin release by isolated islets was slower during glucose stimulation than insulin release by islets of normal rats or mice. Apparently an inherited deficiency in the beta-cell microtubular system results in an inability to release normal quantities of insulin in this species. Granulolysis is also an indication of decreased insulin release in the presence of adequate insulin synthesis.

One variation of the above scheme is seen in the ketotic diabetic spiny mouse. This animal has decreased plasma and pancreatic insulin, which suggests that, in addition to a defective microtubular system, deficient insulin synthesis and storage may also contribute to the problem.

VI. THE BB/WISTAR RAT

A. Introduction

A model of spontaneous diabetes was reported by Nakhooda *et al.* in 1977 (106) in a nonobese Wistar-derived rat from the Bio-Breeding Laboratories of Canada. There are three types of diabetic BB/Wistar rats which develop diabetes between 60 and 120 days of age: stable diabetics, moderately ketotic diabetics, and ketotic diabetics (106,107,108). Many severely ketotic diabetics die shortly after they develop these metabolic abnormalities. Some animals have been reported to remain nondiabetic or to exhibit only transient diabetes.

B. Islet Function

The chemical diabetics (with normal fasting blood sugar levels but abnormal glucose tolerance) had lower plasma insulin levels than BB rats in remission or with renal glycosuria (108). Overt diabetics had lower plasma insulin levels (106,107,108) when measured after onset as compared with preonset and as compared with normal Wistar rats or with nondiabetic BB rats (106,107,108). Ketotic diabetics and moderately ketotics had extremely low plasma insulin levels (106). Plasma insulin was not increased by arginine in any of the diabetics (106).

Pancreatic insulin was lower in stable diabetics and markedly reduced in more severe diabetics (106).

Plasma glucagon was highly elevated in severe diabetics but only slightly in milder ones (106,108). Glucagon did not increase until 4–16 days after the onset of diabetes (107). Glucagon increase with arginine treatment was exaggerated in diabetics as compared with controls as measured by plasma levels. Glucagon secretion by ketotics was considerably more exaggerated than in stable diabetics after arginine (106).

Pancreatic glucagon was about two-thirds of normal in stable and moderately ketotic diabetics and one-third of normal in severely ketotic diabetics (106).

C. Morphology

Morphologically, the spontaneous diabetes in the BB/Wistar rat is characterized by insulitis with infiltration of the pancreatic islets by inflammatory cells mostly of the mononuclear type, beta-cell destruction, and distortion of the islet architecture (107). By the end stage of the disease, the islets are small and rare and consist almost entirely of nonbeta cells (106,107,108). No details of ultrastructural alterations are available at this time.

D. Pathogenesis

Diabetes in this animal is of rapid onset and is characterized by infiltration of the pancreatic islets by inflammatory cells. This results in islet damage which varies in degree. An almost complete loss of beta cells in some animals results in markedly reduced plasma and pancreatic insulin. Other animals can partially recover and show only mild or chemical diabetes with slightly decreased plasma and pancreatic insulin.

Glucagon may contribute to some of the metabolic abnormalities, since it is markedly elevated in severe diabetics and slightly elevated in milder ones. Apparently the release of glucagon from the islets is not under normal control mechanisms, since pancreatic glucagon is decreased in diabetics as plasma glucagon is increased.

The genetics of diabetes in the BB rat are not understood, but the gene(s) involved apparently affects some immunological function related to the beta cells (125). Since some gnotobiotic animals became diabetic, it is assumed that no infectious agent is involved in the pathogenesis of the disease in this model (125).

VII. THE GUINEA PIG

A. Introduction

Spontaneous diabetes in the guinea pig was first described by Munger and Lang (102) and was characterized by hyperglycemia and glycosuria. Not all animals in this particular colony developed diabetes, but those that developed the disease did so within 6 months of age with an average age of onset of 3 months (78). Approximately 50% of the animals develop diabetes characterized by glycosuria and abnormal glucose tolerance (78). In some there is remission of the disease. More severe diabetes may occur, but less than 10% of the diabetics have ketonuria which is mild and often transitory, and exogenous insulin is not required for survival (78). There is some evidence suggesting that diabetes in this species may be the result of an infectious agent (77,78,82,102).

B. Islet Function

There are no data relating to islet function in the diabetic guinea pig.

C. Morphology

Spontaneous diabetes in guinea pigs has been characterized morphologically by four different pathological changes recorded in most of the individual animals: (1) beta-cell degranulation (78,102,109); (2) cytoplasmic inclusions in beta cells (78,102) or vacuolation (109); (3) basement membrane changes (102), hyalinization, and scarring (70,102); and (4) islet neoformation (102) and hyperplasia (78). Electron microscopy has revealed, in addition to the reduction in beta granules, the presence of large RER and Golgi complexes (102).

Vacuolation of beta cells examined by light microscopy was interpreted to correspond to PAS-positive inclusions which were removable by diastase digestion. These inclusions were regarded to consist of a mixture of glycogen and secretory granule cores. However, by electron microscopy, it was found that the material in the inclusions did not resemble typical glycogen particles (102).

Islet neoformation (102), common in guinea pigs, was found in this group of diabetic guinea pigs, in spite of the acute character of the disease. The newly formed islets were small and numerous.

D. Pathogenesis

Diabetes in the guinea pig is probably viral in origin. Susceptibility to the infectious agent may be genetically influenced, since all animals do not develop diabetes although they are apparently exposed to the infectious agent. Those that do develop diabetes exhibit a relatively mild ketosis-resistant type.

The infection causes the beta cells to undergo degranulation, vacuolation, and formation of intracellular inclusions, leading to loss of beta-cell function or destruction which results in insulin deficiency. The guinea pig apparently attempts to counteract the insulin deficiency by islet neoformation and hyperplasia and an increase in the production of insulin by the remaining functional beta cells as evidenced by large RER and Golgi complexes.

VIII. THE SAND RAT (PSAMMOMYS OBESUS)

A. Introduction

Spontaneous diabetes probably does not occur in sand rats while in their natural habitat, since they are essentially normoglycemic when initially captured or maintained on a low-calorie diet (4,10,58,60,62,81,85). When in the wild, sand rats eat exclusively fleshy plants (126) of low caloric content (59,98). When fed laboratory chow, some of these animals develop diabetes ranging from mild to severe fulminating disease with ketosis and early death (13,59,60,62,75,85,93,98).

B. Islet Function

Plasma insulin levels were decreased in sand rats that developed severe diabetes (60,61,62,75), while those with a milder diabetes frequently had normal plasma insulin levels (60,61).

Pancreatic or islet insulin content was decreased in laboratory chow-fed animals (62,93,98).

Release of insulin by pieces of pancreas of severe diabetics was decreased in vitro (93), but the release by pancreatic tissue from mild diabetics was increased (73). Insulin release by isolated islets was increased in mild diabetic or normal glycemic sand rats when exposed to low glucose, high glucose, or arginine (147). Basal insulin release was found to be normal at 60 min but decreased at 120 min (62). In other instances, increased insulin release occurred when stimulated by 15 mM glucose but not 4 mM or less (13). In the perfused pancreas basal secretion of insulin was found to be increased in normoglycemic laboratory chow-fed rats, but at a glucose concentration of 300 mg% insulin release was considerably higher than in Wistar rats (75).

Release of glucagon by isolated islets of sand rats exposed to a low glucose concentration was lower, but when exposed to a high glucose concentration was higher than that released by islets of Wistar rats (13,147). Glucagon released by islets of sand rats, after arginine stimulation, was less than that released by islets of Wistar rats (147).

C. Morphology

Morphological changes in the pancreatic islets of the diabetic sand rat were not remarkable in most animals. Although about 60% of the captive animals fed a high caloric diet developed glycosuria, only one-half of these showed beta-cell degranulation and glycogen deposition (59). Those that showed these changes were the more severe diabetics. When accumulation of glycogen occurred, it produced displacement, compression, and degeneration of beta-cell organelles (93). Protein synthesis was normal in the beta cells in the early stages of diabetes (99), but was increased in severely hyperglycemic animals as evidenced by an enlarged Golgi apparatus and an abundance of coated vesicles (85). In severely hyperglycemic sand rats the simultaneous presence of increased protein synthesis and glycogen deposition was followed by cytoplasmic degeneration, liquification, and beta-cell death (85).

D. Pathogenesis

Variability in the development of diabetes in the sand rat makes it difficult to evaluate the pathogenesis. It must be assumed that genetic heterogeneity exists in the animals studied to date because of the variation in diabetogenic response to a high-calorie diet. But little is known about the inheritance of abnormal glucose metabolism in this species.

Plasma insulin of the mild diabetic was generally normal and, although pancreatic insulin was reported to be reduced, insulin release was increased *in vitro* in response to glucose or arginine. These observations of increased insulin release indicate insulin resistance of peripheral tissues, which creates a continuous demand for elevated insulin levels. Apparently the beta cells, during progression of the diabetic state, cannot continuously meet the increased demand, since the animals develop more severe diabetes, with a resultant decrease in pancreatic and plasma insulin. The morphological changes consisting of beta-cell degranulation, glycogen accumulation, increased protein synthesis, cytoplasmic degeneration, and beta-cell death in severe diabetics correlate with a decreased ability to synthesize, store, and release insulin.

There is no evidence that glucagon or any other pancreatic hormone has a role in the development of diabetes in the sand rat.

IX. CLINICAL DIABETES

A. Introduction

There are at least two distinguishable types of human diabetes, described as type I and type II. Type I is juvenile-onset diabetes which is insulin-dependent and ketosis-prone. The age of onset is characteristically in the juvenile, but it can occur at any age. Type II, maturity-onset diabetes, is not insulin-dependent and may be resistant to the development of ketosis. Type II may or may not require insulin for correction of hyperglycemia, and the age of onset is generally middle or old age although it may occur in the young. There are many phenotypic variations of these two types, which may result from genetic heterogeneity or differences in sensitivity to a variety of environmental factors. (see Chapter 13).

B. Islet Function

One area where the genetic heterogeneity of diabetes is clearly observed is in the function of the cells of the islets of Langerhans.

Fasting plasma insulin levels in human diabetics have been observed to be normal (38,72,74,90,144), higher than normal (63,64), or lower than normal (38,74). The response of beta cells to a glucose challenge also shows considerable variability as measured by plasma insulin levels. Some investigators have observed that the initial response to a glucose load is slow in many maturity-onset diabetics but that after 1–2 hr the plasma insulin level may be normal or even elevated (38,64,74,90,144,145). However, if blood sugar is maintained at the same level in diabetics and normals by glucose infusion, or multiple stimuli over several hours, diabetics generally secrete less insulin (74,135). With progressive deterioration of glucose tolerance, there is usually a progressive decrease in the ability to secrete and maintain plasma insulin levels (63). For example, the severe, nonobese, maturity-onset diabetic exhibits a slow increase in plasma insulin that does not reach a peak as high as that of normal humans during glucose tolerance (145). In the young severe diabetic there are often normal fasting insulin levels with essentially no elevation of plasma insulin following a glucose load (38,64,74).

Heterogeneity of insulin response in diabetics has also been demonstrated in studies on various ethnic groups with diabetes, such as the Navajo, the Pima, the Amish, and a Micronesian population. In general, the diabetic Navajo has a relative insulin deficiency as compared to the normal Navajo (123,124). Diabetic Pima Indians, on the other hand, have elevated fasted insulin levels and a considerably higher than normal insulin response to glucose (42). The Pennsylvania Amish have been reported to be relatively hyperinsulinemic as compared with controls (123,124), but diabetic Amish have low insulin as compared to the Navajo (123). In a Micronesian population, there were six levels of diabetics as defined by insulin response. These ranged from higher than normal, to normal, to a very low insulin response to glucose tolerance test, although all were diabetic (148).

Pancreatic insulin has been reported to be decreased in all diabetics. In the young severe diabetic pancreatic insulin was less than $\frac{1}{30}$ of normal, while in those over 20 pancreatic insulin was 40–50% of normal and was not correlated with duration of diabetes (138).

Fasting plasma glucagon levels of diabetics are generally normal (100,134). Glucagon release was suppressed by glucose in the nondiabetic, but not in the diabetic. Glucagon response as measured by plasma levels following arginine stimulation was greater in adult and juvenile diabetics than in normals (1,133,134). No data exist on pancreatic glucagon levels in human diabetics.

C. Morphology

Since a detailed discussion of islet morphology in diabetic humans is presented in Chapter 13, this subject will not be discussed here. It is sufficient to mention that the pathological changes observed in the pancreatic islets of human diabetics, whether of the juvenile or adult type, are generally nonspecific. The most common changes in the diabetic human islet are hydropic degeneration, hypertrophy, regeneration, ductal proliferation, degranulation of beta cells, atrophy, necrosis, hyalinization, fibrosis, and insulitis. The degree to which the islets and beta cells exhibit morphological changes in human diabetes is extremely variable. However, a considerable number of diabetics have been reported to have histologically normal islets (136).

X. OVERVIEW AND FUTURE RESEARCH NEEDS

The information provided in this chapter clearly shows that there is no typical diabetic if one bases the characterization on glucose metabolism, insulin synthesis, noninsulin pancreatic hormones, or morphological changes in the islets. Further, it is also reasonable to conclude that this variability, at least in part, results from the variety of genetic backgrounds of diabetes. This heterogeniety is seen between diabetic individuals in a single species, as well as between individuals of different species. We will attempt to summarize some of the observations described in this chapter that lead to this conclusion.

Heterogeneity is clearly demonstrated when one attempts to characterize diabetes based on beta-cell function and morphology. Beta-cell function, as measured by plasma insulin response, is not uniform, as is evident from a variety of patterns when comparisons are made under similar conditions. In humans, the plasma insulin response to glucose load or in the fasting state shows considerable variation among individual diabetics. This is particularly true when the response of diabetics of several ethnic groups are compared and one sees both hypo- and hyperresponders. At least in one situation, the Micronesians, the insulin response to glucose varies from hypernormal, to normal, to subnormal. In animals, variation in insulin responses occurs and is observed among individuals of one species, as well as when animals from different species are compared. Animals of different inbred lines of Chinese hamsters respond with hypo- or hyperinsulinemia under conditions designed to challenge the beta cells. The spiny mouse, sand rat, and BB/Wistar rat show individual differences in their ability to respond to a glucose challenge. In other species, such as db and KK mice, the response is relatively uniform and shows that, within these strains of animals, diabetes can be predictable. This uniformity is probably a result of their genetic background.

There is little doubt that genetic factors play an important role in this heterogeneity of diabetes as measured by insulin secretion. Support for genetic influence is obtained from observations that within a given inbred line of Chinese hamsters response is fairly uniform, as it is in the db mouse. However, variability among individual human diabetics and ethnic groups, as well as individual variation in some of the different strains of animal species, also supports the influence of genetic factors on insulin secretory responses. Environmental influences must exist, but their exact role and interaction with the genes in this physiological response is not clear.

Although it is not clear whether the primary genetic problem is in the beta cells or in the peripheral tissues, the fact that in all but two species of animal models the beta cells decrease in the diabetic suggests that beta cells either die early or there is a lack of ability to convert duct cells to beta cells in some species. Supporting this conclusion are observations that in all but two of the diabetic animal species, as well as in man, there is a decrease in pancreatic insulin and in many cases a decreased ability of islets to produce insulin. Information relating to the capacity for neoformation of beta cells has also shown that there is considerable variability in diabetic humans, as well as among different animal species. Islet hypertrophy with reported beta-cell generation from ductal proliferation was described in the early reports on man. Although this is not seen in the Chinese hamster or BB/Wistar rat, neogenesis of beta cells has been reported in the db mouse and guinea pig, and it must occur in the spiny mouse and the KK mouse since their total volume of beta cells markedly increases. Since a decrease in the number of beta cells and in total islet volume occurs in many diabetics, it seems reasonable to conclude that loss of beta cells is a major factor in the inability to maintain sufficient pancreatic insulin production in many diabetics. Exceptions, however, occur in regard to this observed decreased pancreatic insulin storage as well as the total quantity of beta cells. These exceptions are the spiny mouse and the KK mouse, which usually have elevated pancreatic insulin as well as increased mass of beta cells. The ability of these two species to continue to produce an increased number of beta cells and synthesize increased quantities of insulin, and the total inability or only temporary capability of some species to produce beta cells from duct cells, indicate that the control of duct cell transformation into beta cells may be under genetic control.

Most of the morphological changes occurring in beta cells in the islets of diabetic humans have been observed in many diabetic animals. However, hyalinization has not been reported in any of the diabetic animals but is a common finding in diabetic man. Therefore a difference exists between diabetic animals and man as this is the most common finding in clinical diabetes. Since this is seen more frequently in diabetics that are older and presumably have diabetes of longer duration, it may not be seen in the animal models because of their relatively shorter life span, although it may not be an important factor in the disease.

Glycogen infiltration of beta cells commonly described as hydropic degeneration was reported in the early studies in humans prior to the availability of insulin. With the advent of therapy and better control of diabetes, this change is no longer a characteristic morphological alteration in human diabetics. Glycogen deposition is observed more frequently in diabetic animals, since no effort is made to control their hyperglycemia, which is probably the major factor contributing to glycogen deposition. However, these changes are not a constant finding in all diabetic animals. Glycogen infiltration is observed in the beta cells of diabetic Chinese hamsters, guinea pigs, and sand rats, but not in spiny mice or db mice which also have severe blood sugar elevations Consequently, the role of these changes in the pathogenesis of diabetes is not clear. The occurrence of glycogen deposition in some species and not others may indicate a genetic difference in the response of beta cells to hyperglycemia, which might be expected if different genes are involved in diabetes in the different species.

The relative role of the immune process in the pathogenesis of diabetes in man and experimental animals is not clear, although the occurrence of insulitis in some human diabetics and in the BB/Wistar rat suggests that some cases of diabetes may be a result of abnormal immunological processes that affect the beta cell. Evidence available in humans also suggests that some cases of diabetes result from immunologically related damage to beta cells (3) (see Chapter 17). Support for a role of immunological processes in the pathogenesis of diabetes is also obtained from the observation that antilymphocytic serum can prevent diabetes in the BB/Wistar rat. Although infection has also been implicated as the cause of spontaneous diabetes in guinea pigs and in some cases of human diabetes (see Chapter 16), the infectious agent has not been isolated and shown to cause diabetes in the original species. Even if infection agents are implicated as the cause of some cases of diabetes, a genetic influence must exist, since all animals are not susceptible to the same infections.

The diseases diagnosed as diabetes are extremely heterogenic, suggesting that a variety of genes are involved in susceptibility to diabetes and that this contributes to the variability. Since it is difficult to conduct conclusive studies in man due to the long duration of time between generations and the restrictions placed on human research for legal, moral, and ethical reasons, it seems reasonable to conclude that progress in understanding and solving the problems of diabetes in man requires definition of a limited number of end points that have a high probability of being involved in the pathogenesis of this disease. Since there are literally thousands of potential end points in a variety of tissues, without a rational approach to clinical studies designed to limit the number of parameters studied in man, we are probably doomed to failure. Studies with animal models have the greatest potential for leading us in the right direction if we can discover the genetically controlled lesions responsible for the variety of diabetic syndromes and if we can design experimental methods acceptable for human studies. Although many tissues are involved in diabetes, it is difficult to pick the primary one. Since the islets of Langerhans are directly or indirectly involved in the pathogenesis of this disease, it seems reasonable to begin with this organ in an attempt to discover the genetically controlled lesion(s) of diabetes.

The most important research that must be carried out is to understand the genetic basis of diabetes in each species in order to produce predictable genetic diabetics (prediabetics). These prediabetic animals are required if we expect to discover the gene-controlled lesions that result in diabetes. This must be done prior to the phenotypic expression of diabetes, since by that time the metabolic abnormalities are so complex that the genetic lesions are masked. Because the beta cell is the key factor in diabetes, either primary or secondary, it is important to determine why the beta cells of genetic diabetics do not survive. Some of the key areas of study that could lead to identification of the genetic lesions may involve a definition of the role of the immune system, a definition of the cellular origin of beta cells and how it can be controlled, an explanation of why duct cells of some diabetic animals produce new beta cells and others cannot, and an explanation of why alpha cells survive infection or immunological injury but beta cells do not. One basic question that needs an answer is whether the genetic lesion(s) is located only in the beta cells or also in extrapancreatic cells that produce factors required in the pathogenesis of diabetes. In order to study the role of the genetic lesions, a genetic marker(s) is required and methods must be developed for studying their role in the pathogenesis of this disease. Finally, the most important future contribution will be to apply the knowledge gained from these studies in prediabetic and diabetic animal models to the human diabetic in a systematic fashion. Hopefully some of the basic gene-controlled lesions discovered in animals will also exist in man. If we expect to contribute to the understanding of human diabetes and to develop methods for preventing expression of the genes involved in this disease, we must discover well-defined end points in the more easily studied animal models and apply this knowledge to man.

REFERENCES

1. Aguilar-Parada, E., Eisentraut, A. M., and Unger, R. H. (1969). *Am J. Med. Sci.* **257**, 415–418.
2. Amherdt, M., Orci, L., Stauffacher, W., Renold, A. E., and Rouiller, C. (1970). *In* "Proc., Sept. Congr. Intern. de Microscopie Electronique, Grenoble," pp. 501–502. Societe Francaise de Microscopie Electronique, Paris.
3. Anderson, O. O., Deckert, T., and Nerup, J. (1975). *Acta Endocrinologica Suppl.* 205.
4. Appel, M. C., Chang, A. Y., and Dulin, W. E. (1974). *Diabetologia* **10**, 625–632.

5. Baetens, D., Stefan, Y., Ravazzola, M., Malaisse-Lagae, F., Coleman, D. L., and Orci, L. (1978). *Diabetes* **27**, 1–7.
6. Bencosme, S., and Liepa, E. (1955). *Endocrinology* **57**, 588–593.
7. Berglund, O., Frankel, B. J., and Hellman, B. (1978). *Acta Endocrinol.* **87**, 543–551.
8. Boquist, L. (1969). *Acta Pathol. Microbiol. Scand.* **75**, 399–414.
9. Boquist, L. (1973). *Diabetologic* **9**, 61.
10. Boquist, L. (1974). *J. Cell Biol.* **62**, 77–89.
11. Boquist, L., and Falkmer, S. (1970). *Z. Versuchstierkd.* **12**, 96–99.
12. Bowen, R. E., and Swartz, F. J. (1976). *Diabetologia* **12**, 171–180.
13. Brodoff, B. N., and Kagan, A. (1972). *Horm. Metab. Res.* **4**, 310–311.
14. Butler, L., and Gerritsen, G. C (1970). *Diabetologia* **6**, 163–167.
15. Camerini-Davalos, R. A., Oppermann, W., Mittl, R., and Ehrenreich, T. (1970). *Diabetologia* **6**, 324–329.
16. Cameron, D. P., Stauffacher, W., Orci, L., Amherdt, M., and Renold, A. E. (1972). *Diabetes* **21**, 1060–1071.
17. Carpenter, A.-M., Gerritsen, G. C., Dulin, W. E., and Lazarow, A. (1967). *Diabetologia* **3**, 92–96.
18. Carpenter, A.-M., Gerritsen, G. C., Dulin, W. E., and Lazarow, A. (1970). *Diabetologia* **6**, 168–176.
19. Chang, A. Y., (unpublished).
20. Chang, A. Y. (1969). *In* "The Structure and Metabolism of the Pancreatic Islets" (S. Falkmer, B. Hellman, and I.-B. Täljedal, eds.), pp. 515-526. Pergamon, Oxford.
21. Chang, A. Y., Noble, R. E., and Wyse, B. M. (1977). *Diabetes* **26**, 1063–1071.
22. Chang, A. Y., Noble, R. E., and Wyse, B. M. (1976). *In* "Proc. IX Congr. Intern. Diab. Fed" (J. S. Bajaj, ed.), pp. 691–702. Excerpta Medica, Amsterdam.
23. Chang, A. Y., and Schneider, D. I. (1970). *Diabetologia* **6**, 180–185.
24. Chang, A. Y., and Wyse, B. M., (unpublished).
25. Chick, W. L., and Like, A. A. (1970). *Diabetologia* **6**, 243–251.
26. Coleman, D. L. (1978). *Diabetologia* **14**, 141–148.
27. Coleman, D. L., and Hummel, K. P. (1967). *Diabetologia* **3**, 238–248.
28. Coleman, D. L., and Hummel, K. P. (1969). *In* "Diabetes, Proc. VI Congr. Intern. Diab. Fed." (J. Ostman and R. D. G. Milner, eds.), p. 813. Excerpta Medica, Amsterdam.
29. Coleman, D. L., and Hummel, K. P. (1973). *Diabetologia* **9**, 287–293.
30. Coleman, D. L., and Hummel, K. P. (1974). *Diabetologia* **10**, 607–610.
31. Conforti, A. (1972). *Acta Diabetol. Lat.* **9**, 655–687.
32. Deconinck, J. F., Potvliege, P. R., and Gepts, W. (1971). *Diabetologia* **7**, 266–282.
33. Dulin, W. E., Chang, A. Y., and Gerritsen, G. C. (1971). *In* "Diabetes, 7th Congr. Intern. Diabetes Fed." (R. R. Rodriguez and J. Vallance-Owen, eds.), p. 868. Excerpta Medica, Amsterdam.
34. Dulin, W. E., and Gerritsen, G. C. (1972). *Acta Diabetol. Lat.* **9**, 48–84.
35. Dulin, W. E., and Wyse, B. M. (1970a). *Diabetologia* **6**, 317–323.
36. Dulin, W. E., and Wyse, B. M. (1970b). *In* "Early Diabetes" (R. A. Camerini Davalos and H. S. Cole, eds.), pp. 71–77. Academic Press, New York.
37. Ehrie, M. G., and Swartz, F. J. (1976). *Diabetologia* **12**, 167–170.
38. Ehrlich, R. M., and Bambers, G. (1964). *Diabetes* **13**, 177–181.
39. Ehrlich, J. C., and Ratner, J. M. (1961). *Am. J. Pathol.* **38**, 49–59.
40. Frankel, B. J., Gerich, J. E., Hagura, R., Fanska, R. E., Gerritsen, G. C., and Grodsky, G. M. (1974). *J. Clin. Invest.* **53**, 1637–1646.
41. Frankel, B. M., Gerich, J. E., Fanska, R. E., Gerritsen, G. C., and Grodsky, G. M. (1975). *Diabetes* **24**, 272–279.

42. Genuth, S. M., Bennett, P. H., Miller, M., and Burch, T. A. (1967). *Metabolism* **16,** 1010–1015.
43. Gerritsen, G. C., (unpublished).
44. Gerritsen, G. C. (1975). *Compr. Ther.* **1,** 25–29.
45. Gerritsen, G. C., and Blanks, M. C. (1974). *Diabetologia* **10,** 493–499.
46. Gerritsen, G. C., Blanks, M. C., Miller, R. L., and Dulin, W. E. (1974). *Diabetologia* **10,** 559–565.
47. Gerritsen, G. C., and Dulin, W. E., (unpublished).
48. Gerritsen, G. C. (1967). *Diabetologia* **3,** 74–84.
49. Gerritsen, G. C., Needham, L. B., Schmidt, F. L., and Dulin, W. E. (1970). *Diabetologia* **6,** 158–162.
50. Gonet, A. E. (1965). *Diabetologia* **1,** 144 (Abstr. #86).
51. Gonet, A. E. (1969). *In* "Diabetes, Proc. 6th Cong. Intern. Diabetes Fed." (J. Ostman and R. D. G. Milner, eds.), p. 823. Excerpta Medica, Amsterdam.
52. Gonet, A. E., Mougin, J., and Renold, A. E. (1965). *Acta Endocrinol. Suppl.* **100,** 135 (Abstr. 103).
53. Gonet, A. E., Stauffacher, W., Pictet, R., and Renold, A. E. (1965). *Diabetologia* **1,** 162–171.
54. Grodsky, G. M., Frankel, B. M., Gerick, J. E., and Gerritsen, G. C. (1974). *Diabetologia* **10,** 521–528.
55. Gunnarsson, R. (1975). *Diabetologia* **11,** 431–438.
56. Gutzeit, A., Rabinovitch, A., Karakash, C., Stauffacher, W., Renold, A. E., and Cerasi, E. (1974). *Diabetologia* **10,** 661–665.
57. Gutzeit, A., Rabinovitch, A., Studer, P. P., Trueheart, P. A., Cerasi, E., and Renold, A. E. (1974). *Diabetologia* **10,** 667–670.
58. Hackel, D. B., Frohman, L. A., Mikat, E., Lebovitz, H. E., Schmidt-Nielsen, K., and Kinney, T. D. (1965). *Ann. N.Y. Acad. Sci.* **131,** 459–463.
59. Hackel, D. B., Schmidt-Nielsen, K., Haines, H. B., and Mikat, E. (1965). *Lab. Invest.* **14,** 200–207.
60. Hackel, D. B., Frohman, L., Mikat, E., Lebovitz, H. E., Schmidt-Nielsen, K., and Kinney, T. D. (1966). *Diabetes* **15,** 105–114.
61. Hackel, D. B., Mikat, E., Lebovitz, H. E., Schmidt-Nielsen, K., Horton, E. S., and Kinney, T. D. (1967). *Diabetologia* **3,** 130–134.
62. Hahn, H. J., Jutzi, E., Kohler, E., and Schafer, H. (1976). *Endokrinologie* **68,** 338–344.
63. Hales, C. N. (1964). *Endocrinology* **15,** 140–148.
64. Hales, C. N., and Randle, P. J. (1963). *Lancet* **1,** 790–794.
65. Heinze, E., Beischer, W., Keller, L., Winkler, G., Teller, W. M., and Pfeiffer, E. F. (1978). *Diabetes* **27,** 670–676.
66. Hellerstrom, C., Andersson, A., and Gunnarsson, R. (1976). *Acta Endocrinol.* **83,** Suppl. 205, 145–160.
67. Herberg, L., and Coleman, D. L. (1977). *Metabolism* **26,** 59–99.
68. Hummel, K. P., Dickie, M. M., and Coleman, D. L. (1966). *Science* **153,** 1127–1128.
69. Iwatsuka, H., Shino, A., and Suzuoki, Z. (1970). *Endocrinol. Jpn.* **17,** 23–35.
70. Johnson, R. S. (1979). *Res. Resources Reporter* **III,** 1–5.
71. Junod, A., Letarte, J., Lambert, A. E., and Stauffacher, W. (1969). *Horm. Metab. Res.* **1,** 45–52.
72. Karam, J. H., Grodsky, G. M., and Forsham, P. H. (1963). *Diabetes* **12,** 197–204.
73. Kern, H., and Logothetopoulos, J. (1970). *Diabetes* **19,** 145–154.
74. Kipnis, D. M. (1970). *Adv. Int. Med.* **16,** 103–134.

75. Kohler, E., Knospe, S., Schafer, H., Ziegler, B., Blech, W., Bierwolf, B., von Dorsche, H. H., Gottschling, H.-D., Fiedler, H., and Bibergeil, H. (1976). *Endokrinologie* **68**, 198–210.
76. Kondo, K. K., Nozawa, T., Tomida, T., and Ezaki, K. (1957). *Bull. Exp. Anim.* **6**, 107–112.
77. Lang, C. M., and Munger, B. L. (1976). *Diabetes* **25**, 434–443.
78. Lang, C. M., Munger, B. L., and Rapp, F. (1977). *Lab. Anim. Sci.* **27**, 789–805.
79. Larsson, L.-I., Sundler, F., and Hakanson, R. (1976). *Diabetologia* **12**, 211–226.
80. Laube, H., Fussganger, R. D., Maier, V., and Pfeiffer, E. F. (1973). *Diabetologia* **9**, 400–402.
81. Lazarus, H., and Volk, B. (1953). *Arch. Pathol.* **66**, 59–71.
82. Lee, K. J., Lang, C. M., and Munger, B. L. (1978). *Vet. Pathol.* **15**, 663–666.
83. Leiter, E. H., and Eppig. J. J. (1977). *Diabetologia* **13**, 414.
84. Like, A. A. (1977). *In* "The Diabetic Pancreas" (B. W. Volk and K. F. Wellman, eds.), pp. 381–423. Plenum, New York.
85. Like, A. A., and Miki, E. (1967). *Diabetologia* **3**, 143–166.
86. Like, A. A., and Chick, W. L. (1970). *Diabetologia* **6**, 207–215.
87. Like, A. A., and Chick, W. L. (1970). *Diabetologia* **6**, 216–242.
88. Like, A. A., Gerritsen, G. C., Dulin, W. E., and Gaudreau, P. (1974a). *Diabetologia* **10**, 509–508.
89. Like, A. A., Gerritsen, G. C., Dulin, W. E., and Gaudreau, P. (1974b). *Diabetologia* **10**, 509–520.
90. Luft, R., and Efendic, S. (1979). *Horm. Metab. Res.* **11**, 415–423.
91. Luse, S. A., Caramia, F., Gerritsen, G. C., and Dulin, W. E. (1976). *Diabetologia* **3**, 97–108.
92. Makino, H., Matsushima, Y., Kanatsuka, A., Yamamoto, M., Kumagai, A., and Nishimura, M. (1979). *Endocrinology* **104**, 243–247.
93. Malaisse, W. J., Like, A. A., Malaisse-Lagae, F., Gleason, R. E., and Soeldner, J. S. (1968). *Diabetes* **17**, 752–759.
94. Malaisse-Lagae, F., Ravazzola, M., Amherdt, M., Gutzeit, A., Stauffacher, W., Malaisse, W. J., and Orci, L. (1975). *Diabetologia* **10**, 71–76.
95. Malaisse, W., Malaisse-Lagae, F., Gerritsen, G. C., Dulin, W. E., and Wright, P. H. (1967). *Diabetologia* **3**, 109–114.
96. Meier, H., and Yerganian, G. E. (1959). *Proc. Soc. Exp. Biol. Med.* **100**, 810–815.
97. Meier, H., and Yerganian, G. E. (1960). *Diabetes* **10**, 12–21.
98. Miki, E., Like, A. A., Soeldner, J. S., Steinke, J., and Cahill, G. F., Jr. (1966). *Metabolism* **15**, 749–760.
99. Molleson, A. (1973). *Am. J. Pathol.* **73**, 495–509.
100. Muller, W. A., Faloona, G. R., Aguilar-Parada, E., and Unger, R. H. (1970). *N. Engl. J. Med.* **283**, 109–115.
101. Munger, B. L., Caramia, F., and Lacy, P. E. (1965). *Z. Zellforsch.* **67**, 776–798.
102. Munger, B. L., and Lang, C. M. (1973). *Lab. Invest.* **29**, 685–702.
103. Nakamura, M. (1962). *Proc. Jpn. Acad.* **38**, 348–352.
104. Nakamura, M. (1965). *Z. Zellforsch.* **65**, 340–349.
105. Nakamura, M., and Yamada, K. (1967). *Diabetologia* **3**, 212–221.
106. Nakhooda, A. F., Like, A. A., Chappel, C. I., Murray, F. T., and Marliss, E. B. (1977). *Diabetes* **26**, 100–112.
107. Nakhooda, A. F., Like, A. A., Chappel, C. I., Wei, C.-N., and Marliss, E. B. (1978). *Diabetologia* **14**, 199–207.
108. Nakhooda, A. F., Wei, C.-N., Like, A. A., and Marliss, E. B. (1978). *Diabete Metab.* **4**, 255–259.

109. Nevalainen, T. O., White, W. J., Lang, C. M., and Munger, B. L. (1978). *Clin. Exp. Pharmacol. Phys.* **5**, 215–222.
110. Oppermann, W., Ehrenreich, T., Patel, D., Espinoza, T., and Camerini-Davalos, R. A. (1973). *In* "Early Diabetes" (R. A. Camerini-Davalos and H. S. Cole, eds.), pp. 281–290. Academic Press, New York.
111. Orci, L. (1976). *Metabolism* **25**, 1303–1313.
112. Orci, L., Junod, A., Pictet, R., Renold, A. E., and Rouiller, C. (1968). *J. Cell Biol.* **38**, 462–466.
113. Orci, L., Renold, A. E., and Rouiller, C. (1970). *In* "The Structure and Metabolism of the Pancreatic Islets" (S. Falkmer, B. Hellman, and I.-B. Taljedal, eds.), pp. 109–113. Pergamon, Oxford.
114. Patel, Y. C., Orci, L., Bankier, A., and Cameron, D. P. (1976). *Endocrinology* **99**, 1415–1418.
115. Petersson, B., Elde, R., Efendic, S., Hokfelt, T., Johansson, O., Luft, R., Cerasi, E., and Hellerstrom, C. (1977a). *Diabetologia* **13**, 463–466.
116. Petersson, B., Elde, B., Lundquist, G., Efendic, S., Hokfelt, T., Johansson, O., Luft, R., Cerasi, E., and Hellerstrom, C. (1977b). *Acta Endocrinol.* **85**, Suppl. 209, 52.
117. Pictet, R., Orci, L., Gonet, A. E., Rouiller, C., and Renold, A. E. (1967). *Diabetologia* **3**, 188–211.
118. Pohl, M. N., and Swartz, F. J. (1979). *Acta Endocrinol.* **90**, 295–306.
119. Rabinovitch, A., Gutzeit, A., Grill, V., Kikuchi, M., Renold, A. E., and Cerasi, E. (1975). *In* "Contemporary Topics in the Study of Diabetes and Metabolic Endocrinology" (E. Shafrir, ed.), pp. 204–211. Academic Press, New York.
120. Rabinovitch, A., Gutzeit, A., Renold, A. E., and Cerasi, E. (1975). *Diabetes* **24**, 1094–1100.
121. Rabinovitch, A., Renold, A. E., and Cerasi, E. (1976). *Diabetologia* **12**, 581–587.
122. Renold, A. E., Burr, I. M., and Stauffacher, W. (1971). *Proc. R. Soc. Med.* **64**, 613–617.
123. Rimoin, D. L. (1969). *Arch. Intern. Med.* **124**, 695–700.
124. Rimoin, D. L. (1970). *In* "Diabetes Mellitus" (M. Ellenberg and H. Rifkin, eds.), p. 564–581. McGraw-Hill, New York.
125. Rossini, A. A., Williams, R. M., Mordes, JH. P., Appel, M. C., and Like, A. A. (1979). *Diabetes* **28**, 1031–1032.
126. Schmidt-Nielsen, K., Haines, H. B., and Hackel, D. B. (1964). *Science* **143**, 689–690.
127. Shino, A., and Iwatsuka, H. (1970). *Endocrinol. Jpn.* **17**, 459–476.
128. Sims, E. A. H., and Landau, B. R. (1976). *Diabetologia* **3**, 115–123.
129. Solcia, E., Pearse, A. G. E., Grube, D., Kobayashi, S., Bussolati, G., Creutzfeldt, W., and Gepts, W. (1973). *Rend. Gastroenterol.* **5**, 13–16.
130. Soret, M. G., Dulin, W. E., Mathews, J., and Gerritsen, G. C. (1974). *Diabetologia* **10**, 567–579.
131. Stauffacher, W. (1970). *Diabetologia* **6**, 199–206.
132. Stauffacher, W., Orci, L., Amherdt, M., Burr, I. M., Balant, L., Froesch, E. R., and Renold, A. E. (1970). *Diabetologia* **6**, 330–342.
133. Unger, R. H. (1978). *Metabolism* **27**, 1691–1709.
134. Unger, R. H., Aguilar-Parada, E., Muller, W. A., and Eisentraut, A. M. (1970). *J. Clin. Invest.* **49**, 837–848.
135. Vinik, A. I., Kalk, W. J., Botha, J. L., Jackson, W. P. U., and Blake, K. C. H. (1976). *Diabetes* **25**, 11–15.
136. Warren, S., and LeCompte, P. (1952). *In* "The Pathology of Diabetes Mellitus," 3rd ed. Lea & Febiger, Philadelphia, Pennsylvania.

137. Williamson, R. (1960). *Diabetes* **9**, 471.
138. Wrenshall, G. A., Bogoch, A., and Ritchie, R. C. (1952). *Diabetes* **1**, 87–105.
139. Wyse, B. M., and Chang, A. Y. (1972). *Diabetes* **27**, 514.
140. Wyse, B. M., and Dulin, W. E. (unpublished).
141. Wyse, B. M., and Dulin, W. E (1970). *Diabetologia* **6**, 268–273.
142. Wyse, B. M., and Dulin, W. E (1974). *Diabetologia* **10**, 617–623.
143. Wyse, B. M., and Dulin, W. E (1976). *Physiologist* **19**, (Abstr. 417).
144. Yalow, R. S., and Berson, S. A. (1960). *Diabetes* **9**, 254–260.
145. Yalow, R. S., Glick, S. M., Roth, J , and Berson, S. A. (1965). *Ann. N.Y. Acad. Sci.* **131**, 357–373.
146. Yamada, K., and Nakamura, M. (1969). *Experientia* **25**, 878.
147. Ziegler, M., Hahn, H.-J., Ziegler B., Kohler, E., and Fiedler, H. (1975). *Diabetologia* **11**, 63–69.
148. Zimmet, P., Whitehouse, S., Alford, F., and Chisholm, D. (1978). *Diabetologia* **15**, 23–27.

15

Action of Toxic Drugs on Islet Cells

S. J. COOPERSTEIN and D. WATKINS

I. INTRODUCTION

The study of the effect of drugs on the islets of Langerhans had its genesis in the discovery that alloxan exerted a selective cytotoxic effect on the B cells, thereby producing diabetes (Dunn *et al.,* 1943; Dunn and McLetchie, 1943). There have since followed numerous reports of chemical agents which damage the islets of Langerhans. Most of these are B-cell poisons, and of these the two most widely used are alloxan and streptozotocin. Thus this chapter will deal primarily with these two drugs, with particular emphasis on alloxan since study of this agent shows the greatest promise of

The Islets of Langerhans
Copyright © 1981 by Academic Press, Inc.
All rights of reproduction in any form reserved.
ISBN 0-12-187820-1

contributing significantly to our understanding of B-cell physiology. Certain other B-cell toxins are dealt with briefly as they relate to the action of alloxan.

The occasional reports of A-cell toxins, such as Co^{2+} (cf. Hakanson *et al.*, 1974), Cd^{2+} (Von Holt and Von Holt, 1954; Van Campenhout, 1956), iodoacetate (IAA) (Hultquist, 1958), neutral red (Okuda and Grollman, 1966), potassium xanthate, and diethyldithiocarbamate (Kadota and Midorikawa, 1951) will not be discussed, since a selective toxic action of these agents on the A cells is far from a uniform finding (cf. Mohnike *et al.*, 1956; Falkmer, 1961), and in most cases the reports were based solely on the occurrence of hypoglycemia which of course can develop for reasons other than damage to the A cells.

II. ALLOXAN

A. General Actions

The discovery that alloxan was a B-cytotoxic agent came from the studies of Dunn *et al.* (1943) on the etiology of the renal lesions of the crush syndrome. Since uric acid injection was known to produce kidney lesions, Dunn *et al.* injected a number of related compounds, including alloxan, into rabbits. High doses of alloxan produced lesions in the distal convoluted tubules but, more importantly, they also produced necrosis of the islets of Langerhans. Although the animals did not survive long enough to develop established diabetes, permanent hyperglycemia following alloxan injection was subsequently reported in rats, rabbits, dogs, and several other species (cf. Lukens, 1948). Although at high doses alloxan may also damage the kidney and liver (cf. Lukens, 1948), at the proper dose the toxicity of this drug is restricted to the islets of Langerhans.

1. Effect of Alloxan on Islet Tissue Morphology

Studies in rabbits, rats, and dogs (cf. Lukens, 1948), as well as in fish (Falkmer, 1961), have shown similar pathological effects of alloxan. Examination with the light microscope indicated a slight but definite decrease in the number of nuclear and cytoplasmic granules in the B cells within 5 min after a single injection of a diabetogenic dose of alloxan (Bailey *et al.*, 1944); 10–60 min after injection the cytoplasm is vacuolated, the nuclei slightly pycnotic, and the cells shrunken, with a resultant increase in the pericapillary space (Lazarus *et al.*, 1962). Definite pycnosis of the nuclei is seen within 2 hr (Brunschwig and Allen, 1944; Dunn *et al.*, 1944), and after 3 hr some of the B cells are detached from one another, are rounded in shape, and have an eosinophilic cytoplasm. Nuclear karyolysis and disintegration of the nuclear membrane is observed after 5 hr, and at 24 hr most of the B cells are destroyed and the islets are composed primarily of A cells (cf. Lukens, 1948).

Electron microscope studies on the pancreas of the rabbit (Williamson and Lacy, 1959; Wellman *et al.,* 1967) and mouse (Boquist, 1977; Boquist and Lorentzon, 1979), and on the segregated islets of the sculpin (Falkmer and Olsson, 1962), indicate that the earliest B-cell changes in alloxan-treated animals are in the secretion granules, mitochondria, and plasma membrane. In contrast to the earlier report based on light microscopy, electron microscope studies showed that in the rabbit the B-cell granules increased in number during the first 5 min after alloxan injection and only subsequently disappeared (Williamson and Lacy, 1959). Boquist (1977), Boquist and Lorentzon (1979), and Lorentzon and Boquist (1979) reported that the earliest changes (10 min) seen in starved mice were swelling of the endoplasmic reticulum (ER), a decrease in the number, total volume and surface of the secretion granules, mitochondrial swelling, and disruption of the inner mitochondrial membrane; disintegration of mitochondria was seen at 60 min. Using the freeze-fracture technique, Orci *et al.* (1972, 1976) found that rat islets examined 5 min after treatment with alloxan *in vitro,* as well as islets obtained 10 min after injection of alloxan into mice, showed a decrease in the number of intramembranous particles in the plasma membrane and that the decrease was localized to the membrane's A face. Williamson and Lacy (1959) and Wellman *et al.* (1967) also reported deterioration of the plasma membranes of B cells, but at later times (1–2 hr); still later (4–5 hr), the ER and Golgi apparatus became disorganized and the mitochondrial, nuclear, and plasma membranes fragmented (Williamson and Lacy, 1959; Boquist, 1977).

Although there have been occasional reports of slight degenerative changes and necrosis of a few A cells (Dunn *et al.,* 1944; Hughes *et al.,* 1944; Duff and Starr, 1944), for the most part these cells show no visible pathological changes. However, more recent studies (Pagliara *et al.,* 1977; Goto *et al.,* 1978; Tanese *et al.,* 1978) indicate that alloxan may produce at least biochemical effects on A cells as well. Pretreatment of islets with alloxan inhibits glucagon release and suppresses the glucose inhibition of glucagon release. In keeping with the ability of sugars to protect B cells against the action of alloxan (Section II,D) 3-O-methyl-D-glucose likewise protects A cells, leading to the suggestion that alloxan acts on a glucoreceptor site on the A-cell membrane. However, it should be emphasized that A cells are considerably less sensitive to alloxan than B cells.

2. Effect of Alloxan on Blood Sugar

The earliest report of an effect of alloxan on blood sugar, long before its diabetogenic action was known, was that of Jacobs (1937) who showed that the injection of alloxan into rabbits produced initial hyperglycemia followed by severe hypoglycemia, convulsions, and death. Subsequent investigations (Dunn *et al.,* 1944; Duffy, 1945) have clearly established that injection of alloxan produces a triphasic blood sugar curve. There is initial hyperglycemia lasting from 1 to 4 hr after injection, followed by marked hypoglycemia between 6 and 12 hr and permanent hyperglycemia by 12–24 hr. In addition, a short period of hypoglycemia before the initial hyperglycemia (15–30 min after injection) has been sometimes reported (Shipley and Beyer, 1947; Wrenshall *et al.,* 1950; Gaarenstroom and Siderius, 1954).

The initial hyperglycemia may be pancreatic in origin, since it was reduced following alloxan injection into alloxan-diabetic rabbits (Brunfeldt and Iverson, 1950) and since the 12% increase in pancreatic insulin levels found 2 hr after injection of alloxan (Dixit *et al.,* 1962) suggests that there may be a sudden inhibition of insulin secretion (Webb, 1966a; Boquist and Lorentzen, 1980); alloxan is known to inhibit glucose-stimulated insulin release (Section II,D). However, there is also much evidence that the hyperglycemic phase is due to action on the liver, either a direct glycogenolytic effect (Rerup and Lundquist, 1967) or, as originally suggested by Dunn *et al.* (1943), the secretion of glucose from the liver under the influence of epinephrine released from the adrenal medulla. Alloxan produces an epinephrine-like rise in blood pressure (Hard and Carr, 1944), hepatectomy abolishes the hyperglycemic phase (Houssay *et al.,* 1945), and it has been reported that this phase is likewise abolished or decreased by adrenalectomy (Goldner and Gomori, 1944; Gaarenstroom and Siderius, 1954; Boquist and Lorentzen, 1980), although this is not a uniform finding (Houssay *et al.,* 1945).

The most widely held explanation for the subsequent hypoglycemic phase is that insulin is released into the circulation from damaged and dying B cells (Hughes *et al.,* 1944; Howell and Taylor, 1967). This is supported by the findings that (1) blood sugar does not decrease when alloxan is injected into alloxan-diabetic (Kennedy and Lukens, 1944) or depancreatized (Goldner and Gomori, 1944; Ridout *et al.,* 1944) animals, although Houssay *et al.* (1945) have reported that the latter is true only if alloxan is injected 24 hr after pancreatectomy and not if it is injected after 30 min; (2) injection of insulin results in a fall in blood sugar, which resembles that produced by intravenous injection of alloxan (Hughes *et al.,* 1944); (3) injection of antiinsulin serum abolishes the hypoglycemia (Lundquist and Rerup, 1967); and (4) most authors find that plasma insulin levels increase during the hypoglycemic phase (R-Candela *et al.,* 1955; Howell and Taylor, 1967; Lundquist and Rerup, 1967), although contrary findings have recently been reported (Boquist and Lorentzen, 1980).

3. *Possible Role of Alloxan in the Etiology of Human Diabetes*

In view of its chemical relationship to uric acid (Fig. 1), the possibility exists that alloxan may arise in the body from a disturbance in the metabolism of pyrimidines or purines and that it may thereby be an etiological factor in human diabetes (Dunn *et al.*, 1943; Archibald, 1945; Lazarow, 1949). Production of diabetes in rabbits (Griffiths, 1950), but not in rats (Grunert and Phillips, 1951a), by injection of uric acid itself was reported, but very high doses and special conditions were needed, permanent diabetes was rarely produced, and the results could not be confirmed (Collins-Williams and Bailey, 1949). The formation of alloxan from uric acid by horseradish peroxidase (Paul and Avi-Dor, 1954) and by leukocytes (Soberon and Cohen, 1963) in the presence of hydrogen peroxide at acid pH has been demonstrated, but the conditions are clearly not physiological, and attempts to demonstrate this conversion after adding uric acid to liver homogenates under more physiological conditions have failed (Grunert and Phillips, 1951b).

Nevertheless, there have been numerous reports of the presence of alloxan and its derivatives in biological specimens, beginning in the nineteenth century with the report of Liebig (1862) of its presence in the mucus of a patient with intestinal catarrh; this work was followed by the finding by Lang (1867) of murexide (an alloxan derivative) in the urine of a patient with heart disease, and that of Vande Vyver (1876) of alloxantin (a molecule made up of dialuric acid and alloxan) in the intestine of a patient

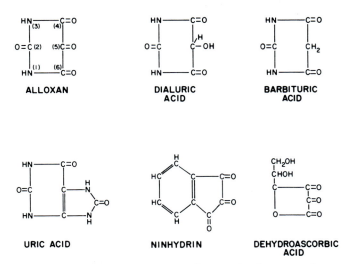

Fig. 1. Structures of alloxan and some related compounds.

poisoned with oxalic acid. In more recent times, alloxan has been reported in tissues of many species (Rubens and Tipson, 1945; Migita, 1963), as well as in the blood of rats after injection or oral administration of glucose (Schioler, 1948; Loubatieres and Bouyard, 1951). In addition, alloxanic acid, the decomposition product of alloxan, has been reported in the urine of both normal and diabetic patients (Seligson et al., 1951), although this could arise by pathways which do not include alloxan as an intermediate (Canellakis, et al., 1955).

These reports, however, cannot be accepted as conclusive evidence for the presence of alloxan in biological material, nor can the negative reports (Archibald, 1945; Bruckmann, 1946) be taken as conclusive evidence against this possibility. Most of the methods used for measuring alloxan are of doubtful specificity and rather insensitive (Karrer et al., 1945; Archibald, 1945; Bruckmann, 1946; Tipson and Cretcher, 1950). Furthermore, attempts to detect alloxan in tissues are complicated by its marked instability under physiological conditions (Richardson and Cannan, 1929; Leech and Bailey, 1945; Archibald, 1945; Patterson et al., 1949a); although it is stable in acid or at low temperature (Watkins et al., 1964a), at pH 7.4 and 37°C the half-life is about 1 min (Patterson et al., 1949a). Therefore in our view, the possible natural occurrence of alloxan remains an open question.

B. Cellular Site of Action

Although early workers suggested that alloxan might damage the B cells indirectly, either by "exhaustion" due to hyperglycemia (Dunn et al., 1943) or by producing a specific spasm of the arterioles supplying the islets (Poulsen, 1946), a large volume of work, including demonstration of selective effects on islet tissue in vitro, has made it clear that alloxan acts directly on the B cell itself. However, there is still not complete agreement on the precise location within the B cell of the target for alloxan.

1. Action on the Plasma Membrane

Considerable evidence points to the B-cell plasma membrane as the primary site of alloxan action. In 1960, Dixon et al. (1960) suggested that alloxan reacts with the surface of the B cell, since they found that after alloxan injection the B cells separated from each other and the surrounding capillaries. More direct evidence was subsequently obtained in a series of studies on the isolated islet of the toadfish. (In this species the islet is a segregated body which can be easily obtained free of pancreatic acinar tissue.) In these studies Watkins et al. (1964b, 1970) showed that as little as 10^{-6} M alloxan markedly increased the penetration of D-[1-^{14}C]mannitol and [^{14}C]inulin (which normally remain in the extracellular compartment) into toadfish islet slices; this increase was apparently due to penetration of the extracellular markers through damaged B-cell plasma membranes, since the leakage of insulin and other protein from the slices into the incubation medium also increased (Watkins *et al.*, 1964b). This *in vitro* action of alloxan resembles its *in vivo* action in that it occurs within 5 min, is selective for islet tissue, and is not duplicated by alloxanic acid, the nondiabetogenic decomposition product of alloxan. Furthermore, the alloxan concentrations most effective *in vitro* (2.5×10^{-4}–10^{-5} M) are well within the range which could reasonably exist in islet tissue following injection of a diabetogenic dose. The latter is subject to considerable uncertainty because of the rapid decomposition of alloxan and the fact that its distribution among different tissues (Section II,E) and between the extracellular and intracellular compartments (see below) is unknown; however, estimates of the maximum amount which could be present in rat islets vary from 4×10^{-4} M if it is uniformly distributed throughout the total water of all organs (Cooperstein and Lazarow, 1958), to 6.25×10^{-4} M if it is distributed among all organs as found in the toadfish (Cooperstein and Lazarow, 1964), to $1.4 \times ^{-3}$ M if it is restricted to the extracellular compartment (Cooperstein and Lazarow, 1964).

Initial studies on mammalian islets (McDaniel *et al.*, 1975a) failed to confirm the finding that alloxan increased the penetration of extracellular markers into islet cells. However, Tomita and Watanabe (1976) subsequently showed that 1.4×10^{-3} M alloxan increased the microscopically observable penetration of horseradish peroxidase into about 50% of the B cells of rat islets, although an increase in overall uptake in each rat islet was not evident. As they point out, this could explain the earlier failure to recognize the increased uptake. In addition, Grankvist *et al.* (1977) more recently showed increased penetration of trypan blue into mouse islet cells treated with alloxan, although a relatively high alloxan concentration (0.02 M) was used.

Numerous other studies on mammalian islets also support the conclusion that alloxan acts primarily on the plasma membrane. For example, as pointed out in Section II,A,1, morphological changes have been demonstrated in B-cell plasma membranes of rat islets incubated in 7×10^{-3} M alloxan (Orci *et al.*, 1976), as well as in those of mice injected with a diabetogenic dose of alloxan (Orci *et al.*, 1972); 5×10^{-3} M alloxan has been shown to depolarize mouse islet plasma membranes (cf. Matthews *et al.*, 1975); pancreatic slices and isolated islets from animals preinjected with alloxan show increased basal insulin release (Howell and Taylor, 1967; Gunnarsson and Hellerstrom, 1973); treatment with 3×10^{-4}–1.4×10^{-3} M alloxan *in vitro* under appropriate conditions increases basal insulin release from the perfused rat pancreas (Goto *et al.,* 1974) and from isolated rat islets (McDaniel *et al.,* 1976a; Weaver *et al.,* 1978a); and treatment with alloxan *in vitro* modifies both Rb$^+$ and Ca^{2+} flux across the plasma membrane (Idahl *et al.,* 1976; Weaver *et al.,* 1978a; Henquin *et al.,* 1979).

Although the increased permeability caused by alloxan suggests a general effect on the integrity of the plasma membrane, the possibility that it reacts more specifically with certain transport systems and/or plasma membrane enzymes has also been explored. This work is described in Section II,D.

2. Action at an Intracellular Site

Although the evidence discussed above and in Sections II,C,2 and II,D suggests that the primary site of action of alloxan is on the B-cell membrane, an intracellular site of action, particularly as a secondary effect, cannot be excluded. Initial investigations showed that tracer doses of [^{14}C]alloxan injected into toadfish did not enter islet cells (Cooperstein and Lazarow, 1964), and the same result was obtained when toadfish islets were incubated with low concentrations of alloxan *in vitro* (Watkins *et al.,* 1964a). However, these experiments did not rule out the possibility that diabetogenic levels of alloxan enter the cells after damaging and increasing the permeability of the membrane. Furthermore, Weaver *et al.* (1978b) have since found that 6.5×10^{-4} M [2-^{14}C]alloxan, but not alloxanic acid, is rapidly taken up by islet cells in a time- and temperature-dependent fashion. Thus, at least at diabetogenic levels, alloxan apparently enters the cells, so that the possibility of an intracellular action must be considered.

If alloxan does act intracellularly, it is reasonable to think that its target is some critical enzyme, although the possibility, for example, that it damages organelle membranes (lysosomes?), thereby disturbing the normal compartmentation of enzymes, cofactors, and ions, also exists. Numerous enzymes and enzyme systems have been shown to be inhibited by alloxan (cf. Webb, 1966a), but virtually all these reports deal with tissues other than islet. Whether or not the corresponding enzymes in islet tissue are inhibited is unknown; studies on islets have been limited largely to the effects of alloxan on overall glucose metabolism. Although Gunnarsson and Hellerstrom (1973) observed no decrease in anaerobic glycolysis or [^{14}C]pyruvate metabolism in islets isolated from obese hyperglycemic mice injected with alloxan 10 min before sacrifice, oxidation of D-[^{14}C]glucose and D-[^{14}C]mannose was strongly inhibited. Furthermore, treatment of islets *in vitro* with 3×10^{-4}–1×10^{-2} M alloxan markedly inhibited D-glucose utilization (Borg *et al.,* 1979; Ishibashi *et al.* 1979), decreased glycolytic flux by 80–85% (Jain *et al.,* 1978), and decreased oxidation of D-glucose by 50% (Henquin *et al.,* 1979).

However, there is considerable doubt that the inhibition of glucose metabolism can explain the rapid cell death produced by alloxan. Cytological changes in the B cell indicative of cell damage are found as early as 5 min after the injection of alloxan (Hughes *et al.,* 1944; Bailey *et al.,* 1944), and it seems unlikely that reaction of this compound with an intracellular enzyme could produce irreversible damage in such a short time. Inhibition of metabolic pathways seldom produces immediate histological changes in tissue, and neither agents known to inhibit major metabolic pathways, nor anoxia for several minutes, produces B-cell damage such as that produced by alloxan (Webb, 1966a). For these reasons, as well as others outlined in Section II,C,2 and II,D, it is felt that the bulk of evidence supports the plasma membrane as the primary site of action of alloxan and that any intracellular effects are probably secondary and not critical to its toxicity.

C. Chemistry of Action

1. Structural Requirements

Numerous studies have attempted to define the specific portions of the alloxan molecule which are responsible for its toxic effects; these have been reviewed previously (Lukens, 1948. Webb, 1966a; Rerup, 1970) and will be summarized briefly here.

The structures of alloxan and some related compounds are shown in Fig. 1. The most critical requirement for producing irreversible B-cell damage appears to be the presence of the CO–CO–CO grouping with the highly reactive central C = O, which is probably hydrated (Bruckmann and Wertheimer, 1947; Tipson and Cretcher, 1951; Lazarow, 1954). Several related compounds lacking the 5-carbonyl group have been studied and shown not to produce diabetes (cf. Bruckmann and Wertheimer, 1945; Webb, 1966a), but the most interesting of these are barbituric acid and dialuric acid, the reduction product of alloxan, since these compounds lack the 5-carbonyl with no change in the rest of the molecule.

Although some islet lesions are seen with barbituric acid, this compound does not produce diabetes (Goldner and Gomori, 1944; Grande-Covian, 1945; Vargus and Mundt, 1948; Schmidt *et al.,* 1968) or duplicate the *in vitro* actions of alloxan on islet tissue (Weaver *et al.,* 1978c). In fact, barbituric acid at least partly protects against both the *in vivo* (Martinez, 1955; Schmidt *et al.,* 1968) and *in vitro* effects of alloxan, although this may be the result of a direct reaction with alloxan (Weaver *et al.,* 1978c).

There is somewhat more uncertainty concerning dialuric acid. Despite occasional negative reports (Goldner and Gomori, 1944), there is little doubt that injection of dialuric acid (Bruckmann and Wertheimer, 1945; Laszt, 1945; Bailey *et al.,* 1946) produces diabetes. However, most workers feel that it does so only because it is rapidly oxidized to alloxan (e.g.,

Lazarow, 1946; Bruckmann and Wertheimer, 1947; Siliprandi and Pisati, 1949; Frerichs and Creutzfeldt, 1971); this conclusion is based largely on the fact that cysteine, which reduces alloxan to dialuric acid, protects animals against alloxan diabetes (Lazarow, 1946). On the other hand, this does not rule out the recent proposal (Section II,C,2) that the active diabetogenic agents may be free radical intermediates formed in the oxidation of dialuric acid and/or the reduction of injected alloxan to dialuric acid by endogenous reducing agents, and that therefore dialuric acid and alloxan are equally diabetogenic. However, methylene blue prevents the reduction of alloxan to dialuric acid and should thereby prevent the production of free radical intermediates, but injection of methylene blue immediately before alloxan in fact potentiates alloxan diabetes (Lazarow and Liambies, 1950). This seems to be strong evidence that alloxan itself is the active agent; while methylene blue might theoretically increase free radical formation by increasing the rate of oxidation of the small amount of dialuric acid formed by endogenous reductants, despite the presence of methylene blue, this seems very unlikely in view of the rapid oxidation of dialuric acid by oxygen itself.

The apparent need for the CO–CO–CO grouping led Patterson (1950) to test dehydroascorbic acid, which is an oxidation product of ascorbic acid and which contains this grouping. He found that this agent produced diabetes in the rat, and the diabetogenic action of dehydroascorbic acid was confirmed by subsequent work in the rabbit (Princiotto, 1951). Furthermore, dehydroascorbic acid behaves like alloxan in many ways. It gives the Strecker reaction (Section II,C,2) (cf. Patterson, 1950); it reacts with SH groups (Drake et al., 1942; cf. Patterson, 1950); its diabetogenic action is prevented by glutathione (GSH) and cysteine (Princiotto, 1951); it accumulates in islets (Hammarstrom, 1966) under the same conditions as alloxan (Section II,E); it produces degenerative changes in B cells similar (but not identical) to those produced by alloxan (Patterson and Lazarow, 1950; MacDonald and Bhattacharya, 1956); it increases the permeability of islet cell membranes in vitro (Pillsbury et al., 1973); it causes a burst of insulin release (Merlini and Caramia, 1965; Pence and Mennear, 1979); and it inhibits subsequent glucose stimulation of insulin release, and this action is partly prevented by high glucose (Pence and Mennear, 1979). On the other hand its action differs from that of alloxan sufficiently to suggest that the CO–CO–CO grouping is not the sole determinant of diabetogenic activity. It is more difficult to produce diabetes with dehydroascorbic acid than with alloxan, as evidenced by several negative reports (Banerjee et al., 1962; Pence and Mennear, 1979); it requires massive doses and repeated injections (Patterson, 1950); and, unlike alloxan, it apparently does not cause significant B-cell necrosis (Patterson and Lazarow, 1950; Merlini and Caramia, 1965).

Among the pyrimidine derivatives, an additional requirement for at least one unsubstituted nitrogen, perhaps because of the need for enolization, has likewise been suggested (cf. Webb, 1966a; Rerup, 1970). Diabetogenic activity is not decreased by the presence of small substituents on one nitrogen but is lost when both nitrogens are substituted.

The requirement for an intact pyrimidine nucleus also seems clear; related compounds lacking this nucleus are not diabetogenic (Lukens, 1948; Rerup, 1970). Ninhydrin is particularly interesting, since it lacks the intact pyrimidine nucleus and the nitrogens, but contains the critical CO–CO–CO grouping with the middle carbon hydrated as in alloxan and has a steric configuration very similar to alloxan (Weaver et al., 1979) (see Chapter 5). Furthermore, ninhydrin is present in the pancreas after injection (Bruckmann and Wertheimer, 1947), is taken up by islets in vitro by an alloxan-sensitive system (McDaniel et al., 1979) and, like alloxan (Section II,D), inhibits glucose-induced insulin release (McDaniel et al., 1977a). Yet, although it has been reported to produce pathological changes in islets (Stoll, 1946; Vargus and Mundt, 1948), it is generally agreed that ninhydrin is not diabetogenic (Bruckmann and Wertheimer, 1945, 1947; Hidy, 1946; Vargus and Mundt, 1948). Perhaps the CO–CO–CO grouping with the particular configuration present in alloxan and ninhydrin is sufficient to damage the insulin release mechanism but, in addition, the intact pyrimidine ring and/or a nitrogen is needed to kill the cell. On the other hand, ninhydrin is very toxic (Bruckmann and Wertheimer, 1945; Stoll, 1946), so that it may be impossible to inject enough to demonstrate diabetogenic activity.

Although these results therefore seem to point clearly to a requirement for an intact pyrimidine nucleus, three adjacent carbonyl groups, and at least one free nitrogen, caution must be used in interpretation, since changes in one substituent can also modify diabetogenic activity indirectly by consequent changes in the reactivity of other parts of the molecule. In particular, Webb (1966a) has pointed out that modifying the carbonyl groups would prevent formation of a quinonoid structure which he feels may be important; none of the inactive compounds reported can form such a structure.

2. Chemical Mechanism of Alloxan Action

Many studies have been carried out in an attempt to determine which of the numerous chemical reactions of alloxan is the specific one underlying its cytotoxicity, and several reviews of this work have appeared (Lazarow,

1949, 1954; Webb, 1966a; Havu, 1969; Frerichs and Creutzfeldt, 1971; Rerup, 1970). None of the theories developed can be considered established, since all the experimental data are subject to reasonable alternate interpretations. In addition to the demonstration that alloxan can carry out the putative critical reaction *in vivo* (a necessary but not sufficient condition), support for each theory has come from two types of approaches: (1) correlating the ability of related compounds to carry out the reaction with their ability to produce B-cell damage, and (2) correlating the ability of agents to prevent the reaction with their ability to prevent the B-cell cytotoxicity of alloxan. While evidence obtained from these approaches can certainly be supportive, neither positive nor negative results are unequivocal. On the one hand, related compounds which carry out the putative critical reaction and are diabetogenic often have other properties in common with alloxan, and some may produce diabetes by a totally different mechanism; compounds which prevent the putative critical reaction and prevent alloxan diabetes could do so by directly inactivating alloxan or by indirectly modifying the cellular site of action rather than by interfering with the critical reaction per se. Conversely, related compounds which carry out the critical reaction may fail to produce B-cell damage, and compounds which interfere with the critical reaction may fail to protect against diabetes because they are too toxic, are not soluble in sufficient concentration, do not reach the crucial cellular site of alloxan action, etc. Furthermore, not all group-specific reagents react with all compounds containing the particular group; very few, if any, SH-containing enzymes react with all SH-binding reagents (Webb, 1966b). A further complication is introduced by the fact that many investigators have used blood sugar changes as their sole criterion of B-cell damage; since it is well known that many other factors can modify blood sugar, these studies shed no real light and will generally not be reviewed in this section.

The theory that alloxan produces B-cell damage by deaminating amino acids to yield ammonia, carbon dioxide, and an aldehyde or ketone with one less carbon (the Strecker reaction) (Strecker, 1862) has been considered (Bruckmann and Wertheimer, 1945, 1947; Said *et al.*, 1977), but it has been rejected by most investigators because this reaction is too slow to account for the rapid action of alloxan (cf. Rerup, 1970; Frerichs and Creutzfeldt, 1971), it requires a higher concentration of alloxan than could reasonably be expected to exist *in vivo* following a diabetogenic dose (Burgen and Lorch, 1947), and many other Strecker reagents do not produce diabetes (Bruckmann and Wertheimer, 1945, 1947; Rerup, 1970).

The theory that alloxan acts at least partly by chelating Zn^{2+} (cf. Kadota, 1950; Maske *et al.*, 1952; Okamoto, 1955) has been supported primarily by reports that alloxan injection results in a loss of histochemically detectable

Zn^{2+} from the B cells and that this loss parallels cell damage (Maske *et al.*, 1952); that a number of metals protect rats against alloxan diabetes (Lazarow, 1954); and that numerous chelators such as oxin (8-hydroxyquinoline), dithizone (diphenylthiocarbazone), and various xanthates and quinoline derivatives produce diabetes with characteristics resembling those of alloxan diabetes (cf. Rerup, 1970; Okamoto, 1970; Frerichs and Creutzfeldt, 1971). However, this theory is not widely accepted for a number of reasons (cf. Lazarow, 1954; Havu, 1969; Lazaris and Babelskyi, 1979). Most importantly, it has been shown that alloxan itself does not complex with Cu^{2+} or Zn^{2+}; it is the nondiabetogenic alloxanic acid which does so (Resnik *et al.*, 1956; Obo, 1960; Tarui, 1963). Furthermore, even the role of chelation in the diabetogenic action of the known chelators is uncertain (Lazarow, 1954); it has been suggested, for example, that 8-hydroxyquinoline may not itself be diabetogenic but may be oxidized to a quinone derivative which, like alloxan, has a highly reactive carbonyl next to a pyridine nitrogen and therefore could also react with SH groups; dithizone likewise has two adjacent reactive groups. This idea takes on added significance in view of reports that dithizone injection decreases GSH levels and that thiol compounds protect rats against dithizone diabetes (cf. Havu, 1969).

The theory that alloxan is toxic by virtue of its ability to react with SH-containing cellular elements, either GSH or an essential SH-containing enzyme or coenzyme (Lazarow, 1949), has been the most widely held view on its mechanism of action. It is well known that alloxan reacts both reversibly and irreversibly with SH groups; the former results in the formation of a disulfide bond with concomitant reduction of alloxan (Labes and Freisburger, 1930) to dialuric acid, and the latter reaction results in the formation of an unidentified complex with GSH and protein SH groups which has a 305-nm absorption maximum (Patterson *et al.*, 1949b; Resnik and Wolff, 1956; Kay and Murfitt, 1960). Although the exact nature of the complex between alloxan and GSH is uncertain, its formation requires the 5-carbonyl group and a free SH group (Patterson *et al.*, 1949b; Resnik and Wolff, 1956). It is further believed that a second bond, in addition to that between $C=O$ and SH, is formed (Lazarow, 1954; Resnik and Wolff, 1956). The nature of this bond is speculative, but it may be with an amino group (Yesair, 1970).

That a reaction between alloxan and SH groups does in fact take place *in vivo* was originally suggested by Lieben and Edel (1933) and now seems clear on the basis of two types of work. First, treatments which lower GSH levels, such as fasting, ascorbic acid injection, and a low-protein diet (cf. Rerup, 1970), increase the susceptibility of animals to alloxan diabetes, whereas various treatments which raise blood GSH (cf. Rerup, 1970) including injection of thiol compounds such as GSH, cysteine, and

2,3-dimercaptopropanol (BAL) (Lazarow, 1946, 1947; Chesler and Tislow, 1947), all protect animals against alloxan diabetes. Second, after alloxan injection the GSH concentration decreases in blood and tissues (Ecker *et al.*, 1939; Leech and Bailey, 1945; Bruckmann and Wertheimer, 1947; Bhattacharya *et al.*, 1956), including the islets (Falkmer, 1961; Havu, 1969); there is likewise a decrease in free SH (detected histochemically) in the B cells (Barnett *et al.*, 1955; MacDonald, 1959). Some investigators also find no change or a concomitant decrease in the level of oxidized GSH (GSSG), indicating that the decrease in GSH involves more than simple oxidation (Falkmer, 1961; Bhattacharya *et al.*, 1956). Since some nondiabetogenic compounds related to alloxan, such as ninhydrin, butyl alloxan, and benzyl alloxan (Bruckmann and Wertheimer, 1947; Griffiths, 1950), also lower blood GSH, not surprisingly other factors must be involved in the production of diabetes as well.

Results of studies designed to determine if other SH-binding reagents produce diabetes have been variable and dependent at least in part on the animal species, making them impossible to evaluate. Damage to B cells has been reported after treatment with IAA and its derivatives, *p*-hydroxymercuribenzoate, methylmercuric chloride, arsenite, Cd^{2+}, and Co^{2+}, but negative results have also been reported for IAA, Co^{2+}, and allylisothiocyanate (cf. Falkmer, 1961; Havu, 1969; Shigenaga, 1976; Boquist, 1979). Nevertheless, Havu (1969) has concluded that SH inhibitors are overtly or potentially diabetogenic and that those agents, such as alloxan and Co^{2+}, which react with both monothiols and dithiols are more effective than those which only react with monothiols (IAA and allylisothiocyanate) or those which react primarily with dithiols (Cd^{2+} and arsenite).

In vitro studies, free of many of the complications of *in vivo* work, strongly support the theory that alloxan damages the B cells by reacting with SH groups and have provided some evidence on the nature and location of these groups. Like alloxan (Section II,B,1), a number of SH-binding reagents increase the permeability of toadfish islet cell membranes to extracellular markers such as mannitol and inulin, and they appear to do so by acting at the same site as alloxan (Watkins *et al.*, 1970, 1973; Cooperstein and Watkins, 1978). Other SH-binding reagents, like alloxan, likewise increase the penetration of trypan blue into mouse islet cells (Grankvist *et al.*, 1979a) and increase basal insulin release from islets (Bloom *et al.*, 1972; Hellman *et al.*, 1974a; Landgraf-Leurs *et al.*, 1978); many (R-Candela *et al.*, 1963; Ghafghazi and Mennear, 1975; Henquin and Lambert, 1975), but not all (Bloom *et al.*, 1972), also inhibit subsequent glucose-induced insulin release. Furthermore, with the exception of their failure to protect against the changes in membrane potential produced by alloxan (Dean and Matthews, 1972), thiol compounds protect islets against the *in vitro* actions of alloxan including the permeability increase produced in toadfish islets (Watkins *et al.*, 1964b, 1971a; Watkins and Cooperstein, 1976) and the alloxan inhibition of glucose-stimulated insulin release (Tomita and Lacy, 1972).

The permeability changes produced by alloxan, and the fact that several SH-binding reagents which increase basal insulin release are nonpenetrating or penetrate membranes very slowly (Bloom *et al.*, 1972; Hellman *et al.*, 1973a, 1974a), suggest that the SH groups with which alloxan reacts are located superficially on the plasma membrane. This is supported by the finding that GSH reverses the effects of GSSG and cystine on toadfish islet cell permeability (Watkins *et al.*, 1971a), yet GSH does not penetrate these cells (unpublished). In this connection it is of interest that Sneer *et al.* (1971) have suggested that GSH maintains membrane SH groups in the reduced form, and when GSH levels are decreased the former are oxidized and permeability thus modified.

Since the SH-binding reagents which increase toadfish islet permeability are generally those capable of reacting with two SH groups to form a ring, since the dose–response curves show an optimum typical of a two-point attachment, since BAL but not GSH reverses the action of alloxan, and since the ability of several dithiols to protect against and reverse the action of alloxan decreases with increased spacing between the two SH groups, it has been suggested that alloxan acts by reacting with two adjacent SH groups (Watkins *et al.*, 1970, 1971a; Watkins and Cooperstein, 1976); however, it is equally possible that only formation of a ring is necessary and that in the case of alloxan the second group is an amino group.

Most recently it has been proposed that alloxan is diabetogenic only because it gives rise to hydrogen peroxide and free radicals such as O_2^- (superoxide) and $\cdot$ OH during reduction to dialuric acid and its reoxidation, and that these are the immediate cytotoxic agents (Heikkila *et al.*, 1974). There is ample evidence that alloxan gives rise to such toxic agents *in vivo*. It has been shown that injected alloxan increases the amount of hydrogen peroxide found in mouse red cells (Heikkila and Cohen, 1975), and a host of earlier studies on the production of hemolysis by dialuric acid and alloxan in vitamin E-deficient animals (Gyorgi and Rose, 1949; Rose and Gyorgi, 1950; Bunyan *et al.*, 1960; Fee and Teitelbaum, 1972) are consistent with the formation of a "reactive intermediate" between dialuric acid and alloxan. The latter studies also suggest that the intermediate is produced during oxidation of dialuric acid rather than reduction of alloxan; dialuric acid is more effective than alloxan *in vivo,* and only the former is effective *in vitro.*

The hypothesis that free radicals are the active agents in the diabetogenic action of alloxan is based on the finding that scavengers of free radicals and hydrogen peroxide, such as various alcohols and urea derivatives (Heikkila *et al.*, 1974, 1976; Heikkila and Cabbat, 1978), protect animals against diabetes. It is also supported by *in vitro* studies. For example, dihydroxyfumarate which, like alloxan, produces superoxide anions and • OH radicals, likewise inhibits glucose stimulation of insulin release from rat islets, and pretreatment of islets with superoxide dismutase, catalase, or dimethylurea (Fischer and Hamburger, 1980a,b) protects against inhibition by both agents. Furthermore, in mouse islets (Grankvist *et al.*, 1979b), superoxide dismutase, catalase, and scavengers of • OH radicals protect against the alloxan-induced inhibition of Rb^+ uptake, and most of them also protect against the alloxan-induced cell membrane damage evidenced by increased trypan blue uptake. In general there is a good correlation between the free radical scavenging ability of various compounds and their ability to protect against the actions of alloxan.

While these data make an impressive case in support of the free radical theory, there are some uncertainties. The possibility that at least the alcohols protect against alloxan diabetes by elevating blood glucose has been discussed (Heikkila *et al.*, 1974, 1976; Schauberger *et al.*, 1977), but it is difficult to imagine that protection against the *in vitro* actions of alloxan could result from the formation of glucose. There are also certain discrepancies in the correlation between the ability of various agents to protect against alloxan and their ability to scavenge free radicals, but these can be rationalized in various ways (Heikkila *et al.*, 1976; McDaniel *et al.*, 1978; Grankvist *et al.*, 1979; Fischer and Hamburger, 1980b). However, two other considerations seem more difficult to explain. First, whereas tocopherol protects against hemolysis by alloxan–dialuric acid (Gyorgi and Rose, 1949), and GSH and cysteine potentiate hemolysis (Rose and Gyorgi, 1950), tocopherol does not protect against alloxan diabetes (Gyorgi and Rose, 1949) while GSH and cysteine do; therefore it seems very likely that different mechanisms are involved. Deamer *et al.* (1971) have acknowledged that, if the thiol reagents reduce alloxan, they should potentiate the action of alloxan rather than protect against it, and suggest that these reagents act by complexing alloxan; however, there is no evidence that cysteine can form such a complex (Patterson *et al.*, 1949b; Kay and Murfitt, 1960). Second, dialuric acid, since it is a better hemolytic agent and is the major source of free radicals, should be at least as effective as alloxan in producing diabetes; yet the weight of evidence appears to support the view that dialuric acid is not diabetogenic (Section II,C,1). At the same time it must be recognized that no satisfactory alternate explanation for the large amount of data consistent with this theory has yet been offered. It should also be recognized that this theory is not inconsistent with the idea that membrane SH groups are the target of alloxan action, since SH groups are certainly affected by free radicals (cf. Pryor, 1976), and Bunyan *et al.* (1960) have suggested that dialuric acid hemolysis results from a product of its oxidation attacking membranes.

D. Relation to Glucose Transport and Insulin Release

There is considerable evidence that alloxan may damage the B cells by reacting with a site involved in glucose transport, insulin release, or both; this is of considerable interest because, if true, alloxan would thereby represent an excellent tool for probing the nature of this site(s) (e.g., see Chapter 5).

It is well known that alloxan treatment modifies insulin release from islets. Injected alloxan increases plasma insulin (Section II,A,2), and islets isolated from preinjected animals, as well as islets incubated with alloxan *in vitro,* show increased basal insulin release (Section II,B,1). This increased insulin release was initially ascribed to cell membrane damage (Watkins *et al.,* 1964b), but it appears to be a more active process since, like glucose stimulation of insulin release, it seems to require Ca^{2+} and is accompanied by increased Ca^{2+} uptake (Weaver *et al.,* 1978a). In addition, pancreatic slices and islets isolated from animals which have been injected with alloxan a short time earlier release less insulin than normal in response to glucose (Howell and Taylor, 1967; Gunnarsson and Hellerstrom, 1973), and pretreatment of islets with low concentrations of alloxan *in vitro* inhibits subsequent D-glucose-induced insulin release (Tomita *et al.,* 1974; Niki *et al.,* 1976; Weaver *et al.,* 1978a).

It is equally well known that injection of sugars protects animals against alloxan diabetes (e.g., Kass and Waisbren, 1945; Sen and Bhattacharya, 1952), and sugars likewise protect islets against the *in vitro* effects of alloxan (Watkins *et al.,* 1968, 1973; Dean and Matthews, 1972; Orci *et al.,* 1976; Idahl *et al.,* 1976; Niki *et al.,* 1976; Weaver *et al.,* 1978a; Ishibashi *et al.,* 1979; Zawalich *et al.,* 1979). Since D-glucose does not hasten alloxan destruction or react chemically with alloxan (Sen and Bhattacharya, 1952; Weaver *et al.,* 1978b), since protection by sugars is competitive (Bhattacharya, 1954; Zawalich and Beidler, 1973: Idahl *et al.,* 1977; Weaver *et al.,* 1978a), and since D-glucose and alloxan are sterically similar (see Chapter 5), it seems most likely that sugars interfere with the action of alloxan at its site of action on the B cell.

If alloxan exerts its effects on islet tissue by interfering with metabolism (Section II,B,2), it is possible that D-glucose, or one of its metabolites, can protect against the action of alloxan by preventing its attachment to the target enzyme. However, while it has been found that sugars protect against alloxan inhibition of D-glucose metabolism by islet tissue (Henquin *et al.,* 1979; Borg *et al.,* 1979; Ishibashi *et al.,* 1979), this explanation seems highly unlikely. Zawalich *et al.* (1979) have concluded from their studies that inhibition of glucose utilization by islets is probably not great enough to account for alloxan inhibition of D-glucose-stimulated insulin release. Furthermore, mannoheptulose, which inhibits glucose metabolism, blocks the protection against alloxan diabetes afforded by glucose even when given after the glucose, when the latter should already have been metabolized (Rossini *et al.*, 1975). In addition, nonmetabolizable sugars and analogues (3-*O*-methyl-D-glucose, D-galactose, phlorizin, 2-deoxy-D-glucose, etc.) protect against both the *in vivo* (Carter and Younathan, 1962; Zawalich and Beidler, 1973; Rossini *et al.*, 1975) and *in vitro* (Watkins *et al.*, 1973; Tomita *et al.*, 1974; Idahl *et al.*, 1976; Tomita, 1976; Weaver *et al.*, 1978a; Henquin *et al.*, 1979) effects of alloxan; although 3-*O*-methyl-D-glucose and D-galactose may protect indirectly, since they apparently stimulate D-glucose metabolism (Tomita *et al.*, 1974), this cannot explain the protective action of phlorizin or 2-deoxy-D-glucose. Finally, both D-glucose and D-mannose facilitate alloxan entry into islet cells (Weaver *et al.*, 1978b) but nevertheless prevent its action.

In view of the considerable evidence that alloxan exerts its primary action on the plasma membrane (Section II,B,1), most workers have considered the latter to be the most likely site of sugar and alloxan interaction. Since transportable sugars protect against the action of alloxan, and since interference with D-glucose uptake could reasonably be presumed to interfere with D-glucose stimulation of insulin release, the sugar transport site was initially considered a likely target (Watkins *et al.*, 1968, 1973). However, evidence that D-glucose may trigger insulin release by reacting with a membrane glucoreceptor, which may be different from the sugar carrier (Matschinsky *et al.*, 1972; Hellman, 1972; Grodsky *et al.*, 1974; McDaniel *et al.*, 1975b), raises the possibility that the glucoreceptor is the binding site of alloxan.

This issue remains undecided. On the one hand there is considerable evidence that alloxan acts at or near the sugar transport site rather than at a site involved in insulin release. For example, the relative abilities of cytochalasin B and cytochalasin D to protect against alloxan inhibition of D-glucose-stimulated insulin release parallel their effects on sugar transport but are not correlated with their relative abilities to potentiate D-glucose stimulation of insulin release (McDaniel *et al.*, 1975B); cytochalasin B protects against alloxan inhibition of D-glucose-stimulated insulin release, inhibits hexose transport and potentiates D-glucose stimulation of insulin release, whereas cytochalasin D potentiates D-glucose stimulation of insulin release but does not inhibit hexose transport and does not protect. Caffeine and theophylline likewise inhibit sugar transport (McDaniel *et al.*, 1977b) and protect against alloxan inhibition of D-glucose-stimulated insulin release (Lacy *et al.*, 1975; Tomita and Scarpelli, 1977). Furthermore, the ability of different sugars to protect against alloxan inhibition of D-glucose-induced insulin release does not parallel their ability to release insulin (Tomita *et al.*, 1974). For example, although it has been reported that 3-*O*-methyl-D-glucose does not protect against the alloxan-induced depolarization of islet cells (Matthews and Dean, 1972), it does protect against most of the *in vitro* actions of alloxan (Watkins *et al.*, 1973; Tomita *et al.*, 1974; Idahl *et al.*, 1976; Pagliara *et al.*, 1977; Zawalich *et al.*, 1979) as well as its diabetogenic effect (Carter and Younathan, 1962; Rossini *et al.*, 1975). However, this sugar does not stimulate insulin release (Coore and Randle, 1964; Hellman *et al.*, 1974b) but is transported by the islet sugar carrier (Cooperstein and Lazarow, 1969; Hellman *et al.*, 1971a) and therefore may compete with alloxan for the latter; this possibility is supported by the finding that 3-*O*-methyl-D-glucose inhibits the transport of alloxan into islet cells by the sugar carrier (Weaver *et al.*, 1978b).

On the other hand there is also considerable evidence supporting the idea that the glucoreceptor which may be involved in insulin release is the site of alloxan binding. For example, the differential abilities of the α and β anomers of D-glucose to protect against alloxan toxicity parallel their actions on insulin release but not their transport by the sugar carrier. The α anomer provides better protection against both the *in vivo* action of alloxan (Rossini *et al.*, 1975) and its *in vivo* effects on membrane permeability (Cooperstein and Watkins, 1973) and D-glucose-stimulated insulin synthesis and release (Niki *et al.*, 1976; McDaniel *et al.*, 1976; Ishibashi *et al.*, 1978). The α anomer is likewise more effective in releasing insulin (Niki *et al.*, 1974; Grodsky *et al.*, 1974) but does not have a greater affinity for the transport system than the β anomer (Miwa *et al.*, 1975; Idahl *et al.*, 1975). The dose-response curve for D-glucose protection against alloxan inhibition of Rb^+ uptake also correlates well with the dose–response curve for D-glucose stimulation of insulin release (Idahl *et al.*, 1977). Furthermore, whereas NADPH (reduced NADP) releases insulin from toadfish islets and protects against and reverses the action of alloxan on these islets, the oxidized form (NADP) does neither. Finally, alloxan does not inhibit sugar transport (McDaniel *et al.*, 1975a), and many of the data supporting the thesis that it acts at this site can be rationalized. The failure of cytochalasin D to protect against alloxan while potentiating insulin release (McDaniel *et al.*, 1975b) could still be explained if it acted on the latter at a step subsequent to the binding of D-glucose to the glucoreceptor, and the argument that the ability of some sugars to protect against alloxan and to release insulin is not correlated is weakened by the fact that the order of their affinity for the sugar carrier is unknown (Tomita *et al.*, 1974). Similarly, the discrepancy between the ability of 3-*O*-methyl-D-glucose to protect against alloxan toxicity and to stimulate insulin release could be explained if this sugar binds to the glucoreceptor in a way which prevents alloxan binding but does not itself stimulate release of insulin (Niki *et al.*, 1976); in addition, as pointed out by Rossini *et al.* (1975), the results with 3-*O*-methyl-D-glucose are equally difficult to incorporate into the thesis that alloxan acts on the sugar carrier, since this sugar provides better protection than D-glucose against the *in vivo* action of alloxan, yet the latter is transported more readily.

There also remains the possibility that alloxan does not bind at either site; this is one alternative proposed by Scheynius and Täljedal (1971), and supported by Rossini *et al.* (1975), in order to explain the effects of mannoheptulose. Mannoheptulose completely blocks at least the first phase of D-glucose-stimulated insulin release (Scheynius and Täljedal, 1971; Tomita *et al.*, 1974), at least partly blocks D-glucose and 3-*O*-methyl-D-glucose protection against alloxan diabetes (Scheynius and Täljedal, 1971; Zawalich and Beidler, 1973), and sensitizes rats to alloxan, presumably by blocking the action of endogenous D-glucose (Rossini *et al.*, 1975); it also blocks sugar protection against alloxan inhibition of D-glucose-stimulated insulin synthesis (Jain and Logothetopoulos, 1976) and release (Tomita *et al.*, 1974) and against alloxan inhibition of Rb^+ accumulation (Idahl *et al.*, 1977). Yet it does not itself protect against alloxan diabetes (Scheynius and Täljedal, 1971), alloxan-induced depolarization of islet cells (Dean and Matthews, 1972), alloxan inhibition of Rb^+ uptake (Idahl *et al.*, 1976, 1977), or alloxan inhibition of glucose-stimulated insulin synthesis (Jain and Logothetopoulos, 1976) and release (cf. Niki *et al.*, 1976).

These results could be explained if binding of D-glucose, to the glucoreceptor or transport site, produced a conformational change which prevented binding of alloxan at some other location, and vice versa (Scheynius and Täljedal, 1971), whereas binding of mannoheptulose to the sugar receptor site prevented D-glucose binding but did not produce this conformational change. At the same time, Scheynius and Täljedal (1971) also entertain the possibility that the site of alloxan binding, like that of mannoheptulose and D-glucose, is the sugar transport site, and that the binding of D-glucose, but not that of mannoheptulose, is associated with a change in the conformation of the carrier, which reduces the latter's affinity for alloxan. They further suggest that the interaction of alloxan with the sugar carrier may occur as alloxan enters the B cell via the carrier subsequently to produce intracellular damage. However, as discussed above, an intracellular site of alloxan action seems highly unlikely, and, as pointed out by Niki *et al.* (1976), the same type of explanation could be invoked to support the hypothesis that sugars and alloxan interact at the glucoreceptor involved in insulin release; this seems more likely than the sugar transport site, since neither alloxan (McDaniel *et al.*, 1975a) nor moderate concentrations of mannoheptulose (Matschinsky *et al.*, 1970; Hellman *et al.*, 1971b) inhibit sugar transport. This implies that mannoheptulose has a greater affinity for the glucoreceptor than D-glucose (since it prevents D-glucose binding) but, unlike D-glucose, does not alter the receptor in a way which prevents alloxan binding or stimulates insulin release (Niki *et al.,* 1976).

More recently, two other sites on the plasma membrane have been proposed as possible targets for alloxan action; one is the Na^+-K^+ pump and the other the cyclic adenosine $3',5'$-monophosphate (cAMP) system. The former was suggested by Idahl *et al.* (1976, 1977) and supported by Henquin *et al.* (1979) on the basis of the finding that alloxan inhibited Rb^+ accumulation by mouse and rat islets and dispersed islet cells and delayed the reduction in Rb^+ efflux normally produced by D-glucose. However, Idahl *et al.* (1977) could not demonstrate inhibition of an ouabain-sensitive ATPase in islets, perhaps because of low control activities. The idea that alloxan acts primarily on the cAMP system was suggested by the finding (Zawalich *et al.,* 1979) that diabetogenic concentrations of alloxan blocked the D-glucose-induced increase in cAMP and that sugars protected against this effect. Furthermore, in contrast to results reported earlier (McDaniel and Lacy, 1975), dibutyryl cAMP, as well as theophylline and caffeine (but not cAMP itself), all protected against alloxan inhibition of D-glucose-stimulated insulin release, suggesting that alloxan may act on adenylate cyclase (Tomita and Scarpelli, 1977). This is supported by the earlier finding of Cohen and Bitensky (1969) that low concentrations of alloxan markedly inhibited adenylate cyclase in washed particles of rat liver, heart, brain, and kidney and in hamster islet adenoma. However, D-glucose protected against the action of alloxan on insulin release and cAMP accumulation even under conditions where the sugar did not stimulate insulin secretion or increase cAMP levels. Furthermore, 3-*O*-methyl-D-glucose protection cannot be mediated by cAMP metabolism, since it does not increase cAMP levels or prevent glucose from doing so (Zawalich *et al.,* 1979). In view of these observations, and since alloxan inhibition of the cAMP increase could be explained as an effect secondary to its blockage of D-glucose binding to the glucoreceptor and/or to a disturbance in normal ion exchange, the cyclase system as a possible primary site of alloxan action does not appear to be well supported.

E. Basis of Selectivity

The basis of the remarkable selectivity of alloxan for the B cells is of intense interest because of the light it may shed on the unique physiology of these cells. Four general types of explanations have been considered:

1. Injected alloxan may accumulate selectively in B cells.
2. Alloxan may be destroyed or detoxified less rapidly in or around B cells than in other tissues.

3. The toxic agent may be a substance derived from alloxan by a reaction which occurs more readily in B cells than elsewhere.

4. The target for alloxan action may be a unique qualitative or quantitative feature of the metabolism or structure of the B cell.

In view of the instability of alloxan and the rapidity of its action, a priori it appears that selective accumulation of alloxan in the islet is unlikely, and most investigations have supported this view. Early workers (Bruckmann and Wertheimer, 1947; Lee and Stetten, 1952; Janes and Winnick, 1952) found that after injection of alloxan lesser amounts accumulated in the pancreas than in other tissues, but it was recognized that, because of the presence of large amounts of acinar tissue, this provided no information on the possible selective accumulation of alloxan in the islets of Langerhans themselves. This problem was circumvented in later work by utilizing either radioautography or a species (toadfish) in which the islet is an isolated structure free of pancreatic acinar tissue. The latter studies (Cooperstein and Lazarow, 1964) showed unequivocally that tracer doses of alloxan were not selectively concentrated in the islet under the conditions used and, although differing from each other in certain details, the radioautographs of Landau and Renold (1954) and Bednik *et al.* (1968) gave similar results for rats and dogs with doses varying from tracer levels to greater than diabetogenic levels. On the other hand, radioautographs prepared 5 min to 24 hr after the injection of tracer doses of alloxan into mice produced clearly contradictory results (Hammarstrom and Ullberg, 1966; Hammarstrom *et al.*, 1967); except for an initial high level in the kidney, the islet always had more radioactivity than any other tissue, and 15 min after injection had 30 times that in the blood. With diabetogenic levels of alloxan, or when a diabetogenic dose was administered 15 min earlier, there was much less or no accumulation in the islet, suggesting that either the islet cells were destroyed so that they could not retain alloxan or the surface receptor sites were saturated by the unlabeled alloxan.

There appears to be no obvious explanation for the discrepancy in the results obtained with low doses of alloxan, except for the unsatisfying one of species differences. Nevertheless, it seems unlikely that selective accumulation is the sole explanation of alloxan's selectivity for the B cell, if indeed it is a factor at all. If the cell membrane damage produced by alloxan *in vitro* is a reflection of the toxicity of alloxan, as appears to be the case (Section II,B,1), selective accumulation cannot be a factor, since the islet is the only tissue whose permeability is affected by alloxan at neutral pH despite the addition of even higher concentrations to other tissues (Watkins *et al.*, 1964).

The concept that alloxan is more stable in B cells than in other cell types has been the basis of several proposals, including the ideas that this results from (1) a lower pH in the B cells than in other cells due to an "acid tide" produced during the secretion of alkaline pancreatic juice (Klebanoff and Greenbaum, 1954a,b); (2) the presence of a uniquely low D-glucose level in the B cell as a result of its content of insulin (Arteta et al., 1954; Bhattacharya, 1953); or (3) a low level of GSH (which if present in high concentrations would reduce and thereby detoxify alloxan) due to the utilization of cysteine for insulin synthesis (Lazarow, 1949) and the lower reducing power of the islets (Lazarow and Cooperstein, 1951; Lazarow, 1954; Lazarow et al., 1964). However, none of these theories appears tenable for many reasons (cf. Webb, 1966a). For example, alloxan diabetes has been produced in a number of species in which the islets are not associated with pancreatic acinar tissue (Lazarow and Berman, 1947; Murrell and Nace, 1959; Falkmer, 1961); preliminary results suggest that the intracellular D-glucose concentration in the islets may in fact be high (Randle et al., 1968); and numerous studies have uniformly failed to find unusually low free SH levels in either the entire islet or in the B cells themselves (MacDonald, 1959; Falkmer, 1961; Havu, 1969; Hellman et al., 1973b).

If, as has been proposed, alloxan is toxic to the B cells only because it produces free radicals during its reduction to dialuric acid and the subsequent reoxidation of the latter (Section II,C,2), it is conceivable that its selectivity may result from a greater ability of the B cells to reduce alloxan (Heikkila and Cohen, 1975; Grankvist et al., 1979b). However, this proposal is inconsistent with the evidence cited above that islets have a low reducing power. It is also inconsistent with reports that reducing agents such as cysteine and GSH (Section II,C,2), as well as sugars (Section II,D) which increase NADPH levels, hence reducing power, protect against the in vivo and in vitro actions of alloxan instead of enhancing them as would be expected.

A number of workers have suggested that the unique susceptibility of B cells to alloxan may result from a unique metabolic and/or structural feature of these cells. Initially it was conceived that B cells may contain a lesser amount of some critical SH-containing enzyme or coenzyme which is damaged by alloxan, and Lazarow (1954) suggested that either GSH or coenzyme A, both of which serve as coenzymes in critical metabolic sequences, might be the key factor. However, as pointed out above, GSH concentrations in the islets are not particularly low, and later work (Cooperstein and Lazarow, 1958) has suggested that coenzyme A is not sufficiently sensitive to alloxan to be a likely target.

More recently a series of studies has suggested that alloxan reacts with SH groups on the B-cell plasma membrane (Watkins et al., 1970, 1971a; Watkins and Cooperstein, 1976), that these groups have different properties than those on other cells, and that they may be unique because of their involvement in insulin release (Cooperstein and Watkins, 1977). A number of SH-binding reagents, like alloxan, increase the permeability of islet tissue *in vitro* (Section II,B,1 and C,2) but, unlike alloxan which affects only islets, the other reagents increase the permeability of other tissues as well (Cooperstein *et al.,* 1964). Since all cells tested therefore apparently have SH groups on their plasma membranes, this is not the determining factor in the unique susceptibility of B cells to alloxan; however, since each tissue showed its own particular pattern of sensitivity to the different SH-binding reagents tested (unpublished), it appeared that the selectivity might result from differences in the nature or location of the critical SH groups, or in the nature of the surrounding groups. In subsequent studies (Watkins *et al.,* 1979) it was found that alloxan increased the permeability of islet slices at pH 7 and 9 but not at pH 5, whereas the other SH-binding reagents which increased islet permeability did so at pH 7 and 5 but not at pH 9. Furthermore, at pH 9, but not at pH 5 or 7, alloxan increased the permeability of other tissues as well. The reaction between GSH and alloxan, which takes place in solution, was affected by pH in the same way as the reaction between alloxan and islet tissue, so that the effect of pH was not due to a change in the conformational state of the membrane and thereby the accessibility and/or reactivity of the membrane components(s) with which alloxan and the other SH-binding reagents reacted. However, evidence was presented that the effect of pH was on the tissue rather than on the SH-binding reagent and that it was reversible, which is consistent with a change in the degree of dissociation of a critical ionizable group on the plasma membrane. Since the reaction between alloxan and GSH involves the SH group of GSH (Section II,C,2), it was concluded that changing the ionization of the SH group changed its reactivity to alloxan, although ionization of neighboring groups which could likewise change the reactivity of the SH group could not be ruled out. On the basis of these results it was proposed that alloxan may interact with the ionized form of the SH group, whereas the other reagents may combine with the un-ionized form, and that the unique susceptibility of B cells to alloxan may be at least partly due to the fact that the critical B-cell plasma membrane groups, because of differences in environment affecting the pK, are largely ionized at neutral pH, whereas those in other tissues are largely un-ionized (Watkins *et al.,* 1979).

Since studies on the effects of SH-binding reagents clearly indicate that SH groups are involved in insulin release (Section II,C,2), since evidence has been presented that these are the same groups with which alloxan reacts, and since lowering the pH, which decreases the degree of ionization of the SH groups, decreases both glucose-stimulated insulin release

(Malaisse *et al.*, 1971; Lernmark, 1971) and the associated uptake of Ca^{2+} (Malaisse-Lagae and Malaisse, 1971), Watkins *et al.* (1979) stated: "It may be that the specialization for insulin secretion mandates the presence of ionized SH groups in the plasma membrane, and that this in turn confers on the B cell its sensitivity to alloxan." While this is far from proven, other workers (Zawalich and Beidler, 1973; Hellman *et al.*, 1973b) have likewise suggested that the basis of the selective action of alloxan will most likely be found in the unique chemical morphology of the B cell required for insulin secretion. Success in this search will both depend upon and aid in the search for the detailed mechanism of insulin secretion, and evidence to date suggests that studies on the interaction of secretagogues and alloxan with the plasma membrane, including characterization of the receptor sites, will be the most fruitful path to follow in solving both problems.

III. STREPTOZOTOCIN

A. General Actions

Streptozotocin, produced by *Streptomyces achromogenes* (Herr *et al.*, 1967), has a wide range of pharmacological properties. It (1) exhibits a broad spectrum of antibacterial activity (White, 1963), (2) possesses both antitumor (Evans *et al.*, 1965) and carcinogenic (Arison and Feudale, 1967; Rakieten *et al.*, 1968) properties, and (3) selectively destroys the B cells in the islets of Langerhans. The initial report of Rakieten *et al.* (1963) that streptozotocin produced diabetes in rats and dogs was confirmed in rats by Evans *et al.* (1965) and Arison and Feudale (1967). Evans *et al.* (1965) attributed the diabetogenic action of streptozotocin to inhibition of the synthesis and/or secretion of insulin. Using light and electron microscopy along with measurements of serum and pancreatic insulin, Junod *et al.* (1967) showed that streptozotocin caused rapid destruction of the B cells in the islets of Langerhans. Subsequent studies have shown that streptozotocin is also diabetogenic in mice and guinea pigs (Brosky and Logothetopoulos, 1969), hamsters (Wilander and Boquist, 1972; Chang *et al.*, 1977), monkeys (Pitkin and Reynolds, 1970), and rabbits (Lazarus and Shapiro, 1973).

1. Effect of Streptozotocin on Islet Morphology

Although injection of streptozotocin produces tumors in various organs, including the pancreas, after prolonged periods (Rakieten *et al.*, 1968), the short-term effects of diabetogenic levels are limited largely to the islets, with little or no damage to other organs (Arison *et al.*, 1967; Junod *et al.*, 1967; Pitkin and Reynolds, 1970; Wilander and Boquist, 1972). The cytological changes in the islets are similar in most species and, although the changes resemble those produced by alloxan, they usually require more time (cf. Fischer and Rickert, 1975). The number of intramembranous particles of the inner leaflet (A face) of the plasma membrane visible with freeze-fracture techniques decreased in B cells within 90 min after injection of streptozotocin (Orci *et al.*, 1972), clumping of nuclear chromatin and decreased nucleolar size were evident at 2 hr (Lazarus and Shapiro, 1972, 1973a), and pycnotic nuclei and disruption of secretion granule membranes were seen within 3–4 hr (Wilander, 1975). In contrast, after alloxan injection, the decrease in the number of intramembranous particles occurred within 10 min (Orci *et al.*, 1972), and pycnotic nuclei were seen after 1 hr (Lazarus *et al.*, 1962). Massive necrosis of the B cells was seen 7 hr after streptozotocin injection (Junod *et al.*, 1967).

Most studies indicate that streptozotocin has little or no effect on A or D cells (Vernon and Tusing, 1967; Brosky and Logothetopoulos, 1969; Lazarus and Shapiro, 1972). The finding that streptozotocin had no significant effect on glucagon secretion from isolated rat islets (Hinz *et al.*, 1971) supports these observations. However, Wilander (1974) observed degenerative changes in A cells in Chinese hamsters injected with a diabetogenic concentration (200 mg/kg intraperitoneally) of streptozotocin, and Lazarus and Shapiro (1972) observed dilated ER, swollen mitochondria, a reduction in interchromatinic nuclear material, and a reduction in the number of secretion granules in rabbit A cells 2–3 hr after injecting 300 mg/kg of streptozotocin. However, as they pointed out, the A-cell effects in this animal may be due to the large doses required to produce consistent B-cell necrosis in rabbits.

2. *Effect of Streptozotocin on Blood Sugar*

Although injection of streptozotocin, like alloxan, produces a triphasic blood glucose curve, the changes, like the effects on tissue morphology, occur later than those found with alloxan. Rerup and Tarding (1969) compared the effects of streptozotocin and alloxan under the same conditions in fed mice and found that, in contrast to the results for alloxan, which produced a sharp increase in blood sugar with a peak at 45 min, there was no change in blood sugar 45 min after streptozotocin injection and the initial hyperglycemic peak was not reached until 2 hr. This delay was also reported to occur in rats (Junod *et al.*, 1967). The hypoglycemia occurring after streptozotocin injection also lasted longer than after alloxan injection and was more severe; however, both drugs produced a similar level of hyperglycemia by 48 hr (Rerup and Tarding, 1969).

Although the mechanism for the early hyperglycemic phase remains unclear, inhibition of insulin release by streptozotocin has been suggested as the cause. Dixit *et al.* (1972) found that injected streptozotocin inhibited the increase in plasma insulin levels in response to glucose. Furthermore, islets treated with streptozotocin *in vitro* released less insulin than normal in response to glucose (Golden *et al.*, 1971; Maldonato *et al.*, 1976). On the other hand, Junod *et al.* (1969) reported that plasma immunoreactive insulin levels changed very little during this phase, and the parellelism between the blood sugar level and the depletion of liver glycogen suggested involvement of the liver (Rerup, 1970). Liver glycogen was unchanged 30 min after streptozotocin injection, but at 90 min (30 min before the peak in hyperglycemia) liver glycogen was depleted (Rerup and Tarding, 1969). However, the mechanism by which streptozotocin may mobilize the glycogen remains unclear.

Since streptozotocin increased plasma free fatty acids, and since hyperglycemia was reduced when the increase in free fatty acid levels was inhibited by antilipolytic agents, Schein *et al.* (1971) suggested that the early hyperglycemia was due to an increase in plasma free fatty acids which indirectly inhibited glucose breakdown.

The proposed mechanism for the hypoglycemic phase following streptozotocin injection is similar to that proposed for alloxan; large amonts of insulin are released into the blood from damaged B cells. Plasma insulin levels increase shortly before and during the streptozotocin-induced hypoglycemic phase and the hypoglycemia can be attenuated by injecting antiinsulin serum (Junod *et al.*, 1967, 1969; Rerup and Tarding, 1969).

B. Chemistry of Action

Streptozotocin consists of 1-methyl-1-nitrosourea attached to the C-2 of D-glucose (Fig. 2) and, because of the glucose moiety, it consists of a mixture of α and β anomers (Herr *et al.*, 1967). Like alloxan, streptozotocin rapidly decomposes in solution at room temperature and neutral pH (Rerup, 1970). The half-life of streptozotocin is reportedly 2.5 min in rat serum and 12 min in an incubation medium containing islets at 37°C (Ritter, 1973). The rate of decomposition can be decreased by lowering the pH to 4.0 and decreasing the temperature to 0°C (Rerup, 1970). After incubation of a streptozotocin solution at 0°C for 60 min virtually all of the reagent is still present, as shown by its absorption at 228 nm (D. Watkins, unpublished).

Changes in the glucose moiety affect the diabetogenic property of streptozotocin. The α- and β-methylglycosides of streptozotocin are ineffective, and the substitution of galactose for glucose destroys the diabetogenic activity of the molecule (Bannister, 1972). Although these studies suggest that the glucose moiety of streptozotocin is essential for its diabetogenic activ-

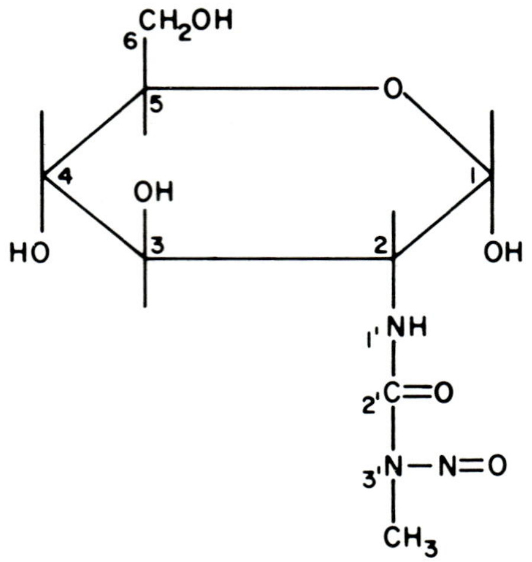

Fig. 2.   Structure of streptozotocin.

ity, recent work has shown that, while the lesions are not as extensive as those produced by streptozotocin, N-nitrosomethylurea, the aglucone derivative of streptozotocin, also damages B cells (Gunnarsson *et al.*, 1974; Wilander and Gunnarsson, 1975). Changing the nitrosourea moiety of the molecule by substituting an N-ethyl group for an N-methyl group reduces but does not eliminate the diabetogenic action of streptozotocin; deoxy-1-[(ethylnitrosoamino)carbonyl amino]-D-glucopyranose is diabetogenic, but 10 times as much is needed to produce the same effect as streptozotocin (Anderson *et al.*, 1975). The presence of the N-methylnitrosourea at position 1 in glucose instead of position 2 destroys the diabetogenic activity (Bannister, 1972).

   Slonim *et al.* (1976) have suggested that streptozotocin, like alloxan, may act as an oxidant and produces its B-cell toxicity by decreasing GSH levels in the B cell, perhaps as a consequence of oxidation of GSH to GSSG. This theory is supported by several findings. Streptozotocin produces a rapid fall in red blood cell GSH levels both *in vivo* and *in vitro,* and reagents which protect the B cell against streptozotocin also prevent the fall in the GSH levels of red blood cells (Slonim *et al.*, 1976). Streptozotocin likewise decreases the levels of GSH in the B cell (Robbins *et al.*, 1980). However, the finding that injection of GSH prior to injection of streptozotocin fails to prevent diabetes (Hoftiezer, 1975) does not support this theory.

   As is the case for alloxan, it has been proposed that streptozotocin may produce its diabetogenic effect by either increasing the concentration of intracellular free radicals or decreasing the ability of the B cell to maintain antioxidants (Robbins *et al.*, 1980). Indirect evidence that streptozotocin may act in this way has been reported. For example, streptozotocin has been shown to inhibit superoxide dismutase, a free radical scavenger, in retina and red blood cells (Crouch *et al.*, 1978). Furthermore, injection of superoxide dismutase prior to administration of a diabetogenic dose of streptozotocin attenuates the diabetogenic effect of the latter (Robbins *et al.*, 1980). However, in contrast to the situation with alloxan, the presence of free radicals in tissues after streptozotocin treatment has not yet to our knowledge been reported.

C. Cellular Site of Action

1. Action on Nicotinamide Adenine Dinucleotide

Although the exact site of action of streptozotocin is unknown, a widely accepted view is that it acts within the B cell to deplete NAD. This has been proposed by Schein and Loftus (1968) on the basis of the finding that injection of nicotinamide into animals either 15 min before or up to 2 hr after streptozotocin treatment prevents its diabetogenic action. In addition, a diabetogenic dose of streptozotocin decreases the levels of NAD in mouse liver (Schein and Loftus, 1968) and pancreatic islets (Schein *et al.*, 1973; Hinz *et al.*, 1973; Hellerstrom *et al.*, 1974), injection of nicotinamide prior to streptozotocin protects the animals against depression of tissue NAD levels (Hinz *et al.*, 1973; Schein *et al.*, 1973), and nicotinamide protects against streptozotocin inhibition of insulin release *in vitro* (Golden *et al.*, 1971). Lazarus and Shapiro (1973b) questioned this theory, since the injection of large amounts of NAD, NADP, or NADPH into mice prior to streptozotocin treatment failed to prevent B-cell necrosis. However, as they pointed out, the NAD levels in the islets after injection of the nucleotides were not measured; this is particularly important in view of the report that neither NADPH nor NADH penetrates islet cell membranes (Watkins *et al.*, 1971b), and it seems unlikely that the oxidized forms would do so.

Several mechanisms have been proposed to explain the decrease in NAD concentration produced by streptozotocin. Schein *et al.* (1973) proposed that it resulted from inhibition of the utilization of nicotinamide in the synthesis of NAD. This is based on their finding that, 1 hr after the intraperitoneal injection of [^{14}C]nicotinamide, the decrease in the incorporation of [^{14}C]nicotinamide into nicotinamide mononucleotide and NAD paralleled the decrease in NAD levels in the liver and islets of streptozotocin-treated mice. Since *N*-alkyl-*N*-nitroso compounds have been shown to methylate DNA, RNA, and proteins and to produce increased excretion of *N*-methylnicotinamide, Karunanayake *et al.* (1976a) considered the possibility that streptozotocin may methylate endogenous nicotinamide in the islets to *N*-methylnicotinamide which would then be unable to serve as a precursor in NAD biosynthesis. However, they pointed out that [^{14}C]*N*-methylnicotinamide was not found in the urine of animals injected with [3′-*methyl*-^{14}C]streptozotocin after prior injection of nicotinamide; in addition, Dulin and Wyse (1969) feel that this mechanism is unlikely, since guanidoacetic acid, which depletes methyl donors, does not protect against streptozotocin-induced diabetes.

Streptozotocin could lower islet NAD content by increasing NAD degradation (Hinz *et al.*, 1973; Yamamoto and Okamoto, 1980). Several observations support this explanation. 5-Methylnicotinamide, a derivative of nicotinamide which does not act as a precursor in NAD synthesis but does prevent NAD degradation by inhibiting NAD glycohydrolase, completely abolished the streptozotocin-induced decrease in NAD levels (Hinz *et al.*, 1973). The facts that streptozotocin increases the activity of islet nuclear poly(ADP-ribose) synthetase, a NAD-degrading enzyme, and that picolinamide, an inhibitor of poly(ADP-ribose) synthetase, completely protects against streptozotocin-induced diabetes and the decrease in islet NAD levels, are consistent with this theory (Yamamoto and Okamoto, 1980).

2. Action on the Plasma Membrane

An alternative theory suggested by several studies is that streptozotocin, like alloxan, acts primarily at the B-cell membrane. *In vitro* studies using toadfish islets (D. Watkins, unpublished) have shown that streptozotocin increases the penetration of D-[1-^{14}C]mannitol into islet slices; since mannitol normally remains in the extracellular space, this suggests that streptozotocin damages the islet cell membranes, thereby increasing their permeability. This effect of streptozotocin is rapid (15 min), occurs at low concentrations (10^{-5} *M*), and cannot be duplicated by its decomposition products. Furthermore, Orci *et al.* (1976) have reported that, as is true with alloxan, the incubation of isolated islets in streptozotocin results in a progressive decrease in the number of intramembranous particles in the inner leaflet of the plasma membrane. The addition of either high glucose (3 mg/ml) or nicotinamide to the incubation medium protects the plasma membrane against the streptozotocin effect. As pointed out above, similar changes in the plasma membrane were seen after alloxan was injected into mice (Orci *et al.*, 1972). Finally, Dean and Matthews (1972) reported that streptozotocin inhibited the production of action potentials in islet cells by D-glucose, D-mannose, L-leucine, and D-glyceraldehyde.

Thus these findings support the theory that streptozotocin, like alloxan, destroys B cells and produces diabetes by damaging the B-cell membrane. Furthermore, the possibility mentioned in Section III,C that streptozotocin, like alloxan, reacts with SH groups, is consistent with the idea that streptozotocin and alloxan act on the same or a similar plasma membrane site. On the other hand several findings are not consistent with this theory. The changes in the plasma membrane seen by Orci *et al.* (1976) with streptozotocin require a longer time than with alloxan; streptozotocin, unlike alloxan, does not itself depolarize islet cells (Dean and Matthews, 1972); streptozotocin does not increase the number of islet cells stained with trypan blue, whereas alloxan does (Grankvist *et al.*, 1979a); and GSH fails to protect against streptozotocin-induced diabetes (Hoftiezer, 1975). In this connection it is of interest to note that to our knowledge no one has yet determined whether alloxan, like streptozotocin, lowers islet NAD levels; this is of potential interest since nicotinamide protects against alloxan diabetes (Lazarow *et al.*, 1950).

D. Basis of Selectivity

The basis of the selectivity of streptozotocin, like that of alloxan, is unknown, but two major possibilities present themselves: (1) streptozotocin selectively accumulates in B cells, and (2) the target for the action of streptozotocin is a unique structural feature of the B cell.

Attempts to demonstrate selective uptake of streptozotocin by islet cells have yielded inconclusive results. The initial studies of Karunanayake *et al.*, (1974) and Ryo *et al.* (1974) showed no selective accumulation of radioactive streptozotocin in rat and dog pancreas; however, since the islets represent only 1–2% of the total weight of the pancreas, these studies provided no information on the possible selective accumulation of streptozotocin in the islets. Using autoradiography, Tjalve *et al.* (1976) found that, 5 min after the injection of $[3'-methyl-^{14}C]$streptozotocin in mice, islet tissue contained the highest level of ^{14}C of any tissue examined. Similar results with this labeled compound were obtained using the Chinese hamster and the rat (Karunanayake *et al.*, 1976b; Johansson and Tjalve, 1978), and Johansson and Tjalve (1978) reported that the centrally located cells in the islets (presumably B cells) were more highly labeled than those at the periphery. By contrast, Ryo *et al.* (1974) found that the isolated islet tissue of the toadfish did not selectively accumulate injected $[3'-methyl-^{14}C]$- or $[3-^3H]$streptozotocin. The autoradiographic studies of Karunanayake *et al.* (1976b) are of particular interest; they found that the injection of $[3'-methyl-^{14}C]$ streptozotocin gave high levels of ^{14}C in islets, whereas much lower levels were found after an injection of either $[1-^{14}C]$- or $[2'-^{14}C]$-streptozotocin. Although the results are not consistent with those of Ryo *et al.* (1974), Karunanayake *et al.* (1976b) have proposed that streptozotocin binds to the cell membrane by way of the glucose moiety and that metabolic degradation results in release of the *N*-methylnitroso portion of the molecule which then penetrates the B cell and produces the cytotoxic effect. This theory is supported by the finding mentioned in Section III,B that *N*-nitrosomethylurea itself induces B-cell necrosis (Gunnarsson *et al.*, 1974).

The alternative idea is that streptozotocin, like alloxan (Section II,D), reacts with a specific glucoreceptor involved in glucose transport and/or insulin release. As pointed out in Section III,A, streptozotocin inhibits insulin release. Furthermore, several investigators (Dulin and Wyse, 1979; Ganda *et al.*, 1976; Rossini *et al.*, 1977) found that 3-*O*-methyl-D-glucose or 2-deoxy-D-glucose completely protectd rats against streptozotocin-induced diabetes. Although Dulin and Wyse (1969) did not obtain protection with glucose itself, Rossini *et al.* (1977) subsequently did, and Orci *et al.* (1976) found that glucose likewise protected against the morphological changes in the plasma membrane produced by streptozotocin. Furthermore, Rossini *et al.* (1977) reported that at doses of 30–40 mg/kg the α anomer of streptozotocin produced more severe B-cell necrosis than the β anomer, although at higher doses there was no difference; this is particularly interesting in that, as has been discussed (Section II,D), the α anomer of D-glucose is the better secretagogue and provides better protection against the actions of alloxan than the β anomer.

These studies thus all show a significant analogy between the results obtained with alloxan and those obtained with streptozotocin, suggesting the same basis for their selectivity. At the same time, in view of the findings of Karunanayake *et al.* (1976b) mentioned above, the two theories for the selectivity of streptozotocin are not mutually exclusive; it may be that the methylnitrosa portion of streptozotocin accumulates in the B cell more than in other cells (and is the toxic agent), but only because the entire molecule binds to a plasma membrane glucoreceptor specific for the B cell.

REFERENCES

Anderson, T., McMenamin, M., and Schein, P. S. (1975). *Biochem. Pharmacol.* **24**, 746–747.

Archibald, R. M. (1945). *J. Biol. Chem.* **158**, 347–373.

Arison, R. N., and Feudale, E. L. (1967). *Nature (London)* **214**, 1254–1255.

Arison, R. N., Ciaccio, E. I., Glitzer, M. S., Cassaro, J. A., and Pruss, M. P. (1967). *Diabetes* **16**, 51–56.

Arteta, J. L., Konig, C., and Carballido, A. (1954). *J. Endocrinol.* **10**, 342–346.

Bailey, O. T., Bailey, C. C., and Hagan, W. H. (1944). *Am. J. Med. Sci.* **208**, 450–461.

Bailey, C. C., Bailey, O. T., and Leech, R. S. (1946). *Proc. Soc. Exp. Biol. Med.* **63**, 502–505.

Banerjee, S., Belavady, B., and Mukherjee, A. K. (1953). *Proc. Soc. Exp. Biol. Med.* **83**, 133–135.

Bannister, B. (1972). *J. Antibiot.* **25**, 377–386.

Barrnett, R. J., Marshall, R. B , and Seligman, A. M. (1955). *Endocrinology* 57, 419–438.
Bekdik, F. C., Farmelant, M. H. and Tyson, I. (1968). *J. Nucl. Med.* 9, 31–34.
Bhattacharya, G. (1953). *Science* 117, 230–231.
Bhattacharya, G. (1954). *Science* 120, 841–843.
Bhattacharya, S. K., Robson, J. 3., and Stewart, C. P. (1956). *Biochem. J.* 62, 12–21.
Bloom, G. D., Hellman, B., Idahl, L.-A., Lernmark, A., Sehlin, J., and Täljedal, I-B. (1972). *Biochem. J.* 129, 241–254.
Boquist, L. (1977). *Acta Pathol. Microbiol. Scand. Sect. A* 85, 219–229.
Boquist, L. (1979). *Acta Diabeto:. Lai.* 16, 35–44.
Boquist, L., and Lorentzon, R. (1979). *Virchows Arch. B* 31, 235–241.
Boquist, L., and Lorentzon, R. (1980). *Diabete Metab.* 6, 55–58.
Borg, L. A. H., Eide, S. J., Andersson, A., and Hellerstrom, C. (1979). *Biochem. J.* 182, 797–802.
Brada, Z. (1951). *Arch. Int. Pharmacodyn.* 85, 497–500.
Brosky, G., and Logothetopoulos, J. (1969). *Diabetes* 18, 606–611.
Bruckmann, G. (1946). *J. Biol. Chem.* 165, 103–113.
Bruckmann, G., and Wertheimer, E. (1945). *Nature (London)* 155, 267–268.
Bruckmann, G., and Wertheimer, E. (1947). *J. Biol. Chem.* 168, 241–256.
Brunfeldt, K., and Iversen, M. (1950) *Acta Physiol. Scand.* 20, 38–45.
Brunschwig, A., and Allen, J. G. (1944). *Cancer Res.* 4, 45–54.
Bunyan, J., Green, J., Edwin, E. E., and Diplock, A. T. (1960). *Biochem. J.* 77, 47–51.
Burgen, A. S. V., and Lorch, J. I. (1947). *Biochem. J.* 41, 223–226.
Canellakis, E. S., Tuttle, A. L., and Cohen, P. P. (1955). *J. Biol. Chem.* 213, 397–404.
Carter, W. J., and Younathan, E. S. (1962). *Proc. Soc. Exp. Biol. Med.* 109, 611–612.
Chang, A. Y., Noble, R. E., and Wyse, B. M. (1977). *Diabetologia* 13, 595–602.
Chesler, A., and Tislow, R. (1947). *Science* 106, 345.
Cohen, K. L., and Bitensky, M. W. (1969). *J. Pharmacol. Exp. Ther.* 169, 80–86.
Collins-Williams, J., and Bailey, C. C. (1949). *Proc. Soc. Exp. Biol. Med.* 71, 583–587.
Cooperstein, S. J., and Lazarow, A. (1958). *J. Biol. Chem.* 232, 695–703.
Cooperstein, S. J., and Lazarow, A. (1964). *Am. J. Physiol.* 207, 423–430.
Cooperstein, S. J., and Lazarow, A. (1969). *Am. J. Physiol.* 217, 1784–1788.
Cooperstein, S. J., and Watkins, D. (1977). *Biochem. Biophys. Res. Commun.* 79, 756–762.
Cooperstein, S. J., and Watkins, D. (1978). *J. Pharmacol. Exp. Ther.* 204, 230–239.
Cooperstein, S. J., Watkins, D., and Lazarow, A. (1964). *In* "The Structure and Metabolism of the Pancreatic Islets" (S. E. Brolin, B. Hellman, and H. Knutson, eds.), pp. 389–410. Pergamon, Oxford.
Coore, H. G., and Randle, P. J. (1964). *Biochem. J.* 93, 66–78.
Crouch, R., Kimsey, G., Priest, D. G., Sarda, A., and Buse, M. G. (1978). *Diabetologia* 15, 53–57.
Deamer, D. W., Heikkila, R. E., Panganamala, R. V., Cohen, G., and Cornwell, D. G. (1971) *Physiol. Chem. Phys.* 3, 426–430.
Dean, D. M., and Matthews, E. K. (1972). *Diabetologia* 8, 173–178.
Dixit, P. K., Lowe, I., and Lazarow, A. (1962). *Nature (London)* 195, 388–389.
Dixit, P. K., Tarn, B. B., and Hernandez, R. E. (1972). *Proc. Soc. Exp. Biol. Med.* 140, 1418–1423.
Dixon, K. C., King, A. J., and Malnin, T. (1960). *Q. J. Exp. Physiol.* 45, 202–212.
Drake, B. B., Smythe, C. V., and King, C. G. (1942). *J. Biol. Chem.* 143, 89–98.
Duff, G. L., and Starr, H. (1944). *Proc. Soc. Exp. Biol. Med.* 57, 280–282.
Duffy, E. (1945). *J. Pathol. Bacteriol.* 57, 199–212.

Dulin, W. E., and Wyse, B. M. (1969). *Diabetes* **18**, 459–466.
Dunn, J. S., and McLetchie, N. G. B. (1943). *Lancet* **245**, II, 384–387.
Dunn, J. S., Sheehan, H. L., and McLetchie, N. G. B. (1943). *Lancet* **244**, I, 484–487.
Dunn, J. S., Duffy, E., Gilmour, M. K., Kirkpatrick, J., and McLetchie, N. G. B. (1944). *J. Physiol. (London)* **103**, 233–243.
Ecker, E. E., Kalina, R., and Pillemer, L. (1939). *Enzymologia* **7**, 307–309.
Evans, J. S., Gerritsen, G. C., Mann, K. M., and Owen, S. P. (1965). *Cancer Chemother. Rep.* **48**, 1–6.
Falkmer, S. (1961). *Acta Endocrinol.* **37**, Suppl. 59, 1–122.
Falkmer, S., and Olsson, R. (1962). *Acta Endocrinol.* **39**, 32–46.
Fee, J. A., and Teitelbaum, H. D. (1972). *Biochem. Biophys. Res. Commun.* **49**, 150–158.
Fischer, L. J., and Hamburger, S. A. (1980a). *Life Sci.* **26**, 1405–1409.
Fischer, L. J., and Hamburger, S. A. (1980b). *Diabetes* **29**, 213–216.
Fischer, L. J., and Rickert, D. E. (1975). *CRC Crit. Rev. Toxicol.* **3**, 231–263.
Frerichs, H., and Creutzfeldt, W. (1971). *Hand. Exp. Pharmacol.* **32**, Part 1, 159–202.
Gaarenstroom, J. H., and Siderius, P. (1954). *In* "Experimental Diabetes, a Symposium" (J. P. Hoet, F. G. Young, J. F. Delafresnaye, and G. H. Smith, eds.) pp. 82–96. Thomas, Springfield, Illinois.
Ganda, O. P., Rossini, A. A., and Like, A. A. (1976). *Diabetes* **25**, 595–603.
Ghafghazi, T., and Mennear, J. H. (1975). *Toxicol. Appl. Pharmacol.* **31**, 134–142.
Golden, P., Baird, L., Malaisse, W. J., Malaisse-Lagae, F., and Walker, M. M. (1971). *Diabetes* **20**, 513–518.
Goldner, M. G., and Gomori, G. (1944). *Endocrinology* **35**, 241–248.
Goto, Y., Seino, Y., Tomohiko, T., Inoue, Y., Kadowaki, S., Mori, K., and Imura, H. (1978). *Endocrinology* **102**, 1496–1500.
Grande-Covian, F., and DeOya, J. C. (1945). *Rev. Clin. Esp.* **17**, 320–327.
Grankvist, K., Lernmark, A., and Täljedal, I-B. (1977). *Biochem. J.* **162**, 19–24.
Grankvist, K., Lernmark, A., and Täljedal, I-B. (1979a). *J. Endocrinol. Invest.* **2**, 139–145.
Grankvist, K., Marklund, S., Sehlin, J., and Täljedal, I-B. (1979b). *Biochem. J.* **182**, 17–25.
Griffiths, M. (1950). *J. Biol Chem.* **184**, 289–298.
Grodsky, G. M., Fanska, R., West, L., and Manning, M. (1974). *Science* **186**, 536–538.
Grunert, R. R., and Phillips, P. H. (1951a). *Proc. Soc. Exp. Biol. Med.* **76**, 642–645.
Grunert, R. R., and Phillips, P. H. (1951b). *J. Biol Chem.* **191**, 633–638.
Gunnarsson, R. and Hellerstrom, C. (1973). *Horm. Metab. Res.* **5**, 404–409.
Gunnarsson, R., Berne, C., and Hellerstrom, C. (1974). *Biochem. J.* **140**, 487–494.
Gyorgi, P., and Rose, C. S. (1949). *Ann. N.Y. Acad. Sci.* **52**, 231–239.
Hakanson, R., Lundquist, I., and Sundler, F. (1974). *Endocrinology* **94**, 318–324.
Hammarstrom, L. (1966). *Acta Physiol. Scand.* **70** Suppl. 289, 1–84.
Hammarstrom, L., and Ullberg, S. (1966). *Nature (London)* **212**, 708–709.
Hammarstrom, L., Hellman, B., and Ullberg, S. (1967). *Diabetologia* **3**, 340–345.
Hard, W. L., and Carr, C. J. (1944). *Proc. Soc. Exp. Biol. Med.* **55**, 214–216.
Havu, N. (1969). *Acta Endocrinol.* **62**, Suppl. 139, 1–231.
Heikkila, R. E., and Cabbat, F. S. (1978). *Eur. J. Pharmacol.* **52**, 57–60.
Heikkila, R. E., and Cohen, G. (1975). *Ann. N.Y. Acad. Sci.* **258**, 221–230.
Heikkila, R. E., Barden, H., and Cohen, G. (1974). *J. Pharmacol. Exp. Ther.* **190**, 501–506.
Heikkila, R. E., Winston, B., and Cohen, G. (1976). *Biochem. pharmacol.* **25**, 1085–1092.
Hellerstrom, C., Andersson, A., Gunnarsson, R., Berne, C., and Asplund, K. (1974). *Endocrinol. Exp.* **8**, 115–126.
Hellman, B. (1972). *Metabolism* **21**, 60–66.
Hellman, B., Sehlin, J., and Täljedal, I-B. (1971a). *Horm. Metab. Res.* **3**, 219–220.
Hellman, B., Sehlin, J., and Täljedal, I-B. (1971b). *Biochim. Biophys. Acta* **241**, 147–154.

Hellman, B., Idahl, L-A., Lernmark, A., Sehlin, J., and Täljedal, I-B. (1973a). *Mol. Phar. macol.* **9**, 792-801.

Hellman, B., Lernmark, A., Sehlin, J., Soderberg, M., and Täljedal, I-B. (1973b). *Arch. Biochem. Biophys.* **158**, 435-441.

Hellman, B., Idahl, L., Lernmark, A., Sehlin, J., and Täljedal, I-B. (1974a). *In* "Diabetes: Proc. Congr. Intern. Diabetes Fed., 8th" (W. J. Malaisse and J. Pirart, eds.), pp. 65-78. Excerpta Medica., Amsterdam.

Hellman, B., Idahl, L-A., Lernmark, A., Sehlin, J., and Täljedal, I-B. (1974b). *Biochem. J.* **138**, 33-45.

Henquin, J. C., and Lambert, A. E. (1975). *Am. J. Physiol.* **228**, 1669-1677.

Henquin, J. C., Malvaux, P., and Lambert, A. E. (1979). *Diabetologia* **16**, 253-260.

Herr, R. R., Jahnke, H. K., and Argoudelis, A. D. (1967). *J. Am. Chem. Soc.* **89**, 4808-4809.

Hidy, P. H. (1946). *J. Biol. Chem.* **163**, 307-311.

Hinz, M., Katsilambros, Y., Abdel Rahman, A., Schatz, H., Maier, V., Schroeder, E., and Pfeiffer, E. F. (1971). *Diabetologia* **7**, 484.

Hinz, M., Katsilambros, N., Maier, V., Schatz, H., and Pfeiffer, E. F. (1973). *FEBS Lett.* **30**, 225-228.

Hoftiezer, V. (1975). *Sci. Biol. J.* **1**, 35-36.

Houssay, B. A., Arias, O., and Sara, I. (1945). *Science* **102**, 197.

Howell, S. L., and Taylor, K. W. (1967). *J. Endocrinol.* **37**, 421-427.

Hughes, H., Ware, L. L., and Young, F. G. (1944). *Lancet* **246**, I, 148-150.

Hultquist, G. T. (1958). *Nature (London)* **182**, 318-319.

Idahl, L-A., Sehlin, J., and Täljedal, I-B. (1975). *Nature (London)* **254**, 75-77.

Idahl, L-A., Lernmark, A., Sehlin, J., and Täljedal, I-B. (1976). *J. Physiol. (Paris)* **72**, 729-746.

Idahl, L-A., Lernmark, A., Sehlin, J., and Täljedal, I-B. (1977). *Biochem J.* **162**, 9-18.

Ishibashi, F., Onari, K., Sato, T., and Kawate, R. (1978). *Hiroshima J. Med. Sci.* **27**, 211-219.

Ishibashi, F., Sato, T., Onari, K., and Kawate, R. (1979). *Endocrinol. Jpn.* **26**, 395-397.

Jacobs, H. R. (1937). *Proc. Soc Exp. Biol. Med.* **37**, 407-409.

Jain, K., and Logothetopoulos, J. (1976). *Biochim. Biophys. Acta* **435**, 145-151.

Jain, K., Asina, S., and Logothetopoulos, J. (1978). *Biochem. J.* **176**, 31-37.

Janes, R. G., and Winnick, T. (1952). *Proc. Soc. Exp. Biol. Med.* **81**, 226-229.

Johansson, E. B., and Tjalve, E. (1978). *Acta Endocrinol.* **89**, 339-351.

Junod, A., Lambert, A. E., Orci, L., Pictet, R., Gonet, A. E., and Renold, A. E. (1967). *Proc. Soc. Exp. Biol. Mea.* **126**, 201-205.

Junod, A., Lambert, A. E., Stauffacner, W., and Renold, A. E. (1969). *J. Clin. Invest.* **48**, 2129-2139.

Kadota, I. (1950). *J. Lab. Clin. Med.* **35**, 568-591.

Kadota, I., and Midorikawa, O. (1951). *J. Lab. Clin. Med.* **38**, 671-688.

Karrer, P., Koller, F., and Sturzinger, H. (1945). *Helv. Chim. Acta* **28**, 1529-1532.

Karunanayake, E. H., Hearse, D. J., and Mellows, G. (1974). *Biochem. Soc. Trans.* **2**, 1006-1009.

Karunanayake, E. H., Hearse, D. J., and Mellows, G. (1976a). *Diabetologia* **12**, 483-488.

Karunanayake, E. H., Baker, J. R. J., Christian, R. A., Hearse, D. J., and Mellows, G. (1976b). *Diabetologia* **12**, 123-128.

Kass, E. H., and Waisbren, B. A. (1945). *Proc. Soc. Exp. Biol. Med.* **60**, 303-306.

Kay, W. W., and Murfitt, K. C. (1960). *Biochem. J.* **74**, 203-208.

Kennedy, W. B., and Lukens, F. D. W. (1944). *Proc. Soc. Exp. Biol. Med.* **57**, 143-149.

Klebanoff, S. J., and Greenbaum, A. L. (1954a). *J. Endocrinol.* **10**, XIX.

Klebanoff, S. J., and Greenbaum, A. L. (1954b). *J. Endocrinol.* **11**, 314-322.

Labes, R., and Freisburger, H. (1930). *Naunyn-Schmeideberg's Arch. Exp. Pathol. Pharmakol.* **156**, 226–252.
Lacy, P. E., McDaniel, M. L., Fink, C. J., and Roth, C. (1975). *Diabetologia* **11**, 501–507.
Landau, B. R., and Renold, A. E. (1954). *Diabetes* **3**, 47–50.
Landgraf-Leurs, M. M. C., Mayer, L., and Landgraf, R. (1978). *Diabetologia* **15**, 337–342.
Lang, G. (1867). *Z. Anal. Chem.* **6**, 294–295.
Laszt, L. (1945). *Experientia* **1**, 234.
Lazaris, J. A., and Babelskyi, F. J. (1979). *Endocrinol. Exp.* **13**, 39–51.
Lazarow, A. (1946). *Proc. Soc. Exp. Biol. Med.* **61**, 441–447.
Lazarow, A. (1947). *Proc. Soc. Exp. Biol. Med.* **66**, 4–7.
Lazarow, A. (1949). *Physiol. Rev.* **29**, 48–74.
Lazarow, A. (1954). *In* "Experimental Diabetes, A Symposium" (J. P. Hoet, F. G. Young, J. F. Delafresnay, and G. H. Smith, eds.), pp. 49–81. Thomas, Springfield, Illinois.
Lazarow, A., and Berman, J. (1947). *Biol. Bull* **92**, 219.
Lazarow, A., and Cooperstein, S. J. (1951). *Biol. Bull.* **100**, 191–198.
Lazarow, A., and Liambies, J. (1950). *Proc. Soc. Exp. Biol. Med.* **73**, 323–326.
Lazarow, A., Liambies, J., and Tausch, A. J. (1950). *J. Lab. Clin. Med.* **36**, 249–258.
Lazarow, A., Dixit, P. K., Lindall, A., Moran, J., Hostetler, K., and Cooperstein, S. J. (1964). *In* "The Structure and Metabolism of the Pancreatic Islets" (S. E. Brolin, B. Hellman, and H. Knutson, eds.), pp. 249–268. Pergamon, Oxford.
Lazarus, S. S., and Shapiro, S. H. (1972). *Diabetes* **21**, 129–137.
Lazarus, S. S., and Shapiro, S. H. (1973a). *Lab. Invest.* **29**, 90–98.
Lazarus, S. S., and Shapiro, S. H. (1973b). *Diabetes* **22**, 499–506.
Lazarus, S. S., Barden, H., and Bradshaw, M. (1962). *Arch. Pathol.* **73**, 210–222.
Lee, J. M., and Stetten, D. (1952). *J. Biol. Chem.* **197**, 205–214.
Leech, R. C., and Bailey, C. C. (1945). *J. Biol. Chem.* **157**, 525–542.
Lernmark, A. (1971). *Acta Diabetol. Lat.* **8**, 649–679.
Lieben, F., and Edel, E. (1933). *Biochem. Z.* **259**, 8–10.
Liebig, J. (1862). *Ann. Chem. Pharmacol.* **121**, 80–82.
Lorentzon, R., and Boquist, L. (1979). *Virchows Archiv B* **31**, 227–233.
Loubatieres, A., and Bouyard, P. (1951). *Seances Soc. Biol. Paris* **145**, 344–348.
Lukens, F. D. W. (1948). *Physiol. Rev.* **28**, 304–330.
Lundquist, I., and Rerup, C. (1967). *Eur. J. Pharmacol.* **2**, 35–41.
McDaniel, M. L., and Lacy, P. E. (1975). *Diabetes* **24**, 400.
McDaniel, M. L., Anderson, S., Fink, J., Roth, C., and Lacy, P. E. (1975a). *Endocrinology* **97**, 68–75.
McDaniel, M. L., Roth, C., Fink, J., Fyfe, G., and Lacy, P. E. (1975b). *Biochem. Biophys. Res. Commun.* **66**, 1089–1096.
McDaniel, M. L., Roth, C. E., Fink, C. J., and Lacy, P. E. (1976). *Endocrinology* **99**, 535–540.
McDaniel, M. L., Roth, C. E., Fink, C. J., Swanson, J. A., and Lacy, P. E. (1977a). *Diabetologia* **13**, 603–606.
McDaniel, M. L., Weaver, D. C., Roth, C. E., Fink, C. J., Swanson, J. A., and Lacy, P. E. (1977b). *Endocrinology* **101**, 1701–1708.
McDaniel, M. L., Roth, C. E., Bry, C. A., Fink, C. J., Swanson, J. A., and Lacy, P. E. (1978). *Biochem. Pharmacol.* **27**, 1749–1751.
McDaniel, M. L., Bry, C. G., Fink, C. J., Homer, R. W., and Lacy, P. E. (1979). *Endocrinology* **105**, 1446–1451.
MacDonald, M. K. (1959). *Q. J. Exp. Physiol.* **44**, 177–182.
MacDonald, M. K., and Bhattacharya, S. K. (1956). *Q. J. Exp. Physiol.* **41**, 153–161.
Malaisse, W. J., Malaisse-Lagae, F., and Brisson, G. (1971). *Horm. Metab. Res.* **3**, 65–70.

Malaisse-Lagae, F., and Malaisse, W. J. (1971). *Endocrinology* **88**, 72–80.

Maldonato, A. Trueheart, P. A., Renold, A. E., and Sharp, G. W. G. (1976). *Diabetologia* **12**, 471–481.

Martinez, C. (1951). *Acta Physiol. Latinamer.* **1**, 135–162.

Martinez, C. (1955). *Am. J. Physiol.* **182**, 267–268.

Maske, H., Wolff, H., Stampfl, B., and Baumgarten, F. (1952). *Naunyn-Schmeideberg's Arch. Exp. Pathol. Pharmakol.* **216**, 457–472.

Matschinsky, F. M., Ellerman, J. E., Landgraf, R., Krzanowski, J., Kotler-Brajtburg, J., and Fertel, R. (1970). *In* "Recent Advances in Quantitative Histo-and Cytochemistry" (U. C. Dubach and U. Schmidt, eds). pp. 143–182. Huber, Bern.

Matschinsky, F. M., Landgraf, R., Ellerman, J., and Kotter-Brajtburg, J. (1972). *Diabetes* **21**, 555–569.

Matthews, E. K., Dean, P. M., and Sakamoto, Y. (1975). *Hand. Exp. Pharmacol.* **32**, Part 2, 157–173.

Merlini, D., and Caramia, F. (1965). *J. Cell Biol.* **26**, 245–262.

Migita, T. (1963). *Kagoshima Daigaku Igaku Zasshi* **15**, 58–60.

Miwa, I., Okuda, J., Niki, H., and Niki, A. (1975). *J. Biochem.* **78**, 1109–1111.

Mohnike, U., Hagemann, U., and Glochner, E. (1956). *Z. Gesamte Exp. Med.* **128**, 115–127.

Murrell, L. R., and Nace, P. F. (1959). *Endocrinology* **64**, 542–550.

Niki, A., Niki, H., Miwa, I., and Okuda, J. (1974). *Science* **186**, 150–151.

Niki, A., Niki, H., Miwa, I., and Lin, B. J. (1976). *Diabetes* **25**, 574–579.

Obo, F. (1960). *Acta Med. Univ. Kagoshima* **3**, 1–4.

Okamoto, K. (1955). *Tohoku J. Exp. Med.* **61**, Suppl. 3, 1–116.

Okamoto, K. (1970). *In* "Diabetes Mellitus: Theory and Practice" (M. Ellenberg, ed.), pp. 230–255. McGraw-Hill, New York.

Okuda, T., and Grollman, A. (1966). *Endocrinology* **78**, 195–203.

Orci, L., Amherdt, M., Stauffache, W., Like, A. A., Rouiller, C., and Renold, A. E. (1972). *Diabetes* **21**, 326.

Orci, L., Amherdt, M., Malaisse-Lagae, F., Ravazzola, M., Malaisse, W. J., Perrelet, A., and Renold, A. E. (1976). *Lab. Invest.* **34**, 451–454.

Pagliara, A. S., Stillings, S. N., Zawalich, W. S., Williams, A. D., and Matschinsky, F. M. (1977). *Diabetes* **26**, 973–979.

Patterson, J. W. (1950). *J. Biol. chem.* **183**, 81–88.

Patterson, J. W., and Lazarow, A. (1950). *J. Biol. Chem.* **186**, 141–144.

Patterson, J. W., Lazarow, A., and Levey, S. (1949a). *J. Biol. Chem.* **177**, 187–196.

Patterson, J. W., Lazarow, A., and Levey, S. (1949b). *J. Biol. Chem.* **177**, 197–204.

Paul, K. G., and Avi-Dor, Y. (1954). *Acta Chem. Scand.* **8**, 637–648.

Pence, L. A., and Mennear, J. H. (1979). *Toxicol. Appl. Pharmacol.* **50**, 57–65.

Pillsbury, S., Watkins, D., and Cooperstein, S. J. (1973). *J. Pharmacol. Exp. Ther.* **185**, 713–718.

Pitkin, R. M., and Reynolds, W. A. (1970). *Diabetes* **19**, 85–90.

Poulsen, J. E. (1946). *Rep. Steno Mem. Hosp. Nord. Insulin Lab.* **1**, 74–77.

Princiotto, J. V. (1951). *J. Clin. Endocrin. Metab.* **11**, 775.

Pryor, W. A. (1976). *In* "Free Radcals in Biology" (W. A. Pryor, ed.), Vol. I, pp. 1–49. Academic Press, New York.

Rakieten, N., Rakieten, M. L., and Nadkarni, M. V. (1963). *Cancer Chemother. Rep.* **29**, 91–98.

Rakieten, N., Gordon, B. S., Cooney, D. A., Davis, R. D., and Schein, P. S. (1968). *Cancer Chemother. Rep.* **52**, 563–567.

Randle, P. J., Ashcroft, S. J. H., and Gill, J. R. (1968). *In* "Carbohydrate Metabolism—Its

Disorders'' (F. Dickens, W. J. Whelan, and P. J. Randle, eds.), Vol. I, pp. 427–447. Academic Press, London.

R-Candela, J. L., Rovira, J., and DeArriba, J. (1955). *Rev. Iber. Endocrinol.* **2**, 783–785.

R-Candela, J. L., Martin-Hernandez, D., and Castilla-Cortazar, T. (1963). *Proc. Soc. Exp. Biol. Med.* **112**, 898.

Rerup, C. C. (1970). *Pharmacol. Rev.* **22**, 485–518.

Rerup, C., and Lundquist, I. (1967). *Acta Endocrinol.* **54**, 514–526.

Rerup, C., and Tarding, F. (1969). *Eur. J. Pharmacol.* **7**, 89–96.

Resnik, R. A., and Cecil, H. (1956). *Arch. Biochem. Biophys.* **61**, 179–185.

Resnik, R. A., and Wolff, A. K. (1956). *Arch. Biochem. Biophys.* **64**, 33–50.

Richardson, G. M., and Cannan, R. K. (1929). *Biochem. J.* **23**, 68–77.

Ridout, J. H., Ham, A. W., and Wrenshall, G. A. (1944). *Science* **100**, 57–58.

Ritter, D. A. (1973). *Diss. Abst. B* **34**, 2826.

Robbins, M. J., Sharp, R. A., Slonim, A. E., and Burr, I. M. (1980). *Diabetologia* **18**, 55–58.

Rose, C. S., and Gyorgy, P. (1950). *Blood* **5**, 1062–1074.

Rossini, A. A., Arcangeli, M. A., and Cahill, G. F., Jr. (1975). *Diabetes* **24**, 516–522.

Rossini, A. A., Like, A. A., Dulin, W. E., and Cahill, G. F., Jr. (1977). *Diabetes* **26**, 1120–1124.

Ruben, J. A., and Tipson, R. S. (1945). *Science* **101**, 536–537.

Ryo, U. Y., Beierwaltes, W.H., Feehan, P., and Ice, R. D. (1974). *J. Nuclear Med.* **15**, 572–576.

Said, A., Fleita, D. H., and Shinouda, H. G. (1977). *Z. Naturforsch Teil. B* **32**, 447–452.

Schauberger, C. W., Thies, R. L., and Fischer, L. J. (1977). *J. Pharmacol. Exp. Ther.* **201**, 450–455.

Schein, P. S., and Loftus, S. (1968). *Cancer Res.* **28**, 1501–1506.

Schein, P. S., Alberti, K. G. M. M., and Williamson, D. H. (1971). *Endocrinology* **89**, 827–834.

Schein, P. S., Cooney, D. A., McMenamin, M. G., and Anderson, T. (1973). *Biochem. Pharmacol.* **22**, 2625–2631.

Scheynius, A., and Täljedal, I-B. (1971). *Diabetologia* **7**, 252–255.

Schioler, P. (1948). *Biochim. Biophys. Acta* **2**, 260–262.

Schmidt, R., Methfessel, J., Schultka, R., and Apel, D. (1968). *Z. Zellforsch.* **84**, 9–23.

Seligson, D., Seligson, H., Shapiro, B., Paley, R. G., Riaboff, T., and Lukens, F. D. W. (1951). *Fed. Proc. Fed. Am. Soc. Exp. Biol.* **10**, 124.

Sen, P. B., and Bhattacharya, G. (1952). *Indian J. Physiol. Allied Sci.* **6**, 112–114.

Shigenaga, K. (1976). *Kumamoto Med. J.* **29**, 67–81.

Shipley, E. G., and Beyer, K. H. (1947). *Endocrinology* **40**, 154–164.

Siliprandi, N., and Pisati, C. (1949). *Boll. Soc. Ital. Biol. Sper.* **25**, 1089–1090.

Slonim, A. E., Fletcher, T., Burke, T., and Burr, I. M. (1976). *Diabetes* **25**, 216–222.

Sneer, A., Stroia, V., Dinu, M., Herscovici, B., and Papp, E. (1971). *Rev. Med. Chir.* **75**, 1005–1010.

Soberon, G., and Cohen, P. P. (1963). *Arch. Biochem. Biophys.* **103**, 331–337.

Stoll, W. (1946). *Z. Naturforsch.* **1**, 592–594.

Strecher, A. (1862). *Ann. Chem.* **123**, 363–365.

Tanese, T., Tajima, N., Yamada, H., Ikeda, Y., and Abe, M. (1978). *Jikeikai Med. J.* **25**, 209–215.

Tarui, S. (1963). *Endocrinol. Jpn.* **10**, 1–8.

Tipson, R. S., and Cretcher, L. H. (1950). *Anal. Chem.* **22**, 822–828.

Tipson, R. S., and Cretcher, L. H. (1951). *J. Org. Chem.* **16**, 1091–1099.

Tjalve, H., Wilander, E., and Johansson, E-B. (1976). *J. Endocrinol.* **69**, 455–456.

Tomita, T. (1976). *FEBS Lett.* **65,** 140–143.

Tomita, T., and Lacy, P. E. (1972). *Diabetes* **21,** 326.

Tomita, T., and Scarpelli, D. G. (1977). *Endocrinology* **100,** 1327–1333.

Tomita, T., and Watanabe, I. (1976) *Virchow's Arch. B* **22,** 217–232.

Tomita, T., Lacy, P. E., Matschinsky, F. M., and McDaniel, M. L. (1974). *Diabetes* **23,** 517–524.

Van Campenhout, E. (1956). *Arch. Biol* **67,** 499–512.

Vande Vyver, E. (1876). *J. Pharmacol. Brux.* **32,** 258–262.

Vargas, L., and Mundt, E. (1948). *Bol. Soc. Biol. Santiago* **5,** 59–62.

Vernon, M. L., and Tusing, T. W. (1967). *U.S. Clearinghouse Report No. PB177067, Dec. 27, 1967.*

Von Holt, C., and Von Holt, L. (1954). *Z. Naturforsch Teil. B* **9,** 319–325.

Watkins, D., and Cooperstein, S. J. (1976). *J. Pharmacol. Exp. Ther.* **199,** 575–582.

Watkins, D., Cooperstein, S. J., and Lazarow, A. (1964a). *Am. J. Physiol.* **207,** 431–435.

Watkins, D., Cooperstein, S. J., and Lazarow, A. (1964b). *Am. J. Physiol.* **207,** 436–440.

Watkins, D., Cooperstein, S. J., and Lazarow, A. (1968). *Anat. Record* **160,** 447.

Watkins, D., Cooperstein, S. J., and Lazarow, A. (1970). *Am. J. Physiol.* **219,** 503–509.

Watkins, D., Cooperstein, S. J., and Lazarow, A. (1971a). *J. Pharmacol. Exp. Ther.* **176,** 42–51.

Watkins, D., Cooperstein, S. J., and Lazarow, A. (1971b). *Endocrinology* **88,** 1380–1384.

Watkins, D., Cooperstein, S. J., and Lazarow, A. (1973). *Am. J. Physiol.* **224,** 718–722.

Watkins, D., Cooperstein, S. J., and Fiel, S. (1979). *J. Pharmacol. Exp. Ther.* **208,** 184–189.

Weaver, D. C., McDaniel, M. L., Naber, S. P., Barry, D., and Lacy, P. E. (1978a). *Diabetes* **27,** 1205–1214.

Weaver, D. C., McDaniel, M. L., and Lacy, P. E. (1978b). *Endocrinology* **102,** 1847–1855.

Weaver, D. C., McDaniel, M. L., and Lacy, P. E. (1978c). *Diabetes* **27,** 71–77.

Weaver, D. C., Barry, C. D., McDaniel, M. L., Marshall, G. R., and Lacy, P. E. (1979). *Mol. Pharmacol.* **16,** 361–368.

Webb, J. L. (1966a). *In* "Enzyme and Metabolic Inhibitors," Vol. III, pp. 367–419. Academic Press, New York.

Webb, J. L. (1966b). *In* "Enzyme and Metabolic Inhibitors," Vol. III, pp. 795–819. Academic Press, New York.

Wellmann, K. F., Volk, B. W., and Lazarus, S. S. (1967). *Diabetes* **16,** 242–251.

White, F. R. (1963). *Cancer Chemother. Rep.* **30,** 49–53.

Wilander, E. (1974). *Acta Pathol. Microbiol. Scand. Sect. A* **82,** 767–776.

Wilander, E. (1975). *Acta Pathol. Microbiol. Scand. Sect. A* **83,** 213–221.

Wilander, E., and Boquist, L. (1972). *Horm. Metab. Res.* **4,** 426–433.

Wilander, E., and Gunnarsson, R. (1975). *Acta Pathol. Microbiol. Scand. Sect. A* **83,** 206–212.

Williamson, J. R., and Lacy, P. E. (1959). *Arch. Pathol.* **67,** 102–109.

Wrenshall, G. A., Collins-Williams, J., and Best, C. H. (1950). *Am. J. Physiol.* **160,** 228–246.

Yamamoto, H., and Okamoto, H. (1980). *Biochem. Biophys. Res. Commun.* **95,** 478–481.

Yesair, D. W. (1970). *Biochem. Pharmacol.* **19,** 687–695.

Zawalich, W. S., and Beidler, L. M. (1973). *Am. J. Physiol.* **224,** 963–966.

Zawalich, W. S., Karl, K. C., and Matschinsky, F. M. (1979). *Diabetologia* **16,** 115–120.

16

Role of Viruses in Diabetes

E. J. RAYFIELD and JI-WON YOON

427

The Islets of Langerhans
Copyright © 1981 by Academic Press, Inc.
All rights of reproduction in any form reserved.
ISBN 0-12-187820-1

For over 100 yr the possibility that certain viruses play a role in the pathogenesis of insulin-dependent diabetes mellitus (IDDM or type I diabetes) has been raised by numerous observations and reports in the literature (Maugh, 1975; Craighead, 1975; Rayfield and Seto, 1978; Notkins, 1979). This chapter will consider mechanisms by which a virus infection can potentially induce diabetes mellitus in a susceptible host, laboratory techniques currently used by investigators to study virus–pancreatic beta-cell interactions, and the available data pointing to a viral etiology of diabetes in man and animal models.

I. MECHANISMS OF VIRUS–INDUCED CELL DISEASE

Before considering specific diabetogenic viruses in terms of the pathogenesis of IDDM, we will give an overview of several possibilities by which a virus infection could lead to cell disease whether in the pancreas or in other tissues (Fig. 1). The first mechanism for the induction of cell disease involves a virus [such as encephalomyocarditis (EMC) or reovirus] attaching to virus-specific receptors on the cell membrane. The genetic background of the host is considered to play an important role in determining the presence or absence of such receptors on the cell membrane (Yoon and Notkins, 1976). The fact that several viruses can share the same receptor on the cell membrane (Longberg-Holm *et al.*, 1976) could explain why certain inbred species of mice are susceptible to both EMC and passaged coxsackie

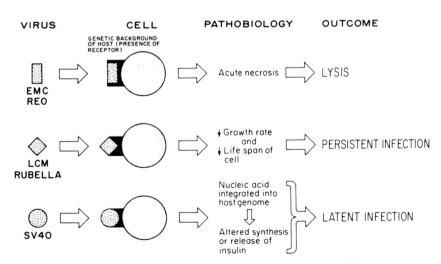

Fig. 1.   General mechanisms by which a virus can lead to cell disease.

B_4 virus-induced beta-cell damage. Once the virus enters the cell, replication begins, and in a matter of hours beta cells show focal areas of cytoplasmic degeneration (Craighead, 1977). Next, actual necrosis of the beta cells occurs, accompanied by an infiltration of mononuclear cells which phagocytize cellular debris (Craighead, 1977). Thus the outcome in this type of infection is cell lysis which leads to diabetes when about 90% of pancreatic beta cells are involved in this process. The next way in which a virus can promote an abnormality in cell function is by causing a persistent infection. Lymphocytic choriomeningitis, rubella, and cytomegalovirus are prototypes of this phenomenon. A persistent infection can be defined as one in which the viral genome (or part of the genome) persists for a prolonged period of time, often the lifetime of the host, irrespective of disease symptoms being manifest after the primary disease process is over. In the case of rubella virus, it is known that chronically infected cells cultured with this virus have a decreased life span (Rawls and Melnick, 1966; Plotkin and Vaheri, 1967), and the same could apply to pancreatic beta cells. The presence of a persistent infection might account for the long time lag between the occurrence of the congenital rubella syndrome and the subsequent development of diabetes mellitus 15–20 yr later (Menser, et al., 1978). A third mechanism by which a virus induces cellular disease is by causing a latent infection. SV–40 virus is an example of a virus which produces a latent infection. Again, the virus first must enter the target cell via membrane receptors. In a latent infection the virus nucleic acid becomes integrated into the host genome; some viral gene products can be detected, but infectious virus particles are not produced. One can postulate a viral infection having the capacity to result in the altered synthesis of or the release of insulin from the beta cell by this means.

II. LABORATORY TECHNIQUES FOR STUDYING VIRUS–PANCREATIC BETA-CELL INTERACTIONS

New methodologies have evolved allowing investigators to study in depth the effect of viruses on beta cells. These include the isolation, cultivation, and characterization of pancreatic beta cells from mice and humans, the double-label antibody technique for determining whether insulin-containing beta cells in vitro and in vivo are infected by specific viruses, and plaque purification of viruses to assess whether original pools of virus contain mixtures of diabetogenic and nondiabetogenic viruses. We describe these methods to enable the reader to understand the techniques better in reviewing papers in the literature as well as to provide a basis for investigators actually to develop these methods in their own laboratories.

A. Murine Pancreatic Beta-Cell Cultures

Pancreases are aseptically removed from 7- to 10-day-old suckling mice (about 70 mice per batch) and washed 10 times in cold phosphate-buffered saline with Ca^{2+} and Mg^{2+} (PBS) and containing penicillin (400 IU/ml) and streptomycin (100 μg/ml). The pancreases are minced into small pieces, and cold PBS is added. The tissue is allowed to settle for 1 min, and the supernatant fluid containing debris is discarded. This procedure is repeated five to seven times. Small pieces of pancreatic tissue are then transferred in an Erlenmeyer flask containing a prewarmed collagenase solution (5 mg/ml PBS) and incubated at 37°C for 15–20 min with vigorous shaking. The collagenase-treated material is then transferred to a conical tube, resuspended in PBS, and centrifuged at 500 rpm for 1–2 min which is just sufficient to allow the islets to settle. The supernatant fluid, which is carefully removed so as not to disturb the pellet, is discarded, and each pellet is resuspended in fresh PBS. The pellet is centrifuged and washed two more times. The resulting material (containing islets, acinar cells, fibroblasts, and other cell types) is transferred to a 35-mm petri dish, and the islets are collected with a Pasteur pipet under a stereomicroscope (Yoon and Notkins, 1976). The islets (100–200 islets per mouse) are disrupted by pipetting or by stirring very gently in a prewarmed collagenase solution (10 mg/ml PBS) for 5–7 min at 37°C. The suspension is filtered through sterile gauze to eliminate large aggregates and to break up small clumps of cells. The filtered cells are centrifuged at 1200 rpm for 5 min. The pellet is suspended in prewarmed chemically defined growth medium (MPNL 65/c) with 7% heat-inactivated fetal calf serum (Yoon, 1978a) and adjusted to 1.0×10^5 viable cells per milliliter. Plastic tissue culture dishes (60 or 35 mm) are then seeded with the cell suspension (5.0 ml for 60-mm dishes or 2.5 ml for 35-mm dishes) and incubated at 37°C in a humidified atmosphere of 5% carbon dioxide. Approximately 12–15 hr later, the nonadherent cells are decanted, thereby eliminating most of the fibroblastoid cells adhering to the dish (Fig. 2A). The decanted cells are seeded in 60- or 35-mm tissue culture dishes as described above and, after 48 hr, the medium is added to fresh MPNL 65/c containing 7% heat-inactivated fetal calf serum plus thimerosal (0.7 mg/liter) (Yoon and Notkins, 1976; Yoon, 1978a). The cells are refed at 2- to 3-day intervals, and at 6–8 days the monolayers are used for the experiments (Fig. 2B).

Cells in cultures prepared by this method are predominantly epithelioid in appearance (Fig. 2C). At 3 days, they contain heavy cytoplasmic granules in the perinuclear region, which generally stain strongly positive with fluorescein-labeled antiinsulin antibody (Fig. 2D). The intensity of staining, however, decreases with the length of time the cells are in culture. A small percentage of fibroblasts is sometimes seen; these cells are morpho-

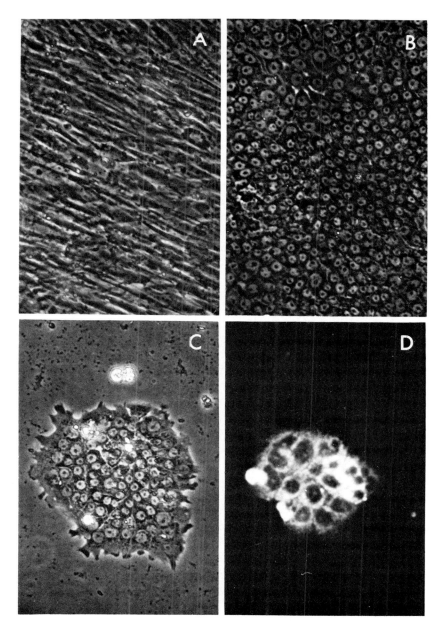

Fig. 2. (A) Confluent monolayer of pancreatic fibroblastoid cells which attached to the tissue culture dish for the first 12–15 hr and then grew for 8 days. × 160. (B) Confluent monolayer of pancreatic islet cells 8 days after seeding. × 160. (C) A colony of pancreatic islet cells 2 days after seeding × 160. Most of fibroblastic cells were eliminated by a decantation step and treatment with thimerosal. (D) Panceatic islet cells, cultured for 2 days, stained with FITC-labeled antiinsulin antibody. × 640.

logically distinct from the epithelioid cells and do not stain with fluo-rescein-labeled antiinsulin antibody. The identification of cultured beta cells is further confirmed by the evaluation of insulin-containing beta granules under the electron microscope (Fig. 3) and by monitoring the functional process of both synthesis and secretion of insulin by radioim-munoassay.

B. Human Pancreatic Beta-Cell Cultures

Monolayer cultures of normal human pancreatic beta cells are extremely valuable for a wide range of endocrinological, biochemical, physiological, and biological studies. Recent attempts to obtain monolayer cultures of normal human beta cells have met with limited success because of large ex-ocrine tissue clumps formed by collagenase treatment. The simple pro-cedure we introduce can yield reproducible cultures of functional human pancreatic beta cells.

About 5 g of tail parts of pancreas from a younger subject (preferably less than 15 yr old) is minced and washed repeatedly to obtain very small, clean pieces of tissue (less than 1 mm in diameter). Crude mincing of pan-creatic tissue can cause large exocrine tissue clumps to form during the col-lagenase treatment. Exhaustive mincing will prevent these clumps from forming, which will result in a much better single-cell yield and facilitate exocrine tissue digestion. The small pieces of pancreatic tissue are then transferred to a flask containing 50 ml of prewarmed collagenase solution (12 mg/ml in PBS). Enzymatic digestion is carried out for 20–25 min at 37°C with vigorous shaking or magnetic stirring. The collagenase-treated material (8 ml) is then transferred to a conical tube containing 35 ml of PBS and centrifuged for 1–2 min at a speed (e.g, 500 rpm) just sufficient to allow the cells to settle. The supernatant fluid is carefully removed, so as not to disturb the pellet, and is discarded. Each pellet is resuspended in fresh PBS. The cells are centrifuged, washed three more times, and then fil-tered through sterile gauze to remove large aggregates of residual exocrine tissue. The filtered cells are centrifuged at 1200 rpm for 7 min. The pellet is suspended in prewarmed chemically defined growth medium and adjusted to 10^5 viable cells per milliliter. The procedures for plating cells and for eliminating fibroblasts by decantation and thimerosol (3.0 μmol) are the same as those described for murine pancreatic beta-cell cultures. Mono-layer cultures prepared by this method yield a high percentage of beta cells that are morphologically and functionally characteristic (Fig. 4).

C. Double-Label Antibody Technique

Studies on the interaction of virus with insulin-containing beta cells have been limited by the difficulty in preparing pure beta-cell cultures. Since

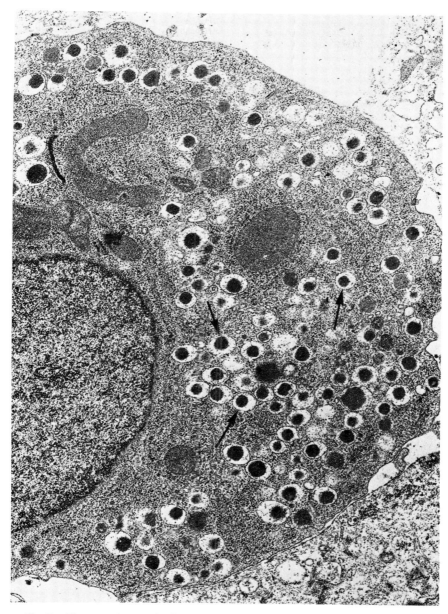

Fig. 3. Electron micrograph of pancreatic beta cell from a 6-day culture shows numerous granules (arrows) in the cytoplasm.

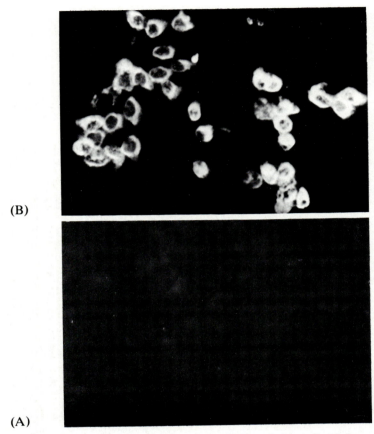

Fig. 4. (A) Confluent monolayer of human pancreatic islet cells 10 days after seeding. × 480. (B) Human pancreatic islet cells, cultured for 7 days stained with FITC-labeled antiinsulin antibody. × 480.

pancreatic monolayer cultures contain a mixed population of several different cell types [e.g., beta cells, alpha cells, D cells, pancreatic polypeptide (PP) cells, fibroblasts, and ductal cells], an increase in viral titer in infected cultures cannot be attributed to replication of the virus in beta cells. To determine if the beta cells in these mixed cultures are susceptible to infection by a specific virus, a double-label antibody technique has been developed (Prince *et al.,* 1978; Yoon *et al.,* 1978).

Antibody to insulin is labeled with tetramethyl rhodamine isothiocyanate (TRITC), and antibody to the virus is labeled with fluorescein isothiocyanate (FITC). To identify virus-infected beta cells, coverslips containing infected cells are fixed in cold acetone and stained with both TRITC-labeled antiinsulin antibody and FITC-labeled antivirus antibody overnight at 4°C. Coverslips are then washed three times for 10 min with cold PBS and mounted with Elvanol (Yoon, 1978). Coverslips are examined with a fluorescence microscope (e.g., a standard universal Zeiss microscope) illuminated by a HBO 200 mercury lamp. Double-labeled cells are identified by examining the coverslips first with rhodamine filters (a BP 546/9 excitation filter and an LP 590 barrier filter) for the detection of TRITC-labeled antiinsulin antibody and then with fluorescein filters (KP 490 and B913 excitation filters and an LP 528 barrier filter) for the detection of FITC-labeled antivirus antibody.

Figure 5A–C are photomicrographs of human pancreatic cell cultures infected with virus (beta-cell-passaged reovirus type 3) and stained 30 hr later with TRITC-labeled antiinsulin antibody and FITC-labeled antivirus antibody. When rhodamine filters are used to examine the cells (Fig. 5A), a diffuse orange color is found in the cytoplasm but not in the nucleus. When the same three cells are examined for viral antigens with fluorescein filters (Fig. 5B), a green color is seen in the cytoplasm. Figure 5B also shows viral antigens in two adjacent cells. The lack of fluorescence in the corresponding position in Fig. 5A, when the rhodamine filters are used, indicates that these cells do not contain insulin and probably represent one of the other cell types (e.g., alpha, D, PP, acinar, ductal, and fibroblast) present in the cultures. Figure 5C shows three insulin-containing beta cells infected with virus identified by the presence of orange and green fluorescence in the cytoplasm.

D. Method for Plaque Purification

The stock pool of some wild-type viruses may contain more than one variant. A recent report has shown that the diabetogenic activity in a virus pool of the M variant of EMC virus may not always be detected when tested *in vivo* because of interference produced by nondiabetogenic variants (Yoon *et al.*, 1980). Moreover, passage in certain tissue culture cell lines of virus pools containing a mixture of variants might favor replication of the interfering or nonbeta tropic variant. This may account for the poor and sometimes changing diabetogenicity of some virus pools (Yoon *et al.*, 1980). To see whether the original virus pool of possible diabetogenic viruses contains a mixture of diabetogenic and nondiabetogenic variants, individual plaques are selected, cloned, and tested *in vivo* as described below.

The stock pool of a virus is diluted to a concentration of one plaque-

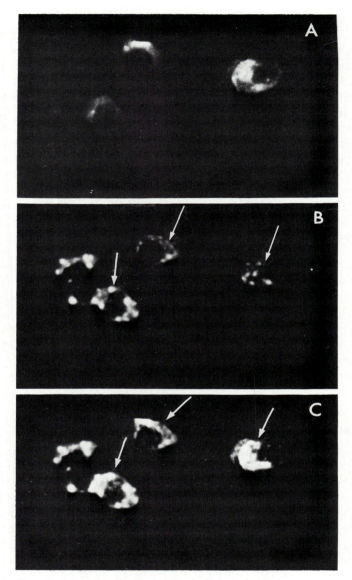

Fig. 5. Human pancreatic cell cultures infected with virus (reovirus type 3) at a virus/cell ratio of 1.0. At the end of 30 hr, the cultures were stained with TRITC-labeled antiinsulin and FITC-labeled antivirus antibody. (A) Photograph taken with rhodamine filters; (B) photograph of same area, but taken with fluorescein filters; (C) photograph of same area, but taken first with rhodamine filters and then with fluorescein filters. × 920.

forming unit (pfu) per milliliter, and 0.1-ml aliquots are allowed to adsorb to monolayers of any susceptible cells (on a 35-mm plate). After adsorption for 1 hr at 37°C, cultures are overlaid with 2% (w/v) methylcellulose in Eagle's minimal essential medium (MEM) containing 5% fetal bovine serum (Yoon, et al., 1977, 1980). Monolayers are stained with a 1:20,000 dilution of neutral red several days later (e.g., 2 days later for EMC and 6 days later for coxsackie B viruses). When examined 24 hr later, some of the plates contain single, distinct, circular plaques, while the rest show either more than one plaque or no plaques. Each of the single plaques is removed using the tip of a micropipet and infected in cell cultures. Several days later (e.g., 2–3 days for EMC and 5–6 days for coxsackie B viruses), infected monolayers show extensive cytopathic effects. Virus is harvested from the medium and cells by standard methods. The selected clones are tested in a susceptible animal to see whether any of them induce diabetes in this animal. The selected clones are usually plaque-purified two more times to obtain a pure diabetogenic variant, as described elsewhere (Yoon et al., 1980).

III. ASSOCIATION OF VIRAL INFECTIONS IN HUMANS WITH INSULIN-DEPENDENT DIABETES MELLITUS

A. Mumps Virus

Following two early case reports of an association of mumps virus infection with diabetes mellitus (Maugh, 1975; Harris, 1899) in the nineteenth century, there have been numerous others (Patrick, 1924; Gunderson, 1927; Kremer, 1947; King, 1962; Hinden, 1962; McCrae, 1963; Messaritakis et al., 1971; Block et al., 1973; Dacou-Voutetakis et al., 1974). Indeed, mumps virus has been the virus most frequently reported in association with diabetes mellitus, with symptoms of diabetes developing from a few days to several months following parotitis or parotitis with pancreatitis. In two separate cases, diabetes developed after mumps in two siblings (King, 1962; Messaritakis et al., 1971) almost simultaneously. While several cases of mumps pancreatitis examined pathologically during autopsy have shown acute inflammation with edema, mononuclear cell infiltration, and degeneration of epithelioid cells, this may not be the rule (Bostrom, 1968).

An epidemiological study performed by Sultz et al. (1975) in Eric County, New York, found a mean lag time of 3.8 yr between mumps infection or vaccination and the development of symptomatic diabetes (Sultz et al. 1975). In contrast a study from southern India showed no correlation between antibody titers to mumps virus in a group of recent-onset juvenile diabetics as compared to juvenile diabetics of long duration, maturity-onset diabetics of short and long duration, and nondiabetic controls (Samantray *et al.,* 1977).

Using the double-label antibody technique described above, Prince and colleagues demonstrated that mumps virus could infect human pancreatic beta cells obtained from autopsy specimens (Prince *et al.,* 1978).

B. Coxsackie Virus

In 1969 Gamble *et al.* reported that insulin-dependent diabetics with a recent onset of disease (within 3 months) had a higher neutralizing antibody titer to coxsackie B_4 virus than either normal subjects or type I diabetics of a duration of longer than 3 months (Gamble *et al.,* 1969). Thus far, other epidemiological studies have not confirmed this finding (Huff *et al.,* 1974; Hierholzer, and Farris, 1974; Dippe *et al.,* 1974, 1975). Two recent case reports have documented the acute onset of insulin-dependent diabetes mellitus (IDDM) in children under 2 yr of age in association with coxsackie B_2 virus (Templeton *et al.,* 1977) and a coxsackie B_5 virus (Champsaur *et al.,* 1980). Lesions in pancreatic islets and insulitis have been described following coxsackie B infections (Gladisch *et al.,* 1976; Sussman *et al.,* 1959). Using the double-label antibody technique, Yoon and co-workers demonstrated that coxsackie B_3 (Nancy strain), which had been passaged 10 times in secondary mouse embryo cells, was capable of infecting human beta cells in an *in vitro* culture system (Yoon *et al.,* 1978). The same laboratory also recently reported the isolation of coxsackie B_4 virus from the pancreas of a 10-yr-old previously healthy boy who died 7 days after admission to the hospital in diabetic ketoacidosis (Yoon *et al.,* 1979). At autopsy, lymphocytic infiltration of islets of Langerhans, beta-cell necrosis, and cerebral edema were noted. Coxsackie B_4 virus was isolated by inoculating mouse, monkey, and human cell cultures with homogenates of the patient's pancreas. Serological testing showed an increase in neutralizing antibody to this virus from < 4 on the second hospital day to 32 on the seventh day. Neutralization studies revealed that the isolated virus was closely related to a diabetogenic mouse-adapted coxsackie B_4 virus but differed antigenically from the nondiabetogenic prototype strain (JVB) of coxsackie B_4. Immunofluorescent staining revealed viral antigen in the patient's brain stem and in SJL mouse pancreatic beta cells 4 days after infection with the human isolate. The inoculation of genetically susceptible SJL mice with the human virus resulted in hyperglycemia, insulinitis, and beta-cell necrosis. While this is certainly an unusual presentation of IDDM, the studies performed in working up this case closely fulfill Koch's postulates and greatly strengthen the notion that in some cases a viral infection can result in IDDM.

C. Rubella Virus

Since 1949, 42 documented cases of diabetes mellitus have been reported in patients with the congenital rubella syndrome (Menser *et al.*, 1967, 1978; Hay, 1949; Forrest *et al.*, 1969, 1971; Plotkin and Kaye, 1970; Johnson and Tudor, 1970; Lundström *et al.*, 1974; Cooper, 1975; Halvorson, 1977; Ginsberg-Fellner *et al.*, 1980). The most extensive studies have been performed by Menser *et al.* in Australia, who have shown that there is a greater than 20% incidence of either clinical diabetes or abnormal glucose tolerance in patients with the congenital rubella syndrome (Menser *et al.*, 1978). In this same group of patients, HLA–B8 was present in 50% of the diabetics in contrast to 24% of a control population (Menser *et al.*, 1974). This antigen is known to be increased in IDDM (Cudworth and Woodrow, 1975). It is interesting to note that these patients did not show an increase in HLA–BW15 which is also associated with type I diabetes (Cudworth and Woodrow, 1975). An ongoing study is investigating the genetic, immunological, and other factors in siblings and their families with type I diabetes alone, the congenital rubella syndrome alone, or a combination of diabetes and the congenital rubella syndrome in order to better understand the interaction of genetic and environmental factors in virus-induced diabetes (Ginsberg-Fellner *et al.*, 1980). Persistent rubella virus infections of the pancreas of infants with the congenital rubella syndrome have been reported (Monif *et al.*, 1965), with mononuclear cell infiltrates in some cases (Bunnell and Monif, 1972). However, some pathological studies on infants dying with the congenital rubella syndrome have not found lesions in the islets of Langerhans (DePrins *et al.*, 1978; Singer *et al.*, 1967). It is clear that long-term prospective studies are needed to follow patients with congenital rubella and their siblings for the subsequent development of subclinical or clinical diabetes mellitus.

D. Other Viruses

Cytomegalovirus (Cappell and McFarlane, 1947), infectious mononucleosis (Wislocki, 1966; Everett *et al.*, 1969), and varicella (Johnson, 1940; Oppenheimer, 1944; Cheatham *et al.*, 1956; Blattner, 1957) can cause pancreatic lesions in man. Furthermore, diabetes mellitus has been associated temporally with viral infections from cytomegalovirus, measles, polio, influenza, tick-borne encephalitis, and infectious hepatitis (John, 1934;

Grishaw *et al.,* 1939; Warfield, 1927; Vizen, 1963: Oli and Nwokolo, 1979).

E. Nucleic Acids

Huang and Maclaren found a significant increase in the incidence of serum antibodies to single-stranded DNA and to both synthetic and native double-stranded RNA in patients with type I diabetes as compared to serum from age- and sex-matched asthmatics and healthy medical students (Huang and Maclaren, 1978). This observation may reflect either an immune response to altered double-stranded RNA of the host, or antibodies as a result of immunization to viral nucleic acids.

F. Insulitis

The presence of a mononuclear infiltration in and surrounding islets of insulin-dependent diabetics, referred to as insulitis, is characteristic of children or young adults with recent-onset diabetes who have come to autopsy (Gepts, 1965; LeCompte, 1958; Junker *et al.,* 1977). While this lesion is consistent with a previous viral infection, it is also consistent with an autoimmune process or a combination of the two.

IV. ANIMAL MODELS OF DIABETES MELLITUS WITH A DEFINITE OR POSSIBLE VIRAL ETIOLOGY

A. Foot-and-Mouth-Disease Virus

Italian workers in 1962 and 1963 reported a diabetes-like syndrome in cattle in which pancreatic pathology showed a severe decrease in islet tissue with insulitis (Barboni and Manocchio, 1962; Pauluzzi, 1963; Pedini, *et al.,* 1962). Platt noted that foot-and-mouth-disease virus (FMDV)-infected mice showed acinar cell necrosis but no islet lesions (Platt, 1959). On the other hand, McVicar *et al.,* using a different strain of FMDV (C type) found no elevation of blood glucose concentrations or of glucose intolerance for more than a month (Notkins, 1977). The discrepancies in the above observations can be accounted for by virus variants having different tropisms for cells or tissues.

B. Spontaneous Diabetes Mellitus in Guinea Pigs

Munger and Lang (Munger and Lang, 1973; Lang and Munger, 1976) described a spontaneous diabetes mellitus in guinea pigs that was contagious and possibly due to a viral infection. The pathology and course of the disease are described in Chapter 14. Guinea pigs exhibited glycosuria and abnormal glucose tolerance tests with variable fasting blood sugars. Pathological examination of the beta cells disclosed degranulation and cytoplasmic inclusions with sparing of alpha and D cells. No necrosis or islet inflammation was noted.

C. Coxsackie B_4

Coleman *et al.* (1973, 1974) observed that coxsackie B_4 virus produced a diabetes-like disease in adult CD_1 mice with pathological evidence of both islet and acinar tissue damage. In contrast, Ross and his associates studied coxsackie B_1–B_5 viruses in as many as six inbred strains of mice and showed increased serum amylase levels and normal or transient hypoglycemic glucose levels (Ross and Notkins, 1974; Ross *et al.*, 1974). These findings were corroborated by pathological evidence of marked destruction of acinar cells with virtually no effect on pancreatic beta cells. The divergence of data from different laboratories might be explained by the vast number of viral variants that exist (some of which are more beta-cytotropic than others) in addition to a spectrum of susceptibility in different inbred strains of animals. Yoon and co-workers reported that coxsackie B_4 virus that had been passaged 14 times (P–14) in cultures enriched for pancreatic beta cells provoked a diabetes-like syndrome after inoculation into SJL/J mice (Yoon *et al.*, 1978b). The infection resulted in insulinitis, beta-cell necrosis, localization of coxsackie B_4 virus in beta cells with the double-label technique described above, hypoinsulinemia, and decreased pancreatic immunoreactive insulin content. Thus serial passage of coxsackie B_4 virus in beta-cell-enriched culture can augment the diabetogenic properties of this virus.

D. Encephalomyocarditis Virus

Encephalomyocarditis virus is a picornavirus, like coxsackie B and FMDV, which produces a diabetes mellitus-like syndrome when the M variant is inoculated into genetically susceptible mice (From *et al.*, 1968; Craighead and McLane, 1968; Craighead and Steinke, 1971; Boucher and Notkins, 1973). Work with this virus involves the most extensively studied animal model for viral diabetes. After EMC infection, murine beta cells exhibit degranulation and coagulation necrosis, whereas alpha cells appear normal (Craighead *et al.*, 1974) and acinar cell necrosis is rare (Craighead *et al.*, 1974; Hayashi *et al.*, 1974). Certain strains, such as DBA/2 mice, have been found to be more susceptible to EMC virus-induced diabetes (Boucher and Notkins, 1973).

Metabolic factors were shown to play a role in beta-cell susceptibility to EMC virus. Male mice were more susceptible to EMC virus-induced hyperglycemia than female mice (Friedman *et al.*, 1972). Castrated male mice developed increased resistance similar to that of female mice (Friedman *et al.*, 1972). The administration of testosterone markedly enhanced susceptibility in both castrated male and female mice, as well as in intact females. Interestingly enough, the increased resistance in castrated males could be eliminated by adrenalectomy (Friedman *et al.*, 1972).

Genetic studies to explain beta-cell susceptibility to EMC virus infection are consistent with a Mendelian inheritance controlled by a single locus influencing two or more alleles (Onodera *et al.*, 1978). With respect to genetic factors influencing the immune response of the host, no differences in anti-EMC neutralizing antibody titers were found in diabetes-susceptible versus diabetes-resistant strains of mice 3–5 days after infection (Boucher *et al.*, 1975). However, susceptible murine strains had higher pancreatic viral titers (Yoon and Notkins, 1976) than resistant strains, as a result of an increased number of beta cells being infected rather than greater amounts of virus replicating per infected cell (Yoon and Notkins, 1976; Yoon *et al.*, 1976). It has been postulated that one mechanism of genetic control is regulation of the presence or absence of EMC virus receptors on the beta-cell membrane, thus allowing viral penetration into selected beta cells (Yoon *et al.*, 1977).

Jansen and co-workers studied the effect of immunosuppression with irradiation or a cyclophosphamide derivative (Jansen *et al.*, 1977). Irradiation protected against the development of hyperglycemia, whereas drug-induced immunosuppression resulted in markedly greater plasma glucose concentrations than in control mice infected with EMC alone. These investigators speculated that the increased insulitis following chemical immunosuppression might be the result of T-lymphocyte-mediated destruction of the beta cells that escaped attack by EMC virus (Jansen *et al.*, 1977).

Recent studies using the plaque purification technique described above for the M variant of EMC virus resulted in the isolation of two stable variants: one diabetogenic (the D variant) and the other nondiabetogenic (the B variant) (Yoon *et al.*, 1980). After inoculation of the D variant into SJL/J mice, hypoinsulinemia and hyperglycemia developed in over 90% of the animals. In contrast, none of the mice inoculated with the B variant developed diabetes. Approximately 10 times more infectious virus was recovered from the islets of animals inoculated with the D variant as compared to those receiving the B variant.

Coinfection experiments showed that the induction of diabetes by the D variant was inhibited by the B variant. When the B and D variants were mixed together at B/D ratios of 1, 9, and 99, diabetes developed in 60, 11, and 0% of the mice, respectively. Tissue culture experiments revealed that the B variant induced considerably more interferon than the D variant. *In vivo* studies demonstrated that interferon appeared earlier and in greater amounts in the circulation of mice infected with the B variant as compared to the D variant. Thus these observations suggest that the induction of interferon by the B variant is at least in part responsible for the inhibition of diabetes by the D variant. The precise role of interferon in the protection of virus-induced diabetes in susceptible mice remains to be determined.

E. Venezuelan Encephalitis Virus

When golden Syrian hamsters were inoculated with the virulent Trinidad strain of Venezuelan encephalitis (VE) virus, mature virions and viral antigens were found in beta cells by electron microscopy and immunofluorescence (Rayfield *et al.*, 1976). Viral replication occurred in the pancreas with both the Trinidad strain and the vaccine (TC–83) strain of VE virus. Metabolic studies performed in TC–83-infected hamsters revealed glucose intolerance lasting for 24 days and severely decreased plasma insulin levels for as long as 90 days following infection. The fact that the pancreatic insulin content was normal in hamsters for 24 days following infection suggested a defect in beta-cell insulin release. Also, TC–83 VE virus was shown to inhibit glucose-stimulated insulin release in three genetic variants of C57B1/Ks mice (*db/db, db/+*, and *+/+*) (Rayfield *et al.*, 1979). These studies were extended to a primate species in collaboration with G. S. Bowen, formerly of the Center for Disease Control, Fort Collins, Colorado (Rayfield and Bowen, 1977). Five young adult healthy male rhesus monkeys were given intravenous glucose tolerance tests (GTT) during a control preinoculation period and for 8 days and 2, 5, and 10 months after inoculation with Trinidad strain VE virus. After the 10-month GTT, monkeys were killed to evaluate pancreatic pathology and extractable hormone content. After VE virus inoculation, glucose intolerance and marked hypoinsulinemia developed in all the monkeys. Since plasma cortisol levels did not change significantly during the studies, it was unlikely that this hypoinsulinemia was induced by nonspecific stress. Light and electron microscopic evaluations of the pancreases were normal after the animals were killed at 10 months. In a second group of rhesus monkeys studied, with six control, six Trinidad strain VE virus-infected, and six TC–83 VE virus-infected monkeys, glucose intolerance did not develop in either the Trinidad or the TC–83 group (Bowen *et al.*, 1979). The only difference between the monkeys in the two studies was that slightly younger (2–3 yr versus 3–4 yr) and lighter (3.3–4.8 kg versus 3.7–7.2 kg) monkeys were used in the first study. One explanation for the different findings in the two studies is that the viral infection in younger monkeys was more severe, as is the case in humans. In this connection, the monkeys in the first experiment were all febrile and exhibited coughing and rhinorrhea, in contrast to the second experiment in which monkeys had no respiratory symptoms and only three were febrile.

In order to understand the mechanism for the inhibition of glucose-stimulated insulin release in TC-83 VE virus-infected islets, a series of experiments were conducted utilizing isolated perifused hamster islets obtained from virus-infected and control animals (Rayfield *et al.*, 1980). These experiments showed an impressive diminution in 20 mM glucose-stimulated insulin release in 3 $\frac{1}{2}$-week-old infected hamster islets in comparison to uninfected controls, similar to *in vivo* experiments. The decrease in 20 mM glucose-stimulated insulin release persisted in 8 mo infected islets.

The glucose-stimulated hypoinsulinemia in virus-infected islets could be corrected by tolbutamide, theophylline, dibutyryl cyclic adenosine 3′,5′-monophosphate (cAMP), and 8-bromo cAMP, all of which increase intraislet cAMP. These data suggest that there may be a virus-induced defect at the level of the putative glucoreceptor on the beta-cell membrane, but that events distal to the cAMP system of the beta cell are intact (Rayfield *et al.*, 1980).

F. Rubella Virus

Menser and associates reported that offspring from rubella virus-infected rabbits exhibited beta-cell degranulation and changes in subcellular organelles, but no evidence of necrosis (Menser *et al.*, 1978).

G. Streptozotocin Model

Like and Rossini found that five daily subdiabetogenic injections of streptozotocin in mice produced pancreatic insulitis with progressive destruction of beta cells and sustained hyperglycemia (Like and Rossini, 1976; Rossini *et al.*, 1977; Like *et al.* 1978; Appel *et al.*, 1978). One explanation of this phenomenon is that streptozotocin in this model initiated a cell-mediated immune response. The presence of type-C viruses within beta cells as demonstrated by electron microscopy suggests that streptozotocin may have activated murine leukemia virus *in vivo* in susceptible hosts. The precise mechanisms for streptozotocin induction of type-C viruses and insulitis, as well as the importance of these viruses pathogenetically, are unclear.

H. Reoviruses

Onodera and his colleagues reported that reovirus type 3, passaged at least seven times in pancreatic beta-cell cultures from SJL/J mice, produced pancreatic islet necrosis and mononuclear leukocyte infiltration after inoculation into 1- to 2-week-old mice (Onodera et al., 1978). The double-label antibody method revealed the presence of reovirus antigens in beta cells from frozen sections of mouse pancreas. Reovirus-infected mice did not exhibit fasting hyperglycemia up to 20 days after infection but did manifest abnormal glucose tolerance.

V. INTERRELATIONSHIP OF VIRAL INFECTION AND AUTOIMMUNITY

At least three mechanisms exist by which a virus infection may trigger the subsequent development of immunological events in the pancreas long after acute viral insult of the tissue (Freytag, 1974). These mechanisms include (1) the formation of new antigenic sites in cellular proteins, (2) the production of cell-specific antibodies directed against the pancreatic islets, and (3) a nonspecific action of virus infection that may lead to a loss of immunological tolerance (Freytag, 1974). The loss of immunological tolerance could promote infections with additional pancreatropic viruses or favor a lingering autoimmune process long after an initial viral infection, the end result being clinical diabetes mellitus. This is discussed further in Chapter 17.

VI. RECENT EPIDEMIOLOGICAL STUDIES

A Danish retrospective epidemiological study concerning the incidence, sex, seasonal, and geographic patterns of IDDM was reported in 1977 and included one-third of the country's population for the period 1970–1974 (Christau et al., 1977). The incidence of the disease remained at about 13.2 per 100,000 per year, with 27% more boys than girls affected. As in the data of Gamble and Taylor (1969), a seasonal variation in the onset of diabetes mellitus was noted, with a reduction in incidence during May, June, and July. One explanation for a seasonal variation in type I diabetes is the associated seasonal fluctuation in viral infections, although other factors such as diet and exercise could also have been at work.

VII. SUMMARY

The mechanisms of virus-induced cell disease have been discussed, including lytic, persistent, and latent infections. Newer laboratory techniques for examining virus–beta cell interactions have been explained in detail, such as murine and human beta-cell tissue culture, the double-label antibody method for identifying virus-infected beta cells, and plaque purification for separating diabetogenic from nondiabetogenic virus variants.

Human viruses associated with type I diabetes include mumps virus, coxsackie B_4, and rubella virus (congenital rubella syndrome). A recent study reported the isolation of a coxsackie B_4 virus from the pancreas of a 10-yr-old child who died in diabetic ketoacidosis. Inoculation of this human isolate into genetically susceptible SJL mice resulted in hyperglycemia, insulitis, and beta-cell necrosis, closely fulfilling Koch's postulates with respect to a viral etiology of type I diabetes in man. Animal models for virus-induced diabetes include EMC, coxsackie, VE, and rubella viruses, EMC virus being the most extensively studied. One site of genetic control in mice might relate to differences in number of viral receptors on the beta-cell membrane that can confer susceptibility or resistance to EMC-virus-induced diabetes. Recent data suggest that the induction of interferon by the nondiabetogenic B variant of EMC virus plays a role in the inhibition of diabetes by the D variant of EMC virus. Primate models could offer a unique opportunity for careful study of the evolution of diabetic complications.

A viral infection and an autoimmune process may interrelate as follows: a virus can precipitate an autoimmune event, and an autoimmune process can augment susceptibility to a pancreatropic virus, leading to the development of type I diabetes.

Epidemiological studies show a relationship of IDDM with seasonal patterns, which could be the result of viral infections, although dietary, exercise, and other factors might also account for such patterns.

REFERENCES

Appel, M. C., Rossini, A. A., Williams, R. M., and Like, A. A. (1978). Viral studies in streptozotocin-induced pancreatic insulitis. *Diabetologia* **15**, 327–336.

Barboni, E., and Manocchio, I. (1962). Alterazionia pancreatiche in bovini con diabete mellito post-aftoso. *Arch Vet. Ital* **13**, 477–489.

Blattner, R. J. (1957). Serious complications of varicella including fatalities. *J. Pediatr.* **50**, 515–517.

Block, M. B., Berk, J. E., Fridhandler, L. S., Steiner, D. F., and Rubenstein, A. H. (1973). Diabetic ketoacidosis asociated with mumps virus infection: Occurrence in a patient with macroamylasemia. *Ann. Intern. Med.* **78**, 633–667.

Bostrom, K. (1968). Patho-anatomic findings in a case of mumps with pancreatitis, myocarditis, orchitis, epididymitis, and seminal vesiculitis. *Virchows Arch.* **344**, 111–117.

Boucher, D. W., and Notkins, A. L. (1973). Virus-induced diabetes mellitus. I. Hyperglycemia and hypoinsulinemia in mice infected with encephalomyocarditis virus. *J. Exp. Med.* **137**, 1226–1239.

Boucher, D. W., Hayashi, K., Rosenthal, J., and Notkins, A. L. (1975). Virus-induced diabetes mellitus. III. Influence of the sex and strain of the host *J. Infect. Dis.* **131**, 462–466.

Bowen, G. S., Rayfield, E. J., Monath, T. P., and Kemp, G. E. (1981). Studies of Glucose Metabolism in Rhesus Monkeys After Venezuelan Equine Encephalitis Virus Infection. *J. Med. Virol.* (in press).

Bunnell, C. E., and Monif, G. R. G. (1972). Interstitial pancreatitis in the congenital rubella syndrome. *J. Pediatr.* **80**, 465–465.

Cappell, D. F., and McFarlane, M. N. (1947). Inclusion bodies (protozoan-like cells) in the organs of infants. *J. Pathol. Bacteriol.* **59**, 385–398.

Champsaur, H., Dussaix, E., Samolyk, D., Fabre, M., Bach, C., and Assan, R. (1980). Diabetes and Coxsackie B$_5$ infection. *Lancet* **1**, 251.

Cheatham, W. J., Weller, T. H., Dolan, T. F., and Dower, J. C. (1956). Varicella: Report of two fatal cases with necropsy, virus isolation, and serologic studies. *Am. J. Pathol* **32**, 1015–1036.

Christau, B., Kromann, H., Andersen, O. O., Christy, M., Buschard, K., Arnung, K., Kristensen, I. H., Peitersen, B., Steinrud, J., and Nerup, J. (1977). Incidence, seasonal and geographical patterns of juvenile-onset insulin-dependent diabetes mellitus in Denmark. *Diabetologia* **13**, 281–284.

Coleman, T. J., Gamble, D. R., and Taylor, K. W. (1973). Diabetes in mice after Coxsackie B$_4$ virus infection. *Br. Med. J.* **3**, 25–27.

Coleman, T. J., Taylor, K. W., and Gamble, D. R. (1974). The development of diabetes following Coxsackie B virus infection in mice. *Diabetologia* **10**, 755–759.

Cooper, L. Z. (1975). Congenital rubella in the United States. *In* "Infections of the Fetus and Newborn Infant." (S. Krugman and A. A. Gershon, eds.) p 1. Alan R. Liss, New York.

Craighead, J. E. (1975). The role of viruses in the pathogenesis of pancreatic disease and diabetes mellitus. *Prog. Med. Virol.* **19**, 161–214.

Craighead, J. E. (1977). "The Diabetic Pancreas" (B. W. Volk and K. F. Wellman, eds.), pp. 467–488. Plenum, New York.

Craighead, J. E., and McLane, M. F. (1968). Diabetes mellitus: Induction in mice by encephalomyocarditis virus. *Science* **162**, 913–914.

Craighead, J. E., and Steinke, J. (1971). Diabetes mellitus-like syndrome in mice infected with encephalomyocarditis virus. *Am. J. Pathol.* **63**, 119–130.

Craighead, J. E., Kanich, R. E., and Kessler, J. B. (1974). Lesions of the islets of Langerhans in encephalomyocarditis virus-infected mice with diabetes-like disease. I. Acute lesions. *Am. J. Pathol.* **74**, 287–300.

Cudworth, A. G., and Woodrow, J. C. (1975). HL-A system and diabetes mellitus. *Diabetes* **24**, 345–349.

Dacou-Voutetakis, C., Constantinidis, M., Moschos, A., Vlachou, C., and Matsaniotis, N. (1974). Diabetes mellitus following mumps: Insulin reserve. *Am. J. Dis. Child.* **127**, 890–891.

DePrins, F., Van Assche, F. A., Desmyter, J., DeGroote, G., and Gepts, W. (1978). Congenital rubella and diabetes mellitus. *Lancet* **1**, 440.

Dippe, S. E., Bennett, P. H., and Miller, M. (1974). Coxsackie B virus and diabetes. *Br. Med. J.* **2**, 443–444.

Dippe, S. E., Bennett, P. H., and Miller, M. (1975). Lack of causal association between Coxsackie B4 virus infection and diabetes. *Lancet* **1**, 1314–1317.

Everett, E. D., Volpe, J. A., and Bergin, J. J. (1969). Pancreatitis in infectious mononucleosis. *South. Med. J.* **62**, 359–360.

Forrest, J. M., Menser, M. A., and Harley, S. S. (1969). Diabetes mellitus and congenital rubella. *Pediatrics* **44**, 445–446.

Forrest, J. M., Menser, M. A., and Burgess, J. A. (1971). High frequency of diabetes mellitus in young adults with congenital rubella. *Lancet* **2**, 332–334.

Freytag, G. (1974). Do viruses serve as mediators of immunological reactions? *In* "Immunity and Autoimmunity in Diabetes" (P. A. Bastenie and W. Gepts, eds.), pp. 247–251. Excerpta Medica, Amsterdam.

Friedman, S. F., Grota, L. J., and Glasgow, L. A. (1972). Differential susceptibility of male and female mice to encephalomyocarditis virus: Effects of castration, adrenalectomy, and the administration of sex hormones. *Infect. Immun.* **5**, 637–644.

From, G. L. A., Craighead, J. E., McLane, M. F., and Steinke, J. (1968). Virus-induced diabetes in mice. *Metabolism* **17**, 1154–1158.

Gamble, D. R., and Taylor, K. W. (1969). Seasonal incidence of diabetes mellitus *Br. Med. J.* **3**, 631–633.

Gamble, D. R., Kinsley, M. L., FitzGerald, M. G., Bolton, R., and Taylor, K. W. (1969). Viral antibodies in diabetes mellitus. *Br. Med. J.* **3**, 627–630.

Gepts, W. (1965). Pathologic anatomy of the pancreas in juvenile diabetes mellitus. *Diabetes* **14**, 619–633.

Ginsberg-Fellner, F., Klein, E., Dobersen, M., Jenson, A. B., Rayfield, E. J., Notkins, A. L., Rubinstein, P., and Cooper, L. Z. (1980). The interrelationship of congenital rubella (CR) and insulin-dependent diabetes mellitus (IDDM). *Ped. Res.* **14**, 572 (Abstr.).

Gladisch, R., Hofmann, W., and Waldherr, R. (1976). Myocarditis and insulitis in Coxsackie virus infection. *Z. Kardiol* **65**, 837–849.

Grishaw, W. H., West, H. F., and Smith, B. (1939). Juvenile diabetes mellitus. *Arch. Intern. Med.* **64**, 787–799.

Gundersen, E. (1927). Is diabetes of infectious origin? *J. Infect. Dis.* **41**, 197–202.

Halvorson, E. P. (1977). Diabetes mellitus and congenital rubella: Report of a case. *Mt. Sinai J. Med. N.Y.* **44**, 566–567.

Harris, H. F. (1899). A case of diabetes mellitus quickly following mumps. *Boston Med. Surg. J.* **140**, 465–469.

Hay, D. R. (1949). Studies in preventive hygiene from the Otago Medical School. I. The relation of maternal rubella to congenital deafness and other abnormalities in New Zealand. *N.Z. Med. J.* **48**, 604–608.

Hayashi, K., Boucher, D. W., and Notkins, A. L. (1974). Virus-induced diabetes mellitus. II. Relationship between beta cell damage and hyperglycemia in mice infected with encephalomyocarditis virus. *Am. J. Pathol* **75**, 91–102.

Hinden, E. (1962). Mumps followed by diabetes. *Lancet* **1**, 1381.

Hierholzer, J. C., and Farris, W. A. (1974). Follow-up of children infected in a Coxsackie B3 and B4 outbreak: No evidence of diabetes. *J. Infect. Dis.* **129**, 741–746.

Huang, S-W., and Maclaren, N. K. (1978). Antibodies to nucleic acids in juvenile-onset diabetes. *Diabetes* **27**, 1105–1111.

Huff, J. C., Hierholzer, J. C., and Farris, W. A. (1974). An "outbreak" of juvenile diabetes mellitus: Consideration of a viral etiology. *Am. J. Epidemiol.* **100**, 277–287.

Jansen, F. K., Münterfering, H., and Schmidt, W. A. K. (1977). Virus induced diabetes and the immune system. I. Suggestion that appearance of diabetes depends on immune reactions. *Diabetologia* **13**, 545–549.

John, H. J. (1934). The diabetic child: Etiologic factors. *Ann. Intern. Med.* **8**, 198–213.

Johnson, H. N. (1940). Visceral lesions associated with varicella. *Arch. Pathol.* **30**, 292–307.

Johnson, G. M., and Tudor, R. B. (1970). Diabetes mellitus and congenital rubella infection. *Am. J. Dis. Child.* **120**, 453–455.

Junker, K., Egeberg, J., Kromann, H., and Nerup, J. (1977). An autopsy study of the islets of Langerhans in acute-onset juvenile diabetes mellitus. *Acta Pathol. Microbiol. Scand. A.,* **85**, 699–706.

King, R. C. (1962). Mumps followed by diabetes. *Lancet* **2**, 1055.

Kremer, H. V. (1947). Juvenile diabetes as a sequel to mumps. *Am. J. Med.* **3**, 257–258.

Lang, C., M., and Munger, B. L. (1976). Diabetes mellitus in the guinea pig. *Diabetes* **25**, 434–443.

LeCompte, P. M. (1958). "Insulitis" in early juvenile diabetes. *Arch. Pathol.* **66**, 450–457.

Like, A. A., and Rossini, A. A. (1976). Streptozotocin-induced pancreatic insulitis: New model of diabetes mellitus. *Science* **193**, 415–417.

Like, A. A., Appel, M. C., Williams, R. M., and Rossini, A. A. (1978). Streptozotocin-induced pancreatic insulitis in mice: Morphologic and physiologic studies. *Lab. Invest.* **38**, 470–486.

Lonberg-Holm, K., Crowell, R. L., and Philipson, L. (1976). Unrelated animal viruses share receptors. *Nature (London)* **259**, 679–681.

Lundström, R., Ahnsjö, S., Berczy, J., Blomqvist, B., and Eklund, G. (1974). "Proc. XIV Intern. Congr. Pediatr.," Vol 4, p 61, Buenos Aires. *Pediatria* **14**.

McCrae, W. (1963). Diabetes mellitus following mumps. *Lancet* **1**, 1300–1301.

Maugh, T. H. (1975). Diabetes: Epidemiology suggests a viral connection. *Science* **188**, 347–351.

Menser, M. A., Dods, L., and Harley, J. D. (1967). A twenty-five year follow-up of congenital rubella. *Lancet* **2**, 1347–1350.

Menser, M. A., Forrest, J. M., and Honeyman, M. C. (1974). Diabetes, HL-A antigens and congenital rubella. *Lancet* **2**, 1508–1509.

Menser, M. A., Forrest, J. M., and Bransby, R. D. (1978). Rubella infection and diabetes mellitus. *Lancet* **1**, 57–60.

Messaritakis, J., Karabula, C., Kattamis, C., and Matsaniotis, N. (1971). Diabetes following mumps in sibs. *Arch. Dis. Child.* **46**, 561–562.

Monif, G. R. G., Avery, B. G., Koromes, S. B., and Sever, J. L. (1965). Isolation of the rubella virus from the organs of three children with rubella syndrome defects. *Lancet* **1**, 723–724.

Munger, B. L., and Lang, C. M. (1973). Spontaneous diabetes mellitus in guinea pigs: The acute cytopathology of the islets of Langerhans. *Lab. Invest.* **29**, 685–702.

Notkins, A. L. (1977). Virus-induced diabetes: Brief review. *Arch Virol.* **54**, 1–17.

Notkins, A. L. (1979). The causes of diabetes. *Sci. Am.* **241**, 62–73.

Oli, J. M., and Nwokolo, C. (1979). Diabetes after infectious hepatitis: A follow-up study. *Br. Med. J.* **1**, 926–927.

Onodera, T., Yoon, J-W., Brown, K. A., and Notkins, A. L. (1978a). Evidence for a single locus controlling susceptibility to virus-induced diabetes mellitus. *Nature (London)* **274**, 693–696.

Onodera, T., Jenson, A. B., Yoon, J-W., and Notkins, A. L. (1978b). Virus-induced diabetes mellitus: Reovirus infection of pancreatic B cells in mice. *Science* **201**, 529–531.

Oppenheimer, E. H. (1944). Congenital chickenpox with disseminated visceral lesions. *Johns Hopkins Hosp. Bull.* **74**, 240–249.

Patrick, A. (1924). Acute diabetes following mumps. *Br. Med. J.* **2**, 802.

Pauluzzi, L. (1963) Sindrome diabetica post-aftosa nel bovino e nel caprino. *Clin Vet.* **86**, 113–132.

Pedini, B., Avellini, G., Morettini, B., and Comodo, N. (1962). Diabete mellito post-aftoso nei bovini. *Atti Soc. Ital Sci. Vet.* **16**, 443–450.

Platt, H. (1959). The occurrence of pancreatic lesions in adult mice infected with the virus of FMD. *Virology* **9**, 484–486.

Plotkin, S. A., and Kaye, R. (1970). Diabetes mellitus and congenital rubella. *Pediatrics* **46**, 650–651.

Plotkin, S. A., and Vaheri, A. (1967). Human fibroblasts infected with rubella virus produce a growth inhibitor. *Science* **156**, 659–661.

Prince, G., Jenson, A. B., Billups, L., and Notkins, A. L. (1978). Infection of human pancreatic beta cell cultures with mumps virus. *Nature (London)* **271**, 158–161.

Rawls, W. E., and Melnick, J. L. (1966). Rubella virus carrier cultures deriveed from congenitally infected infants. *J. Exp. Med.* **123**, 795–816.

Rayfield, E. J., and Bowen, G. S. (1977). The evolution of Venezuelan encephalitis virus induced carbohydrate abnormalities in rhesus monkeys. *Clin. Res.* **25**, 398–A (Abstr.).

Rayfield, E. J., and Seto, Y. (1978). Viruses and the pathogenesis of diabetes mellitus. *Diabetes* **27**, 1126–1142.

Rayfield, E. J., Gorelkin, L., Curnow, R. T., and Jahrling, P. B. (1976). Virus-induced pancreatic disease by Venezuelan encephalitis virus: Alterations in glucose tolerance and insulin release. *Diabetes* **25**, 623–631.

Rayfield, E. J., Seto, Y., Goldberg, S. L., Schulman, R. H., and Walker, G. F. (1979) Venezuelan encephalitis virus-induced alterations in carbohydrate metabolism in genetically diabetic mice. *Diabetes* **28**, 799–803.

Rayfield, E. J., Seto, Y., and Walsh, S. B. (1980). Virus induced abnormalities in insulin release in perifused hamster islets. *Diabetes* **29**, Suppl. 2, 131–A (Abstr.).

Ross, M. E., and Notkins, A. L. (1974). Coxsackie B viruses and diabetes mellitus. *Br. Med. J.* **2**, 226.

Ross, M. E., Hayashi, K., and Notkins, A. L. (1974). Virus-induced pancreatic disease: Alterations in concentration of glucose and amylase in blood. *J. Infect. Dis.* **129**, 669–676.

Rossini, A. A., Like, A. A., Chick, W. L., Appel, M. C., and Cahill, G. F., Jr. (1977) Studies of streptozotocin-induced insulitis and diabetes. *Proc. Natl. Acad. Sci. U.S.A.* **74**, 2485–2489.

Samantray, S. K., Christopher, S., Mukundan, P., and Johnson, S. C. (1977). Lack of relationship between viruses and human diabetes mellitus. *Aust. N. Z. J. Med.* **7**, 139–142.

Singer, D. B., Rudolph, A. J., Rosenberg, H. S., Rawls, W. E., and Boniuk, M. (1967) Pathology of the congenital rubella syndrome. *J. Pediatr.* **71**, 665–675.

Sultz, H. A., Hart, B. A., Zielezny, M., and Schlesinger, E. R. (1975). Is mumps virus an etiologic factor in juvenile diabetes mellitus? *J. Pediatr.* **86**, 654–656.

Sussman, M. L., Strauss, L., and Hodes, H. L. (1959). Fatal Coxsackie group B virus infection in the newborn. *Am. J. Dis. Child.* **97**, 483–492.

Templeton, A. A., Kerr, M. G., Cole, R. A., and Less, M. M., (1977). Coxsackie B_2 virus infection and acute-onset diabetes in a child. *Br. Med. J.* **1**, 1007–1008.

Vizen, E. M. (1963). On the atypical forms of tick-borne encephalitis (In Russian) *Zh. Nevropatol. Psikhiatr. Im. S. S. Korsakova* **63**, 1462–1466.

Warfield, I. M. (1927). Acute pancreatitis followed by diabetes. *J. Am. Med. Assoc.* **89**, 654–658.

Wislocki, L. C. (1966). Acute pancreatitis in infectious mononucleosis. *N. Engl. J. Med.* **275**, 322–323.

Yoon, J-W. (1978). Method for cultivation and identification of human pancreatic beta cells. *T. C. A. Manual* **4**, 885–888.

Yoon, J-W., and Notkins, A. L. (1976) Virus-induced diabetes mellitus. VI. Genetically determined host differences in the replication of encephalomyocarditis virus in pancreatic beta cells. *J. Exp. Med.* **143**, 1170–1185.

Yoon, J-W., Lesniak, M. A., Fussganger, R., and Notkins, A. L. (1976) Genetic differences in susceptibility of pancreatic B cells to virus-induced diabetes mellitus. *Nature (London)* **264**, 178–180.

Yoon, J-W., Onodera, T., and Notkins, A. L. (1977). Virus-induced diabetes mellitus. VIII. Passage of encephalomyocarditis virus and severity of diabetes in susceptible and resistant strains of mice. *J. Gen. Virol* **37**, 225.

Yoon, J-W., Onodera, T., Jenson, A. B , and Notkins, A. L. (1978a). Virus-induced diabetes mellitus. XI. Replication of Coxsackie virus B$_3$ in human pancreatic beta cell cultures. *Diabetes* **27**, 778–781.

Yoon, J-W., Onodera, T., and Notkins, A. L. (1978b). Virus-induced diabetes mellitus. XV. Beta cell damage and insulin-dependent hyperglycemia in mice infected with Coxsackie virus B4. *J. Exp. Med.* **148**, 1068–1080.

Yoon, J-W., Austin, M., Onodera, T., and Notkins, A. L. (1979). Virus-induced diabetes mellitus: Isolation of a virus from the pancreas of a child with diabetic ketoacidosis. *N. Engl. J. Med.* **300**, 1173–1179.

Yoon, J-W., McClintock, P. R., Onodera, T., and Notkins, A. L. (1980) Virus-induced diabetes mellitus. XVIII. Inhibition by a non-diabetogenic variant of encephalomyocarditis virus. *J. Exp. Med.* **152**, 878–892.

17

Autoimmunity and Diabetes

N. K. MACLAREN

I. INTRODUCTION

A. IDDM as an Autoimmune Disease

There is much circumstantial evidence supporting the concept that insulin-dependent diabetes mellitus (IDDM) has an autoimmune basis. Among the most compelling observations are:

1. The specific lymphocytic infiltration of the pancreatic islets, or "insulitis," seen near the onset of IDDM (see Gepts, Chapter 13).

453

The Islets of Langerhans
Copyright © 1981 by Academic Press, Inc.
All rights of reproduction in any form reserved.
ISBN 0-12-187820-1

2. The identification of islet cell-reactive autoantibodies (ICA) in patients with IDDM (Section II,B).

3. The association of IDDM with thyroid and adrenal endocrinopathies and with pernicious anemia, diseases which have features suggestive of autoimmunity (Section II,C).

4. Indirect evidence of active cell-mediated immunity (CMI) toward pancreatic islet cells and islet cell antigens (Section II,D).

5. The association with the disease of certain antigens of the human leukocyte antigen (HLA) system which are the same as those associated with other autoimmune organ-specific and nonorgan-specific disorders (Section III).

Notwithstanding, there are some experimental deficiencies which must be overcome before IDDM can be considered unequivocally to be an autoimmune disease. These are:

6. Lack of good animal models for autoimmune IDDM. (The BB rat may be one such model.)

7. Failure to transfer IDDM immunologically.

8. Failure to demonstrate that any immunotherapy could either prevent the onset of IDDM or reverse its clinical manifestations.

This chapter will deal with the "state of the art" as related to autoimmune aspects of IDDM. Since this reflects the general state of medical knowledge of autoimmune diseases as a whole, some review of the latter will first be attempted.

B. Autoimmunity—The State of the Art

1. Immune Response and Tolerance

The *immune response* depends upon a host of mechanisms, including macrophage processing of antigens, macrophage–T lymphocyte interactions involving presentation of the immunizing antigen with HLA-DR antigens (Ia in the mouse), B–T lymphocyte interaction, and B lymphocyte transformation to mature committed lymphocytes and plasma cells. The latter usually results in small, relatively nonspecific immunoglobin M (IgM) elevations, followed by large specific IgG responses which require participation from helper T lymphocytes. Human T helper cells can be identified by the Leu 3 or OKT4 monoclonal antibodies. T lymphocytes may also become cytotoxic to antigenically transformed self-cells, e.g., virus-infected cells, and this response is strongly enhanced by the commonality of effector and target cells for surface HLA-A -B, and -(C) (D and K in the mouse) in a process of "dual recognition." Activated T lymphocytes also produce various lymphokines such as interferon, macrophage inhibitory factor, and others, depending on the nature of the immunizing antigen.

The magnitude of an immune response is also regulated by several *feedback machanisms* including specific T lymphocyte suppression. Human T suppressor cells can be identified by the Leu 2 or OKT8 monoclonal antibodies. Effector lymphocytes have limited life spans, and continued antigenic stimulation is required to prolong the immune response. In a recent review Jerne (1973) expanded on his "network theory of immunological regulation" in which the idiotypic determinants of responder immunoglobulin molecules and immunocytes may be immunogenic themselves, and in turn induce antiidiotypic responses from both T and B lymphocytes which inhibit lymphocytes expressing the idiotype.

Vertebrates have the necessary prerequisites to generate self-reactive antibodies, however, contact with self-antigens at a precursor stage of lymphocyte development may eliminate them or render them quiescent. This theory of *clonal abortion* (Burnet, 1957) seems to be especially applicable to fetuses or newborn animals in their acquisition of tolerance to self, although maintainence of tolerance to many self-antigens depends on their continued presence. Aggregate protein antigens are more immunogenic than soluble monomeric forms, and it seems probable that self-antigens are often presented at sufficient concentrations in the latter manner to maintain tolerance. Experimentally, mature lymphocytes are more difficult to make tolerant than immature lymphocytes. T lymphocyte tolerance is more readily induced and more prolonged than B-lymphocyte tolerance. Whereas B lymphocytes with surface IgD molecules need exposure to large amounts of antigens for tolerance to occur, B lymphocytes with monomeric IgM surface immunoglobulins, can become tolerant to low antigen concentrations. Induction and perhaps maintenance of tolerance in later life depends on selective activation of *suppressor T lymphocytes* with specificities for immunogenic antigen (Allison, 1971). Notwithstanding, several workers have concluded that active lymphocyte suppression is not obligatory for the maintenance of unresponsiveness (Doyle, 1976; Basten, 1975).

It seems probable that some autoimmune disorders may result from the breakdown of suppressor T-cell functioning (Gershon, 1977). In mice, a factor which has antigen specificity and contains histocompatibility determinants coded for by the *I* region (*I-J*) of chromosome 17, is found on cells and has suppressor activities (Murphy, 1976). There are also soluble suppressor factors such as the one released by exposure of lymphocytes to the mitogen concanavalin A (Cantor, 1977).

2. Breakdown of Tolerance in Autoimmunity

It was once considered that many self-antigens were *sequestered* from the immune system and that autoimmunity might result from their exposure to the immune system. Some self-immunogens, however, have been found to be constantly present in the circulation, e.g., thyroglobulin (Torrigiani, 1969), and not sequestered as previously thought. For others, such as the microsomal membrane antigens to which autoantibodies are commonly found in autoimmune endocrinopathies, the case for sequestration remains open. Postulating a central role for autoantibodies in the majority of autoimmune diseases, Allison (1977) has reviewed the ways in which tolerant *T cells* may be *bypassed* to allow the emergence of sensitized B lymphocytes:

1. Drug induction, by acting as carriers for self-antigens.
2. Viruses, by acting as T-lymphocyte stimulants for helper T-cell activities or by inducing nonspecific B-lymphocyte proliferation which could unmask self-reactive clones.
3. Release of sequestered self-antigens as above, e.g., ICA (?) formation in IDDM.
4. Bacterial antigens, by serving as immunological adjuvants and stimulating B lymphocytes polyclonally or by crossreacting with self-antigens, e.g., as in rheumatic fever.
5. Lymphotoxic antibodies produced in some autoimmunities like systemic lupus erythematosus (SLE), which could reduce suppressor activities.

In addition, foreign immunogens such as drugs (or viruses) could complex with self-antigens and lead to autosensitization through a hapten effect.

It is apparent that nonantibody-dependent T-lymphocyte cytolysis may mediate autoimmune disease also. Such has been well shown in two experimental autoimmune models. Allergic encephalitis is induced by immunization with basic myelin protein. Experimental lymphocytic choriomeningitis (LCM) in mice is a T-lymphocyte-mediated autoimmune disease induced by a virus (Doherty and Zinkernagal, 1974). The LCM model has appeal for translation to IDDM, and so is briefly described. When LCM virus is administered intravenously to mice, mild disease results together with evidence of parallel immunity. Virus elimination is by T lymphocytes, especially by specific cytotoxic T cells. Immunity to LCM can be transferred by T cells to uninfected mice. However, if immunocompetent mice are innoculated intracerebrally with LCM virus, they develop acute, rapidly fatal LCM. Procedures that reduce T lymphocytes prior to innoculation protect the animals from fatal disease and allow them to become chronic carriers. For effective T-lymphocyte cytolysis of virus-infected cells, both effector T and the target cells must share at least one common K or D histocompatibility antigen. These antigens are analogous to HLA-A, -B, and -(C) in man. Ia (or D equivalent) antigens are not directly involved. Thus T-lymphocyte cytolysis in LCM was dependent on dual recognition of viral antigens budding from the surface of infected cells, plus commonality of histocompatibility antigens (Zinkernagal and Doherty, 1977). As pointed out by Zinkernagel and Doherty, autoimmunity results from the very same mechanisms that were important in protecting the animal from LCM virus. In other immune models involving budding viruses, the level of the immune response is dictated in part by genes of the I subregions of the major histocompatibility complex which are analogous to human MLA-DR genes.

3. Possible Mechanisms of Immune Self-Destruction

There are several possible ways in which pancreatic β cells could be eliminated in IDDM.

1. Antibody mediated cytolysis involving complement activation.

2. Antibody-dependent CMI, in which armed macrophages or nonspecific killer (K) cells attack target cells coated with specific immune complexes (Allison, 1977).

3. Antibody-independent CMI by cytolytic T lymphocytes as exemplified by the LCM model above.

4. Combinations of the above.

II. EVIDENCE FOR AUTOIMMUNITY IN DIABETES

A. Heterogeneity of Diabetes

It is clear that diabetes defined as a state of abnormal glucose tolerance comprises a multiplicity of defects as reviewed by Zonana and Rimoin (1976). In general, distinguishing IDDM from noninsulin-dependent diabetes mellitus (NIDDM) serves the purpose of largely separating diabetes associated with autoimmunity (IDDM) from those without such features. Notwithstanding, IDDM and NIDDM are heterogeneous diseases, and some patients with clinical NIDDM have underyling autoimmunity, whereas some patients with IDDM lack any evidence of autoimmune manifestations.

B. IDDM-Associated Autoimmunity

It has been known for years that organ-specific autoimmunities have increased frequency in IDDM. The list includes chronic lymphocytic thyroiditis and/or Grave's disease, pernicious anemia, and Addison's disease (Review, Maclaren, 1977). The combination of lymphocytic infiltrations and organ-specific autoantibodies to the thyroid gland, pancreatic islets, and adrenal glands may be termed Schmidt's or Carpenter's syndrome. Organ-specific autoantibodies to cytoplasmic antigens (microsomal lipoproteins) in these specific cells are common in IDDM. In a recent study on over 500 children with IDDM we obtained the results shown in Table I (Neufeld *et al.*, 1980). It is probable that the frequency of thyrogastric autoantibodies will increase in this population with advancing age (Irvine, *et al.*, 1970). No increase in thyroglobulin-reactive autoantibodies among patients with IDDM was observed. Notable were the lower frequency of thyroid microsomal antibodies in black patients with IDDM. For the 20% of IDDM Caucasian patients with thyroid microsomal antibodies, overt disease was evident in about 1 in 3 indicating the need for routine screening. More will be expected to develop overt thyroid disease eventually, although we have seen hypothyroidism in IDDM resolve over time due to compensatory thyroid cell hyperplasia. Since Addison's disease is potentially life threatening, Riley *et al.* (1980a) examined patients with IDDM for adrenal autoantibodies and Addison's disease and found 2.0% of the Caucasian patients to be positive. About 25% of those with adrenal autoantibodies had adrenal insufficiency. Whereas the frequency of this association was sufficiently low probably not to warrant screening for it (1 in 200–250), about 6.5% of those with associated thyroid autoimmunity were adrenal antibody-positive, making screening of the latter group more reasonable.

Gastric parietal cell autoantibodies occur in more than 8% of younger patients with IDDM of whom more than half had achlorhydria following pentagastrin infusion and smaller numbers had defective secretion of in-

TABLE I

Frequency of Organ-Specific Autoantibodies According to Sex and Race in 504 Patients with IDDM and in Normal Controls[a,b]

	No. of patients, N	ICAs		TMAs		PCAs		AAs	
		Percent	N	Percent	N	Percent	N	Percent	N
Total	504	33.0	168	17.0	84	9.0	44	1.6	8
Females	268	34.0	92	22.0	59	11.0	28	1.9	5
Males	236	32.0	76	11.0	25	7.0	16	1.2	3
Blacks	100	22.0	22	4.0	4	10.0	10	0	0
Caucasians	404	36.1	146	20.0	80	8.5	34	2.0	8
Controls	162	0	0/162	2.1	2/95	1.4	2/147	0.6	1/144

[a] ICAs, Islet cell antibodies; TMAs, thyroid microsomal antibodies; PCAs, gastric parietal cell antibodies; AAs, adrenocortical antibodies.

[b] Reproduced with permission from The American Diabetes Association, Inc.

trinsic factor and overt iron and vitamin B$_{12}$ deficiency (W. J. Riley and
N. Maclaren, unpublished).

While the above organ specific autoimmunities are unquestionably increased in IDDM (not NIDDM), there is little or no association with connective tissue autoimmune diseases. Huang and Maclaren (1978), however,
found increased antibodies to polynucleotides in IDDM, including that to
single-stranded DNA. From the author's experience to date, there also appears to be a small increase in autoantibodies to tissue DNA in IDDM when
compared to matched controls, however, the clinical significance of such
findings, if any is not known.

C. Islet Cell Autoantibodies and IDDM

Bottazzo and colleagues (1974) first described cytoplasmic reactive ICA in
patients with polyendocrinopathies, while Lendrum found ICA to be common in patients with IDDM expecially near clincial onset. Such ICA reacts
by indirect immunofluorescerce to all cells of the human pancreatic islet,
which is in contrast to the rather specific loss of β cells seen in IDDM (see
Chapter 13), making a direct role for the autoantibody unlikely. These antibodies are exclusively of the IgG class and are often complement-fixing.
Although published studies vary somewhat in the frequency of ICA after
diagnosis, there is accord that about three of every four newly diagnosed
children and young adults with IDDM have circulating ICA, and that the
frequency falls with disease duration. In our laboratory, 82% of the patients were ICA-positive at diagnosis, about 50% were ICA positive 1-2
years after onset and about 1 in 5 had persistent ICA for up to 10 yr
(Neufeld, et al. 1980) (Fig. 1). Of interest was the lower frequency of ICA
found in black patients. This is in agreement with our finding of a reduced
frequency of thyroid microsomal antibodies in black IDDM patients, and
suggests that there may be underlying heterogeneity of IDDM in black patients complicated by Caucasian–black racial admixture. Among nondiabetics, ICA is relatively rare (0.5%). The ICAs react specifically to all
islet cell types in that they do not cross-react with gastrointestinal cells
secreting glucagon and somatostatin as they do in the islets. The antigen is
believed to be a membrane lipoprotein of the microsomes analogous to that
seen in thyroid or adrenal autoimmunity (Bottazzo and Lendrum, 1976).
The clinical usefulness of ICA determinations depends on the length of
time they are present before clinical IDDM appears. According to Irvine et
al. (1976), some ICA-positive relatives (2%) of IDDM probands tend to
progress to overt diabetes, while the minority of patients with NIDDM who
are ICA positive (8%) tend to become insulin-requiring over time.

Irvine et al. (1977) also have shown that IDDM patients who have persis-

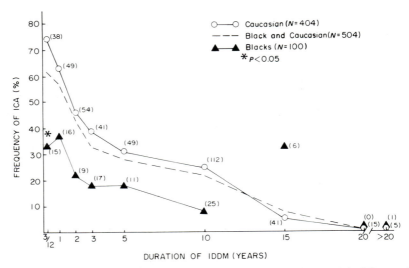

Fig. 1. Frequency of ICAs in black and Caucasian patients in the United States after diagnosis of IDDM. (Reproduced with permission from The American Diabetes Association.)

tent ICA may form a subgroup in that they also tended to have high frequencies of associated thyrogastric and adrenal autoimmunities as well as high frequencies of HLA-B8- but not HLA-B15-bearing haplotypes. We found that IDDM patients with persisting ICA had increased thyroid autoimmunity, while patients with IDDM and adrenal autoimmunity seemed to have exclusively HLA-B8-bearing haplotypes (Neufeld, *et al.* 1980; Riley, *et al.*, 1980). More recently, Bottazzo and Lendrum (1976) have shown the existence of separate ICAs which react only to glucagon- or somatostatin-secreting cells of the islets. The significance of these ICAs which may be of IgA and IgM as well as IgG subclasses, is unknown (Bottazzo and Lendrum, 1976). They have not been associated with glucagon or somatostatin deficiencies to date.

ICAs exist in low titers in comparison to those seen for thyroid or other autoimmunities. By analogy with thyroiditis (Urbaniak, *et al.,* 1973), it may be supposed that ICA arises mainly from pancreatically located lymphocytes. Placental passage of ICA has not been shown to affect neonatal insulin secretion, and to date it is unknown whether ICAs have any functional significance. Most recently, complement-fixing ICA has been demonstrated to be a subspecies of ICA which may be more closely related to the actual damage of β cells than non-complement-fixing ICA (Bottazzo, 1980). In our hands, ICA as detected by complement fixation appeared to be a less-sensitive method of detecting ICA and was of no increased significance (Riley, 1980c).

Besides ICA, autoantibodies reactive to surface antigens on pancreatic islet cells (ICSA) have also been described by Maclaren (1975) and Lernmark *et al.* (1978). The latter group (Soderstrom *et al.,* 1979) suggested that ICSA might inhibit metabolic functions of cultured islet cells and thus could have an *in vivo* pathogenic role in IDDM. Doberson and colleagues (1980) as well as at least two other groups of investigators have been able to demonstrate that ICSA are indeed cytotoxic to cultured rodent islet cells *in vitro*. That such antibodies exist, also raises the possibility that nonspecific killer K-cell activity might account for the β-cell destruction seen in IDDM. Such a mechanism has already been suggested for chronic active hepatitis (Cochrane, *et al.* 1976).

D. Cell-Mediated Autoimmunity in IDDM

Evidence for cell-mediated autoimmunity to pancreatic islet cells in IDDM has been accumulating since Nerup (1971) first reported, in patients with diabetes, *in vitro* inhibition of leukocyte migration in the presence of porcine islet-rich panceatic homogenates. Similar observations were made by other groups using various pancreatic sources as antigen, as reviewed by Christy *et al.* (1977). The latter commented on the lack of standardization and the complexity of such systems. In our laboratory, Huang and Maclaren (1976) demonstrated enhanced cytoadherence and positive cytotoxicity when lymphocytes from children with IDDM were incubated with human insulinoma cells in *in vitro* cultures. Positive results were not obtained using lymphocytes from patients with SLE, Graves' disease, or thyroiditis together with insulinoma cells, or by using of different target cells with IDDM lymphocytes (Maclaren and Huang, 1980). Since the target cells were cancer cells with abnormal antigens, these studies need to be confirmed using normal islet cells, preferably of human origin. Buschard *et al.* reported that leukocytes enriched for T lymphocytes from patients with recent-onset IDDM induced hyperglycemia when placed intraperitoneally in nude, thymus-deficient mice. This exciting finding could not be confirmed by us (Neufeld *et al.,* 1980) or by other investigators. Others have recently described raised levels of circulating mononuclear K cells in 57% of children with recent-onset IDDM. The levels of K cells returned to normal within 1 yr (Pozzilli, *et al.* 1979). Since mechanisms for clonal abortion of self-reactive cells may be confined to fetal and infant life, mechanisms which influence helper T-lymphocyte function may be increasingly important in latter life (Teale and MacKay, 1979). Thus it seems reasonable to examine suppressor cell functions in autoimmune diseases (Waldman, *et al.* 1978) such as IDDM. Were such an abnormality to underlie IDDM, then soluble suppressor-inducing factors might prove to be therapeutically useful. Such a therapy has proved to be efficacious in the New Zealand hybrid "autoimmune" mouse. At least one group to date has reported abnormal T-lymphocyte suppression functions in patients with IDDM (Horowitz, 1977).

Diabetes may induce abnormalities of the immune system, and observations involving such functions in relation to the cause of diabetes, may be only a secondary consequence of it. For example, reversible, defective phagocytosis has been reported in diabetes and suggested to be a function of blood glucose (Bagdade, *et al.*, 1974). Other workers (Selam, 1979) have shown a reversible defect in T lymphocytes, dependent on diabetes control, however, defective numbers of cells bearing the receptors for the Fc fragment of IgG (cells considered to have suppressor functions) were found even in well-controlled patients.

III. THE GENETICS OF IDDM

A. Diabetes in Identical Twins

In the classical studies of Pyke and colleagues, Nelson and Pyke (1975) reported that concordance for NIDDM was usually found between identical twins, whereas discordance for IDDM between other identical twins reached approximately 50%. Although genetic factors were of great importance in NIDDM, this group showed no disturbances in HLA frequencies. In contrast, the twins with IDDM had increased HLA-B15, while only concordant twins had increased HLA-B8 as well, suggesting that two alleles related to HLA might be involved in susceptibility.

B. Human Leukocyte Antigens and Diabetes

Singal and Blajchman (1973) first reported that IDDM was associated with disturbed HLA frequencies and noted an increase in HLA-B15 in these patients. There have been multiple reports since, which have been well summarized by Christy *et al.* (1979) as modified below:

1. Disturbed HLA frequencies are associated with IDDM and not with NIDDM.
2. There is a primary association of IDDM with HLA-D3 (or -DR3), with increased frequency of HLA-B8, -B18, and -A1 by linkage disequilibrium of these antigens to HLA-D3. These antigens are associated with a broader tendency for autoimmunity, e.g., Graves' disease and autoimmune Addison's disease.
3. There is also a primary association between IDDM and HLA-D4 (or -DR4) and -B15 in disequilibrium with HLA-D4. This association does not

seem to be related to an autoimmune predisposition, although HLA-D4 has been found to be increased in rheumatoid arthritis.

4. There is a protective role for HLA-D2 (or HLA-DR2) in disequilibrium with HLA-B7, in IDDM, which must be dominant in that few patients with IDDM have had a HLA-D2-bearing haplotype despite a general Caucasian frequency for HLA-D2 of about 25%. The strength of HLA-D2 protection in IDDM, however, is controversial.

5. Families with multiple members affected by IDDM tend to show HLA-D3/D4-bearing haplotypes, notably among siblings with IDDM.

Parenthetically, it may be added that HLA genes reside in a small region of the short arm of chromosome 6. Typing for HLA-A, -B, -C, and -DR may be carried out using serological methods with type-specific antisera. Several of the polymorphic types of the HLA-B and -DR series appear to have common determinants, since apparently monospecific antisera react with several antigens in constant patterns (supratypic). Typing for HLA-D determinants is done in mixed lymphocyte cultures using homozygous HLA-D lymphocytes as panel cells. An absence of response as determined by radiolabeled thymidine uptake denotes like specificities, while positive responses indicate unlike HLA-D in responder and panel target cells. HLA-D and HLA-DR antigens are thought to be coded for by separate but closely linked loci, and there is good but not complete agreement between HLA-D and HLA-DR specificities. HLA-DR molecules consist of a transmembrane α chain (constant) and a β chain (variable). The HLA-DR (HLA-D) series has strong analogies to the Ia series in the mouse and is important in macrophage presentation of antigens and in the proliferative response following immunization. Antigens of the HLA-D/HLA-DR series are present on B lymphocytes, monocytes, and macrophages and may be expressed on proliferating T lymphocytes which by analogy with mouse systems may have helper or suppressor functions. The association of IDDM with antigens of the HLA-DR series at present suggests that immune response (*Ir*) genes are involved. Recently, Baum (1979) has reported that IDDM is also related to increased frequency of fast-migrating properdin factor B (BfFi) of the alternative complement pathway. It has been suggested that this factor is associated with IDDM because of disequilibrium with nearby HLA-D3 genes (Deschamps *et al.*, 1979).

Several studies have attempted to elicit the mode(s) of genetic transmission of IDDM by HLA haplotype inheritance in multiplex families. Rubenstein (1978) claimed IDDM to be a recessive disease with a 50% penetrance rate and a high HLA recombinant frequency. Spielman's studies (1979), like our own (McLaughlin, 1979), suggest that the principal mode is as a dominant or codominant with reduced penetrance, however, doubts about the random rate for diabetic genes in the population and the crossover rates between HLA and the IDDM gene loci, confound estimations. The subject is complex, and genetic heterogeneity seems probable. Thomsen and colleagues (as reported by Christy *et al.*, 1979) believe that there are two HLA IDDM-related susceptibility genes which, when inherited together, cause increased risk for IDDM by a process of "overdominance." Rubenstein (1981) and colleagues refute this possibility.

IV. ENVIRONMENTAL TRIGGERS FOR AUTOIMMUNE IDDM

From the work of Pyke and colleagues mentioned above, in which it was shown that discordance for IDDM between identical twins reached 50%, the need for an environmental influence against a background of genetic susceptibility to explain the results seems likely. The reduced penetrance necessary for any Mendelian explanation of IDDM among pedigrees also seems to indicate a role for addition factors. Viruses (Chapter 16) and beta-cell toxins (Chapter 15) are the leading candidates. In this respect, it seems likely that some IDDM will be the direct result of these agents, whereas for others the agent(s) may alter self-antigens of the islet cells, leading to autoimmune β-cell destruction in the genetically susceptible. Whereas the latter course of events is speculative, the LCM model of Zinkernagal (Section I) provides a basis for its feasibility.

We have shown that single low doses of streptozotocin, especially in young male mice, result in a delayed-onset type of diabetes associated with variable insulitis. Like and Rossini demonstrated greater degrees of insulitis after multiple small doses of the drug (Chapter 16). Overdoses of the rat poison Vacor, a drug like streptozotocin which results in lowered available NAD to β cells, has been associated with diabetes and ICA in man. Yoon *et al.* (1979) recently isolated coxsackie B_4 virus, which is diabetogenic in mice, from the pancreas of a patient with recent-onset IDDM (Chapter 16). In a joint study of household members of newly diagnosed children with IDDM, we and Yoon could not find evidence for recent coxsackie virus infection in the patients as a group, suggesting that the case reported by Yoon above might represent a rare event (Riley, 1980b). Further, Rand (1981) could show no amelioration in the clinical course of two patients with newly diagnosed IDDM after "immune" interferon therapy.

V. FUTURE DIRECTIONS

It still remains to be shown that β-cell autoimmunity plays a primary role in IDDM instead of that of a secondary phenomenon of little pathogenic consequence. My prejudice is with the former and, if correct, the mechanisms need further elucidation. Possible therapies include treatment with idiotypic anti-ICA or ICSA, specific antilymphocyte antisera, or soluble mediators of suppressor cell activity if IDDM is shown to be associated with defective suppression of self-immunization. The possibility of β-cell transplantation has been enhanced by the demonstration of Lacy *et al.* (1979) that the rejection process across a major histocompatibility barrier in rats can be attenuated by maintaining islet cells in culture for periods sufficient to reduce the content of contained lymphocytes. It is not clear whether such transplants in man with IDDM would result in renewed autoimmunity to the transplants.

ACKNOWLEDGMENTS

Supported by National Institutes of Health grant AM 25403-02. The assistance of Patricia Johnson, Oonagh Kater, and Enea Hyden in preparing the manuscript is gratefully acknowledged.

REFERENCES

Allison, A. C. (1971). *Lancet* 2, 1401–1403.
Allison, A. C. (1977). *In* "Autoimmunity" (N. Talal, ed.), pp. 92–133. Academic Press, New York.
Bagdade, J. D., Root, R. K., and Bulger, R. J. (1974). *Diabetes* 23, 9–15.
Basten, A., Miller, J. F., and Johnson, P. (1975). *Transplant, Rev.* 26, 130–169.
Bottazzo, G. F., and Lendrum, R. (1976). *Lancet* 2, 873–876.
Bottazzo, G. F., Florin-Christensen, A., and Doniach, D. (1974). *Lancet* 2, 1279–1282.
Bottazzo, G. F., Dean, B., Gorsuch, A. N., Cudworth, A. G., and Doniach, D. (1980). *Lancet* 1, 668–672.
Burnet, F. M. (1957). *Aust. J. Exp. Biol. Med. Sci.* 20, 67–72.
Buschard, K., Masbad, S., and Rygaard, J. (1978). *Lancet* 1, 908–910.
Christy, M., Deckert, T., and Nerup, J. (1977). *Clin. Endocrinol. Metab.* 6, 305–327.
Cochrane, A. M. G., Moussouros, A., Thompson, A. D., Eddleston, A. L., and Williams, R. (1976). *Lancet* 1, 441–444.
Deschamps, I., Lestradet, H., Marcelli-Barge,A., Benajam, A., Busson, M., Hors, J., and Dausset, J. (1979). *Lancet* 2, 793.
Dobeson, M. J., Schartt, J. E., Ginsberg-Fellner, F., and Notkins, A. L. (1981). *N. Engl. J. Med.* 304, 1493–1498.
Doherty, P. C., and Zinkernagel, R. M. (1974). *Transplant, Rev.* 19, 89–210.
Doyle, M. V., Parks, D. E., and Weigle, W. P. (1976). *J. Immunol.* 117, 1152–1158.
Gershon, R. K. (1977). *In* "Autoimmunity" (KN. Talal, ed.), pp. 171–180. Academic Press, New York.
Horowitz, S. D., Borcherding, W., and Bargman, C. J. (1978). *Ped. Res.* 86, 507.
Huang, S. W., and Maclaren, N. K. (1976). *Science* 192, 64–66.
Huang, S. W., and Maclaren, N. K. (1978). *Diabetes* 27, 1105–1111.

Irvine, W. J., Clarke, B. F., Scarth, L., Cullen, D. R., and Duncan, L. J. P. (1970). *Lancet* **2**, 163–168.

Irvine, W. J., Gray, R. S., and MacCallum, (1976). *Lancet* **2**, 1097–1102.

Irvine, W. J., MacCallum, C. J., Gray, R. S., Campbell, C. J., Duncan, L. J. P., Farquhar, J. W., Vaughan, H., and Morris, P. J. (1977). *Diabetes* **26**, 138–147.

Jerne, N. K. (1973). *Sci. Am.* **229**, 52.

Kim, C., Taylor, G., Maclaren, N., Jones, R., Huang, S. W., and McLaughin, J. (1977). *Diabetes* **26**, 380.

Lacy, P. E., Davis, J. M., and Fink, E. H. (1979). *Science* **204**, 312–313.

Lendrum, R., Walker, G., and Gamble, D. R. (1975). *Lancet* **1**, 880–883.

Lernmark, A., Freedman, Z. R., Hofman, C., Rubenstein, A. H., Steiner, D. F., Jackson, R. L., Winter, R. J, and Traisman, H. (1978). *N. Engl. J. Med.* **229**, 375–377.

Maclaren, N., (1977). *Am. J. Dis. Child.* **131**, 1149–1152.

Maclaren, N., and Huang, S. W. (1980). *In* "The Immunology of Insulin Dependent Diabetes" (W. J. Irvine, ed.) Teviot Scientific Publications, Edinburgh, pp. 185–194.

Maclaren, N., Huang, S. W., and Fogh, J. (1975). *Lancet* **1**, 997–998.

McLaughlin, J., Maclaren, N., Neufeld, M., Krupp, BN., Bruck, E., and Huang, S. W. (1979). *Pediatr. Res.* **13**, 442, Abstr. 581.

Murphy, D. B., Herzenberg, L. A., Okumura, K., and McDevitt, H. O. (1976). *J. Exp. Med.* **144**, 699–712.

Nelson, P. G., Pyke, D. A. (1975). *Lancet* **2**, 193–195.

Nerup, J., Anderson, O. O., Bendixen, G., Egeberg, J., and Poulsen, J. E. (1971). *Diabetes* **20**, 424–427.

Neufeld, M., Maclaren, N., Riley, W., Lezotte, D., McLaughlin, J., Silverstein, J., and Rosenbloom, A. (1980). *Diabetes* **29**, 589–594.

Neufeld, M., McLaughlin, J., Maclaren, N., Donnelly, W., and Rosenbloom, E. (1980). *N. Engl. J. Med.* **301**, 665.

Pozzilli, P., Sensi, M., Gorsuch, A., and Bottazzo, G. F. (1979). *Lancet* **2**, 173–175.

Rand, K., Rosenbloom, A., Maclaren, N., Silverstein, J., Riley, W., Butterworth, B., Yoon, J., Rubenstein, A., and Menigan T., (1981). *Diabetologia* (in press).

Riley, W. J., Maclaren, N., and Neufeld, M. (1980a). *J. Pediatr. Ped. Res.* **97**, 191–196.

Riley, W. J., Maclaren, N., Rand, K., and Bejar, R. (1980b). **54a**. 211.

Riley, W. J., Neufeld, M., and Maclaren, N. (1980c). *Lancet* **1**, 1133.

Rubenstein, P., Suciu-Foca, N., and Nicholson, J. F. (1977). *N. Engl. J. Med.* **297**, 1036–1040.

Rubenstein, P., Walker, M., Krassner, J., Carrier, C., Carpenter, C., Doberson, M., Notkins, A., and Ginsberg. F. (1981). *AACHT. Seventh Annu. Meet.* p. 10.

Selam, J. L., Clot, J., Andary, M., and Mirouze, J. (1979). *Diabetologia* **16**, 35–40.

Singal, D. P., and Blajchman, M. A. (1973). *Diabetes* **22**, 429–432.

Soderstrum, W. K., Fredman, Z. R., and Lernmark, A. (1979). *Diabetes* **28**, 379–399.

Spielman, R. S., Baker, L., and Zmijewski, C. M. (1978). *In* "Genetic Analysis to Common Diseases: Applications to Predictive Factors in Coronary Heart Disease" (C. F. Sing and M. H. Skdnick, eds.), pp. 567–585. Alan R. Liss, New York.

Teale, J. M., and MacKay, I. R. (1979). *Lancet* **2**, 284–286.

Torrigiani, D., Doniach, D., and Roitt, I. M. (1969). *J. Clin. Endocrinol. Metab.* **29**, 305–314.

Urbaniak, S. J., Penhale, W. J. and Irvine, W. J. (1973). *Clin. Exp. Immunol.* **15**, 345–353.

Waldman, T. A., Blaese, R. M., Broder, S., and Krakaner, R. S. (1978A). *Ann. Int. Med.* **88**, 226–238.

Yoon, J. W., Austin, M., Onodera, T., and Notkins, A. L. (1979). *N. Engl. J. Med.* **300**, 1173–1179.

Zinkernagal, R. M., and Doherty, P. C. (1977). *Contemp. Top. Immunobiol.* **7**, 179–220.

Zonana, J., and Rimoin, D. (1976). *N. Engl. J. Med.* **295**, 603–605.

18

Insulin, Glucagon, and Somatostatin Interaction in Diabetes

P. RASKIN*

I. INTRODUCTION

During the past several years the interaction of islet cell hormones in the pathophysiology of diabetes mellitus has been of considerable interest. Of particular interest has been the contribution of the alpha-cell hormone glucagon to the diabetic syndrome. Although there is considerable controversy regarding the exact quantitative contribution made by abnormal glucagon physiology in the pathogenesis of the metabolic abnormalities of diabetes mellitus, (7,36) there is no question regarding the fact that alpha-cell function is indeed disordered in human diabetes. In fact, it is generally agreed that diabetes mellitus is a bihormonal disease—one of insulin deficiency and glucagon excess (33,34). Glucagon is a powerful glycogenolytic, gly-

---

* Done during the tenure of Dr. Raskin as a Clinical Investigator, Dallas Veterans Administration Medical Center, Dallas, Texas

The Islets of Langerhans
Copyright © 1981 by Academic Press, Inc.
All rights of reproduction in any form reserved.
ISBN 0-12-187820-1

coneogenic, lipolytic, and ketogenic hormone, and its actions are intensified by insulin deficiency. Its potential contribution to the metabolic abnormalities of diabetes is clear.

This chapter will cover three issues directed toward a description of the interaction of three islet cell hormones, insulin, glucagon, and somatostatin, in diabetes. I will describe in detail the abnormalities of alpha-cell function occurring in human diabetes which I consider to be of major pathogenic import in this disease. The second issue to be addressed is one which as yet is not completely resolved. This issue deals with the question of the etiology of the alpha-cell dysfunction in diabetes. In particular, what is the relationship between insulin deficiency and glucagon excess in diabetes? Is the disordered alpha-cell function merely a reflection of insulin deficiency, as seems to be the case in experimental alloxan-induced diabetes in the dog, or is it a primary, perhaps inherent, abnormality of the diabetic alpha cell? Finally, brief mention will be made of the possible interaction of the third islet cell hormone, somatostatin, in human diabetes.

II. NORMAL ALPHA–CELL FUNCTION

Before presenting a description of the abnormal alpha-cell function that occurs in diabetes it seems appropriate to describe alpha-cell physiology in the nondiabetic. The alpha cell does not function independently but works as a part of a unit, being coupled to its neighboring insulin-secreting beta cell within the islets of Langerhans. In fact, the islets of Langerhans may be viewed as the microorgan responsible for managing the fuel distribution of the organism. This microorgan directs the flow of nutrients to various tissues of the body in response to varying needs. In order to be maximally effective the islets must be able to "sense" the availability of various fuels as well as the needs of the various tissues and to respond in two directions. It must be able to direct the storage of fuels when they are present in excess and to mobilize fuel from storage sites at times of need.

The islets of Langerhans are remarkable in their ability to perform this feat. It is accomplished simply by varying the amount of two biological antagonists—insulin, the fuel storage hormone, and glucagon, the hormone of fuel recall. The alpha- and beta-cell function as a coupled unit. Thus, during times of exogenous fuel excess, such as after meals, the islets release into the circulation a secretion mixture in which insulin is present in high concentrations relative to glucagon. This circumstance favors the synthesis of glycogen, fat, and protein. Conversely, at times when endogenous fuel production is needed for survival by the organism, such as during prolonged fasting, the islets secrete a mixture which has a high glucagon concentration relative to insulin. This circumstance favors production of glucose from the breakdown of hepatic glycogen as well as from gluconeogenic precursors. It also results in increased production of free fatty acids, glycerol, and ketones for use as alternative substrates.

Glucose is the primary fuel the organism uses to provide energy for life. Why this is the case is not clear, however, because it is, its concentration in the extracellular space varies considerably less than that of other circulating substrates (6). It is apparent that the primary regulator of the alpha–beta cell couplet in the islets of Langerhans is the arterial glucose concentration. Small changes in plasma glucose concentration are immediately sensed by the islet which immediately changes the relative concentration of the two hormones in its secretion mixture so as to keep the glucose concentration within the normal range. Increases in plasma glucose levels, such as would be seen after a glucose meal, trigger a secretion mixture high in insulin relative to glucagon. The increased concentration of circulating insulin promotes glucose efflux from the extracellular space, so that the plasma glucose concentration increases only slightly despite the fact that relatively large amounts of glucose may enter the circulation from the gut. On the other hand, when glucose efflux from the extracellular space is increased, as occurs with exercise or because of the aminogenic insulin secretion from a protein meal, secretion of a hormone mixture by the islets, which is high in glucagon relative to insulin, promotes an increase in hepatic glucose production so as to provide the necessary fuel for the exercising muscles and prevent hypoglycemia.

This push–pull arrangement of the secretion products of the alpha and beta cells is demonstrated graphically in Fig. 1 which shows the response of nondiabetics to a protein meal (25). Plasma glucose levels remain relatively constant despite the fact that plasma insulin levels rise. Hypoglycemia is prevented by the simultaneous increase in circulating immunoreactive glucagon (IRG) levels in response to the oral protein. Since the plasma glucose concentration is the primary regulator of glucagon secretion, if one experimentally produces hyperglycemia with a glucose infusion in nondiabetic subjects prior to the ingestion of a protein meal, the hyperglycemia actually inhibits IRG secretion and blocks the protein-induced increase in IRG as shown in Fig. 2. In these experiments in which the protein meal was preceded by a glucose infusion, the hyperglycemia actually suppressed IRG levels and of course there was no increase following protein ingestion (25).

Maintenance of a balance between glucose production and glucose utilization so that the extracellular glucose concentration is kept normal requires a coordinated relationship between the glucagon-producing alpha cell and the insulin-producing beta cell. This relationship is carefully orchestrated under the direction of a ''glucose sensor.'' This sensor must re-

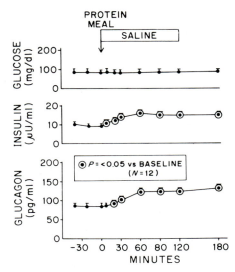

Fig. 1. Plasma glucose, insulin, and glucagon response to a protein meal in nondiabetic subjects (25).

spond to changes in extracellular glucose concentration and also must vary secretion in response to other nonglucose influences in accordance with glucose needs. In the nondiabetic individual this sensor, which relays information to the islet, maintains meticulous control of the plasma glucose concentration.

III. DISORDERED ALPHA–CELL FUNCTION IN DIABETES MELLITUS

The defects in alpha-cell function in diabetes can be divided into two major categories. The first is a loss of its glucose-sensing ability and the second is hypersecretion in response to various aminogenic stimuli.

From the preceding discussion it seems quite clear that the primary regulator of hormone secretion from the islets of Langerhans is the circulating plasma glucose concentration. Thus, in nondiabetic individuals, elevation of the plasma glucose level by whatever means results in an immediate secretion of insulin and a prompt decline in plasma glucagon levels. Figure 3 shows this response graphically (25).

Conversely, should the plasma glucose level fall to hypoglycemic levels, as might occur if one administered exogenous insulin to a nondiabetic, then there would be a marked increase in the secretion of glucagon so as to in-

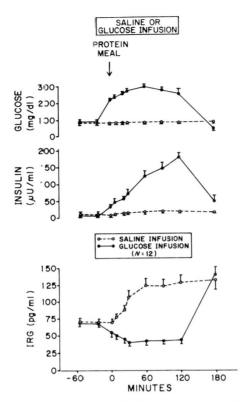

Fig. 2. Plasma glucose, insulin, and the IRG response to a protein meal in nondiabetic subjects (25). The meal was preceded by either a saline infusion or a glucose infusion at a rate of 1.0 g/kg/hr.

crease hepatic glucose production in an attempt to maintain normoglycemia. Thus the nondiabetic alpha cell can sense changes in plasma glucose levels and respond appropriately to either increased or decreased secretion. In human diabetes the alpha cell has lost its ability to sense changes in plasma glucose levels. In fact, the responses to both hyperglycemia and hypoglycemia are defective. As originally described by Unger and his colleagues, patients with diabetes mellitus exhibit fasting hyperglucagonemia despite an elevated plasma glucose level which if induced in nondiabetic subjects would result in a fall in circulating glucagon levels of approximately 50% (31). In fact, not only is there fasting hyperglucagonemia in human diabetes, but hyperglucagonemia is present throughout the entire day in both juvenile- and adult-onset-type diabetes (24).

Hyperglucagonemia is present not only in all human diabetics but in

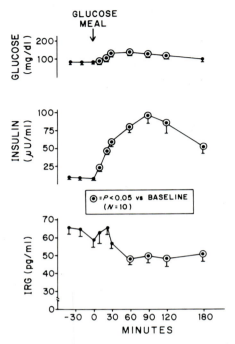

Fig. 3. Plasma glucose, insulin, and glucagon response to a glucose meal (100 g) in nondiabetic subjects (25).

most forms of experimental diabetes as well. That is, plasma IRG levels are either absolutely elevated or elevated relative to the plasma glucose level. Because the sine qua non of diabetes is hyperglycemia, even a normal plasma glucagon level under these circumstances can be thought of as relative hyperglucagonemia since in the nondiabetic individual plasma glucagon levels fall whenever hyperglycemia occurs. Thus the presence of basal hyperglucagonemia in diabetics is clearly a reflection of the abnormal glucose-sensing ability of the diabetic alpha cell.

In addition to basal hyperglucagonemia diabetics have an abnormal response to the ingestion of carbohydrate. Muller *et al.* (14) and later Buchanan and McCarroll (5) showed that the diabetic alpha cell responded abnormally following the ingestion of a carbohydrate meal. Whereas in nondiabetics plasma IRG levels are suppressed after such meals, diabetics fail to suppress and in some instances even show a paradoxical increase in plasma glucagon levels. In nondiabetics, hyperglycemia produced by any means, be it a glucose or a carbohydrate meal or intravenous glucose administration (40), results in immediate glucagon suppression. All diabetics show failure of glucagon suppression by oral glucose, although there are differences in the abnormal alpha-cell response to oral glucose in patients with insulin-deficient diabetes (type I, hypoinsulinemic, or juvenile-onset-type diabetes) and those with the obese hyperglycemic diabetic syndrome (type II, hyperinsulinemic, or maturity-onset diabetes). Patients with hypoinsulinemic diabetes actually have a paradoxical increase in IRG levels in response to oral glucose (2) similar to the response seen in an insulin-deprived alloxan-diabetic dog given intravenous glucose (3). However, patients with type II diabetes (hyperinsulinemic) have a biphasic IRG response. There is an initial increase in IRG levels with a late fall to levels below the baseline (2,14).

The diabetic alpha cell is also unable to sense hypoglycemia. In nondiabetics, when hypoglycemia is produced with intravenous insulin, there is a fourfold increase in circulating IRG levels. In diabetics this response to hypoglycemia is defective. Gerich showed that in juvenile-onset-type diabetics insulin hypoglycemia failed to produce any rise in plasma glucagon levels (8).

Thus the diabetic alpha-cell fails to recognize changes in the plasma glucose concentration in either direction. Hyperglycemia fails to produce the expected fall in IRG levels, and hypoglycemia fails to produce the expected increase.

The other major category of disordered alpha-cell function in human diabetes relates to alpha-cell hypersecretion in response to various aminogenic stimuli. In nondiabetics IRG levels rise in response to intravenous arginine and alanine or following the ingestion of a protein meal. In diabetics these responses are exaggerated (2,31,38,23). Figure 4 shows the response to a protein meal in juvenile-onset-type diabetic patients. Despite the fact that these patients are hyperglycemic, they demonstrate basal hyperglucagonemia and an exaggerated response to oral protein (25). This hyperresponsiveness of the alpha cell is responsible for the increase in plasma glucose that also follows the meal.

IV. ISLET CELL HORMONE INTERACTION IN DIABETES

Because of the many abnormalities in alpha-cell function in human diabetes much has been written about its etiology. Some workers suggested that the problem was related to insulin deficiency and that hyperglucagonemia was a consequence of insulin deficiency. Thus alpha-cell function might be affected by either a local or a systemic absence of its neighboring beta-cell hormone insulin. This concept seemed appropriate in patients with hypoinsulinemic diabetes, but how could one explain the abnormali-

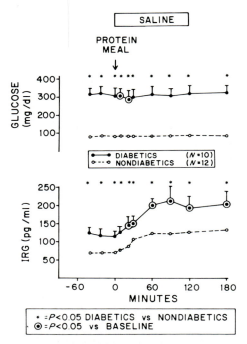

Fig. 4. Plasma glucose and IRG response to a protein meal in spontaneously hyperglycemic juvenile-onset diabetics compared to nondiabetics. (25).

ties of alpha-cell function in the type II diabetic who often had normal or even elevated levels of circulating insulin? Thus Unger suggested that the abnormal alpha-cell function in human diabetes mellitus was not the simple consequence of insulin deficiency, as in alloxan diabetes, but rather was a more complex disorder perhaps even primary in the pathogenesis of diabetes (32).

Further studies have caused some modification of this initial view and have pointed out different features in the alpha-cell response to insulin in the two forms of human diabetes. Table I shows a summary of studies specifically designed to evaluate this question. In general it may be said that in type I or hypoinsulinemic diabetes, whereas the abnormality of alpha-cell function in the untreated state is often considerably more severe than may be seen in the type II (hyperinsulinemic) form of the disease (e.g., the paradoxical rise in plasma IRG levels after oral glucose in untreated type I diabetes, whereas in type II diabetes IRG levels rise initially but later fall to levels below baseline), it can be modified and in some cases even normalized with the administration of exogenous insulin. However, insulin must

TABLE I

Alpha-Cell Function in Diabetes Mellitus: The Response to Insulin

Type of diabetes	Treatment	Basal IRG levels	24-hr IRG profile	Oral glucose and carbohydrate	Oral protein			Intravenous glucose	Intravenous arginine
					Spontaneous hyperglycemia	Induced hyperglycemia			
Type I diabetes (juvenile-onset type)	Untreated	Abnormal	Abnormal	Abnormal	Abnormal	Abnormal		—	Abnormal
	Insulin-treated	Normal	Lower but not normal	Normal	Normal	Abnormal		Normal	Normal
Type II diabetes (maturity-onset type	Untreated	Abnormal	Abnormal	Abnormal	Abnormal	Abnormal		Normal	Abnormal
	Insulin-treated	Normal	Normal	Abnormal	Abnormal	Abnormal		Normal	Abnormal

be given in supraphysiological amounts, which raises plasma insulin levels to values well above those seen in nondiabetics undergoing a similar study. There are two exceptions to this general statement. We have been able to lower but not completely normalize the 24-hr IRG profile of type I diabetics treated with conventional but aggressive insulin treatment program periods of from 5 to 10 days (24) and to show in juvenile diabetics, made normoglycemic by overnight insulin infusion, complete suppression of the IRG response to oral protein when hyperglycemia is induced by glucose infusion prior to the start of the meal (2). It must be pointed out that IRG profiles in type I diabetics can be normalized within 4–5 weeks of treatment with continuous subcutaneous insulin infusion given via portable insulin infusion pumps (27). Thus in juvenile diabetics the elevated plasma IRG levels can be lowered into the normal range under most circumstances, but under rare circumstances alpha-cell function is not always made normal.

Despite these exceptions which suggest that alpha-cell abnormality in type I diabetes is not completely correctable by exogenous insulin, it is difficult to accept the idea that the defect in alpha-cell function in type I diabetes is not merely the consequence of insulin deficiency, as it is usually normalized by the administration of exogenous insulin, albeit in supraphysiological amounts. In a pure sense one may not be able to say that alpha-cell function is made normal in juvenile-onset-type diabetes by the administration of exogenous insulin under any circumstances. Normality implies that all aspects under study are identical to those of the nondiabetic. Since the alpha cell responds only to supraphysiological levels of exogenous insulin, an exact definition of normality may never be fulfilled.

In the maturity-onset form of the disease things are quite different. Exogenous insulin normalizes both basal IRG levels in fasting adult-onset diabetics (35) and the 24-hr IRG profile in conventionally treated adult-onset diabetics (24). However, all tests of alpha-cell function such as the response to oral glucose (2,32) and protein (25) and the response to intravenous arginine (23) are abnormal and are completely unaffected by even pharmacological doses of exogenous insulin. In this form of human diabetes it seems apparent that disordered alpha-cell function is in no way related to insulin deficiency.

A brief look at the anatomical structure of the islet provides some insight into the possible mechanism of the alpha-cell abnormality in type I diabetes. In most species, including humans, the various cell types in the nondiabetic islet are arranged as depicted in Fig. 5a (35). There is an outer layer of glucagon-containing alpha (A) cells which envelope a large central mass of insulin-containing beta (B) cells. Located strategically between the alpha and beta cells are the somatostatin-containing D cells (16). This structural arrangement allowing cell-to-cell contact may be important in the "within-

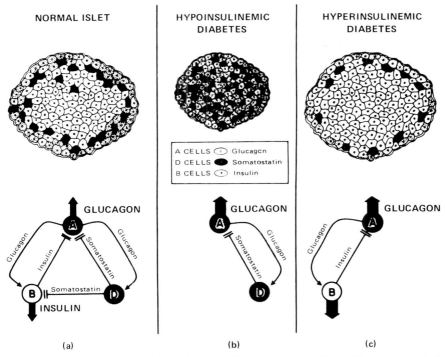

NORMAL ISLET

HYPOINSULINEMIC
DIABETES

HYPERINSULINEMIC
DIABETES

A CELLS ⊙ Glucagon
D CELLS ● Somatostatin
B CELLS ⊙ Insulin

GLUCAGON

GLUCAGON

GLUCAGON

INSULIN

(a)   (b)   (c)

Fig. 5. (a) Arrangement of the major islet cell types in a normal islet. (b) Arrangement of islet cell types in insulin-dependent (type I) diabetes. (c) Arrangement of islet cell types in hyperinsulinemic (type II) diabetes (35).

islet'' regulation of hormone secretion from each of the cell types. It is clear that the secretory product of each islet cell type can influence the secretion of both of its neighbors. For example, insulin can directly inhibit the secretion of glucagon (29) and somatostatin (41). Glucagon stimulates the secretion of insulin (28) and may possibly also stimulate somatostatin release (21). Finally, somatostatin inhibits the release of both insulin and glucagon (13,17).

The islets of the juvenile-onset diabetic (17), as well as of several forms of experimental hypoinsulinemic diabetes in animals (10,11,12,18), lack beta cells (Fig. 5b). Instead, the islets of these forms of insulinopenic diabetes are made up entirely of alpha cells and somatostatin-containing D cells. Thus this intraislet insulin deficiency as proposed by Weir *et al.* (39) may explain the disordered function of the type I diabetic alpha cell. Restoration of the relatively high intraislet insulin concentration present under normal circumstances within the nondiabetic islet with exogenous insulin requires the supraphysiological insulin doses given to these patients in order to affect changes in alpha-cell function. With regard to the somatostatin content of these islets, it has been found that it is often increased (17), and Schusdziarra *et al.* (30) have described elevated somatostatin-like radio-immunoreactivity in the plasma of alloxan-diabetic dogs.

On the other hand, in the maturity-onset form of the disease (although islets from this type of patient have not yet been studied and we are at a bit of a disadvantage in this regard) most of the patients have an endogenous insulin secretory capacity; in fact, they often have hyperinsulinemia. Thus they probably do not have an intraislet insulin deficiency and therefore might not be expected to show any effect of exogenous insulin administration on their alpha-cell function. Clearly, alpha-cell abnormalities in this form of diabetes must be independent of insulin deficiency and must have another etiology. It is of considerable interest that in animal models of the human obese hyperinsulinemic syndrome it has been demonstrated that there is a decrease in both islet D cells (4) as well as diminished islet somatostatin-like radioimmunoactivity (19,20), suggesting possibly that this syndrome results from a somatostatin deficiency (37).

V. THERAPEUTIC IMPLICATIONS

In the previous sections I have tried to point out the interaction of islet hormones in diabetes mellitus and how these interactions differ from those in the nondiabetic individual. This information is certainly important from a theoretical point of view, but can this knowledge be translated into improved therapy for diabetic patients?

The fact that most diabetic patients have hyperglucagonemia has led many workers to suggest that attempts to reduce the elevated plasma glucagon levels might have merit in regard to improving diabetic control. Most of the studies have been carried out in type I diabetics where plasma glucagon levels might be expected to be normalized with the administration of insulin. In practical terms it is not possible to normalize plasma glucagon levels completely with conventionally administered insulin (24), and thus investigators have attempted to use somatostatin, which directly suppresses alpha-cell function in combination with insulin treatment.

Figure 6 shows the plasma glucose and glucagon response and urinary glucose excretion in type I diabetic patients treated with insulin alone, insulin plus somatostatin, or insulin, somatostatin, and glucagon. The patients were hyperglucagonemic and hyperglycemic and had glycosuria when only insulin was given. Administration of somatostatin in combination with the same dose of insulin, which markedly reduced plasma glucagon

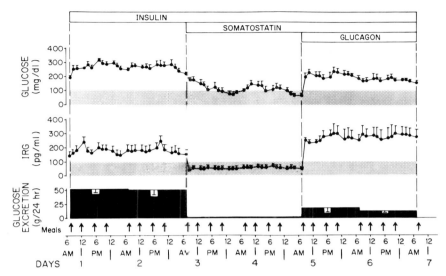

Fig. 6. Effects of somatostatin and somatostatin with glucagon on the daily profiles of mean (± SEM) levels of glucose, IRG, and on glucose excretion in four patients with type I diabetes receiving a continuous insulin infusion and a diet containing 150 g/day of carbohydrate (26).

levels, resulted in normal plasma glucose profiles. When an exogenous glucagon infusion was added to the infusion mixture, returning plasma glucagon levels to their original elevated levels, hyperglycemia and glucosuria returned. Thus this study clearly showed that diabetic control was better using a combination of insulin and somatostatin than when insulin was used alone. The improvement in diabetic control seems to be the direct result of glucagon suppression (26). Other investigators obtained similar results (9).

Because of these observations suggesting that a specific reduction in the hyperglucagonemia in type I diabetes may offer an adjunct to the present conventional methods of diabetes treatment, much work is being done on finding an analogue for somatostatin which is glucagon-specific, has a longer duration of action, and might be given by some route other than intravenously. Only time will tell if these problems can be overcome so that this form of therapy can be offered on a routine basis to diabetic patients.

ACKNOWLEDGMENTS

Supported by National Institutes of Health grants 1-R01-AM18179 and 1-M01-RR00633, American Diabetes Association, North Texas Affiliate, American Heart Association.

P. Raskin

REFERENCES

1. Alberti, K. G. M. M., Christensen, N. J., Christensen, S. E., Hansen, S. E., Iverson, A. P., Lundbeck, J., Sayer-Hansen, K., and Orskov. H. (1973). *Lancet* **2**, 1299–1301.
2. Aydin, I., Raskin, P., and Unger, R. H. (1977). *Diabetologia* **13**, 629–636.
3. Baetens, J. T., Faloona, G. R., and Unger, R. H. (1974). *J. Clin. Invest.* **53**, 1017–1028.
4. Baetens, D., Stefan, Y., Ravazzola, M., Malaisse-Lagae, F., Coleman, D. L., and Orci, L. (1978). *Diabetes* **27**, 1–7.
5. Buchanan, K. D., and McCarroll, A. M. (1972). *Lancet* **2**, 1394–1395.
6. Cahill, G. F., Jr. (1971). *Diabetes* **10**, 785–799.
7. Felig, P., Wahren, J., Sherwin, R., and Hendler R. (1976). *Diabetes* **25**, 1091–1099.
8. Gerich, J. E., Langlois, M., Noacco, C., Karam, J. H., and Forsham, P. H. (1973). *Science* **182**, 171–172.
9. Gerich, J. E., Schultz, T. A., Lewis, S. B., and Karam, J. H. (1977). *Diabetologia* **13**, 537–544.
10. Makino, H., Matsushima, Y., Kanatsuka, A., Yamamoto, M., Kumagai, A., and Nishimura, M. (1979). *Endocrinology* **104**, 243–247.
11. Matsushima, Y., Makino, H., Kanatsuka, A., Yamamoto, M, and Kumagai, A. (1978). *Endocrinol. Jpn.* **25**, 111–115.
12. McEvoy, R. C., and Hegre, O. D. (1977). *Diabetes* **26**, 1140–1146.
13. Mortimer, C. H., Trunbridge, W. M. G., Yeomans, L., Lind, T., Coy, D. H., Bloom, S. R., Kastin, A., Mallison, C. H., Besser, G. M., Schally, A. V., and Hall, R. (1974). *Lancet* **1**, 697–701.
14. Muller, W. A., Faloona, G. R., Aquilar-Parada, E., and Unger, R. H. (1970). *N. Engl. J. Med.* **283**, 109–115.
15. Muller, W. A., Faloona, G. R., and Unger, R. H. (1971). *J. Clin. Invest.* **50**, 1992–1999.
16. Orci, L., and Unger, R. H. (1975). *Lancet* **2**, 1243–1244.
17. Orci, L., Baetens, D., Rufener, C., Amherdt, M., Ravazzola, M., Studer, P., Malaisse-Lagae F., and Unger, R. H. (1976). *Proc. Natl. Acad. Sci. U.S.A.* **73**, 1338–1342.
18. Patel, Y. C., and Weir, G. C. (1976a). *Clin. Endocrinol.* **5**, 191–194.
19. Patel, Y. C., Orci, L., Bankier, A., and Cameron, D. P. (1976b). *Endocrinology* **99**, 1415–1418.
20. Patel, Y. C., Cameron, D. P., Stefan, Y., Malaisse-Lagae, F., and Orci, L. (1977). *Science* **198**, 930–931.
21. Patton, G. S., Ipp, E., Dobbs, R. E., Orci, L., Vale, W., and Unger, R. H. (1977). *Proc. Natl. Acad. Sci. U.S.A.* **74**, 2140–2143.
22. Raskin, P., Fujita, Y., and Unger, R. H. (1975). *J. Clin. Invest.* **56**, 1132–1138.
23. Raskin, P., Aydin, I., and Unger, R. H. (1976). *Diabetes* **25**, 227–229.
24. Raskin, P., and Unger, R. H. (1978a). *Diabetes* **27**, 411–419.
25. Raskin, P., Aydin, I., Yamamoto, T., and Unger, R. H. (1978b). *Am. J. Med.* **64**, 988–997.
26. Raskin, P., and Unger, R. H. (1978c). *N. Engl. J. Med.* **299**, 433–436.
27. Raskin, P., Pietri A., and Unger, R. H. (1979). *Diabetes* **28**, 1033–1037.
28. Samols, E., Tyler, J. M., and Marks. V. (1972). *In* "Glucagon: Molecular physiology, clinical and therapeutic implications" (P. J. Lefebvre and R. H. Unger, eds.) pp. 151–173. Pergamon, Oxford.
29. Samols, E., and Harrison, J. (1976). *Metabolism* **25**, Suppl. 1, 1443–1447.
30. Schusdziarra, V., Ipp, E., Harris, V., Dobbs, R. Raskin, P., Orci, L., and Unger, R. H. (1978). *Metabolism* **27**, Suppl. 1, 1227–1232.

31. Schusdziarra, V., Rouoiller, D., Arimura, A., Boden, G., Brown, J., and Unger, R. H. (1979). *Diabetes* **28**, 380 (Abstr.).
32. Unger, R. H., Aguilar-Parada, E. Muler, W. A., and Eisenstraut, A. M. (1970). *J. Clin. Invest.* **49**, 837–848.
33. Unger, R. H., Madison, L. L., and Muller, W. A. (1972). *Diabetes* **21**, 301–307.
34. Unger, R. H., and Orci, L. (1975). *Lancet* **1**, 14–16.
35. Unger, R. H. (1976). *Diabetes* **25**, 136–151.
36. Unger, R. H., and Orci, L. (1977a). *Ann. Rev. Med.* **28**, 119–130.
37. Unger, R. H., and Orci, L. (1977b). *Diabetes* **26**, 241–244.
38. Unger, R. H. (1978). *Metabolism* **27**, 1691–1709.
39. Weir, G. C., Knowlton, S. D., Atkins, R. F., McKennan, K. X., and Martin, D. B. (1976). *Diabetes* **25**, 275–282.
40. Wise, J. K., Hendler, R., and Felig, P. (1972). *Science* **178**, 153–154.
41. Yamamoto, T., Raskin, P., Aydin, I., and Unger, R. H. (1979). *Metabolsim* **28**, 568–574.

Index